The Sociology of Health and Illness
Critical Perspectives

The Sociology of Health and Illness

Critical Perspectives

Edited by

Peter Conrad & Rochelle Kern
Brandeis University   *New York University*

BIP-89, 2idud., 1985

St. Martin's Press
New York

Acknowledgments

Acknowledgments and copyrights continue at the back of the book on page 634 and following pages, which constitute an extension of the copyright page.

John B. McKinlay and Sonja M. McKinlay, "Medical Measures and the Decline of Mortality." Under the title "The Questionable Contribution of Medical Measures to the Decline of Mortality in the United States in the Twentieth Century," this article originally appeared in *Milbank Memorial Fund Quarterly/Health and Society,* Summer 1977, pp. 405–428. Reprinted by permission of the Milbank Memorial Fund and John B. McKinlay.

S. Leonard Syme and Lisa F. Berkman, "Social Class, Susceptibility, and Sickness." Reprinted by permission from *The American Journal of Epidemiology,* vol. 104, pp. 1–8, 1976.

Ingrid Waldron, "Why Do Women Live Longer Than Men?" Reprinted with permission from *Social Science and Medicine,* vol. 10. Copyright 1976, Pergamon Press, Ltd.

Victor R. Fuchs, "A Tale of Two States." Reprinted with permission of the author and Basic Books, Inc., from *Who Shall Live? Health Economics and Social Change.*

Samuel S. Epstein, "The Political and Economic Basis of Cancer." Reprinted with permission from *Technology Review,* July/August 1976. Copyright © 1976 by the Alumni Association of M.I.T. This article is based on material appearing in *The Politics of Cancer* by Samuel S. Epstein (Anchor/Doubleday, 1979).

James S. House, "Occupational Stress and Coronary Heart Disease: A Review and Theoretical Integration." Reprinted and excerpted with permission of the American Sociological Association from *Journal of Health and Social Behavior,* vol. 15, March 1974, pp. 17–21.

Peter L. Schnall and Rochelle Kern, "Hypertension in American Society: An Introduction to Historical Materialist Epidemiology," was written for this volume. Reprinted by permission of the authors.

Mark Zborowski, "Cultural Components in Response to Pain." Reprinted and excerpted with permission of the Society for the Psychological Study of Social Issues and the author from the *Journal of Social Issues,* vol. 8, no. 4 (1952), pp. 16–30.

Anselm Strauss, "Chronic Illness." Published by permission of Transaction, Inc. from *Society,* vol. 10, no. 6. Copyright © 1973 by Transaction, Inc.

Contents

Preface

Medical sociology has grown very rapidly from a subspecialty taught occasionally in graduate departments to a major area of scholarly activity and student interest. Along with this growth we have witnessed a major shift of emphasis: Medical sociology has increasingly become the sociology of health and illness. For where sociologists once focused on the role of the physician, they are now examining the societal bases of health and illness. These developments reflect, in part, growing concern among both specialists and the public about a crisis in American health care—a crisis evident in the rapid development of chronic illness as our central medical and social problem, in the skyrocketing of medical costs, and in the "medicalization" of what were until recently considered social problems or life's natural contingencies. Although by some standards the present American medical system and profession may be considered among the best in the world, a health care crisis exists in such crucial areas as primary care, national distribution of medical services, and prevention of disease and illness.

In this volume we have sought to show students that both disease and medical care are related to the structure of society and that, accordingly, a sociology of medicine cannot exclude a sociology of health. For the readings collected here we draw on diverse sources. The articles are not only by sociologists but also by public health specialists, health activists, and social critics. We also include a number of original articles written especially for this book. Taken together, the readings place the relationship between society's institutions and its medical care system in a critical perspective. By "critical" we mean a perspective which assumes neither that the present organization of medicine is sacred or inviolable nor that any particular organization would solve all of the problems.

Following a General Introduction, the readings are arranged in four major sections. Section 1 examines "The Social Production of Disease and Illness"; Section 2 analyzes "The Social Organization of Medical Care"; Section 3 presents "Contemporary Critical Debates"; and Section 4, "Toward Alternatives in Health Care," suggests solutions. Introductions to each section set the readings in context and highlight the critical issues, focusing attention on both the structural and interactional aspects of the health care crisis. While the four sections are related and follow naturally from each other, they can be read or referred to in any order the instructor desires.

This book is the product of both excitement and frustration: our excitement about teaching in a field so enlivened by controversy and ferment; our frustration, term after term, in trying to make conveniently accessible to our own students a collection of materials that accurately conveyed the dynamic condition of the field. As we have worked to bring these materials together in a single volume we have been helped by many people who supported the project in various ways. Joseph Behar, Sandra Klein Danziger, Eliot Freidson, Kim Hopper, and Michael Radelet reacted favorably and helpfully to our early ideas about the book. John McKinlay, Peter Schnall, Irving Kenneth Zola, Nancy Zeman-Paul, and several anonymous reviewers read most of the manuscript and made valuable suggestions. Sharon Grosfeld and Linda Cushman cheerfully and capably completed the many clerical tasks necessary to prepare the manuscript. We thank Emily Berleth and Bob Woodbury of St. Martin's Press for their enthusiasm, help, and patience. Nina Schnall contributed in her own very special way; we thank you, Nina. Finally, we thank Libby and Peter, the doctors who share our lives, for their love and encouragement and for their visions of a better health care system.

General Introduction

Three major themes underlie the organization of this book: that the conception of medical sociology must be broadened to encompass a sociology of health and illness; that medical care in the United States is presently in crisis; and that the solution of that crisis requires that our health care and medical systems be reexamined from a critical perspective.

Toward a Sociology of Health and Illness

The increase in "medical sociology" courses and the number of medical sociological journals now extant are but two indicators of rapid development in this field.[1] The knowledge base of medical sociology has expanded apace so that this discipline has moved in less than two decades from an esoteric subspecialty taught in a few graduate departments to a central concern of sociologists and sociology students. The causes of this growth are too many and too complex to be within the scope of this present work. However, a few of the major factors underlying this development may be noted.

The rise of chronic illness as a central medical and social problem has led physicians, health planners, and public health officials to look to sociology for help in understanding and dealing with this major health concern. In addition, the increase of governmental involvement in medical care has created research opportunities (and funding) for sociologists to study the organization and delivery of medical care. Sociologists have also become increasingly involved in medical education (as evidenced by the large number of sociologists currently on medical school faculties). Further, since the 1960s, the social and political struggles over health and medical care have become major social issues, thus drawing additional researchers and students to the field. Indeed, some sociologists have come to see the organization of medicine and the way medical services are delivered as social problems in themselves.

Traditionally, the sociological study of illness and medicine has been called, simply, medical sociology. Strauss (1957) differentiated between sociology "of" medicine and sociology "in" medicine. Sociology *of* medicine focuses on the study of medicine to illuminate some *sociological concern* (e.g., patient-practitioner relationships, the role of professions in society). Sociology *in* medicine, on the other hand, focuses primarily on *medical problems* (e.g., the sociological causes of disease and illness, reasons for delay in seeking medical aid, patient compliance or noncompliance with medical regimens). As one might expect, the conceptual dichotomy between these two approaches is more distinct than in actual sociological practice. Be that as it may, sociologists who have concentrated on a sociology of medicine have tended to focus on the profession of medicine and on doctors and to slight the social basis of health and illness. Today, for example, our understanding of the sociology of medical practice and the organization of medicine is much further developed than our understanding of the relationship between social structure and health and illness.

One purpose of this book is to help redress this imbalance. In it, we shift from a focus on the physician and the physician's work to a more general concern with how health and illness are dealt with in our society. This broadened conceptualization of the relationship between sociology and medicine encourages us to examine problems such as the social causation of illness, the economic basis of medical services, and the influence of medical industries, and to direct our primary attention to the social production of disease and illness and the social organization of the medical care system.

Both disease and medical care are related to the structure of society. The social organization of society influences to a significant degree the type and distribution of disease. It also shapes the organized response to disease and illness—the medical care system. To analyze either disease or medical care without investigating its connection with social structure and social interaction is to miss what is unique about the sociology of health and illness. To make the connection between social structure and health, we must investigate how social factors such as the political economy, the corporate structure, the distribution of resources, and the uses of political, economic, and social power influence health and illness and society's response to health and illness. To make the connection between social interaction and health we need to examine people's experiences, how "reality" is constructed, cultural variations within society, and face-to-face relationships. Social structure and interaction are, of course, interrelated, and it is central to the sociological task to make this linkage clear. Both health and the medical system should be analyzed as integral parts of society. In short, instead of a "medical sociology," in this book we posit and profess a *sociology of health and illness*.[2]

The Crisis in American Health Care

It should be noted at the outset that, by any standard, the American medical system and the American medical profession are among the best in the world. Our society invests a great amount of its social and economic resources in medical care; has some of the world's finest physicians, hospitals, and medical schools; is no longer plagued by deadly infectious diseases; and is in the forefront in developing medical and technological advances for the treatment of disease and illness.

This being said, however, it must also be noted that American health care is in a state of crisis. It has been judged to be so, not simply by a small group of social and political critics, but by concerned social scientists, thoughtful political leaders, leaders of labor and industry, and members of the medical profession itself. Although there is general agreement that a health-care crisis exists, there is, as one would expect, considerable disagreement as to the cause of this crisis and how the crisis should be dealt with.

What are some of the major elements and manifestations of this crisis as reflected in the concerns expressed by the contributors to this volume?

Medical costs have risen exponentially; in three decades the amount Americans spend annually on medical care increased from 4 percent to nearly 10 percent of the nation's gross national product. In 1980, the total cost was over $200 billion. Indeed, medical costs have become the leading cause of personal bankruptcy in the United States.

The increasing specialization of medicine has made *primary-care* medicine scarce. Less than one out of four doctors can be defined as primary-care physicians (general and family practitioners, and some pediatricians, internists, and obstetrician-gynecologists). In many rural and inner-city areas, the only primary care available is in hospital emergency rooms, where waits are long, treatment often impersonal, and continuity of care minimal (and the cost of service delivery very high).

Although it is difficult to measure the quality of health and medical care, a few standard measures are helpful. *Life expectancy,* the number of years a person can be expected to live, is at least a crude measure of a nation's health. According to United Nations data, the U.S. ranks nineteenth among nations in life expectancy for males and ninth for females. *Infant mortality,* generally taken to mean infant death in the first year, is one of our best indicators of health and medical care (particularly prenatal care). The U.S. ranks fifteenth in infant mortality, behind such countries as Sweden, Finland, Canada, Japan, the German Democratic Republic (East Germany), and the United Kingdom (United Nations Demographic Yearbook, 1974).

Our medical system is organized to deliver "medical care" (actually, "sick care") rather than "health care." Medical care is that part of the system "which deals with individuals who are sick or who think they may be sick." Health care is that part of the system "which deals with the promotion and protection of health, including environmental protection, the protection of the individual in the workplace, the prevention of accidents, [and] the provision of pure food and water. . . ." (Sidel and Sidel, 1977: xxi–xxii).

Very few of our resources are invested in "health care"—that is, in *prevention* of disease and illness. Yet, with the decrease in infectious disease and the subsequent increase in chronic disease, prevention is becoming ever more important to our nation's overall health and would probably prove more cost-effective than "medical care" (Department of Health, Education and Welfare, 1979).

There is little *public accountability* in medicine. Recent innovations such as Health Systems Agencies, regional organizations designed to coordinate medical services, and Professional Standards Review Organizations, boards mandated to review the quality of (mostly) hospital care, have had limited success in their efforts to control the quality and cost of medical care. (The recent incredible rise in malpractice suits may be seen not as an indication of an increase in poor medical practice but as an indication that such suits are about the only form of medical accountability presently available to the consumer.)

Another element of our crisis in health care is the *"medicalization"* of society. Many, perhaps far too many, of our social problems have been redefined as medical problems (e.g., alcoholism, drug addiction, child abuse, etc.). Many, again perhaps far too many, of life's normal and natural events have also come to be seen as "medical problems," regardless of pathology (e.g., birth, death, sexuality, etc.). It is by no means clear that such matters constitute appropriate medical problems per se. Indeed, there is evidence that the medicalization of social problems and life's natural events has now itself become a social problem (Zola, 1972).

Many other important elements and manifestations of our crisis in health care are described in the works contained in this volume, including the uneven distribution of disease and health care, the role of the physical environment in disease and illness, the monopolistic nature of the medical profession, the role of government in financing health care, sexism and racism in medical care, and the challenge of self-help groups. The particularities of America's health crisis aside, however, most of the contributors to this volume reflect the growing conviction that the social organization of medicine in the United States has been central to its perpetuation.

Critical Perspectives on Health and Illness

The third major theme of this book is that we must examine the relationship between our society's organization and institutions and its medical care system from a "critical perspective." What do we mean by a critical perspective?

A critical perspective is one that does not consider the present fundamental organization of medicine as sacred and inviolable. Nor does it assume that some other particular organization would necessarily be a panacea for all our health-care problems. A critical perspective accepts no "truth" or "fact" merely because it has hitherto been accepted as such. It examines what is, not as something given or static, but as something out of which change and growth can emerge. Moreover, any theoretical framework that claims to have all the answers to understanding health and illness is not a critical perspective. The social aspects of health and illness are too complex for a monolithic approach.

Further, a critical perspective assumes that a sociology of health and illness entails societal and personal values, and that these values must be considered and made explicit if illness and health-care problems are to be satisfactorily dealt with. Since any critical perspective is informed by values and assumptions, we would like to make ours explicit. (1) The problems and inequalities of health and medical care are connected to the particular historically located social arrangements and the cultural values of any society. (2) Health care should be oriented toward the prevention of disease and illness. (3) The priorities of any medical system should be based on the needs of the consumers and not the providers. A direct corollary of this is that the socially based inequalities of health and medical care must be eliminated. (4) Ultimately, society itself must be changed for health and medical care to improve.

Bringing critical perspectives to bear on the sociology of health and illness has informed the selection of articles contained in this volume. It has also informed editorial comments that introduce and bind together the book's various parts and subparts. Explicitly and implicitly, the goal of this work is toward the awareness that informed social change is a prerequisite for the elimination of socially based inequalities in health and medical care.

Notes

1. Until 1960 only one journal, *Milbank Memorial Fund Quarterly* (now called *Health and Society*), was more or less devoted to medical sociological writings (although many articles on medicine and illness were published in other sociological journals). Today there are five more journals, all of which specifically focus on sociological work on health, illness, and medicine: *The Journal of Health and Social Behavior; Social Science and Medicine; International Journal of Health Services; Sociology of Health and Illness;* and a new annual volume, *Research in the Sociology of Health Care.* Such medical journals as *Medical Care* and *American Journal of Public Health* frequently publish medical sociological articles, as do various psychiatric journals.
2. Inasmuch as we define the sociology of health and illness in such a broad manner, it is not possible to cover adequately all the topics it encompasses in one volume. Although we attempt to touch on most important sociological aspects of health and illness, space limitations precluded presenting all potential topics. For instance, we do not include sections on professional socialization, the social organization of hospitals, and the utilization of services. Discussions of these are easily available in standard medical sociology textbooks. We have made a specific decision not to include materials on mental health

and illness. While mental and physical health are not as separate as was once thought, the sociology of mental health comprises a separate literature and raises some different issues from the ones developed here.

References

Sidel, Victor W. and Ruth Sidel. 1977. A Healthy State. New York: Pantheon Books.

Straus, Robert. 1957. "The nature and status of medical sociology." American Sociological Review 22 (April): 200–204.

U.S. Department of Health, Education and Welfare. 1979. Healthy People: The Surgeon General's Report on Health Promotion and Disease Prevention. Washington, D.C.: U.S. Government Printing Office.

Zola, Irving Kenneth. 1972. "Medicine as an institution of social control." Sociological Review 20: 487–504.

Part One

The Social Production of Disease and Illness

Part One of this book is divided into four sections. While the overriding theme is "the social production of disease and illness," each section develops a particular aspect of the sociology of disease production. For the purposes of this book we define *disease* as the biophysiological phenomena which manifest themselves as changes in and malfunctions of the human body. *Illness,* on the other hand, is the experience of being sick or diseased. Accordingly, we can see disease as a physiological state and illness as a social psychological state presumably caused by the disease. Thus, pathologists and public health doctors deal with disease, patients experience illness, and, ideally, clinical physicians treat both. (Cf. Cassell, 1979.) Furthermore, such a distinction is useful for dealing with the possibility of people feeling ill in the absence of disease or being "diseased" without experiencing illness. Obviously disease and illness are related, but separating them as concepts allows us to explore the objective level of disease and the subjective level of illness. The first three sections of Part One focus primarily on disease, the final one focuses on illness.

All the articles in Part One consider how disease and illness are socially produced. The so-called *medical model* focuses on organic pathology in individual patients, rarely taking societal factors into account. Clinical medicine locates disease as a problem in the individual body, and although this is clearly important and useful, it provides an incomplete and sometimes distorted picture. With the increased concern about chronic disease and its prevention (U.S. DHEW, 1979), the articles suggest that a shift in focus from the internal environment of individuals to the interaction between external environments in which people live and the internal environment of the human body will yield new insights into disease causation and prevention.

The Social Nature of Disease

WHEN WE LOOK HISTORICALLY at the extent and patterns of disease in Western society we see enormous changes. In the early nineteenth century the infant mortality rate was very high, life expectancy was short (approximately forty years), and life-threatening epidemics were common. Infectious diseases, especially those of childhood, were often fatal. Even at the beginning of the twentieth century, the United States' annual death rate was 28 per 1000 population compared with 9 per 1000 today, with the cause of death usually pneumonia, influenza, tuberculosis, typhoid fever, and various forms of dysentery (Cassell, 1979: 72). But patterns of *morbidity* (disease rate) and *mortality* (death rate) have changed. Today we have "conquered" most infectious diseases; they are no longer feared and few people die from them. Chronic diseases such as heart disease, hypertension and stroke, and cancer are now the major causes of death in the United States (see Figure 3, p. 20).

Medicine is usually credited for the great victory over infectious diseases. After all, certain scientific discoveries (e.g., germ theory) and medical interventions (e.g., vaccinations and drugs) had been developed and used to combat infectious diseases and, so the logic goes, must have been responsible for reducing deaths from them. While this view may seem reasonable from a not too careful reading of medical history, it is contradicted by some important social scientific work.

René Dubos (1959) was one of the first to argue that it was social changes in the environment rather than medical interventions that led to the reduction of mortality by infectious diseases. He viewed the nineteenth-century Sanitary Movement's campaign for clean water, air, and proper sewage disposal as a particularly significant "public health" measure. Thomas McKeown (1971) showed that biomedical interventions were not the cause of the decline in mortality in England and Wales in the nineteenth century. This viewpoint has become known as the "limitations of modern medicine" argument (Powles, 1973) and is now well known in public health circles. The argument is essentially a simple one: Discoveries and interventions by *clinical medicine* were not the cause of the decline of mortality for various populations. Rather, it seems that social and environmental factors such as (1) sanitation, (2) improved housing and nutrition, and (3) a general rise in the standard of living were the most significant contributors. This does not mean that clinical medicine did not reduce people's sufferings or prevent or cure diseases in some people; we know it did. But social factors appear much more important than medical interventions in the "conquest" of infectious disease.

In the keynote article of this book, John B. McKinlay and Sonja M. McKinlay assess "Medical Measures and the Decline of Mortality." They offer empirical evidence to support the limitations of medicine argument and point to the social nature of disease. We must note that mortality rates, which are the data on which they base their analysis, only crudely measure "cure" and don't measure "care" at all. But it is important to understand that much of what is attributed to "medical intervention" seems not to be the result of clinical medicine per se.

The limitations of medicine argument underlines the need for a broader, more comprehensive perspective to understanding disease and its treatment (see also Turshen, 1977); a perspective that focuses on the significance of social structure and change in disease causation and prevention.

References

Cassell, Eric J. 1979. The Healer's Art. New York: Penguin Books.

Dubos, René. 1959. Mirage of Health. New York: Harper and Row.

McKeown, Thomas. 1971. "A historical appraisal of the medical task." Pp. 29–55 in G. McLachlan and T. McKeown (Eds.), Medical History and Medical Care: A Symposium of Perspectives. New York: Oxford University Press.

Powles, John. 1973. "On the limitations of modern medicine." Science, Medicine and Man 1: 1–30.

Turshen, Meredeth. 1977. "The political ecology of diseases." The Review of Radical Political Economics 9 (Spring): 45–60.

U.S. Department of Health, Education and Welfare. 1979. Healthy People: The Surgeon General's Report on Health Promotion and Disease Prevention.

1

Medical Measures and the Decline of Mortality

John B. McKinlay and Sonja M. McKinlay

... by the time laboratory medicine came effectively into the picture the job had been carried far toward completion by the humanitarians and social reformers of the nineteenth century. Their doctrine that nature is holy and healthful was scientifically naive but proved highly effective in dealing with the most important health problems of their age. When the tide is receding from the beach it is easy to have the illusion that one can empty the ocean by removing water with a pail.
R. Dubos, Mirage of Health, *New York: Perennial Library, 1959, p. 23*

Introducing a Medical Heresy

The modern "heresy" that medical care (as it is traditionally conceived) is generally unrelated to improvements in the health of populations (as distinct from individuals) is still dismissed as unthinkable in much the same way as the so-called heresies of former times. And this is despite a long history of support in popular and scientific writings as well as from able minds in a variety of disciplines. History is replete with examples of how, understandably enough, self-interested individuals and groups denounced popular customs and beliefs which appeared to threaten their own domains of practice, thereby rendering them heresies (for example, physicians' denunciation of midwives as witches, during the Middle Ages). We also know that vast institutional resources have often been deployed to neutralize challenges to the assumptions upon which everyday organizational activities were founded and legitimated (for example, the Spanish Inquisition). And since it is usually difficult for organizations themselves to directly combat threatening "heresies," we often find otherwise credible practitioners, perhaps unwittingly, serving the interests of organizations in this capacity. These historical responses may find a modern parallel in the way the everyday practitioners of medicine, on their own altruistic or "scientific" grounds and still perhaps unwittingly, serve present-day institutions (hospital complexes, university medical centers, pharmaceutical houses, and insurance companies) by spearheading an assault on a most fundamental challenging heresy of our time: *that the introduction of specific medical measures and/or the expansion of medical services are generally not responsible for most of the modern decline in mortality.*

In different historical epochs and cultures, there appear to be characteristic ways of explaining the arrival and departure of natural viscissitudes. For salvation from some plague, it may be that the gods were appeased, good works rewarded, or some imbalance in nature corrected. And there always seems to be some person or group (witch doctors, priests, medicine men) able to persuade others, sometimes on the basis of acceptable evidence for most people at that time, that they have *the* explanation for the phenomenon in question and may even claim responsibility for it. They also seem to benefit most from common acceptance of the explanations they offer. It is not uncommon today for biotechnological knowledge and specific medical interventions to be invoked as *the major reason* for most of the modern (twentieth century) decline in mortality.[1] Responsibility for this decline is often claimed by, or ascribed to, the present-day major beneficiaries of this prevailing explanation. But both in terms of the history of knowledge and on the basis of data presented in this paper, one can reasonably wonder whether the supposedly more sophisticated explanations proffered in our own time (while seemingly distinguishable from those accepted in the past) are really all that different from those of other cultures and earlier times, or any more reliable. Is medicine, the physician, or the medical profession any more entitled to claim responsibility for the decline in mortality that obviously has occurred in this century than, say, some folk hero or aristocracy of priests sometime in the past?

Aims

Our general intention in this paper is to sustain the ongoing debate on the questionable contribution of specific medical measures and/or the expansion of medical services to the observable decline in mortality in the twentieth century. More specifically, the following three tasks are addressed: (a) selected studies are reviewed which illustrate that, far from being idiosyncratic and/or heretical, the issue addressed in this paper has a long history, is the subject of considerable attention elsewhere, attracts able minds from a variety of disciplines, and remains a timely issue for concern and research; (b) age- and sex-adjusted mortality rates (standardized to the population of 1900) for the United States, 1900–1973, are presented and then considered in relation to a number of specific and supposedly effective medical interventions (both chemotherapeutic and prophylactic). So far as we know, this is the first time such data have been employed for this particular purpose in the United States, although reference will be made to a similar study for England and Wales; and (c) some policy implications are outlined.

Background to the Issue

The beginning of the serious debate on the questionable contribution of medical measures is commonly associated with the appearance, in Britain, of Talbot Griffith's (1967) *Population Problems in the Age of Malthus.* After examining certain medical activities associated with the eighteenth century—particularly the growth of hospital, dispensary, and midwifery services, additions to knowledge of physiology and anatomy, and the introduction of smallpox inoculation—Griffith concluded that they made important contributions to the observable decline in mortality at that time. Since then, in Britain and more recently in the United States, this debate has continued, regularly engaging scholars from economic history, demography, epidemiology, statistics, and other disciplines. Habakkuk (1953), an economic historian, was probably the first to seriously challenge the prevailing view that the modern increase in population was due to a fall in the death rate attributable to medical interventions. His view was that this rise in population resulted from an increase in the birth rate, which, in turn, was associated with social, economic, and industrial changes in the eighteenth century.

McKeown, without doubt, has pursued the argument more consistently and with greater effect than any other researcher, and the reader is referred to his recent work for more detailed background information. Employing the data and techniques of historical demography, McKeown (a physician by training) has provided a detailed and convincing analysis of the major reasons for the decline of mortality in England and Wales during the eighteenth, nineteenth, and twentieth centuries (McKeown et al., 1955, 1962, 1975). For the eighteenth century, he concludes that the decline was largely attributable to improvements in the environment. His findings for the nineteenth century are summarized as follows:

> . . . the decline of mortality in the second half of the nineteenth century was due wholly to a reduction of deaths from infectious diseases; there was no evidence of a decline in other causes of death. Examination of the diseases which contributed to the decline suggested that the main influences were: (a) rising standards of living, of which the most significant feature was a better diet; (b) improvements in hygiene; and (c) a favorable trend in the relationship between some micro-organisms and the human host. *Therapy made no contributions, and the effect of immunization was restricted to smallpox which accounted for only about one-twentieth of the reduction of the death rate.* (Emphasis added. McKeown et al., 1975, p. 391)

While McKeown's interpretation is based on the experience of England and Wales, he has examined its credibility in the light of the very different circumstances which existed in four other European countries: Sweden, France, Ireland, and Hungary (McKeown et al., 1972). His interpretation appears to withstand this cross-examination. As for the twentieth century

(1901–1971 is the period actually considered), McKeown argues that about three-quarters of the decline was associated with control of infectious diseases and the remainder with conditions not attributable to microorganisms. He distinguishes the infections according to their modes of transmission (air- water- or food-borne) and isolates three types of influences which figure during the period considered: medical measures (specific therapies and immunization), reduced exposure to infection, and improved nutrition. His conclusion is that:

> The main influences on the decline in mortality were improved nutrition on air-borne infections, reduced exposure (from better hygiene) on water- and food-borne diseases and, less certainly, immunization and therapy on the large number of conditions included in the miscellaneous group. Since these three classes were responsible respectively for nearly half, one-sixth, and one-tenth of the fall in the death rate, it is probable that the advancement in nutrition was the major influence. (McKeown et al., 1975, p. 422)

More than twenty years of research by McKeown and his collegues recently culminated in two books—*The Modern Rise of Population* (1976a) and *The Role of Medicine: Dream, Mirage or Nemesis* (1976b)—in which he draws together his many excellent contributions. That the thesis he advances remains highly newsworthy is evidenced by recent editorial reaction in *The Times* of London (1977).

No one in the United States has pursued this thesis with the rigor and consistency which characterize the work by McKeown and his collegues in Britain. Around 1930, there were several limited discussions of the questionable effect of medical measures on selected infectious diseases like diphtheria (Lee, 1931; Wilson and Miles, 1946; Bolduan, 1930) and pneumonia (Pfizer and Co., 1953). In a presidential address to the American Association of Immunologists in 1954 (frequently referred to by McKeown), Magill (1955) marshalled an assortment of data then available—some from England and Wales—to cast doubt on the plausibility of existing accounts of the decline in mortality for several conditions. Probably the most influential work in the United States is that of Dubos who, principally in *Mirage of Health* (1959), *Man Adapting* (1965), and *Man, Medicine and Environment* (1968), focused on the nonmedical reasons for changes in the health of overall populations. In another presidential address, this time to the Infectious Diseases Society of America, Kass (1971), again employing data from England and Wales, argued that most of the decline in mortality for most infectious conditions occurred prior to the discovery of either "the cause" of the disease or some purported "treatment" for it. Before the same society and largely on the basis of clinical experience with infectious diseases and data from a single state (Massachusetts), Weinstein (1974), while conceding there are some effective treatments which seem to yield a favorable outcome (e.g., for poliomyelitis, tuberculosis, and possibly smallpox), argued that despite the presence of supposedly effective treatments some conditions may have increased (e.g., subacute bacterial endocarditis, streptococcal pharyngitis, pneumococcal pneumonia, gonorrhea, and syphilis) and also that mortality for yet other conditions shows improvement in the absence of any treatment (e.g., chickenpox). With the appearance of his book, *Who Shall Live?* (1974), Fuchs, a health economist, contributed to the resurgence of interest in the relative contribution of medical care to the modern decline in mortality in the United States. He believes there has been an unprecedented improvement in health in the United States since about the middle of the eighteenth century, associated primarily with a rise in real income. While agreeing with much of Fuchs' thesis, we will present evidence which seriously questions his belief that "beginning in the mid '30s, major therapeutic discoveries made significant contributions independently of the rise in real income."

Although neither representative nor exhaustive, this brief and selective background should serve to introduce the analysis which follows. Our intention is to highlight the following: (a) the debate over the questionable contribution of medical measures to the modern decline of mortality has a long history and remains topical; (b) although sometimes popularly associated with dilettantes such as Ivan Illich (1976), the debate continues to preoccupy able scholars from a variety of disciplines and remains a matter of concern to the most learned societies; (c) although of emerging interest in the United States, the issue is already a matter of concern and considerable research elsewhere; (d) to the extent that the subject has been pursued in the United States, there has been a restrictive tendency to focus on a few selected diseases, or to employ only statewide data, or to apply evidence from England and Wales directly to the United States situation.

How Reliable are Mortality Statistics?

We have argued elsewhere that mortality statistics are inadequate and can be misleading as indicators of a nation's overall health status (McKinlay and McKinlay, forthcoming). Unfortunately, these are the only types of data which are readily accessible for the examination of time trends, simply because comparable morbidity and disability data have not been available. Apart from this overriding problem, several additional caveats in the use of mortality statistics are: (a) difficulties introduced by changes in the registration area in the United States in the early twentieth century; (b) that often no single disease, but a complex of conditions, may be responsible for death (Krueger, 1966); (c) that studies reveal considerable inaccuracies in recording the cause of death (Moriyama et al., 1958); (d) that there are changes over time in what it is fashionable to diagnose (for example, ischaemic heart disease and cerebrovascular disease); (e) that changes in disease classifications (Dunn and Shackley, 1945) make it difficult to compare some conditions over time and between countries (Reid and Rose, 1964); (f) that some conditions result in immediate death while others have an extended period of latency; and (g) that many conditions are severely debilitating and consume vast medical resources but are now generally non-fatal (e.g., arthritis and diabetes). Other obvious limitations could be added to this list.

However, it would be foolhardy indeed to dismiss all studies based on mortality measures simply because they are possibly beset *with known limitations*. Such data are preferable to those the limitations of which are either unknown or, if known, cannot be estimated. Because of an overawareness of potential inaccuracies, there is a timorous tendency to disregard or devalue studies based on mortality evidence, even though there are innumerable examples of their fruitful use as a basis for planning and informed social action (Alderson, 1976). Sir Austin Bradford Hill (1955) considers one of the most important features of Snow's work on cholera to be his adept use of mortality statistics. A more recent notable example is the study by Inman and Adelstein (1969) of the circumstantial link between the excessive absorption of bronchodilators from pressurized aerosols and the epidemic rise in asthma mortality in children aged ten to fourteen years. Moreover, there is evidence that some of the known inaccuracies of mortality data tend to cancel each other out.[2] Consequently, while mortality statistics may be unreliable for use in individual cases, when pooled for a country and employed in population studies, they can reveal important trends and generate fruitful hypotheses. They have already resulted in informed social action (for example, the use of geographical distributions of mortality in the field of environmental pollution).

Whatever limitations and risks may be associated with the use of mortality statistics, they obviously apply equally to all studies which employ them—both those which attribute the decline in mortality to medical measures and those which argue the converse, or something else entirely. And, if such data constitute acceptable evidence in support of the presence of medicine, then it is not unreasonable, or illogical, to employ them in support of some opposing position. One difficulty is that, depending on the nature of the results, double standards of rigor seem to operate in the evaluation of different studies. Not surprisingly, those which challenge prevailing myths or beliefs are subject to the most stringent methodological and statistical scrutiny, while supportive studies, which frequently employ the flimsiest impressionistic data and inappropriate techniques of analysis, receive general and uncritical acceptance. Even if all possible "ideal" data were available (which they never will be) and if, after appropriate analysis, they happened to support the viewpoint of this paper, we are doubtful that medicine's protagonists would find our thesis any more acceptable.

Figure 1. *The Trend in Mortality for Males and Females Separately (Using Age-Adjusted Rates) for the United States, 1900–1973.**

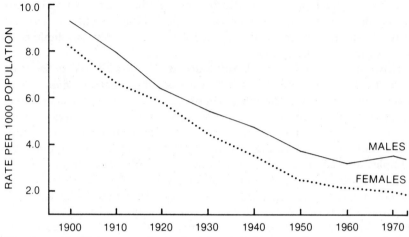

*For these and all other age- and sex-adjusted rates in this paper, the standard population is that of 1900.

The Modern Decline in Mortality

Despite the fact that mortality rates for certain conditions, for selected age and sex categories, continue to fluctuate, or even increase (U.S. Dept. HEW, 1964; Moriyama and Gustavus, 1972; Lilienfeld, 1976), there can be little doubt that a marked decline in overall mortality for the United States has occurred since about 1900 (the earliest point for which reliable national data are available).

Just how dramatic this decline has been in the United States is illustrated in Fig. 1 which shows age-adjusted mortality rates for males and females separately.[3] Both sexes experienced a marked decline in mortality since 1900. The female decline began to level off by about 1950, while 1960 witnessed the beginning of a slight increase for males. Figure 1 also reveals a slight but increasing divergence between male and female mortality since about 1920.

Figure 2 depicts the decline in the overall age-and sex-adjusted rate since the beginning of this century. Between 1900 and 1973, there was a 69.2 percent decrease in overall mortality. The average annual rate of decline from 1900 until 1950 was .22 per 1,000, after which it became an almost negligible decline of .04 per 1,000 annually. Of the total fall in the standardized death rate between 1900 and 1973, 92.3 percent occurred prior to 1950. Figure 2 also plots the decline in the standardized death rate *after* the total number of deaths in each age and sex category has been

Figure 2. *Age- and Sex-Adjusted Mortality Rates for the United States 1900–
1973, Including and Excluding Eleven Major Infectious Diseases,
Contrasted with the Proportion of the Gross National Product
Expended on Medical Care.*

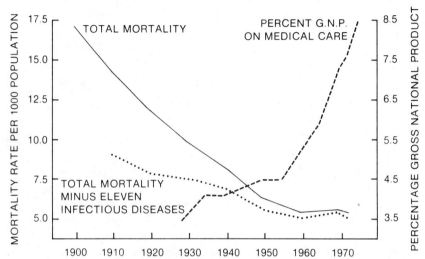

reduced by the number of deaths attributed to the eleven major infectious
conditions (typhoid, smallpox, scarlet fever, measles, whooping cough,
diphtheria, influenza, tuberculosis, pneumonia, diseases of the digestive
system, and poliomyelitis). It should be noted that, although this latter rate
also shows a decline (at least until 1960), its slope is much more shallow
than that for the overall standardized death rate. A major part of the
decline in deaths from these causes since about 1900 may be attributed to
the virtual disappearance of these infectious diseases.

An absurdity is reflected in the third broken line in Fig. 2 which also
plots the increase in the proportion of Gross National Product expended
annually for medical care. *It is evident that the beginning of the precipitate
and still unrestrained rise in medical care expenditures began when nearly
all (92 percent) of the modern decline in mortality this century had already
occurred.*[4]

Figure 3 illustrates how the proportion of deaths contributed by infectious and chronic conditions has changed in the United States since the
beginning of the twentieth century. In 1900, about 40 percent of all deaths
were accounted for by eleven major infectious diseases, 16 percent by three
chronic conditions, 4 percent by accidents, and the remainder (37 percent)
by all other causes. By 1973, only 6 percent of all deaths were due to these
eleven infectious diseases, 58 percent to the same three chronic conditions,
9 percent to accidents, and 27 percent were contributed by other causes.[5]

Now to what phenomenon, or combination of events can we attribute

Figure 3. *Pictorial Representation of the Changing Contribution of Chronic and Infectious Conditions to Total Mortality (Age- and Sex-Adjusted), in the United States, 1900–1973.*

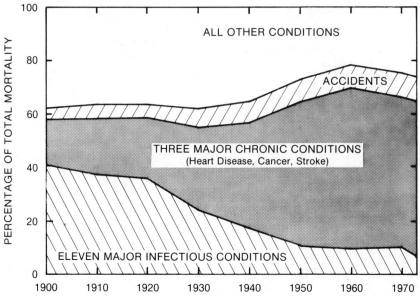

this modern decline in overall mortality? Who (if anyone), or what group, can claim to have been instrumental in effecting this reduction? Can anything be gleaned from an analysis of mortality experience to date that will inform health care policy for the future?

It should be reiterated that a major concern of this paper is to determine the effect, if any, of specific medical measures (both chemotherapeutic and prophylactic) on the decline of mortality. It is clear from Figs. 2 and 3 that most of the observable decline is due to the rapid disappearance of some of the major infectious diseases. Since this is where most of the decline has occurred, it is logical to focus a study of the effect of medical measures on this category of conditions. Moreover, for these eleven conditions, there exist clearly identifiable medical interventions to which the decline in mortality has been popularly ascribed. No analogous interventions exist for the major chronic diseases such as heart disease, cancer, and stroke. Therefore, even where a decline in mortality from these chronic conditions may have occurred, this cannot be ascribed to any specific measure.

The Effect of Medical Measures on Ten Infectious Diseases Which Have Declined

Table 1 summarizes data on the effect of major medical interventions (both chemotherapeutic and prophylactic) on the decline in the age- and

Table 1.
The Contribution of Medical Measures (Both Chemotherapeutic and Prophylactic) to the Fall in the Age- and Sex-Adjusted Death Rates (S.D.R.) of Ten Common Infectious Diseases, and to the Overall Decline in the S.D.R., for the United States, 1900–1973

Disease	Fall in S.D.R. per 1,000 Population, 1900-1973 (a)	Fall in S.D.R. as % of the Total Fall in S.D.R. $(b)=\frac{(a)}{12.14}\times100\%$	Year of Medical Intervention (Either Chemotherapy or Prophylaxis)	Fall in S.D.R. per 1,000 Population After Year of Intervention (c)	Fall in S.D.R. After Intervention as % of Total Fall for the Disease $(d)=\frac{(c)}{(a)}\times100\%$	Fall in S.D.R. After Intervention as % of Total Fall in S.D.R. for All Causes $(e)=\frac{(b)(c)}{(a)}\%$
Tuberculosis	2.00	16.48	Izoniazid/ Streptomycin, 1950	0.17	8.36	1.38
Scarlet Fever	0.10	0.84	Penicillin, 1946	0.00	1.75	0.01
Influenza	0.22	1.78	Vaccine, 1943	0.05	25.33	0.45
Pneumonia	1.42	11.74	Sulphonamide, 1935	0.24	17.19	2.02
Diphtheria	0.43	3.57	Toxoid, 1930	0.06	13.49	0.48
Whooping Cough	0.12	1.00	Vaccine, 1930	0.06	51.00	0.51
Measles	0.12	1.04	Vaccine, 1963	0.00	1.38	0.01
Smallpox	0.02	0.16	Vaccine, 1800	0.02	100.00	0.16
Typhoid	0.36	2.95	Chloramphenicol, 1948	0.00	0.29	0.01
Poliomyelitis	0.03	0.23	Vaccine, Salk/ Sabin, 1955	0.01	25.87	0.06

sex-adjusted death rates in the United States, 1900–1973, for ten of the eleven major infectious diseases listed above. Together, these diseases accounted for approximately 30 percent of all deaths at the turn of the century and nearly 40 percent of the total decline in the mortality rate since then. The ten diseases were selected on the following criteria: (a) some decline in the death rate had occurred in the period 1900–1973; (b) significant decline in the death rate is commonly attributed to some specific medical measure for the disease; and (c) adequate data for the disease over the period 1900–1973 are available. The diseases of the digestive system were omitted primarily because of lack of clarity in diagnosis of specific diseases such as gastritis and enteritis.

Some additional points of explanation should be noted in relation to Table 1. First, the year of medical intervention coincides (as nearly as can be determined) with the first year of widespread or commercial use of the appropriate drug or vaccine.[6] This date does *not* necessarily coincide with the date the measure was either first discovered, or subject to clinical trial. Second, the decline in the death rate for smallpox was calculated using the death rate for 1902 as being the earliest year for which this statistic is readily available (U.S. Bureau of the Census, 1906). For the same reasons, the decline in the death rate from poliomyelitis was calculated from 1910. Third, the table shows the contribution of the decline in each disease to the total decline in mortality over the period 1900–1973 (column b). The overall decline during this period was 12.14 per 1,000 population (17.54 in 1900 to 5.39 in 1973). Fourth, in order to place the experience for each disease in some perspective, Table 1 also shows the contribution of the relative fall in mortality after the intervention to the overall fall in mortality since 1900 (column e). In other words, the figures in this last column represent the percentage of the total fall in mortality contributed by each disease after the date of medical intervention.

It is clear from column b that only reductions in mortality from tuberculosis and pneumonia contributed substantially to the decline in total mortality between 1900 and 1973 (16.5 percent and 11.7 percent, respectively). The remaining eight conditions *together* accounted for less than 12 percent of the total decline over this period. Disregarding smallpox (for which the only effective measure had been introduced about 1800), only influenza, whooping cough, and poliomyelitis show what could be considered substantial declines of 25 percent or more after the date of medical intervention. However, even under the somewhat unrealistic assumption of a constant (linear) rate of decline in the mortality rates, only whooping cough and poliomyelitis even approach the percentage which would have been expected. The remaining six conditions (tuberculosis, scarlet fever, pneumonia, diphtheria, measles, and typhoid) showed negligible declines in their mortality rates subsequent to the date of medical intervention. The seemingly quite large percentages for pneumonia and diphtheria (17.2 and

Table 2.
Pair-Wise Correlation Matrix for 44 Countries, Between Four Measures of Health Status and Three Measures of Medical Care Input

Matrix of Coefficients

Variable	1	2	3a	3b	4a	4b	5	6
1. Infant Mortality Rate (1972)								
2. Crude Mortality Rate (1970–1972)	−0.14							
3.(a) Life Expectancy (Males) at 25 years	−0.14	−0.12						
3.(b) Life Expectancy (Females) at 25 years	−0.12	0.04	0.75					
4.(a) Life Expectancy (Males) at 55 Years	−0.01	0.10	0.74	0.93				
4.(b) Life Expectancy (Females) at 55 Years	−0.13	0.01	0.75	0.98	0.95			
5. Population per Hospital Bed (1971–1973)	0.64	−0.30	0.05	−0.02	0.17	0.0		
6. Population per Physician (1971–1973)	0.36	−0.30	0.11	0.04	0.16	0.07	0.70	
7. Per Capita Gross National Product: In $U.S. Equivalent (1972)	−0.66	0.26	0.16	0.18	0.07	0.22	−0.56	−0.46
Variable (by number)	1	2	3a	3b	4a	4b	5	6

SOURCES: 1. *United Nations Demographic Yearbook: 1974*, New York, United Nations Publications, 1975. (For the Crude and Infant Mortality Rates). 2. *World Health Statistics Annual: 1972*, Vol. 1, Geneva, World Health Organization, 1975, pp. 780–783. (For the Life Expectancy Figures). 3. *United Nations Statistical Yearbook, 1973 and 1975*. New York, United Nations Publications, 25th and 27th issues, 1974 and 1976. (For the Population bed/physician ratios). 4. *The World Bank Atlas*. Washington, D.C., World Bank, 1975. (For the per capita Gross National Product).

13.5, respectively) must of course be viewed in the context of relatively early interventions—1935 and 1930.

In order to examine more closely the relation of mortality trends for these diseases to the medical interventions, graphs are presented for each disease in Fig. 4. Clearly, for tuberculosis, typhoid, measles, and scarlet fever, the medical measures considered were introduced at the point when the death rate for each of these diseases was already negligible. Any change in the rates of decline which may have occurred subsequent to the interventions could only be minute. Of the remaining five diseases (excluding smallpox with its negligible contribution), it is only for poliomyelitis that the medical measure appears to have produced any noticeable change in the trends. Given peaks in the death rate for 1930, 1950 (and possibly for 1910), a comparable peak could have been expected in 1970. Instead, the death rate dropped to the point of disappearance after 1950 and has remained negligible. The four other diseases (pneumonia, influenza, whooping cough, and diphtheria) exhibit relatively smooth mortality trends which are unaffected by the medical measures, even though these were introduced relatively early, when the death rates were still notable.

It may be useful at this point to briefly consider the common and dubious practice of projecting estimated mortality trends (Witte and Axnick, 1975). In order to show the beneficial (or even detrimental) effect of some medical measure, a line, estimated on a set of points observed prior to the introduction of the measure, is projected over the period subsequent to the point of intervention. Any resulting discrepancy between the projected line and the observed trend is then used as some kind of "evidence" of an effective or beneficial intervention. According to statistical theory on least squares estimation, an estimated line can serve as a useful predictor, but the prediction is only valid, and its error calculable, within the range of the points used to estimate the line. Moreover, those predicted values which lie at the extremes of the range are subject to much larger errors than those nearer the center. It is, therefore, probable that, even if the projected line was a reasonable estimate of the trend after the intervention (which, of course, it is not), the divergent observed trend is probably well within reasonable error limits of the estimated line (assuming the error could be calculated), as the error will be relatively large. In other words, this technique is of dubious value as no valid conclusions are possible from its application, and a relatively large prediction error cannot be estimated, which is required in order to objectively judge the extent of divergence of an observed trend.

With regard to the ten infectious diseases considered in this paper, when lines were fitted to the nine or ten points available over the entire period (1900–1973), four exhibited a reasonably good fit to a straight line (scarlet fever, measles, whooping cough, and poliomyelitis), while another four (typhoid, diphtheria, tuberculosis, and pneumonia) showed a very

Figure 4. *The Fall in the Standardized Death Rate (per 1,000 Population) for Nine Common Infectious Diseases in Relation to Specific Medical Measures, for the United States, 1900–1973.*

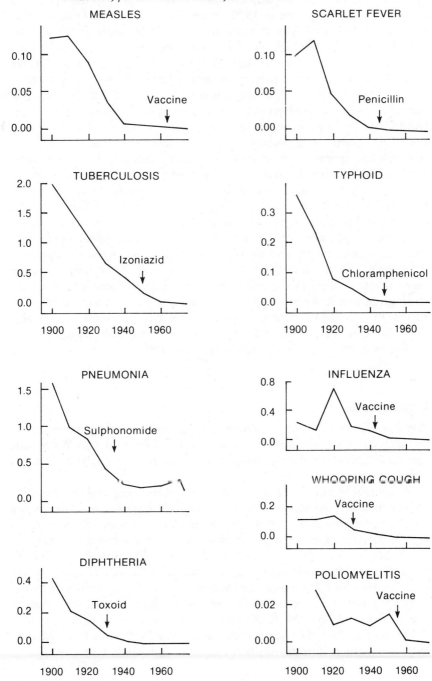

good quadratic fit (to a curved line). Of the remaining two diseases, small-pox showed a negligible decline, as it was already a minor cause of death in 1900 (only 0.1 percent), and influenza showed a poor fit because of the extremely high death rate in 1920. From Fig. 4 it is clear, however, that the rate of decline slowed in more recent years for most of the diseases considered—a trend which could be anticipated as rates approach zero.[7]

Now it is possible to argue that, given the few data points available, the fit is somewhat crude and may be insensitive to any changes subsequent to a point of intervention. However, this can be countered with the observation that, given the relatively low death rates for these diseases, any change would have to be extremely marked in order to be detected in the overall mortality experience. Certainly, from the evidence considered here, only poliomyelitis appears to have had a noticeably changed death rate subsequent to intervention. Even if it were assumed that this change was entirely due to the vaccines, then only about one percent of the decline following interventions for the diseases considered here (column d of Table 1) could be attributed to medical measures. Rather more conservatively, if we attribute some of the subsequent fall in the death rates for pneumonia, influenza, whooping cough, and diphtheria to medical measures, then perhaps 3.5 percent of the fall in the overall death rate can be explained through medical intervention in the major infectious diseases considered here. Indeed, given that it is precisely for these diseases that medicine claims most success in lowering mortality, 3.5 percent probably represents a reasonable upper-limit estimate of the total contribution of medical measures to the decline in mortality in the United States since 1900.

Conclusions

Without claiming they are definitive findings, and eschewing pretentions to an analysis as sophisticated as McKeown's for England and Wales, one can reasonably draw the following conclusions from the analysis presented in this paper:

In general, medical measures (both chemotherapeutic and prophylactic) appear to have contributed little to the overall decline in mortality in the United States since about 1900—having in many instances been introduced several decades after a marked decline had already set in and having no detectable influence in most instances. More specifically, with reference to those five conditions (influenza, pneumonia, diphtheria, whooping cough, and poliomyelitis) for which the decline in mortality appears substantial after the point of intervention—and on the unlikely assumption that all of this decline is attributable to the intervention—it is estimated that at most 3.5 percent of the total decline in mortality since 1900 could be ascribed to medical measures introduced for the diseases considered here.

These conclusions, in support of the thesis introduced earlier, suggest issues of the most strategic significance for researchers and health care legislators. Profound policy implications follow from either a confirmation or a rejection of the thesis. If one subscribes to the view that we are slowly but surely eliminating one disease after another because of medical interventions, then there may be little commitment to social change and even resistance to some reordering of priorities in medical expenditures. If a disease X is disappearing primarily because of the presence of a particular intervention or service Y, then clearly Y should be left intact, or, more preferably, be expanded. Its demonstrable contribution justifies its presence. But, if it can be shown convincingly, and on commonly accepted grounds, that the major part of the decline in mortality is unrelated to medical care activities, then some commitment to social change and a reordering of priorities may ensue. For, if the disappearance of X is largely unrelated to the presence of Y, or even occurs in the absence of Y, then clearly the expansion and even the continuance of Y can be reasonably questioned. Its demonstrable ineffectiveness justifies some reappraisal of its significance and the wisdom of expanding it in its existing form.

In this paper we have attempted to dispel the myth that medical measures and the presence of medical services were primarily responsible for the modern decline of mortality. The question now remains: if they were not primarily responsible for it, then how is it to be explained? An adequate answer to this further question would require a more substantial research effort than that reported here, but is likely to be along the lines suggested by McKeown which were referred to early in this paper. Hopefully, this paper will serve as a catalyst for such research, incorporating adequate data and appropriate methods of analysis, in an effort to arrive at a more viable alternative explanation.

Notes

1. It is obviously important to distinguish between (a) advances in knowledge of the cause and natural course of some condition and (b) improvements in our ability to effectively treat some condition (that is, to alter its natural course). In many instances these two areas are disjoint and appear at different stages of development. There are, on the one hand, disease processes about which considerable knowledge has been accrued, yet this has not resulted (nor necessarily will) in the development of effective treatments. On the other hand, there are conditions for which demonstrably effective treatments have been devised in the absence of knowledge of the disease process and/or its causes.

2. Barker and Rose cite one study which compared the ante-mortem and autopsy diagnoses in 9,501 deaths which occurred in 75 different hospitals. Despite

lack of a concurrence on *individual* cases, the *overall* frequency was very similar in diagnoses obtained on either an ante-mortem or post-mortem basis. As an example they note that clinical diagnoses of carcinoma of the rectum were confirmed at autopsy in only 67 percent of cases, but the incorrect clinical diagnoses were balanced by an almost identical number of lesions diagnosed for the first time at autopsy (Barker and Rose, 1976).

3. All age and sex adjustments were made by the "direct" method using the population of 1900 as the standard. For further information on this method of adjustment, see Hill (1971) and Shryock et al. (1971).

4. Rutstein (1967), although fervently espousing the traditional view that medical advances have been largely responsible for the decline in mortality, discussed this disjunction and termed it "The Paradox of Modern Medicine." More recently, and from a perspective that is generally consistent with that advanced here, Powles (1973) noted the same phenomenon in England and Wales.

5. Deaths in the category of chronic respiratory diseases (chronic bronchitis, asthma, emphysema, and other chronic obstructive lung diseases) could not be included in the group of chronic conditions because of insurmountable difficulties inherent in the many changes in disease classification and in the tabulation of statistics.

6. In determining the dates of intervention we relied upon: (a) standard epidemiology and public health texts; (b) the recollections of authorities in the field of infectious diseases; and (c) recent publications on the same subject.

7. For this reason, a negative exponential model is sometimes used to fit a curved line to such data. This was not presented here as the number of points available was small and the difference between a simple quadratic and negative exponential fit was not, upon investigation, able to be detected.

References

Alderson, M. 1976. *An Introduction to Epidemiology.* London: Macmillan Press. pp. 7–27.

Barker, D.J.P., and Rose, G. 1976. *Epidemiology in Medical Practice.* London: Churchill Livingstone. p. 6.

Bolduan, C.F. 1930. *How to Protect Children From Diphtheria.* New York: N.Y.C. Health Department.

Dubos, R. 1959. *Mirage of Health.* New York: Harper and Row.

Dubos, R. 1965. *Man Adapting.* New Haven, Connecticut: Yale University Press.

Dubos, R. 1968. *Man, Medicine and Environment.* London: Pall Mall Press.

Dunn, H.L., and Shackley, W. 1945. *Comparison of cause of death assignments by the 1929 and 1938 revisions of the International List: Deaths in the United States, 1940 Vital Statistics—Special Reports* 19:153–277, 1944, Washington, D.C.: U.S. Department of Commerce, Bureau of the Census.

Fuchs, V.R. 1974. *Who Shall Live?* New York: Basic Books. p. 54.

Griffith, T. 1967. *Population Problems in the Age of Malthus.* 2nd ed. London: Frank Cass.

Habakkuk, H.J. 1953. English Population in the Eighteenth Century. *Economic History Review,* 6.

Hill, A.B. 1971. *Principles of Medical Statistics.* 9th ed. London: Oxford University Press.

Hill, A.B. 1955. Snow—An Appreciation. *Proceedings of the Royal Society of Medicine* 48:1008–1012.

Illich, I. 1976. *Medical Nemesis.* New York: Pantheon Books.

Inman, W.H.W., and Adelstein, A.M. 1969. Rise and fall of asthma mortality in England and Wales, in relation to use of pressurized aerosols. *Lancet* 2:278–285.

Kass, E.H. 1971. Infectious diseases and social change. *The Journal of Infectious Diseases* 123 (1):110–114.

Krueger, D.E. 1966. New enumerators for old denominators—multiple causes of death. In *Epidemiological Approaches to the Study of Cancer and Other Chronic Diseases,* edited by W. Haenszel. National Cancer Printing Office. pp. 431–443.

Lee, W.W. 1931. Diphtheria Immunization in Philadelphia and New York City. *Journal of Preventive Medicine* (Baltimore) 5:211–220.

Lilienfeld, A.M. 1976. *Foundations of Epidemiology.* New York: Oxford University Press. pp. 51–111.

McKeown, T. 1976a. *The Modern Rise of Population.* London: Edward Arnold.

McKeown, T. 1976b. *The Role of Medicine: Dream, Mirage or Nemesis.* London: Nuffield Provincial Hospitals Trust.

McKeown, T.; Brown, R.G.; and Record, R.G. 1972. An interpretation of the modern rise of population in Europe. *Population Studies* 26:345–382.

McKeown, T., and Record, R.G. 1955. Medical evidence related to English population changes in the eighteenth century. *Population Studies* 9:119–141.

McKeown, T., and Record, R.G. 1962. Reasons for the decline in mortality in England and Wales during the nineteenth century. *Population Studies* 16:94–122.

McKeown, T.; Record, R.G.; and Turner, R.D. 1975. An interpretation of the decline of mortality in England and Wales during the twentieth century, *Population Studies* 29:391–422.

McKinlay, J.B., and McKinlay, S.M. *A refutation of the thesis that the health of the nation is improving.* Forthcoming.

Magill, T.P. 1955. The immunologist and the evil spirits. *Journal of Immunology* 74:1–8.

Moriyama, I.M.; Baum, W.S.; Haenszel, W.M.; and Mattison, B.F. 1958. Inquiry into diagnostic evidence supporting medical certifications of death. *American Journal of Public Health* 48:1376–1387.

Moriyama, I.M., and Gustavus, S.O. 1972. *Cohort Mortality and Survivorship: United States Death—Registration States, 1900–1968.* National Center for Health Statistics, Series 3, No. 16. Washington, D.C.: U.S. Government Printing Office.

Pfizer, C. and Company. 1953. *The Pneumonias, Management with Antibiotic Therapy.* Brooklyn.

Powles, J. 1973. On the limitations of modern medicine. *Science, Medicine and Man.* 1:2–3.

Reid, O.D., and Rose, G.A. 1964. Assessing the comparability of mortality statistics. *British Medical Journal* 2:1437–1439.

Rutstein, D. 1967. *The Coming Revolution in Medicine*. Cambridge, Massachusettes: MIT Press.

Shryock, H., et al. 1971. *The Methods and Materials of Demography*. Washington, D.C.: U.S. Government Printing Office.

The Times (London). 1977. The Doctors Dilemma: How to Cure Society of a Life Style That Makes People Sick. Friday, January 21.

U.S. Department of Health, Education and Welfare. 1964. *The Change in Mortality Trend in the United States*. National Center for Health Statistics, Series 3, No. 1. Washington, D.C.: U.S. Government Printing Office.

U.S. Bureau of the Census. 1906. *Mortality Statistics 1900–1904*. Washington, D.C.: Government Printing Office.

Weinstein, L. 1974. Infectious Disease: Retrospect and Reminiscence, *The Journal of Infectious Diseases*. 129 (4):480–492.

Wilson, G.S., and Miles, A.A. 1946. In Topley and Wilson's *Principles of Bacteriology and Immunity*. Baltimore: Williams and Wilkins.

Witte, J.J., and Axnick, N.W. 1975. The benefits from ten years of measles immunization in the United States. *Public Health Reports* 90 (3):205–207.

This paper reports part of a larger research project supported by a grant from the Milbank Memorial Fund (to Boston University) and the Carnegie Foundation (to the Radcliffe Institute). The authors would like to thank John Stoeckle, M.D. (Massachusetts General Hospital) and Louis Weinstein, M.D. (Peter Bent Brigham Hospital) for helpful discussions during earlier stages of the research.

Who Gets Sick? The Unequal Social Distribution of Disease

DISEASE IS NOT DISTRIBUTED EVENLY throughout the population. Certain groups of people get sick more often, and some populations die at higher rates than others. The study of what groups of people get sick with what diseases is called *epidemiology* and has been defined by one expert as ". . . the study of the distributions and determinants of states of health in human populations" (Susser, 1973: 1). By studying populations rather than individuals, epidemiologists seek to identify characteristics of groups of people or their environments which make them more or less vulnerable to disease. Recently, the term *social epidemiology* has been used by some researchers to emphasize the importance of social variables in the patterning of disease. For the social scientist, the study of social epidemiology is central to the understanding of the connections between society and physical well-being. This section presents information about the distribution of disease in the United States and explores the possible explanations for specific differences in health according to social class, gender, and life style.

The early nineteenth century saw the emergence of a "social medicine" with a number of important studies in Western Europe. In England, Edwin Chadwick studied population death rates to identify the connections of disease with social problems, such as poverty, laying an important foundation for the developing Public Health Movement (Chadwick, 1842, in Susser, 1973). Another early investigator in social medicine, Rudolf Virchow, was asked by the Prussian government to study the causes of a terrible typhus epidemic. His pioneering work identified a relationship between disease and particular features of society, including the economy, conditions of work, and the organization of agriculture (Virchow, 1868, 1879, in Waitzkin, 1978). The success of social efforts like sanitary reform were discussed in the previous section in the context of the limitations of modern medicine argument. In this section we present selected studies on the distribution of death and sickness in the United States and point to the relevance of a social epidemiological perspective for understanding those patterns.

In the United States one of the most striking features about the distribution of disease is its relationship to poverty. By and large, death and disease vary *inversely* with social class; that is, the poorer the population, the more sick people and the higher the death rates. For example,

> Low income people in general have worse health than people with higher incomes. In 1976, about half of the population 45–64 years of age with family incomes of less than $5,000 were limited in their usual activity because of a chronic condition compared with about a sixth of the population with incomes of $15,000 or more. Similarly people 45–64 years of age with low family incomes had more than three times as many bed-disability days per person as with people with higher incomes (19 days versus 6 days). (DHEW, 1978: ix.)

While it has been known for well over a century that poor people suffer from more disease than others, just how poverty influences health is not completely understood. In their article, "Social Class, Susceptibility and Sickness," S. Leonard Syme and Lisa F. Berkman explore what is known about the relationship of social class and sickness, including the influence of stress, living conditions, nutrition, and medical services on the patterns of death and disease among the poor. They particularly focus on how life in the lower class may compromise "disease defense systems" and engender greater vulnerability to disease.

Another consistent and puzzling difference exists between the disease and death patterns of women and men. Women have higher *morbidity* (disease) rates than men, but men have higher *mortality* (death) rates. There is a great deal of disagreement as to the explanation for these differences. Among the issues being debated is whether women actually do get sick more often than men or whether they are more likely to report symptoms or seek medical care. Some investigators suggest that women have been socialized to experience or accept a definition of their problems as personal ones requiring medical care (e.g., Nathanson, 1977; Verbrugge, 1979). Others claim that these different socialization processes, while important, do not account for the systematic differences in disease patterns between women and men (Gove and Hughes, 1979). Ingrid Waldron's article in this section asks "Why Do Women Live Longer Than Men?" and presents a range of evidence that suggests the importance of social and psychological socialization factors involved in being raised as a man or a woman in our society on physical vulnerability to accidents and disease. Her article argues for the importance of an interaction between these social-psychological characteristics and the consequent patterns of biological disease.

In a fascinating little article, "A Tale of Two States," Victor R. Fuchs compares the health of the populations of two neighboring states: Nevada and Utah. While similar in many ways, these populations have very different patterns of death. Fuchs argues that the explanation for this difference is to be found in the life styles of each of the populations; these life style differences emerge from the cultural environments, values, and norms of each of the populations.

The research represented by these articles challenges the traditional medical model, at least to the degree that it points to social and sociological factors in the production of disease. A recent nine-year follow-up study (Berkman and Syme, 1979) provides evidence that groups with weaker "social networks" (neighborhood, family, or community ties) have two to four times the relative mortality risk of groups with strong social networks. Research in social epidemiology, stress, and social networks has demonstrated again and again that diseases are unequally distributed in society. There is a need for a new and broader conceptualization of disease production than the medical model provides; one that can account for social causes of disease differentiation in various populations. Although this model is still in the embryonic stage, several analysts propose the notion of *general susceptibility* as useful for reorienting our analysis (Najman, 1980; and also the Syme and Berkman article in this section). General susceptibility holds that social position, "stress," life style, or some combination of these make certain groups more vulnerable or susceptible to disease and death. These factors may not directly cause disease, but they are central in disease production. As one proponent of this view suggests: ". . . it would appear that some combination of situations, experiences and behaviors either predispose or precipitate poor health and death in a small proportion of the persons exposed." (Najman, 1980: 235) This type of reconceptualization of disease causation shifts our analytic attention from the individual to the social and physical environment. Development of such a model could go a long way in explaining disease production as a social process and, ultimately, in pointing toward new directions for intervention and prevention.

References

Berkman, Lisa F., and S. L. Syme. 1979. "Social networks, host resistance, and mortality: A nine-year follow-up study of Alameda County residents." American Journal of Epidemiology. 109:(July) 186–204.

Chadwick, Edwin. 1842. Report on the Sanitary Condition of the Labouring Population of Great Britain. Reprinted 1965. Edinburgh: Edinburgh University Press.

Department of Health, Education, and Welfare. 1978. Health United States 1978. Public Health Service, Office of the Assistant Secretary for Health, National Center for Health Statistics, National Center for Health Statistics Research Center Building, 3700 East-West Highway, Hyattsville MD 20782. DHEW Publication No. (PHS) 78-1232, December.

Gove, Walter, and Michael Hughes. 1979. "Possible causes of the apparent sex differences in physical health: An empirical investigation." American Sociological Review. 44: 126–146.

Najman, Jackob M. 1980. "Theories of disease causation and the concept of general susceptibility: A review." Social Science and Medicine. 14A:(May) 231–237.

Nathanson, Constance. 1977. "Sex, illness and medical care: A review of data, theory and method." Social Science and Medicine. 11:13–25.

Susser, Mervyn. 1973. Causal Thinking in the Health Sciences, Concepts and Strategies in Epidemiology. New York: Oxford University Press.

Verbrugge, Lois. 1979. "Marital status and health." Journal of Marriage and Family. (May): 267–285.

Virchow, Rudolf. 1958. Disease, Life and Man. Tr. Lelland J. Rather. Stanford: Stanford University Press.

Waitzkin, Howard. 1978. "A Marxist view of medical care." Annals of Internal Medicine. 89:264–278.

2

Social Class, Susceptibility, and Sickness

S. Leonard Syme and Lisa F. Berkman

Social class gradients of mortality and life expectancy have been observed for centuries, and a vast body of evidence has shown consistently that those in the lower classes have higher mortality, morbidity, and disability rates. While these patterns have been observed repeatedly, the explanations offered to account for them show no such consistency. The most frequent explanations have included poor housing, crowding, racial factors, low income, poor education and unemployment, all of which have been said to result in such outcomes as poor nutrition, poor medical care (either through non-availability or non-utilization of resources), strenuous conditions of employment in non-hygienic settings, and increased exposure to noxious agents. While these explanations account for some of the observed relationships, we have found them inadequate to explain the very large number of diseases associated with socioeconomic status. It seemed useful, therefore, to reexamine these associations in search of a more satisfactory hypothesis.

Obviously, this is an important issue. It is clear that new approaches must be explored emphasizing the primary prevention of disease in addition to those approaches that merely focus on treatment of the sick (1). It is clear also that such preventive approaches must involve community and environmental interventions rather than one-to-one preventive encounters (2). Therefore, we must understand more precisely those features of the environment that are etiologically related to disease so that interventions at this level can be more intelligently planned.

Of all the disease outcomes considered, it is evident that low socioeconomic status is most strikingly associated with high rates of infectious and parasitic diseases (3–7) as well as with higher infant mortality rates (8, 9). However, in our review we found higher rates among lower class groups of a very much wider range of diseases and conditions for which obvious explanations were not as easily forthcoming. In a comprehensive review of over 30 studies, Antonovsky (10) concluded that those in the lower classes invariably have lower life expectancy and higher death rates from all causes of death, and that this higher rate has been observed since the 12th century when data on this question were first organized. While differences in infectious disease and infant mortality rates probably accounted for much of this difference between the classes in earlier years, current differences must primarily be attributable to mortality from non-infectious disease.

Kitagawa and Hauser (11) recently completed a massive nationwide study of mortality in the United States. Among men and women in the 25–64-year age group, mortality rates varied dramatically by level of education, income, and occupation, considered together or separately. For example, . . . white males at low education levels had age-adjusted mortality rates 64 per cent higher than men in higher education categories. For white women, those in lower education groups had an age-adjusted mortality rate 105 per cent higher. For non-white males, the differential was 31 per cent and, for non-white females, it was 70 per cent. These mortality differentials also were reflected in substantial differences in life expectancy, and . . . for most specific causes of death. . . . White males in the lowest education groups have higher age-adjusted mortality rates for every cause of death for which data are available. For white females, those in the lowest education group have an excess mortality rate for all causes except cancer of the breast and motor vehicle accidents.

These gradients of mortality among the social classes have been observed over the world by many investigators (12–18) and have not changed materially since 1900 (except that non-whites, especially higher status non-whites, have experienced a relatively more favorable improvement). This consistent finding in time and space is all the more remarkable since the concept of "social class" has been defined and measured in so many different ways by these investigators. That the same findings have been obtained in spite of such methodological differences lends strength to the validity of the observations; it suggests also that the concept is an imprecise term encompassing diverse elements of varying etiologic significance.

In addition to data on mortality, higher rates of morbidity also have been observed for a vast array of conditions among those in lower class groups (19–28). This is an important observation since it indicates that excess mortality rates among lower status groups are not merely attributable to a higher case fatality death rate in those groups but are accompanied also by a higher prevalence of morbidity. Of special interest in this regard are data on the various mental illnesses, a major cause of morbidity. As shown by many investigators (29–35), those in lower as compared to higher socioeconomic groups have higher rates of schizophrenia, are more depressed, more unhappy, more worried, more anxious, and are less hopeful about the future.

In summary, persons in lower class groups have higher morbidity and mortality rates of almost every disease or illness, and these differentials have not diminished over time. While particular hypotheses may be offered to explain the gradient for one or another of these specific diseases, the fact that so many diseases exhibit the same gradient leads to speculation that a more general explanation may be more appropriate than a series of disease-specific explanations.

In a study reported elsewhere (36), it was noted that although blacks had higher rates of hypertension than whites, blacks in the lower classes had higher rates of hypertension than blacks in the upper classes. An identical social class gradient for hypertension was noted among whites in the sample. In that report, it was concluded that hypertension was associated more with social class than with racial factors, and it was suggested that the greater prevalence of obesity in the lower class might be a possible explanation. The present review makes that earlier suggestion far less attractive since so many diseases and conditions appear to be of higher prevalence in the lower class groups. It seems clear that we must frame hypotheses of sufficient generality to account for this phenomenon.

One hypothesis that has been suggested is that persons in the lower classes either have less access to medical care resources or, if care is available, that they do not benefit from that availability. This possibility should be explored in more detail, but current evidence available does not suggest that differences in medical care resources will entirely explain social class gradients in disease. The hypertension project summarized above was conducted at the Kaiser Permanente facility in Oakland, California, which is a pre-paid health plan with medical facilities freely available to all study subjects. The data in this study showed that persons in lower status groups had utilized medical resources more frequently than those in higher status categories (37). To study the influence of medical care in explaining these differences in blood pressure levels, all persons in the Kaiser study who had ever been clinically diagnosed as hypertensive, or who had ever taken medicine for high blood pressure, were removed from consideration. Differences in blood pressure level between those in the highest and lowest social classes were diminished when hypertensives were removed from analysis, but those in the lowest class still had higher (normal) pressures. Thus, while differences in medical care may have accounted for some of the variation observed among the social class groups, substantial differences in blood pressures among these groups nevertheless remained. Similar findings have been reported from studies at the Health Insurance Plan of New York (38).

Lipworth and colleagues (39) also examined this issue in a study of cancer survival rates among various income groups in Boston. In that study, low-income persons had substantially less favorable one and three-year survival rates following treatment at identical tumor clinics and hospitals; these differences were not acounted for by differences in stage of cancer at diagnosis, by the age of patients, or by the specific kind of treatment patients received. It was concluded that patients from lower income areas simply did not fare as well following treatment for cancer. While it is still possible that lower class patients received less adequate medical care, the differences observed in survival rates did not seem attributable to the more obvious variations in quality of treatment. Other studies support this general conclusion but not enough data are available to assess clearly the role of medical care in explaining social class gradients in morbidity and mortality; it would seem, however, that the medical care hypothesis does not account for a major portion of these gradients.

Another possible explanation offered to explain these consistent differences is that persons in lower socioeconomic groups live in a more toxic, hazardous and non-hygienic environment resulting in a broad array of disease consequences. That these environments exert an influence on disease outcome is supported by research on crowding and rheumatic fever (5), poverty areas and health (40), and on air pollution and respiratory illnesses (41). While lower class groups certainly are exposed to a more physically noxious environment, physical factors alone are frequently unable to explain observed relationships between socioeconomic status and disease outcome. One example of this is provided by the report of Guerrin and Borgatta (16) showing that the proportion of people who are illiterate in a census tract is a more important indicator of tuberculosis occurrence than are either economic or racial variables. Similarly, the work of Booth (42) suggests that perceived crowding which is not highly correlated with objective measures of crowding may have adverse effects on individuals.

There can be little doubt that the highest morbidity and mortality rates observed in the lower social classes are in part due to inadequate medical care services as well as to the impact of a toxic and hazardous physical environment. There can be little doubt, also, that these factors do not entirely explain the discrepancy in rates between the classes. Thus, while enormous improvements have been made in environmental quality and in medical care, the mortality rate gap between the classes has not diminished. It is true that mortality rates have been declining over the years, and it is probably true also that this benefit is attributable in large part to the enormous improvements that have been made in food and water purity, in sanitary engineering, in literacy and health education, and in medical and surgical knowledge. It is important to recognize, however, that these reductions in mortality rates have not eliminated the gap between the highest and the lowest social class groups; this gap remains very substantial and has apparently stabilized during the last 40 years. Thus, while improvements in the environment and in medical care clearly have been of value, other factors must be identified to account for this continuing differential in mortality rate and life expectancy.

The identification of these new factors might profitably be guided by the repeated observation of social class gradients in a wide range of disease distributions. That so many different kinds of diseases are more frequent in lower class groupings directs attention to generalized susceptibility to disease and to generalized compromises of disease defense systems. Thus, if something about life in the lower social classes increases vulnerability to illness in general, it would not be surprising to observe an increased prevalence of many different types of diseases and conditions among people in the lower classes.

While laboratory experiments on both humans and animals have established that certain "stressful events" have physiologic consequences, very little is known about the nature of these "stressful events" in nonlaboratory settings. Thus, while we may conclude that "something" about the lower class environment is stressful, we know much less about what specifically constitutes that stress. Rather than attempting to identify *specific* risk factors for *specific* diseases in investigating this question, it may be more meaningful to identify those factors that affect *general* susceptibility to disease. The specification of such factors should rest on the identification of variables having a wide range of disease outcomes. One such risk factor may be life change associated with social and cultural mobility. Those experiencing this type of mobility have been observed to have higher rates of diseases and conditions such as coronary heart disease (43–46), lung cancer (47), difficulties of pregnancy (48, 49), sarcoidosis (50), and depression (30). Another risk factor may be certain life events; those experiencing what are commonly called stressful life events have been shown to have higher rates of a wide variety of diseases and conditions (51-57).

Generalized susceptibility to disease may be influenced not only by the impact of various forms of life change and life stress, but also by differences in the way people cope with such stress. Coping, in this sense, refers not to specific types of psychological responses but to the more generalized ways in which people deal with problems in their everyday life. It is evident that such coping styles are likely to be products of environmental situations and not independent of such factors. Several coping responses that have a wide range of disease outcomes have been described. Cigarette smoking is one such coping response that has been associated with virtually all causes of morbidity and mortality (58); obesity may be another coping style associated with a higher rate of many diseases and conditions (59, 60); pattern A behavior is an example of a third coping response that has been shown to have relatively broad disease consequences (61). There is some evidence that persons in the lower classes experience more life changes (62) and that they tend to be more obese and to smoke more cigarettes (63, 64).

To explain the differential in morbidity and mortality rates among the social classes, it is important to identify additional factors that affect susceptibility and have diverse disease consequencs; it is also important to determine which of these factors are more prevalent in the lower classes. Thus, our understanding would be enhanced if it could be shown not only that those in the lower classes live in a more toxic physical environment with inadequate medical care, but also that they live in a social and psychological environment that increases their vulnerability to a whole series of diseases and conditions.

In this paper, we have emphasized the variegated disease consequences of low socioeconomic status. Any proposed explanations of this phenomenon should be capable of accounting for this general outcome. The proposal offered here is that those in the lower classes consistently have higher rates of disease in part due to compromised disease defenses and increased general susceptibility. To explore this proposal further, systematic research is needed on four major problems:

(1) The more precise identification and description of subgroups within the lower socioeconomic classes that have either markedly higher or lower rates of disease: Included in what is commonly called the "lower class" are semi-skilled working men with stable work and family situations, unemployed men with and without families, the rural and urban poor, hard core unemployed persons, and so on. The different disease experiences of these heterogeneous subgroups would permit a more precise understanding of the processes involved in disease etiology and would permit a more precise definition of social class groupings.

(2) The disentanglement of socio-environmental from physical-environmental variables: It is important to know whether high rates of illness and discontent in a poverty area, for example, are due to the poor physical circumstances of life in such an area, to the social consequences of life in such an area, or to the personal characteristics of individuals who come to live in the area.

(3) The clarification of "causes" and "effects": The implication in this paper has been that the lower class environment "leads to" poor health. Certainly, the reverse situation is equally likely. Many measures of social class position may be influenced by the experience of ill health itself. Further research is needed to clarify the relative importance of the "downward drift" hypothesis. One way of approaching such study is to use measures of class position that are relatively unaffected by illness experience. An example of one such measure is "educational achievement" as used by Kitagawa and Hauser (11). In this study, educational level was assumed to be relatively stable after age 20 and was felt to be a measure relatively unaffected by subsequent illness experience.

(4) The more comprehensive description of those psycho-social variables that may compromise bodily defense to disease and increase susceptibility to illness: The possible importance of life events, life changes, and various coping behavior has been suggested but systematic research needs to be done to provide a more complete view of the factors involved in this

process. Of particular interest would be research on the ways in which social and familial support networks (48,55) mediate between the impact of life events and stresses and disease outcomes.

The research that is needed should not be limited to the study of the specific risk factors as these affect specific diseases. Instead, the major focus of this research should be on those general features of lower class living environments that compromise bodily defense and thereby affect health and well-being in general. This research should go beyond the superficial description of demographic variables associated with illness and should attempt the identification of specific etiologic factors capable of accounting for the observed morbidity and mortality differences between the social classes.

The gap in mortality and life expectancy between the social classes has stabilized and may be increasing; the identification of those factors that render people vulnerable to disease will hopefully provide a basis for developing more meaningful prevention programs aimed toward narrowing the gap.

References

1. Winkelstein W Jr, French FE: The role of ecology in the design of a health care system. Calif Med 113:7–12, 1970.
2. Marmot M, Winkelstein W Jr: Epidemiologic observations on intervention trials for prevention of coronary heart disease. Am J Epidemiol 101:177–181, 1975
3. Tuberculosis and Socioeconomic Status. Stat Bull, January 1970
4. Terris M: Relation of economic status to tuberculosis mortality by age and sex. Am J Public Health 38:1061–1071, 1948
5. Gordis L, Lilienfeld A, Rodriguez R: Studies in the epidemiology and preventability of rheumatic fever. II. Socioeconomic factors and the incidence of acute attacks. J Chronic Dis 21:655–666, 1969
6. Influenza and Pneumonia Mortality in the U.S., Canada and Western Europe. Stat Bull, April 1972
7. Court SDM: Epidemiology and natural history of respiratory infections in children. J Clin Pathol 21:31, 1968
8. Chase HC (ed): A study of risks, medical care and infant mortality. Am J Public Health 63: supplement, 1973
9. Lerner M: Social differences in physical health. *In:* Poverty and Health. Edited by J Kozsa, A Antonovsky, IK Zola. Cambridge, Harvard University Press, 1969, pp 69–112
10. Antonovsky A: Social class, life expectancy and overall mortality. Milbank Mem Fund Q 45:31–73, 1967
11. Kitagawa EM, Hauser PM: Differential Mortality in the United States. Cambridge, Harvard University Press, 1973.

12. Nagi MH, Stockwell EG: Socioeconomic differentials in mortality by cause of death. Health Serv Rep 88:449–465, 1973
13. Ellis JM: Socio-economic differentials in mortality from chronic disease. *In:* Patients, Physicians and Illness. Edited by EG Jaco. Glencoe, Ill, The Free Press, 1958, pp 30–37
14. Yeracaris J: Differential mortality, general and cause-specific in Buffalo, 1939–1941. J Am Stat Assoc 50:1235–1247, 1955
15. Brown SM, Selvin S, Winkelstein W Jr: The association of economic status with the occurrence of lung cancer. Cancer 36:1903–1911, 1975
16. Guerrin RF, Borgatta EF: Socio-economic and demographic correlates of tuberculosis incidence. Milbank Mem Fund Q 43:269–290, 1965
17. Graham S: Socio-economic status, illness, and the use of medical services. Milbank Mem Fund Q 35:58–66, 1957
18. Cohart EM: Socioeconomic distribution of stomach cancer in New Haven. Cancer 7:455–461, 1954
19. Socioeconomic Differentials in Mortality. Stat Bull, June 1972
20. Hart JT: Too little and too late. Data on occupational mortality, 1959–1963. Lancet 1:192–193, 1972
21. Wan T: Social differentials in selected work-limiting chronic conditions. J Chronic Dis 25:365–374, 1972
22. Hochstim JR, Athanasopoulos DA, Larkins JH: Poverty area under the microscope. Am J Public Health 58:1815–1827, 1968
23. Burnight RG: Chronic morbidity and socio-economic characteristics of older urban males. Milbank Mem Fund Q 43:311–322, 1965
24. Elder R, Acheson RM: New Haven survey of joint diseases. XIV. Social class and behavior in response to symptoms of osteoarthritis. Milbank Mem Fund Q 48:499–502, 1970
25. Cobb S: The epidemiology of rheumatoid disease. *In:* The Frequency of Rheumatoid Disease. Edited by S Cobb. Cambridge, Harvard University Free Press, 1971, pp 42-62
26. Graham S: Social factors in the relation to chronic illness. *In:* Handbook of Medical Sociology. Edited by HE Freeman, S Levine, LG Reeder. Englewood Cliffs, NJ, Prentice-Hall Inc, 1963, pp 65–98
27. Wan T: Status stress and morbidity: A sociological investigation of selected categories of working-limiting conditions. J Chronic Dis 24:453–468, 1971
28. Selected Health Characteristics by Occupation, U.S. July 1961–June 1963. National Health Center for Health Statistics, Series 10 21:1–16, 1965
29. Abramson JH: Emotional disorder, status inconsistency and migration. Milbank Mem Fund Q 44:23-48, 1966
30. Schwab JJ, Holzer CE III, Warheit GJ: Depression scores by race, sex, age, family income, education and socioeconomic status. (Personal communication, 1974)
31. Srole L, Langner T, Michael S, et al: Mental Health in the Metropolis: the Midtown Study. New York, McGraw-Hill, 1962
32. Jackson EF: Status consistency and symptoms of stress. Am Sociol Rev 27:469–480, 1962

33. Hollingshead AB, Redlich FC: Social Class and Mental Illness. New York, John Wiley and Sons Inc. 1958
34. Gurin G, Veroff J, Feld S: Americans View Their Mental Health. New York, Basic Books Inc. 1960
35. Langner TS: Psychophysiological symptoms and the status of women in two Mexican communities. *In:* Approaches to Cross-cultural Psychiatry. Edited by AH Leighton, JM Murphy. Ithaca, Cornell University Press, 1965. pp 360–392
36. Syme SL, Oakes T, Friedman G, et al: Social class and racial differences in blood pressure. Am J Public Health 64:619–620, 1974
37. Oakes TW, Syme SL: Social factors in newly discovered elevated blood pressure. J Health Soc Behav 14:198–204, 1973
38. Fink R, Shapiro S, Hyman MD, et al: Health status of poverty and non-poverty groups in multiphasic health testing. Presented at the Annual Meeting of the American Public Health Association, November 1972
39. Lipworth L, Abelin T, Connelly RR: Socioeconomic factors in the prognosis of cancer patients. J Chronic Dis 23:105–116, 1970
40. Hochstim JR: Health and ways of living. *In:* Social Surveys. The Community as an Epidemiological Laboratory. Edited by I Kessler, M Levine. Baltimore, Johns Hopkins Press, 1970, pp 149–176
41. Winkelstein W Jr, Kantor S, Davis EW, et al: The relationship of air pollution and economic status to total mortality and selected respiratory system mortality in men. I. Suspended particulates. Arch Environ Health 14:162–171, 1967
42. Booth A: Preliminary Report: Urban Crowding Project. Canada, Ministry of State for Urban Affairs, August 1974 (mimeographed)
43. Syme SL, Hyman MM, Enterline PE: Some social and cultural factors associated with the occurrence of coronary heart disease. J Chronic Dis 17:277–289, 1964
44. Tyroler HA, Cassel J: Health consequences of cultural change. II. The effect of urbanization on coronary heart mortality in rural residents. J Chronic Dis 17:167–177, 1964
45. Nesser WB, Tyroler HA, Cassel JC: Social disorganization and stroke mortality in the black populations of North Carolina. Am J Epidemiol 93:166–175, 1971
46. Shekelle RB, Osterfeld AM, Paul O: Social status and incidence of coronary heart disease. J Chronic Dis 22:381–394, 1969
47. Haenszel W, Loveland DB, Sirken N: Lung-cancer mortality as related to residence and smoking histories. I. White males. J Natl Cancer Inst 28:947–1001, 1962
48. Nuckolls KB, Cassel J, Kaplan BH: Psychosocial assets, life crisis, and the prognosis of pregnancy. Am J Epidemiol 95:431–441, 1972
49. Gorusch RL, Key MK: Abnormalities of pregnancy as a function of anxiety and life stress. Psychosom Med 36:352–362, 1974
50. Terris M, Chaves AD: An epidemiologic study of sarcoidosis. Am Rev Respir Dis 94:50–55, 1966
51. Rahe RH. Gunderson EKE, Arthur RJ: Demographic and psychosocial factors in acute illness reporting. J Chronic Dis 23:245–255, 1970

52. Wyler AR, Masuda M, Holmes TH: Magnitude of life events and seriousness of illness. Psychosom Med 33:115–122, 1971

53. Rahe RH, Rubin RT, Gunderson EKE, et al: Psychological correlates of serum cholesterol in man: A longitudinal study. Psychosom Med 33:399–410, 1971

54. Spilken AZ, Jacobs MA: Prediction of illness behavior from measures of life crisis, manifest distress and maladaptive coping. Psychosom Med 33:251–264, 1971

55. Jacobs MA, Spilken AZ, Martin MA, et al: Life stress and respiratory illness. Psychosom Med 32:233–242, 1970

56. Kasl SV, Cobb S: Blood pressure changes in men undergoing job loss; A preliminary report. Psychosom Med 32:19–38, 1970

57. Hinkle LE, Wolff HG: Ecological investigations of the relationship between illness, life experiences, and the social environment. Ann Intern Med 49:1373–1388, 1958

58. US Dept of Health, Education, and Welfare: The Health Consequences of Smoking. National Communicable Disease Center, Publication No 74-8704, 1974

59. US Public Health Service, Division of Chronic Diseases: Obesity and Health. A Source Book of Current Information for Professional Health Personnel. Publication No 1485. Washington DC, US GPO, 1966

60. Build and Blood Pressure Study. Chicago, Society of Actuaries, Vol I and II, 1959

61. Rosenman RH, Brand RH, Jenkins CD, et al: Coronary heart disease in the Western collaborative group study: Final follow-up experience of 8½ years. (Manuscript)

62. Dohrenwend BS (ed): Stressful Life Events: Their Nature and Effects. New York, Wiley-Interscience, 1974.

63. US Dept of Health, Education, and Welfare: Adult Use of Tobacco 1970, Publication No HSM-73-8727, 1973

64. Khosla T, Lowe CR: Obesity and smoking habits by social class. J Prev Soc Med 26:249–256, 1972

3

Why Do Women Live Longer Than Men?

Ingrid Waldron

Part I

The sex differential in mortality has increased strikingly over the past half century in the U.S. In 1920, the life expectancy for women was 56, only two years longer than that for men (1). By 1970, women's life expectancy was 75, almost eight years longer than men's (2). In 1920, male death rates were no more than 30 percent higher than female death rates at any age. By 1970, male death rates exceeded female death rates by as much as 180 percent for 15–24-year-olds and 110 percent for 55–64-year-olds.

Among young adults the excess of mortality for males is due primarily to accidents (3). At older ages, cardiovascular-renal diseases make the largest contribution to higher mortality among men. Rising male mortality for these causes of death and for lung cancer has been a major component of the increase in the sex differential in mortality (4). These trends were due in part to the sizeable increase in cigarette smoking by men during the first third of the twentieth century (5,6). Another substantial component of the increase in the sex differential in mortality has been the decline in maternal mortality and uterine cancer due to improvements in medical care. These data suggest that a wide variety of cultural factors, including automobile use, cigarette smoking and health care, contributes to the contemporary sex differential in mortality.

Further evidence of the importance of cultural factors is provided by international comparisons, which show that higher male death rates, although common, have not been universal. In many countries female death rates have exceeded male death rates at ages between one and forty and in some cases at older ages as well (7). Higher mortality among females has been observed most frequently in nonindustrial countries.

The sex differential in mortality also varies for different groups within the United States. For example the excess of male mortality is lowest among married adults, it is 10 percent greater among single and widowed adults, and it is 50 percent greater among divorced adults (data from 8). The excess of mortality for males who are not married is particularly large for causes like cirrhosis of the liver which are strongly influenced by behavior, and for diseases like tuberculosis in which health habits and care play an important role. Gove (9) has argued that the major reasons why the sex mortality differential is higher among males who are not married are that men do not adjust as well as women do to being unmarried, and that men derive greater advantages from being married, both in care received and in psychological well-being.

Genetic factors apparently also contribute to higher male mortality, although the evidence for this is not as strong as commonly has been believed. Males have higher mortality than females in many different species, and this has been cited as evidence for a genetic contribution to the higher mortality of men (10). However, although higher male mortality is widespread among insects, other Arthropoda and fishes (10), higher female mortality appears to be just as common as higher male mortality among our closer relatives, the birds and mammals (10–12). Among humans, higher female mortality is also common at certain ages, as described above. However, it is striking that, wherever statistics are available, males have had higher mortality during the first year of life (7). Males also have been found to have higher fetal mortality in most studies (13), although fetal mortality during late pregnancy is as high for females as for males in pairs of twins of opposite sex (14), in multiple births of triplets or more (15), and in a few geographical areas, for example Scotland (16). Male mortality is higher for many different causes of death (see Table 1). Several authors (10,17) have inferred from these observations that genetically determined metabolic differences may contribute to the higher mortality of males.

Another study which has been cited widely as evidence of the importance of genetic factors is Madigan's (18) comparison of life expectancy for Roman Catholic Sisters and Brothers in teaching Orders. Madigan found that the differential in life expectancy between Sisters and Brothers has been almost as large as the differential between women and men in the general population, even though the Sisters and Brothers had more similar adult roles. However, the higher mortality of the Brothers cannot be attributed solely to genetic causes, since the Brothers smoked and drank more than the Sisters and probably were socialized differently as children, and each of these differences would contribute to higher male mortality (as discussed in detail below).

This earlier work suggests that both cultural and genetic factors contribute to the longer life expectancy of women (19–21). Therefore, we have considered both cultural and genetic factors in our analysis of the specific causes of the sex differential in mortality in the contemporary U.S.

Table 1.
Sex mortality ratios for all major causes of death, U.S., 1967*

Ratio of male to female death rates	Cause of death	Male death rate	Female death rate†
		(Deaths/100,000 population)	
5.9	Malignant neoplasm of respiratory system, not specified as secondary	50.1	8.5
4.9	Other bronchopulmonic disease (71% emphysema)	24.4	5.0
2.8	Motor vehicle accidents	39.4	14.2
2.7	Suicide	15.7	5.8
2.4	Other accidents	41.1	17.4
2.0	Cirrhosis of liver	18.5	9.1
2.0	Arteriosclerotic heart disease, including coronary disease	357.0	175.6
1.8	Symptoms, senility and ill-defined conditions	14.9	8.3
1.7	Pneumonia, except of newborn	32.3	19.5
1.6	Other diseases of heart	17.9	11.1
1.6	Other diseases of circulatory system	18.2	11.1
1.5	Malignant neoplasm of digestive organs and peritoneum, not specified as secondary	53.0	36.2
1.4	All other diseases (residual)	32.4	22.4
1.4	Malignant neoplasm of other and unspecified sites	20.5	14.7
1.4	Birth injuries, postnatal asphyxia, and atelectasis	11.9	8.4
1.4	Certain diseases of early infancy	29.2	21.6
1.3	Other diseases peculiar to early infancy, and immaturity, unqualified	15.3	11.7
1.3	Nonrheumatic chronic endocarditis and other myocardial degeneration	26.8	20.5
1.2	General arteriosclerosis	17.2	14.8
1.2	Vascular lesions affecting central nervous system	96.3	83.3
1.0	Hypertensive heart disease	22.3	22.2
0.89	Malignant neoplasm of genital organs	17.9	20.1
0.89	Diabetes mellitus	14.9	16.8
0.008	Malignant neoplasm of breast	0.2	24.6
1.6	All causes	1081.7	657.0

The causes of death with the highest sex mortality ratios all have major behavioral components (calculated from data in ref. 98).

*All causes of death were included, except those responsible for less than 1% of the deaths (e.g. homicide).
†Female death rates have been age-adjusted to the male age distribution.

Our analysis is based on the identification of the causes of death which make a large contribution to the sex differential in mortality in the United States. . . . For each of these causes of death we considered all the major factors believed to contribute to its etiology and selected for analysis those factors which appeared to be relevant to the sex difference in mortality.

Behavioral factors emerge as important determinants of the sex differential for . . . death. . . . The importance of behavioral factors is obvious in the case of accidents and suicide, and also for the respiratory diseases, which largely are due to smoking (22) as well as for cirrhosis of the liver, which is related to alcohol consumption (23). These causes of death with clear behavioral components are responsible for one-third of the excess of male mortality. Arteriosclerotic heart disease is responsible for an additional 40 percent of the excess deaths among males. The data presented in the next section suggest that men have higher death rates for arteriosclerotic heart disease in large part because they smoke cigarettes more and because they more often develop the aggressive, competitive Coronary Prone Behavior Pattern.

Arteriosclerotic Heart Disease

Death rates for arteriosclerotic heart disease, which is primarily coronary heart disease (CHD), are twice as high for men as for women. Cigarette smoking is associated with an elevation of CHD death rates ranging from 100 percent or more among middle-aged adults to 20 percent at the oldest ages (24). The elevated risk of CHD among smokers is probably due in part to the correlation between smoking and other risk factors (such as the Coronary Prone Behavior Pattern discussed below), but it is almost certainly also a direct consequence of the pharmacological effects of smoking (22). A rough quantitative estimate of the contribution of smoking habits to the sex differential in CHD death rates can be obtained by comparing the sex differential among nonsmokers to the sex differential for the general population. The contribution of cigarette smoking appears to be substantial, paticularly for adults under age 65. Among middle-aged adults who have never smoked regularly, the CHD mortality for men exceeds that for women by 350 percent while for the total sample (including smokers) men's CHD mortality exceeds women's by 650 percent.

A variety of evidence suggests that another important cause of higher rates of coronary heart disease in men may be their involvement in paid jobs and in aggressive, competitive roles, in contrast to the greater orientation of women toward family and less competitive, more supportive roles. For example several studies have found that among men the risk of coronary heart disease is higher for those who have worked many hours overtime or who have held two jobs simultaneously (25). Also, in a projective test, men who subsequently developed CHD were more likely to locate their stories in a "socioprofessional" setting and not in a family or recreational setting (26).

A more specific formulation of the proposed hypothesis can be derived from studies of the "Coronary Prone Behavior Pattern." A person shows the Coronary Prone Behavior Pattern if he or she is work-orientated, ambitious, aggressive, competitive, hurried, impatient and preoccupied with deadlines (27). Large prospective studies have shown that men who display this Coronary Prone Behavior Pattern are twice as likely as other men to develop or die of coronary heart disease (27,28). Smaller retrospective studies (29–31) have also established that women who have coronary heart disease are more likely to display the Coronary Prone Behavior Pattern than controls.

Behavior pattern may make a larger contribution to the risk of coronary heart disease than does sex *per se* . . . for samples of men (32) and women (31) who have clear Coronary Prone Behavior Pattern (called Type A in these studies) or clear Type B (the opposite of Type A). These data must be interpreted with caution since the samples were small and were not obtained by systematic or even strictly comparable methods. Nevertheless, it is striking that Type B men had the same low prevalence of CHD as did Type B women. This suggests that men who adopt a less competitive and rushed style of life are just as likely to avoid CHD as comparable women. At older ages, Type A men and women had the same high prevalence of CHD. The only category in which women had substantially lower rates of CHD was the younger Type A's, but even in this age range Type A women had more CHD than Type B men.

These data suggest the hypothesis that men have more coronary heart disease than women in part because the Type A or Coronary Prone Behavior Pattern is more prevalent among men. In a large sample of employed adults women were slightly less Type A than men (Shekelle, personal communication). Housewives may be even less Type A than employed women (31) and about half of adult women are housewives (33). Aggressiveness and competitiveness are two key components of the Coronary Prone Behavior Pattern. Maccoby and Jacklin, in their review of nearly 2000 studies of sex differences in behavior (34), conclude that, on the average, males are more aggressive and competitive than females.

Why do males develop more aggressiveness and competitiveness—more of the Coronary Prone Behavior Pattern—then females? Genetic factors make some contribution to the sex differences in aggressiveness (34), but the extent of aggressiveness among males varies enormously, depending on child-rearing and cultural conditions (35). Sex differences in competitiveness are fostered by parents and schools who push boys to achieve in the occupational world and girls to seek success in the family sphere (34,36–38). Occupational achievement apparently requires competitiveness, since in our society there are seldom as many jobs (particularly rewarding, high status jobs) as there are people who want and can do them (39,40). In the family sphere, on the other hand, warmth and love are believed to be much more appropriate and aggressive competitiveness much less appropriate than in the business world (37). Evidence that cultural pressures and expectations do have a substantial influence on the development of the Coronary Prone Behavior Pattern comes from the observation that this Behavior Pattern rarely develops in the social environment of many nonindustrial societies (27,35).

Thus, a variety of evidence suggests that cultural and socioeconomic pressures related to the role of men in our society push them to develop the Coronary Prone Behavior Pattern, and that this makes a major contribution to men's higher risk of coronary heart disease. Many aspects of this hypothesis need further testing; some of this testing has been started.

Although smoking and the Coronary Prone Behavior Pattern appear to be the most important behavioral factors contributing to the sex differential in arteriosclerotic heart disease, other behavioral differences also may play a role. For example women attend church more often than men do (41) and frequent church attenders of either sex have substantially lower death rates for arteriosclerotic heart disease, at least in one Protestant community studied (42). Extrapolating the risk differential nationally leads to a prediction that men's death rates for arteriosclerotic heart disease would be 7 percent higher than women's, based on sex differences in church attendance and exclusive of related differences in smoking.

Bengtsson and co-workers (3) reach conclusions similar to ours in their study of sex differences in coronary heart disease in 50–54 year-old Swedish women and men. They conclude that men's higher rates of CHD are related to their higher rates of smoking and drinking alcohol, higher aggression and achievement scores and greater self-reported stress. These authors believe that additional factors also contribute to the observed sex differences in CHD.

Further evidence for the substantial contribution of cultural factors to the sex differential in coronary heart disease is provided by the wide cross-cultural variation in the size of this differential. In some countries the sex differential is much smaller than in the U.S. (17,43). For example, in 1960 in Greece and Hungary, arteriosclerotic heart disease mortality was only 30 percent higher for males than for females (44). The age trend of the male excess also varies widely, with a peak at premenopausal ages in the U.S. and many European countries but a peak at postmenopausal ages in Japan and Colombia (data from [44]). On the other hand, men do have higher arteriosclerotic heart disease death rates in all countries studied, and this suggests that genetic factors also contribute to the sex differential.

Sex Hormones and CHD

Most previous discussions of the sex differential in coronary heart disease have focused primary attention on the hypothesis that this sex differential is a result of the physiological effects of the sex hormones. The evidence for this hypothesis is suggestive, but it is ambiguous and inconsistent. Castration of men apparently does not reduce deaths due to cardiovascular disease (45), and castration of older men does not seem to reduce atherosclerosis (46). The data of Gertler and White (47) suggest that androgen levels of male coronary patients do not differ from androgen levels in a control group. Thus male hormones do not appear to increase the risk of coronary heart disease.

Do female hormones lower the risk of coronary heart disease? Several studies have found that oophorectomy of young women is associated with increased atherosclerosis and CHD (43,48–51) but other studies have not found a relationship (43,52,53).

. . . .

Women who use oral contraceptives have an increased risk of death due to myocardial infarction (55,56), cerebral thrombosis, deep vein thrombosis and pulmonary embolism (57,58). High doses of estrogen given to men produce increased rates of pulmonary embolism and thrombophlebitis (70) and cerebral thrombosis (54). We did not find data on the effects of male hormones on thrombosis.

. . . .

Respiratory Diseases and Smoking

For "malignant neoplasm of the respiratory system" (primarily lung cancer), men's death rates are six times higher than women's. For "other bronchiopulmonic diseases" (primarily emphysema), men's death rates are five times higher than women's. These mortality ratios are higher than for any other major cause of death (Table 1). Men have higher mortality for these diseases primarily because men smoke more and cigarette smoking is the major cause of both lung cancer and emphysema (6,22). If men and women who have never smoked regularly are compared, the sex mortality ratios for lung cancer and emphysema are drastically reduced. These data suggest that cigarette smoking is the primary cause of men's excess lung cancer and emphysema mortality.

Comparing those who have ever smoked cigarettes to nonsmokers of the same sex, lung cancer death rates are elevated ninefold for men, but only twofold for women. Similarly, emphysema death rates are elevated sevenfold among men smokers, but only fivefold for women smokers. The elevation of death rates is less for women smokers than for men in large part because women smokers inhale less, smoke fewer cigarettes and less of each cigarette and, in the past, women have begun smoking at older ages (22,24). In addition, industrial hazards aggravate the effects of cigarette smoking for many men (as discussed below).

The total pathological effect of smoking, particularly the elevation of coronary heart disease, lung cancer and emphysema, makes a major contribution to the sex differential in total death rates. For middle-aged adults who never have smoked regularly, men's mortality exceeds women's by only 30 percent compared to a male excess of 120 percent for the total sample. For older nonsmokers, men's mortality exceeds women's by 60–70 percent, compared to 100–150 percent for the total sample. Retherford (5) (in a similiar analysis which was published while this manuscript was in the final stages of preparation) estimates that as much as half of the sex differential in life expectancy from the ages of 37 to 87 may be due to the effects of higher rates of cigarette smoking in men.

Why do more men than women smoke? Smoking by women was strongly discouraged by the social mores of the early twentieth century. The conventions of that period continue to influence the smoking patterns of people who were teenagers at that time, since relatively few people begin smoking cigarettes after age 20. As a consequence, the sex differential in cigarette smoking is largest for older people who were over 60 in 1970 and who thus were teenagers before 1930 (59). Many other social and motivational factors have been shown to influence cigarette smoking (60,61). Among these, the factor which probably contributes most to the sex differential in smoking is the strong component of rebelliousness which cigarette smoking has had for many teenagers. In general, girls tend to be less rebellious and more conforming to adult standards, probably in part because parents and teachers of schoolaged children allow boys more independence and expect girls to be more obedient (34, 62–64). Girls' lesser rebelliousness is probably one reason why, until very recently, fewer teenage girls than boys have begun smoking.

Although cigarette smoking is the major cause of the higher rates of lung cancer in men, industrial carcinogens also make a substantial contribution. Men who work with asbestos have up to eight times higher a risk of (bronchogenic) lung cancer than other men (65). This elevated risk affects primarily cigarette smokers. Asbestos is widely used in construction and insulation materials, and about one man in 100 is now or has been exposed to asbestos dust at his work (66). Thus, asbestos may be responsible for one in 20 male lung cancer deaths in this country. Metallic dusts and fumes elevate lung cancer risk between 20 percent and 130 percent for various categories of metal workers (67). About one man in 30 works or has worked in such an occupation (68). Thus, metallic dusts and fumes may be responsible for one in 50 male lung cancer deaths. Taken together, the established and suspected industrial carcinogens appear to be a factor in roughly one out of every 10 male lung cancer deaths (67, 69).

PART II

Accidents, Alcohol and Cirrhosis

Death rates for motor vehicle accidents are almost three times higher for males than for females. This is due in part to the fact that men drive more, but the major cause appears to be that men drive less safely. Male drivers are involved in 30 percent more accidents per mile driven, and 130 percent more fatal accidents per mile driven (71). These higher accident rates are correlated with driving habits that are less safe than those of women. For example among 917 drivers observed at an intersection in a large town and another intersection in a large city, 15 percent of the male drivers entered the intersection when the light was yellow or red compared to only 10 percent of the female drivers. Among the 283 drivers making a turn, 47 percent of the males and only 20 percent of the females failed to signal the turn (Naomi Sullam and Susan Johnston, unpublished observations). It is possible that men drive more at times when roads are crowded or under other hazardous conditions and this also may contribute to their higher accident rates.

For accidents other than motor vehicle accidents, death rates for females are less than half the rates for males. About half of the male excess is due to accidents "while at work." The rate of work accidents is higher for men because more men work and because their jobs are physically more hazardous (calculated from data in 70, 72). An additional third of the male excess is due to accidental drownings and accidents caused by firearms, which are five times as common among males (70).

It is evident from these statistics that men's higher accident fatalities are a result of behaviors which are encouraged in boys and men: driving, working at sometimes hazardous jobs, using guns, being adventurous and acting unafraid. The expectation that boys and men will be more adventurous and take more risks than girls and women is conveyed by the stories children read (36–39). In addition, males are expected to be brave, not to cry, and, as a result, males are generally less able to respond to a risky situation by admitting fear and backing out (34). Because of these attitudes males are more likely to be involved in fatal auto accidents, accidental drownings, etc.

Another cause of men's higher accidental death rates is their greater consumption of alcohol (73). Half of all fatal motor vehicle accidents involve drunken drivers. Other accidents and suicide also are associated with alcohol use. Most drinking drivers responsible for a fatal accident were alcoholics or at least had serious drinking problems (74). Men are particularly likely to be heavy drinkers, four times as likely as women (75). Since excessive alcohol consumption and the malnutrition which is a concomitant are major contributors to cirrhosis of the liver (23, 76), it is not surprising that men's death rates for cirrhosis of the liver are twice as high as women's.

Cross-cultural comparisons show that sex differences in alcohol consumption are influenced by cultural factors (77). In one-third of nonindustrial societies studied, both sexes consume alcohol equally. Which of the cultural factors known to influence alcohol consumption might contribute to the sex differential in drinking in this country? One factor of possible importance is suggested by cross-cultural studies which show that heavy use of alcohol is correlated with greater socialization pressures to achieve and with lower tolerance of dependent behavior (77). As discussed in Part I, males in our society are under more pressure than females to achieve in careers and to be independent. Another factor which may contribute to sex differences is suggested by prospective studies in this country which show that disobedient, dishonest, impulsive adolescents are more likely to become alcoholics (78). These characteristics may be more common and more tolerated in males. Finally, attitudes toward alcohol are a major concomitant of heavy drinking (75), and more favorable attitudes are apparently fostered in males by the generally greater acceptance of drinking among men (75, 79).

Psychoactive drugs other than alcohol make a much smaller contribution to death rates, but their pattern of use confirms our description of men taking more risks and as therefore being more likely to have fatal accidents. At the turn of the century when opiates were widely available from legal sources and relatively safe to use, two-thirds of addicts were women. Now, when opiates are illegal and generally associated with a dangerous life style, more than 80 percent of the addicts are men (80). Today, more women use the relatively safe and socially acceptable mood-altering drugs (81). For example twice as many women as men use minor tranquilizers (82), drugs which do not appear to be associated with any notable elevation in risk of death (76). When men do use prescription psychoactive drugs, they are more likely to obtain them from non-medical sources (83).

Suicide

One cause of the higher suicide rates among men is the stress of competition for jobs. The suicide rates of men are more strongly correlated with unemployment rates than are the suicide rates of women (84, 85). During the recession phase of business cycles, men's suicide rates have risen an average of 9.5 percent per year, whereas women's suicide rates have risen only 2.9 percent per year (86). In addition, some occupations seem to be associated with higher suicide rates than the housewife role. Women physicians (87) and psychologists (88) have suicide rates about three times higher than women in general and as high as the suicide rates of men in their professions.

Although three times more men than women actually commit suicide, twice as many women as men attempt suicide without killing themselves (89). Suicidal men are particularly prone to use guns, with consequences which are often irreversible and fatal, whereas women are more likely to use poisons, which can be treated by the use of stomach pumps and antidotes (90). For every method, however, there are more male than female suicides, so some additional explanation must be sought for the preponderance of male suicides and female suicide attempts. The suicide attempt has been widely interpreted as a desperate, last ditch cry for help, rather than an actual attempt to end life (91). Women apparently are better able to use a suicide attempt as a cry for help, and it seems likely that this ability to some extent protects them from the need to actually kill themselves (92). In contrast, males "see themselves as strong, powerful, dominant, " 'potent' " (34) and find it difficult to seek help; thus, they are more likely to use guns rather than poisons and to carry a suicidal act through to a fatal conclusion.

Cancer

Males have higher death rates for many additional causes of death. We will not analyze each in detail, but will, in the next three sections, present some general observations.

The sex ratios for different types of cancer vary widely (Table 1). At one extreme, malignant neoplasms of the respiratory system are six times more common among men, primarily because men smoke cigarettes more (6). At the other extreme, deaths due to malignant neoplasms of the breast are 100 times more common among women. The normal stimulatory action of estrogens on breast growth seems to extend to stimulation of the development of breast cancers; removal of the ovaries before age 35 results in a decrease of over two-thirds in breast cancer rates at older ages (93).

. . . .

While no precise estimate can be made of the contribution of sex hormones and genetic differences to the sex differential in total cancer mortality, it is nevertheless clear that hormonal and other genetic differences make little if any net contribution to men's higher total cancer mortality. Even if, as an extreme assumption, the entire excess of digestive, peritoneal and "other" cancers among males were attributed to hormonal and other genetic factors, this excess is approximately balanced by the hormonally related excess of deaths due to breast and genital cancers among females (Table 1). Thus, there would be little sex differential in total cancer mortality were it not for men's excess of respiratory system cancers, and this excess is due primarily to greater cigarette smoking among men.

Sex Chromosome-Linked Conditions

Males generally have less resistance than females to infectious disease. . . .

Various . . . genetically determined biological differences apparently make only a small contribution to the sex differential in death rates. There are more than fifty pathological conditions which occur almost exclusively in males because they are caused by X-linked recessive mutations (94). Most of these pathologies are not common and the few common ones are rarely lethal. Deaths due to all of these conditions constitute less than 2 percent of the excess of deaths experienced by males up to the end of the reproductive years (calculated from data in 94, 70). Deaths due to "deliveries and complications of pregnancy, childbirth, and the puerperium" are also now uncommon, equivalent to less than 1 percent of the sex differential in death rates (data from 70). Sex hormones have differential effects which result in numerous other physiological differences between the sexes, such as more fat deposition in women (95) and differences in liver enzymes (96, 97). However, these physiological differences have not been shown to make any substantial contribution to higher male death rates.

Health Care

A striking paradox in the study of sex differences in health is the fact that men have higher mortality but women have higher morbidity. Specifically, women report more symptoms, visit doctors more often and more often restrict their usual activities or spend a day in bed because of illness (19, 98–101). Several authors have proposed that this seeming paradox may be resolved by the following hypothesis. Men may tend to ignore minor somatic illnesses and not seek rest or medical help unless more serious illness develops; this failure to care for their health may contribute to their higher mortality (19, 101). This tendency on the part of men may be due in part to more stoic and self-reliant attitudes and in part to the pressures men feel not to miss work since they are usually the chief bread-winners for their families (102). An examination of the more detailed evidence available provides support for some, but not all aspects of this hypothesis.

When self-reported illness is compared with evaluations based on clinical examination, both men and women omit mention of many of the conditions found clinically. Men generally underestimate their illness more than women do (103–106). However, there is little sex difference in the extent of agreement between the specific conditions found clinically and the specific conditions reported by a respondent (103, 104).

For people who report having a symptom, there is little if any consistent sex difference in the proportion who go to see a doctor (99, 100, 107, 108). Women delay as long as men before seeking medical attention after the first symptoms of cancer (109, 110) or a myocardial infarction (111–113). However, women do visit doctors more on the average, corresponding to their higher rates of reporting symptoms (98–100). Women also make more use of preventive services than men do (19, 107, 114).

Most studies find no sex differences in the proportion of patients who comply with doctor's recommendations (115).

Such sex differences in health care as are observed do not seem to originate with experiences of early childhood. Under the age of about ten, boys have more illness than girls, more days of restricted activity, and slightly more doctor visits (19, 98, 99, 114). Studies of social attitudes have revealed no significant sex differences in estimation of which types of illness justify the adoption of the sick role (116, 117).

Thus, there seems to be no sex difference in the readiness to see a doctor once symptoms are perceived or in the willingness to comply with doctor's recommendations. On the other hand, women make greater use of preventive services, perceive more symptoms and apparently as a consequence visit doctors more often, and also more frequently reduce their activity because they feel poorly. In these ways women appear to take better care of their health, and this may contribute to their lower mortality.

Recent Trends

In recent years the ratio of male to female death rates has continued the steady upward trend which began around 1920 (4, 21). However, there is some evidence which suggests that a reversal of this trend may develop in the future. For the causes of death with the greatest excess of males deaths, the ratio of male to female death rates has fallen recently over much of the adult age span. From 1958 to 1967 (the span of use for the Seventh Revision of the International List of causes of death) the ratio of male to female death rates fell for motor vehicle accidents at all ages above 5, for suicide at ages 15–84, for malignant neoplasm of the respiratory system at ages 15–65, for emphysema at ages 25–74, for other accidents and arteriosclerotic heart disease at ages 15–54, and for cirrhosis of the liver at ages 45–74 (calculated from data in 70, 118). In most of these cases, the decline in the ratio of male to female death rates was due to a rise in female death rates.

These rising female death rates reflect a trend for more and more women to include in their life style various life-endangering habits which formerly have been more common among men. Probably the most important trend is the long-term rise in women's cigarette smoking (6), since this habit alone may be responsible for over a third of the sex differential in adult mortality. Another factor contributing to the relative rise of arteriosclerotic heart disease in women may be the increased time pressures (119) and role conflicts (120) that have resulted as an increasing proportion of women have taken jobs while still carrying primary responsibility for housework and care of children (121). Additional trends are indicated by the types of accidents for which females have shown the greatest rise relative to males, namely accidents involving firearms, drowning and aircraft (calculated from data in 70, 118). Finally, there has been an increase in the proportion of women who drink (79) which undoubtedly has contributed to the increase in women's death rates for cirrhosis of the liver, motor vehicle and other accidents.

Conclusions

Male mortality exceeds female mortality by 100 percent or more for seven major causes of death: coronary heart disease, lung cancer, emphysema, motor vehicle and other accidents, cirrhosis of the liver and suicide. Together these causes of death account for three-quarters of the sex differential in mortality in the contemporary U.S.

In the preceding sections we have analyzed the causes of higher male mortality for each of these causes of death. On the basis of these analyses we have made estimates of the proportion of the total sex differential in mortality which may be attributed to each of several major proximal causes. Very roughly, we estimate that one-third of the difference between male and female death rates may be due to men's higher cigarette smoking (with the major contribution via increased coronary heart disease, lung cancer and emphysema); one-sixth may be due to a greater prevalence of the aggressive, competitive Coronary Prone Behavior Pattern among men (with the major contribution via increased coronary heart disease); one-twelfth may be due to men's higher alcohol consumption (with the major contribution via increased accidents and cirrhosis of the liver); and one-twentieth may be due to physical hazards related to employment (with the largest contributions via increased accidents and lung cancer). Other factors which probably contribute to higher male mortality have been discussed in previous sections and some of these may make as large a contribution as one or more of the factors listed above.

. . . .

Each of the factors which we have identified as a major contributor to men's excess mortality involves a behavior which is more socially acceptable for males than for females, for example aggressive competitiveness, working at physically hazardous jobs, drinking alcohol and, especially in the early part of the century, smoking cigarettes. The sex differential in smoking and alcohol consumption seems also to be linked to underlying attitudes, such as rebelliousness and achievement striving, which are fostered to a greater extent in males.

Similar conclusions emerge from a brief examination of the minor causes of death, each of which is responsible for less than 1 percent of total deaths and is therefore excluded from our main analysis (data from 70). Male mortality exceeds female mortality by 100 percent or more for eight of these minor causes of death. Three of these eight have well-known behavioral components related to the male role (homicide, syphilis, and ulcers). Four are elevated in cigarette smokers and appear to increase as a result of cigarette smoking (bronchitis, buccal and pharyngeal cancers, urinary tract cancers and ulcers). Taken together, these minor causes of death account for an additional 6 percent of the excess of male mortality.

We conclude that sex differences in behavior are a more important cause of higher male mortality than are any inherent sex differences in physiology. Furthermore, although these sex differences in behavior may be due in part to genetic differences, cross-cultural and developmental studies clearly show that child-rearing practices and cultural factors strongly influence behavioral differences in both children and adults (34, 122, 123).

These results point to a hopeful and exciting conclusion: substantial reductions in men's excess mortality can be achieved by cultural and behavioral changes. Many possibilities can be imagined, ranging from changes in child-rearing practices and individual behavior to changes in institutions, laws and the physical environment. We will mention only a few examples with a demonstrated potential to reduce the behaviors which contribute to men's excess mortality or to reduce the lethal effects of these behaviors. In the last few years deaths due to motor vehicle accidents have been reduced by improved safety features of cars and by reductions in speed limits (124). Behavioral modification and group support techniques have been used in programs to help cigarette smokers stop smoking. Many programs have had a high relapse rate, with only a quarter or a third of enrollees not smoking at the end of a year (125). However, long-term success rates have been doubled by several improved methodologies developed recently (125). An alternative approach has been to attempt to reduce smoking in an entire community, not just among those who come to special programs. One recent effort, using mass media and personal instruction, succeeded in reducing cigarette consumption in the community by 24 percent over a period of two years (126).

Very little information is available about attempts to change the Coronary Prone Behavior Pattern, but preliminary results indicate that a program to train Coronary Prone cardiac patients to recognize and to reduce anxiety states resulted in a significant decrease in their serum lipid levels (127). We believe that efforts to change or to avert the Coronary Prone Behavior Pattern will be more successful and beneficial if directed at teenagers and young adults, rather than at middle-aged cardiac patients whose coronary arteries already have suffered considerable irreversible damage. Many young people appear to adopt the Coronary Prone Behavior Pattern only at times when they are under pressure, especially pressure arising from competition for the limited number of highly rewarding jobs available (Waldron, Butensky, Faralli and Heebner, unpublished data). Thus, a major cause of the development of the Coronary Prone Behavior Pattern appears to be the scarcity of satisfying jobs and the large differentials in pay and intrinsic rewards for the jobs which are available. This suggests that fewer people would develop this behavior pattern if more institutions were restructured along the lines already accomplished by a variety of businesses, with substantial increases in the sharing of responsibility and profits. This type of restructuring leads to increased satisfaction for most employees and a decrease in hierarchical differentials (40). Such changes could reduce the competitive pressures which currently contribute to men's excess mortality; they could also open the way for women to obtain the benefits which more and more of them are seeking in jobs, without the excessive pressures and elevated mortality which men currently suffer.

These are but some examples of the types of social and behavioral changes which are suggested by our analysis. Many of these changes will be difficult to achieve; however the potential benefits include not only decreased mortality but also improvements in the quality of life.

Note

This article was written with the assistance of SUSAN JOHNSTON.

Acknowledgements—We are happy to thank Joseph Eyer, Jean Gerth, Deborah Heebner, and Kimberly Schmidt for their help in finding useful materials. We are grateful to many friends and colleagues, particularly C. D. Jenkins, for their helpful comments on an earlier version of the manuscript.

References

1. Keyfitz N. and Flieger W. *World Population—An Analysis of Vital Data.* University of Chicago Press, Chicago, 1968.
2. United States Department of Health, Education and Welfare, Public Health Service. *Vital Statistics of the United States, 1970,* Vol. II—*Mortality.* Government Printing Office, Washington, D.C., 1974.
3. Yerushalmy J. Factors in human longevity. *Am. J. publ. Hlth* 53, 148, 1963.
4. Enterline P. E. Causes of death responsible for recent increases in sex mortality differentials in the United States. *Millbank Mem. F. Q.* 39, 312, 1961.
5. Retherford R. D. *The Changing Sex Differential in Mortality.* Studies in Population and Urban Demography #1. Greenwood Press, Westport, CT, 1975.

6. Burbank F. U.S. lung cancer death rates begin to rise proportionately more rapidly for females than for males: a dose-response effect? *J. chron. Dis.* **25**, 473, 1972.
7. Stolnitz G. J. A century of international mortality trends: II *Pop. Stud.* **10**, 17, 1956.
8. United States Department of Health, Education and Welfare, National Center for Health Statistics. *Mortality from Selected Causes by Marital Status: U.S. Vital and Health Statistics,* Series 20, Nos. 8a and 8b. Government Printing Office, Washington, D.C., 1963.
9. Gove W. R. Sex marital status and mortality. *Am. J. Sociol.* **79**, 45, 1973.
10. Hamilton J. B. The role of testicular secretions as indicated by the effects of castration in man and by studies of pathological conditions and the short life span associated with maleness. *Recent Prog. Horm. Res* **3**, 257, 1948.
11. Ricklefs R. E. Fecundity, mortality and avian demography. *Breeding Biology of Birds* (Edited by D. S. Farner), pp. 370–390. National Academy of Science, Washington, 1973.
12. Caughley G. Mortality patterns in mammals. *Ecology* **47**, 906, 1966.
13. Tricomi V., Serr O. and Solish C. The ratio of male to female embryos as determined by the sex chromatin. *Am. J. Obstet. Gynecol.* **79**, 504, 1960.
14. Donaldson R. S. and Kohl S. G. Perinatal mortality in twins by sex. *Am. J. publ. Hlth* **55**, 1411, 1965.
15. Hammoud E. I. Studies in fetal and infant mortality. *Am. J. publ. Hlth* **55**, 1152, 1965.
16. Teitelbaum M. S. Male and female components of perinatal mortality: international trends, 1901–63. *Demography* **8**, 541, 1971.
17. Scheinfeld A. The mortality of men and women. *Scient. Am.* **198**, 22, 1958.
18. Madigan F. C. Are sex mortality differentials biologically caused? *Milbank Mem. F. Q.* **35**, 202, 1957.
19. Sowder W. T., Bond J.O., Williams, Jr., E.H. and Flemming E. L. *Man to Man Talk about Women . . . and Men.* Florida State Board of Health, Monograph Series 10, Jacksonville, 1966.
20. Potts D. M. Which is the weaker sex? *J. Biosoc. Sci.* Suppl. **2**, 147, 1970.
21. Sex differentials in mortality. *Stat. Bull. Metropol. Life Ins. Co.,* pp. 2–5. August, 1974.
22. Report of the Royal College of Physicians. *Smoking and Health Now.* Pitman, London, 1971.
23. Lelbach W. K. Organic Pathology related to volume and pattern of alcohol use. *Research Advances in Alcohol and Drug Programs* I, 93, 1974.
24. Hammond E. C. Smoking in relation to the death rates of one million men and women. *Nat. Cancer Inst. Monogr.* **19**, 127, 1966.
25. Jenkins C. D. The coronary-prone personality. *Psychological Aspects of Myocardial Infarction and Coronary Care* (Edited by W. D. Gentry and R. B. Williams), pp. 5–23. Mosby, St. Louis, 1975.
26. Bonami M. and Rime B. Approche exploratoire de la personalité pre-coronarienne par analyse standardisée de données projectives thematiques. *J. psychosom. Res.* **16**, 103, 1972.
27. Rosenman R. H. The role of behavior patterns and neurogenic factors in the

pathogenesis of coronary heart disease. *Stress and the Heart* (Edited by R. S. Eliot), pp. 123–141. Futura Publ., Mount Kisco, N.Y., 1974.

28. Rosenman R. H., Brand R. J., Jenkins C. D. *et al.* Coronary heart disease in the western collaborative group study. *J.A.M.A.* **233,** 872, 1975.

29. Kenigsberg D., Zyzanski S. J., Jenkins C. D. *et al.* The coronary-prone behavior pattern in hospitalized patients with and without coronary heart disease. *Psychosom. Med.* **36,** 344, 1974.

30. Bengtsson C. Ischaemic heart disease in women. *Acta Med. Scand.* Suppl. 549, pp. 1–128, 1973.

31. Rosenman R. H. and Friedman M. Association of specific behavior pattern in women with blood and cardiovascular findings. *Circulation* **24,** 1173, 1961.

32. Friedman M. and Rosenman R. H. Association of specific overt behavior pattern with blood and cardiovascular findings. *J.A.M.A.* **169,** 1286, 1959.

33. U.S. Department of Labor, Bureau of Labor Statistics, *Employment and Earnings* **19,** 30, 1973.

34. Maccoby E. E. and Jacklin C. N. *The Psychology of Sex Differences.* Stanford University Press, Stanford, 1974.

35. Dentan R. K. *The Semai—A Nonviolent People of Malaya.* Holt, Rinehart & Winston, New York, 1968.

36. Saario T. N., Jacklin C. N. and Tittle C. K. Sex role stereotyping in the public schools. *Harvard Educ. Rev.* **43,** 386, 1973.

37. Bart P. Why women see the future differently from men. *Learning for Tomorrow: The Role of the Future in Education* (Edited by A. Toffler), pp. 33–55. Random House, New York, 1972.

38. U'Ren M. B. The image of woman in textbooks. *Woman in Sexist Society* (Edited by V. Gornick and B. K. Moran), pp. 318–328. New American Library, New York, 1971.

39. Chinoy E. *The Automobile Worker and the American Dream.* Doubleday, New York, 1955.

40. Report of a Special Task Force to the Secretary of Health, Education and Welfare. *Work in America.* MIT Press, Cambridge, 1973.

41. U.S. Churchgoing 40% in '71 Poll, *New York Times,* p. 59, January 9, 1972.

42. Comstock G. W. and Partridge K. B. Church attendance and health. *J. chron. Dis.* **25,** 665, 1972.

43. Furman R. H. Endocrine factors in atherogenesis. In *Atherosclerosis* (Edited by F. G. Schettler and G. S. Boyd), pp. 375–409. Elsevier, Amsterdam, 1969.

44. Segi M., Kurihara M. and Tsukahara Y. *Mortality for Selected Causes in 30 Countries (1950–1961).* Kosei Tokei Kyokai, Tokyo, 1966.

45. Hamilton J. B. and Mestler G. E. Mortality and survival: comparison of eunuchs with intact men and women in a mentally retarded population. *J. Gerontol.* **24,** 395, 1969.

46. London W. T., Rosenberg S. E., Draper J. W. and Almy T. P. The effect of estrogens on atherosclerosis. *Ann. intern. Med.* **55,** 63, 1961.

47. Gertler M. M. and White P. D. *Coronary Heart Disease in Young Adults.* Harvard University Press, Cambridge, 1954.

48. Berkson D. M., Stamler J. and Cohen D. B. Ovarian function and coronary atherosclerosis. *Clin. Obstet. Gynecol.* **7,** 504, 1964.

49. Ask-Upmark E. Life and death without ovaries. *Acta med. scand.* **172**, 129, 1962.
50. Parrish H., Carr C. A., Hall D. G. and King T. M. Time interval from castration in premenopausal women to development of excessive coronary atherosclerosis. *Am. J. Obstet. Gynecol.* **99**, 155, 1967.
51. Higano N., Robinson R. W. and Cohen W. D. Increased incidence of cardiovascular disease in castrated women. *N. Engl. J. Med.* **268**, 1123, 1963.
52. Ritterband A. B., Jaffe I. A., Densen P. M. *et al.* Gonadal function and the development of coronary heart disease. *Circulation* **27**, 237, 1963.
53. Williams T. J. and Novak E. R. Effect of castration and hysterectomy on the female cardiovascular system. *Geriatrics* **18**, 852, 1963.
54. Blackard C. E., Doe R. P., Mellinger G. T. and Byar D. P. Incidence of cardiovascular disease and death in patients receiving diethylstilbestrol for carcinoma of the prostrate. *Cancer* **26**, 249, 1970.
55. Mann J. I., Vessey M. P., Thorogood M. and Doll R. Myocardial infarction in young women with special reference to oral contraceptive practice. *Br. med. J.* **2**, 241, 1975.
56. Mann J. I. and Inman W. H. W. Oral contraceptives and death from myocardial infarction. *Br. med. J.* **2**, 245, 1975.
57. Vessey M. P. Thromboembolism, cancer and oral contraceptives. *Clin. Obstet. Gynecol.* **17**, 65, 1974.
58. Stolley P. D., Tonascia J. A., Tockman M. S. *et al.* Thrombosis with low-estrogen oral contraceptives. *Am. J. Epidemiol.* **102**, 197, 1975.
59. United States Department of Health, Education and Welfare, Public Health Service, National Clearinghouse for Smoking and Health. *Adult Use of Tobacco—1970.* U.S. Government Printing Office, Washington, D.C., 1973.
60. Borgatta E. F. and Evans R. R. Social and psychological concomitants of smoking behavior and its change among university freshmen. *Smoking, Health and Behavior* (Edited by E. F. Borgatta and R. R. Evans), pp. 206–219. Aldine, Chicago, 1968.
61. Mausner B. and Platt E. S. with assistance of Mausner J. S. *Smoking: A Behavioral Analysis.* Pergamon Press, Oxford, 1971.
62. Fischer J. L. and Fischer A. F. The New Englanders of Orchardtown. *Six Cultures-Studies of Child-Rearing* (Edited by B. B. Whiting). Wiley, New York, 1963.
63. Hoffman L. W. Early childhood experiences and women's achievement motives. *J. soc. Issues* **28**, 129, 1972.
64. Levitin T. E. and Chananie J. D. Responses of female primary school teachers to sex-typed behaviors in male and female children. *Child Dev.* **43**, 1309, 1972.
65. Selikoff I. J., Hammond E. C. and Churg J. Asbestos exposure, smoking and neoplasia. *J.A.M.A.* **204**, 104, 1968.
66. Stellman J. M., and Daum S. M. *Work Is Dangerous to Your Health.* Vintage Books, New York, 1973.
67. Hueper W. C. Occupational and environmental cancers of the respiratory system. *Recent Results Cancer Res.* **3**, 1, 1966.

68. U.S. Department of Commerce, Social and Economic Statistics Administration. *Subject Reports Final Report PC(2)-7A, Occupational Characteristics.* Government Printing Office, Washington, D.C., 1973.
69. Breslow L., Hoaglin L., Rasmussen G. and Abrams H. K. Occupations and cigarette smoking as factors in lung cancer. *Am. J. publ. Hlth* 44, 171, 1954.
70. United States Department of Health, Education and Welfare, Public Health Service. *Vital Statistics of the United States, 1967,* Vol. II—*Mortality.* Government Printing Office, Washington, D.C., 1969.
71. National Safety Council. *Accident Facts, 1972.* National Safety Council, Chicago, 1972.
72. United States Department of Health, Education and Welfare, Public Health Service. *Vital and Health Statistics,* Series 10, No. 58. Government Printing Office, Washington, D.C., 1970.
73. Blum R. H. assisted by Braunstein L. Mind-altering drugs and dangerous behavior: alcohol, Appendix B, pp. 29–49. *Task Force Report: Drunkeness.* President's Commission on Law Enforcement and Administration of Justice, Government Printing Office, Washington, D.C., 1967.
74. Fine E. W. and Scoles P. Alcohol, alcoholism and highway safety. *Publ. Hlth Rev.* 3, 423, 1974.
75. Cahalan D. *Problem Drinkers.* Jossey-Bass, Inc., San Francisco, 1970.
76. Goodman L. S. and Gilman A. *The Pharmacological Basis of Therapeutics,* 4th ed. Macmillan, New York, 1970.
77. Bacon M. K. Cross-cultural studies of drinking. *Alcoholism* (Edited by P. G. Bourne), pp. 171–194. Academic Press, New York, 1973.
78. Loper R. G., Kammeier M. L. and Hoffmann H. MMPI characteristics of college freshman males who later became alcoholics. *J. abn. Psychol.* 82, 159, 1973.
79. Cahalan D., Cisin I. and Crossley H. *A National Study of Drinking Behavior and Attitudes.* College and University Press, New Haven, Conn., 1969.
80. Brecher E. M. *Licit and Illicit Drugs.* Consumer Reports, Little-Brown, Boston, 1972.
81. Cooperstock R. Sex differences in the use of mood-modifying drugs: an explanatory model. *J. Hlth Soc. Behav.* 12, 238, 1971.
82. Parry H. J., Balter M. B., Mellinger G. D. *et al.* National patterns of psychotherapeutic drug use. *Archs gen. Psychiat.* 28, 769, 1973.
83. Mellinger G. D., Balter M. B., Manheimer D. I. Patterns of psychotherapeutic drug use among adults in San Francisco. *Archs gen. Psychiat.* 25, 385, 1971.
84. MacMahon B., Johnson S. and Pugh T. F. Relation of suicide rates to social conditions. *Publ. Hlth Rep.* 78, 285, 1963.
85. Dublin L. I. and Bunzel B. *To Be or Not To Be.* Harrison Smith & Robert Haas, Inc., New York, 1933.
86. Henry A. F. and Short J. F. *Suicide and Homicide.* Free Press, New York, 1968.
87. Steppacher R. C. and Mausner J. S. Suicide in male and female physicians. *J.A.M.A.* 228, 323, 1974.
88. Mausner J. S. and Steppacher R. C. Suicide in professionals: a study of male and female psychologists. *Am. J. Epid.* 98, 436, 445, 1973.

89. Schneidman E. S. and Farberow N. L. Statistical comparisons between attempted and committed suicides. *The Cry for Help* (Edited by N. L. Farberow and E. S. Schneidman), pp. 19–47. McGraw-Hill, New York, 1961.
90. Kramer M., Pollack E. S., Redick R. W. *et al. Mental Disorders/Suicide.* Harvard Univ. Press, Cambridge, Mass., 1972.
91. Stengel E., Cook N. G. and Kreeger I. S. *Attempted Suicide. (Maudsley)* (Maudsley Monographs, No. 4), Chapman & Hall, London, 1958.
92. Peck M. L. and Schrut A. Suicidal behavior among college students. *HSMHA Hlth Reports* 86, 149, 1971.
93. MacMahon B., Cole P. and Brown J. Etiology of human breast cancer: a review. *J. natn. Cancer Inst.* 50, 21, 1973.
94. Stevenson A. C. and Kerr C. B. On the distributions of frequencies of mutation to genes determining harmful traits in man. *Mutation Res.* 4, 339, 1967.
95. Mountcastle V. B. (Editor) *Medical Physiology,* Vol. II. Mosby, St. Louis, 1974.
96. Denef C. and DeMoor P. Sexual differentiation of steroid metabolizing enzymes in the rat liver: further studies on predetermination by testosterone at birth. *Endocrin.* 91, 374, 1971.
97. Song C. S., Rifkind A. B., Gillette P. N. *et al.* Hormones and the liver. *Am. J. Obstet. Gynecol.* 105, 813, 1969.
98. United States Department of Health, Education and Welfare, Public Health Service. *Current Estimates from Health Interview Survey: U.S. 1971: Vital and Health Statistics.* Series 10, No. 79. Government Printing Office, Washington, D.C., 1973.
99. Committee for the Special Research Project in the Health Insurance Plan of Greater New York. *Health and Medical Care in New York City.* Harvard Univ. Press, Cambridge, 1957.
100. White K. L., Williams F. and Greenberg B. G. The ecology of medical care. *N. Engl. J. Med.* 265, 885, 1961.
101. Hinkle L. E., Redmont R., Plummer N. *et al.* II. An examination of the relation between symptoms, disability, and serious illness, in two homogeneous groups of men and women. *Am. J. publ. Hlth* 50, 1327, 1960.
102. United States Department of Labor, Wage and Labor Standards Administration, Women's Bureau. Facts about women's absenteeism and labor turnover. In *Woman in a Man-Made World* (Edited by N. Glazer-Malbin and H.Y. Waehrer), pp. 265–271. Rand McNally, Chicago, 1972.
103. Commission on Chronic Illness. *Chronic Illness in the United States.* Vol. IV. *Chronic Illness in a Large City.* Harvard Univ. Press, Cambridge, 1957.
104. Trussell R. E. and Elinson J. *Chronic Illness in the United States.* Vol. III. *Chronic Illness in a Rural Area.* Harvard Univ. Press, Cambridge, 1959.
105. Maddox G. L. Self-assessment of health status. *J. chron. Dis.* 17, 449, 1964.
106. Leo R. G., Dysterheft, A. H. and Merkel G. G. Health profile of lumber mill employees. *Ind. Med. Surg.* 26, 377, 1957.
107. Andersen R. and Anderson O. W. *A Decade of Health Services.* Univ. Chicago Press, Chicago, 1967.

108. Phillips D. L. and Segal B. E. Sexual status and psychiatric symptoms. *Am. sociol. Rev.* **34,** 58, 1969.
109. Hackett T. P., Cassem N. H. and Raker J. W. Patient delay in cancer. *New Engl. J. Med.* **289,** 14, 1973.
110. Worden J. W. and Weisman A. D. Psychosocial components of lagtime in cancer diagnosis. *J. Psychosom. Res.* **19,** 69, 1975.
111. Simon A. B., Feinleib M. and Thompson, Jr., H. K. Components of delay in the pre-hospital setting of acute myocardial infarction. *Am. J. Cardiol.* **30,** 475, 1972.
112. Hackett T. P. and Cassem N. H. Factors contributing to delay in responding to the signs and symptoms of acute myocardial infarction. *Am. J. Cardiol.* **24,** 651, 1969.
113. Moss A. J., Wynar B. and Goldstein S. Delay in hospitalization during the acute coronary period. *Am. J. Cardiol.* **24,** 659, 1969.
114. Kasl S. V. and Cobb S. Health behavior, illness behavior and sick role behavior. *Archs envir. Hlth* **12,** 246, 1966.
115. Marston M. V. Compliance with medical regimens. A Review of the Literature. *Nursing Res.* **19,** 312, 1970.
116. Petroni F. A. The influence of age, sex and chronicity in perceived legitimacy to the sick role. *Sociol. Social*
117. Apple D. How laymen define illness. *J. Hlth hum. Behav.* **1,** 219, 1960.
118. United States Department of Health, Education and Welfare, Public Health Service. *Vital Statistics of the United States, 1958,* Vol. II—*Mortality.* Government Printing Office, Washington, D.C., 1960.
119. Robinson J. P., Converse P. E. and Szalai A. Everyday life in twelve countries. *The Use of Time* (Edited by A. Szalai), pp. 113–144. Mouton, The Hague, 1972.
120. Gove W. R. The relationship between sex roles, marital status and mental illness. *Social Forces* **51,** 34, 1972.
121. Waldman E. and Gover K. R. Marital and family characteristics of the labor force. *Monthly Labor Rev.* **95** (April), 4, 1972.
122. Chodorow N. Being and doing: a cross-cultural examination of the socialization of males and females. *Woman in Sexist Society* (Edited by V. Gornick and B. K. Moran), pp. 259–291. New American Library, New York, 1971.
123. Money J. and Ehrhardt A. A. *Man and Woman—Boy and Girl.* Johns Hopkins Univ. Press, Baltimore, 1972.
124. Waldron I. and Eyer J. Socioeconomic causes of the recent rise in death rates for 15–24-year-olds. *Soc. Sci. & Med.* **9,** 383, 1975.
125. McAlister A. Helping people quit smoking: current progress. *Applying Behavioral Science to Cardiovascular Disease* (Edited by A. Enelow *et al.*), American Heart Association, New York, 1975.
126. McAlister A., Meyer A. and Maccoby N. Results of a two-year health education campaign on smoking behavior: Stanford three community study. *Circulation* (Suppl. II) **51** and **52,** 117, 1975.
127. Suinn R. M. Behavior therapy for cardiac patients. *Behav. Therapy* **5,** 569, 1974.

4

A Tale of Two States

Victor R. Fuchs

In the western United States there are two contiguous states that enjoy about the same levels of income and medical care and are alike in many other respects, but their levels of health differ enormously. The inhabitants of Utah are among the healthiest individuals in the United States, while the residents of Nevada are at opposite end of the spectrum. Comparing death rates of white residents in the two states, for example, we find that infant mortality is about 40 percent higher in Nevada. And lest the reader think that the higher rate in Nevada is attributable to the "sinful" atmosphere of Reno and Las Vegas, we should note that infant mortality in the rest of the state is almost exactly the same as it is in these two cities. Rather, . . . infant death rates depend critically upon the physical and emotional condition of the mother.

The excess mortality in Nevada drops appreciably for children because, as shall be argued below, differences in life-style account for differences in death rates, and these do not fully emerge until the adult years. As the following figures indicate, the differential for adult men and women is in the range of 40 to 50 percent until old age, at which point the differential naturally decreases.

The two states are very much alike with respect to income, schooling, degree of urbanization, climate, and many other variables that are frequently thought to be the cause of variations in mortality. (In fact, average family income is actually higher in Nevada than in Utah.) The numbers of physicians and of hospital beds per capita are also similar in the two states.

What, then, explains these huge differences in death rates? The answer almost surely lies in the different life-styles of the residents of the two states. Utah is inhabited primarily by Mormons, whose influence is strong throughout the state. Devout Mormons do not use tobacco or alcohol and in general lead stable, quiet lives. Nevada, on the other hand, is a state with high rates of cigarette and alcohol consumption and very high in-

Table 1.
Excess of Death Rates in Nevada
Compared with Utah, Average for
1959–61 and 1966–68

Age Group	Males	Females
<1	42%	35%
1–19	16%	26%
20–29	44%	42%
30–39	37%	42%
40–49	54%	69%
50–59	38%	28%
60–69	26%	17%
70–79	20%	6%

dexes of marital and geographical instability. The contrast with Utah in these respects is extraordinary.

In 1970, 63 percent of Utah's residents 20 years of age and over had been born in the state; in Nevada the comparable figure was only 10 percent; for persons 35–64 the figures were 64 percent in Utah and 8 percent in Nevada. Not only were more than nine out of ten Nevadans of middle age born elsewhere, but more than 60 percent were not even born in the West.

The contrast in stability is also evident in the response to the 1970 census question about changes in residence. In Nevada only 36 percent of persons 5 years of age and over were then living in the same residence as they had been in 1965; in Utah the comparable figure was 54 percent.

The differences in marital status between the two states are also significant in view of the association between marital status and mortality discussed in the previous section. More than 20 percent of Nevada's males ages 35–64 are single, widowed, divorced, or not living with their spouses. Of those who are married with spouse present, more than one-third had been previously widowed or divorced. In Utah the comparable figures are only half as large.

The impact of alcohol and tobacco can be readily seen in the following comparison of death rates from cirrhosis of the liver and malignant neoplasms of the respiratory system. For both sexes the excess of death rates from these causes in Nevada is very large.

The populations of these two states are, to a considerable extent, self-selected extremes from the continuum of life-styles found in the United States. Nevadans, as has been shown, are predominantly recent immigrants from other areas, many of whom were attracted by the state's permissive mores. The inhabitants of Utah, on the other hand, are evidently willing to remain in a more restricted society. Persons born in

Table 2.
Excess of Death Rates in Nevada
Compared with Utah for Cirrhosis of
the Liver and Malignant Neoplasms of
the Respiratory System, Average for
1966–68

Age	Males	Females
30–39	590%	443%
40–49	111%	296%
50–59	206%	205%
60–69	117%	227%

Utah who do not find these restrictions acceptable tend to move out of the state.

Summary

This dramatic illustration of large health differentials that are unrelated to income or availability of medical care helps to highlight the [following] themes . . .

1. From the middle of the eighteenth century to the middle of the twentieth century rising real incomes resulted in unprecedented improvements in health in the United States and other developing countries.
2. During most of this period medical care (as distinct from public health measures) played an insignificant role in health, but, beginning in the mid-1930s, major therapeutic discoveries made significant contributions independently of the rise in real income.
3. As a result of the changing nature of health problems, rising income is no longer significantly associated with better health, except in the case of infant mortality (primarily post-neonatal mortality)—and even here the relationship is weaker than it used to be.
4. As a result of the wide diffusion of effective medical care, its marginal contribution to health is again small (over the observed range of variation). There is no reason to believe that the major health problems of the average American would be significantly alleviated by increases in the number of hospitals or physicians. This conclusion might be altered, however, as the result of new scientific discoveries. Alternatively, the *marginal* contribution of medical care might become even smaller as a result of such advances.
5. The greatest current potential for improving the health of the American people is to be found in what they do and don't do to and for themselves. Individual decisions about diet, exercise, and smoking are of critical importance, and collective decisions affecting pollution and other aspects of the environment are also relevant.

These conclusions notwithstanding, the demand for medical care is very great and growing rapidly. As René Dubos has acutely observed, "To ward off disease or recover health, men as a rule find it easier to depend on the healers than to attempt the more difficult task of living wisely."[1]

Note

1. René Dubos, *The Mirage of Health* (New York: Harper, 1959), p. 110.

Our Sickening Social and Physical Environments

THE PAST DECADE HAS SEEN increasing public awareness of the importance of eliminating dangerous substances from our physical environment and improving the quality of our social environment through efforts to reduce stress. We are only beginning to understand the significant health consequences for many people—sometimes occurring decades after initial exposure—of the dumping of industrial wastes into water supplies and land fills, additives in foods, the exhaust of chemicals into the air we breathe, and the use of nuclear power as a source of energy. Health and environmentalist groups have also alerted us to the dangers of working or living in physical and social environments which make us anxious, uncomfortable or angry (Stellman and Daum, 1973; Page and O'Brien, 1973). Today's major diseases are often slow-developing, chronic and incurable disorders. This section explores the relation of chronic diseases to the social and physical environments in which they develop.

In the previous section we began exploring the relationship between society and the distribution of disease and death. We saw that in American society diseases are patterned by socio-cultural variables, including social class, gender, and life style. Here we continue to search for an understanding of the interface between diseases and society by examining three serious and widespread health disorders in the United States today: coronary heart disease, cancer, and hypertension (high blood pressure).

Social scientists have little difficulty analyzing the social nature of such problems as homicide, suicide, and automobile accidents. However, only rarely have they applied sociological perspectives to understanding the causes and prevention of diseases such as cancer or hypertension. The articles in this section share the theme that at least some of these chronic diseases have developed as a result of modern industrialization, and so are deeply connected to the organization and characteristics of social life.

The Department of Health, Education and Welfare estimates that in the first nine months of 1979, about 49.9 percent of all deaths were from major cardio-vascular diseases—diseases of the heart and circulatory system. These include heart disease, hypertension, and stroke. Another 21.2 percent of all deaths in that period were from some form of cancer (DHEW, 1979). These data give us a general picture of the significant impact of chronic disease on our population's health. Chronic diseases generally develop and persist over a long period of time. Their signs often go unnoticed or unidentified until serious damage is done to the victim's body, and they usually have complex rather than simple or single causes. Medical treatment generally aims to alleviate symptoms, prevent or slow down further organic damage, or minimize physical discomfort, primarily through treatments with medications or surgery. Treatment rather than prevention is the dominant medical approach to these diseases.

Although *prevention* of chronic diseases would seem to be the most logical, safe, and perhaps the most moral approach, few financial resources have been devoted in the United States to the elimination of the physical and social causes of chronic health disorders. (To the contrary, the federal government continues to subsidize the tobacco industry in the United States despite the Surgeon General's warnings that cigarette smoking is the leading cause of death from lung cancer.) As Samuel S. Epstein notes in "The Political and Economic Basis of Cancer" which follows, little commitment has been made to research into the physical and social factors which cause cancer. The growing recognition of the environmental component in many chronic diseases has led some critics to question the priorities of our current medical care system, as well as the limits of its approach to the treatment, let alone prevention, of these disorders.

Epstein's article analyzes what the author terms the growing "epidemic" of cancer in American society. He points to a range of physical substances that have been identified as cancer-causing or carcinogenic, and questions why those substances were not tested properly, or eliminated once identified as dangerous. He sees cancer as both a medical and social issue, involving as it does a range of political and economic factors, including the use of chemicals in manufacturing to increase profits, the economic and political pressures on industry scientists, and the relatively low priority given to cancer prevention research. If many cancers are environmentally produced—and the federal government has estimated that as many as 90 percent may be so—why has medical research and treatment focused on cure rather than prevention?

The second article in this section is "Occupational Stress and Coronary Heart Disease: A Review and Theoretical Integration," by James S. House. It examines the relationship between occupational stress and coronary heart disease. The development of many chronic disorders, including heart disease, seems to be related to both biophysiological and psycho-social processes. Increasingly there is evidence that the distinction between "physical" and "mental" health may not be helpful because it masks the important social and interactional components of disease by isolating physical health from its social components. However, many people get sick because they are physically *and* emotionally stressed, and House reviews the literature on the impact of stress caused by work. He points out the severe limitations in the research and data available in this area. For example, certain groups of people, particularly women and working class people of both sexes, have been overlooked in the research which has examined the impact of work on health. Some studies make the mistake of examining small populations, such as executive level, white men, and generalizing their findings to all populations. House's article suggests the importance of studying stress directly and in all populations in order to learn more about the relationship among stress, work, and health. What we do know, he argues, is that there is considerable evidence that stress contributes to the cause of coronary heart disease and probably to other chronic diseases as well. It is important, therefore, that we unravel the complexities of physical and social variables in order to understand better the impact of stress on health.

These issues are placed within a broader conceptual framework in the article by Peter L. Schnall and Rochelle Kern entitled "Hypertension in American Society: An Introduction to Historical Materialist Epidemiology." In considering the particular problem of hypertension, the authors present the concept of "historical materialist epidemiology" (HME). HME, as one approach to social epidemiology, is " . . . the study of disease as it spreads and involves large groups of people within the context of the social organization of any particular society" (Gaynor et al., 1976:ME/1). HME differs from standard social epidemiology in that it focuses on the disease producing consequences of the social and economic organization of society—an organization which changes historically and differs from society to society—rather than demographic variables. Schnall and Kern expand on this view and use it to examine the problem of hypertension as well as the way that disease has been conceptualized, studied, and treated by medicine. HME provides one approach to integrating an understanding of society with our knowledge of disease, and in so doing makes an important contribution to the critical perspective encouraged throughout this book.

References

Department of Health, Education and Welfare (DHEW). 1980. "Births, marriages, divorces and deaths for October 1979" Monthly Vital Statistics Report. Provisional Statistics from the National Center for Health Statistics. 28, 10, January: 9–10.

Gaynor, David, Joseph Eyer, and Howard Berliner. 1976. "Materialist epidemiology." Health Marxist Organization (HMO) Packet #1. (Unpublished paper available from Health/PAC, 17 Murray St., New York, NY 10007).

Page, Joseph, and M. O'Brien. 1973. Bitter Wages. New York: Grossman.

Stellman, Jeanne M., and Susan M. Daum. 1973. Work Is Dangerous to Your Health. New York: Random House.

5

The Political and Economic Basis of Cancer

Samuel S. Epstein

Cancer is now a killing and disabling disease of epidemic proportions. More than 53 million people in the U.S. (over a quarter of the population) will develop some form of cancer in their lifetimes, and approximately 20 percent will die of it.

It is estimated that in 1975, 665,000 new cancer cases were diagnosed, and that there were 365,000 cancer deaths. Thus, cancer deaths in 1975 alone were approximately five times higher than the total U.S. military deaths in the Viet Nam and Korean war years combined.

Cancer spares no age, sex, or ethnic group. It is a leading cause of death at all ages, including infancy and childhood. Susceptibility to cancer has been induced even before birth, as demonstrated in post-adolescent girls whose mothers had been treated in pregnancy with the anti-abortant diethylstilbestrol.

Cancer has a major economic impact. In 1969, the estimated direct costs for hospitalization and medical care of cancer patients exceeded $500 million. It appears that the total direct costs for any patient range between $5,000 and over $20,000. The direct and indirect costs of cancer, including loss of earnings during illness and during the balance of normal life expectancy, were estimated by the U.S. Department of Health, Education and Welfare (H.E.W.) at $15 billion for 1971.

Increasing Incidence

Only three major causes of death have increased significantly in the recent past: cancer, homicide, and cirrhosis of the liver. Overall, deaths from most other causes are decreasing. This increase in the incidence of cancer is real, over and above that due to an increase in life expectancy, and has occurred despite advances in diagnosis and cure. Interestingly, the last major inprovements in five-year cancer survival rates occurred prior to 1955, and appear to reflect the first half of the century's advances in surgery, blood transfusion, and antibiotic therapy, rather than advances in cancer chemotherapy and treatment. (Greenberg, 1975)

Cancer death rates for the U.S. are available only from 1900. Early rate estimates are crude: they are not adjusted for age, and are based on less than half of the population living in 153 cities and ten states. Overall crude cancer death rates since 1933 have increased annually by about 1 percent until 1975, when the rate appears to have increased to approximately 2.3 percent, according to provisional estimates.

Standardized cancer death rates, adjusted for age and based on the total U.S. population, have been available since 1933, the year the National Center for Health Statistics was established. These more reliable data also show an overall increase in cancer death rates. Standardized cancer death rates have increased overall by approximately 11 percent in the last four decades.

Much of the overall increase in cancer mortality since 1933 is attributable to lung cancer, and is due to smoking. Similar large increases in the incidence of cancer have been noted in other organs, particularly among blacks. Some of this increase may reflect access to improved diagnostic facilities.

At the same time, the incidence of cancer for other organs such as stomach and cervix has declined significantly (Cutler and Devesa, 1973). In fact, the decrease in the incidence of cervical cancer rates may be the source of the overall decrease in standardized cancer mortality rates for white females. On the other hand, recent evidence suggests an increasing incidence of endometrial (uterine lining) cancer, which is possibly associated with the popularity of prescribing estrogens to post-menopausal women. "Spotty" changes in cancer incidence, of which endometrial cancer is an example, and in death rates over the past few decades have, in fact, provided important epidemiological clues to environmental causes of cancer in various organs.

A recent National Cancer Institute (N.C.I.) publication, an atlas of cancer mortality rates compiled by county, shows marked geographical clustering of high cancer rates in white men and women (for various organs) in heavily industrialized areas. Such data correlate cancer rates in the general community with living near certain industries.

Apart from the importance of occupational factors in the incidence of "neighborhood" cancer in the population at large, specific occupational exposures are also an important cause of cancer deaths, particularly in males. Various estimates indicate that 5 to 15 percent of all current cancer deaths in males are occupational in origin. These include lung cancer and pleural mesotheliomas (cancer of the chest lining) in insulation workers, construction workers, and others exposed to asbestos, bladder cancer in aniline dye and rubber industry workers, induced by such chemicals as 2-naphthylamine, benzidine, 2-aminobiphenyl, and 2-nitrobiphenyl (used in dyes and resins); lung cancer in uranium miners of Colorado, in coke oven workers, and in workers even briefly exposed to bischloromethyl ether; skin cancer in cutting and shale oil workers; nasal sinus cancer in woodworkers; cancer of the pancreas and lymphomas in organic chemists; and angiosarcoma of the liver in workers involved in the manufacture and fabrication of polyvinyl chloride.

The toll of workers stricken by cancer in particular occupational exposures is overwhelming. For instance, an estimated 50 percent of long-term asbestos-insulation workers die of cancer, and 20 percent of all long-term asbestos workers die of lung cancer. Approximately 30 percent of all premature deaths in uranium miners is due to lung cancer. The many other occupations that involve a high risk of cancer, include steel workers, miners and smelters, rubber workers, and workers in a wide range of petrochemical industries.

Environmental Chemical Carcinogens

The consensus is growing that most human cancers are environmental in origin, and thus ultimately preventable. Numerous estimates by expert national and international committees suggest that 70 to 90 percent of human cancers are environmentally induced or related; Dr. Frank Rauscher, the Director of the N.C.I., recently placed the incidence of environmental cancer at 90 percent. The basis for such estimates largely derives from epidemiological studies in large community populations over extended periods. These reveal that the incidence of cancer varies geographically. It must be noted, however, that the role of specific environmental carcinogens so far has been implicated or identified in relatively few of the studies.

There is also general agreement now that the U.S. population and workforce has been—and is being—continuously exposed to countless known and unknown chemical carcinogens in their air, water, and food. Potent new chemical agents are being synthesized and introduced into commerce and the workplace, generally without prior, adequate testing for carcinogenicity or for other adverse public health and ecological effects.

Detecting Carcinogens

A particular chemical or mixture is determined to be carcinogenic by toxicological testing in experimental animals, or epidemiological observations in large, exposed human populations. While each approach has problems, the results of animal testing can help pinpoint carcinogens before they are introduced to commerce and the workplace. Epidemiological studies can identify only carcinogens which have already affected the human population; they are generally based on identifying temporal or geographical clustering of specific organ cancers.

Toxicological techniques currently used on laboratory animals are relatively insensitive. Their ability to detect carcinogens—individually and in various combinations—in concentrations which reflect the low or changing patterns of actual environmental exposure is limited. In the same vein, epidemiological techniques are unlikely to detect weak carcinogens, unless there are sharp differentials in the general population's exposure, as with cigarette smoking. Even for smoking, the single largest cause of cancer deaths, several decades of investigation were required before cause and effect could be established. For widely dispersed agents, including unintentional or accidental food additives such as dieldrin and DDT, to which the population-at-large is generally and ubiquitously exposed, human experience and epidemiological observations are unlikely to provide any meaningful or immediate indication of safety or hazard.

A majority of the qualified scientific community agrees that valid and well conducted animal experiments yield carcinogenicity data with a high degree of presumptive human relevance. Indeed, every chemical known to be carcinogenic to humans, with the possible exception of tri-valent arsenic, is also carcinogenic to animals. Many chemicals now recognized as carcinogenic to humans were first identified by animal testing. These include diethylstilbestrol, bischloromethyl ether, vinyl chloride, and aflatoxins. There can be no possible justification, scientific or otherwise, for leading industrial representatives' or regulatory agency officials' continued insistence that animal data must be validated by human experience before regulatory action can be taken. Legislation has already recognized the scientific validity of data derived from animal testing: in the 1958 Delaney Amendment to the Federal Food Drug and Cosmetic Act; in such recent regulatory actions as the suspension of the major agricultural uses of dieldrin; and, still more recently, in the suspension of major agricultural uses of chlordane and heptachlor, whose carcinogenicity has been clearly demonstrated in animals, but not yet in humans.

In carcinogenicity tests, animals must be subjected to relatively high concentrations of the test substance. This is an attempt to reduce the gross insensitivity imposed on these tests by the relatively small size of animal groups tested, when compared to the millions of people who are presumed to be at risk. This insensitivity also applies to the numerous possible synergistic interactions between individual carcinogens, such as DDT and dieldrin, or between carcinogenic and noncarcinogenic chemicals.

Thus, safe levels of human exposure to chemical carcinogens cannot be predicted, either on the basis of animal or epidemiological data. That fact underlies the 1958 Delaney Amendment, which imposes a zero tolerance for carcinogenic food additives. The Amendment states: " . . . no additive shall be deemed to be safe if it is found, after tests which are appropriate for the evaluation of the safety of food additives, to induce cancer in man or animals. . . ."

This position was restated by H.E.W. Secretary Casper W. Weinberger in June, 1974: "At present, the Department of Health, Education and Welfare lacks the scientific information necessary to establish no-effect levels for carcinogenic substances in animals in general and in man in particular. In the absence of such information, we do not believe that detectable residues of carcinogenic animal drugs should be allowed in the food supply"

Constraints to Reducing Cancer

I believe there are reasonable *a priori* grounds for associating recent cancer death rate increases with the increase of industrial chemicals in our environment, and concurrent exposure of large populations to these chemicals over the last four decades.

Such increases are likely to have occurred in other industrialized countries, although perhaps later and less dramatically than in the U.S.

Aside from some special purpose regulations of pesticides, food additives, and drugs, post-war petrochemical technology has burgeoned largely unrestricted by national or international controls. There are no general requirements for pre-testing chemicals for carcinogenic or other adverse effects prior to manufacture or use. Consequently, many carcinogens whose effects may become manifest only now, in the next few years, or in decades, may have been used extensively. The case of vinyl chloride may be only a portent of similar disasters. Now a recognized occupational carcinogen, vinyl chloride was originally introduced into large-scale production in the 1950s. Manufacture of the substance grew at about 15 percent per year, culminating in 1970 when about 4 billion pounds were manufactured in the U.S. Of the vinyl chloride workers identified by June, 1974, with confirmed diagnoses of hepatic angiosarcoma (a rare form of liver cancer), more than half were first exposed before 1950.

Toxic substances legislation is required to mandate requirements for toxicological testing in general, and for carcinogenicity testing in particular, of new chemical agents before their introduction to commerce and the workplace. Failure to enact such legislation, largely due to intensive lobbying by the chemical industry, is likely to result in still further increases in the incidence of cancer in the coming decades. Various adverse economic impact analyses of such legislation, procured by the chemical industry, have in general ignored the very substantial, and hitherto externalized, costs of human cancer, while exaggerating the financial cost.

Several thousand new compounds are now being introduced into commerce each year. Using appropriate systems of priorities and registration, and with the possible judicious use of short-term screening tests (McCann, *et al,* 1975), it has been estimated that approximately 500 new compounds would have to be tested each year, and that this would necessitate some four- to five-fold expansion of current facilities. This should not represent any great problem, particularly as there are abundant untapped resources in the private sector, including universities and the chemical and pharmaceutical industries. The national laboratories, such as Brookhaven, Oak Ridge, and Argonne, also represent important potential facilities.

In many cases, the federal government is meeting the bill for carcinogenicity testing of potentially profitable chemicals and products. Following an injunction to "reduce cancer rates," the N.C.I. has initiated a bioassay program, largely on industrial chemicals, and a program on "safe cigarette testing." Limited federal intramural programs are also being carried out, such as the F.D.A. tests on food additives. Clearly, national policies should be established to shift these costs from the public to the private sector, allowing industry to pay for testing in approved laboratories under contract to the N.C.I.

Even within allotted federal resources, low priority has been accorded to research on environmental carcinogens and on the prevention of human cancer. The N.C.I.'s expenditure on environmental carcinogens has been estimated at between 5 and 20 percent of the total budget. For the 1975 budget of $691 million, for example, direct expenditures on environmental carcinogens appear to be only 10 percent. This low priority for environmental carcinogenesis by the N.C.I. shows up in the January, 1974, subject index of current N.C.I. grants. Only one of a total of 307 pages deals with epidemiological and population studies on cancer. Further, none of the three members of the President's Cancer Panel or of the approximately 23 members of the 1975 National Cancer Advisory Board appears to have significant professional qualifications or experience in epidemiology and preventive medicine, and only one is authoritative in chemical carcinogenesis. Industrial representation on the Board and Panel, in the absence of labor and consumer representation, also seems disproportionately strong.

N.C.I. expenditures on anti-smoking propaganda are relatively low, while research on "safe cigarettes" is well supported. The latter costs should perhaps more properly be borne by the tobacco industry, which now spends about $250 million annually on advertising. Similar considerations apply to costs of the N.C.I. bioassay program on profitable chemicals, costs which should also be borne by the private sector. It is also significant that the U.S.D.A. spends approximately $50 million annually on various tobacco support programs, and that its Agricultural Research Service (A.R.S.) assigns more laboratory space to research on tobacco than to research on food distribution. What's more, the A.R.S.'s concern is to produce a more marketable product, not a safer product. These federal policies are not consistent with very high national costs from the current epidemic of lung cancer, apart from bladder cancer and cardio-respiratory disease, all due to smoking.

. . . .

The Barriers Ahead

Certain sectors of industry have a standard response to regulatory agencies' attempts to promulgate standards limiting environmental and occupational exposure to chemical carcinogens and other toxic agents. They forecast, generally on the basis of procured reports, major economic disruption and unemployment attending compliance with the suggested regulations. These forecasts, apart from their questionable validity, do not address themselves to the externalized costs, economic and otherwise, of the carcinogenic and other toxic effects of human exposure to carcinogens.

Estimates in the summer of 1974 (by A. D. Little, under contract to the Society of Plastics Industry [S.P.I.], and by Foster D. Snell, under contract to O.S.H.A.) on the impact of proposed occupational standards for vinyl chloride, predicted costs as high as $65 billion and losses of up to 1.6 million jobs. Such estimates are clearly gross distortions, as most PVC producers are now in compliance, in the absence of major economic disruptions (Rattner, 1975). For example, capital costs of B.F. Goodrich Co. for compliance were approximately $34 million. This industry now is considering leasing its "clean-up" technology, and has found that the installed compliance technology actually cuts labor costs. It is of interest, however, that B.F. Goodrich has recently increased the prices of its PVC products, alleging higher production costs from compliance with regulatory standards.

Only experiences such as the ability of the PVC industry to meet occupational standards for vinyl chloride at relatively low costs can prove that safeguarding the health of consumers and workers is compatible with its primary interests. Yet the problem is clear, the evidence incontrovertible:
—The incidence of some human cancer is rising. Cancer is killing one in five Americans. And the economic costs of cancer are a minimum of $15 billion a year.
—The majority of human cancers are environmental in origin, and therefore preventable.
—In addition to a number of chemical carcinogens already contaminating our air, water, food, and workplace, new carcinogens are being synthesized and introduced into commerce in increasing numbers and in a largely unregulated manner.

The solution is clear, and remains to be implemented. Its constraints appear to be mainly political and economic, rather than scientific. Toxic substances legislation must be a critical element of national policies to reduce the incidence of human cancers. Such legislation should also update current policies for regulation of environmental carcinogens by federal agencies.

Moreover, scientific research on chemical carcinogenesis conducted by industry, the N.C.I., and other federal agencies must be insulated from political and economic pressures if the principles of chemical carcinogenesis are not to be subverted further by such considerations as short-term marketing interests and alleged regulatory requirements.

The regulation of environmental and occupational carcinogens is clearly consistent with long-term industrial and national interests. The nation's interests cannot be served by economic analyses that distort and exaggerate the costs and unemployment which may attend compliance with responsible standards.

References

Cutler, S. J., and S. S. Devesa, "Trends in Cancer Incidence and Mortality in the U.S.A." in R. Doll and I. Vodopija, eds., *Host Environmental Interactions in the Etiology of Cancer in Man.* International Agency for Research on Cancer, Scientific Publication No. 7, Lyon, 1973.

Edsall, J. T., "Report of the A.A.A.S. Committee on Scientific Freedom and Responsibility," *Science,* Vol. 188, p. 687, 1975.

Epstein, S. S. "Environmental Determinants of Human Cancer," *Cancer Research,* Vol. 34, p. 2425, 1974. (This provides further information and references on many topics discussed in the present article.)

Epstein, S. S., "Public Health Hazards from Chemicals in Consumer Products," in S. S. Epstein and R. Grundy, eds., *Consumer Health and Product Hazards: The Legislation of Product Safety,* Vol. 1. M.I.T. Press, Cambridge, Mass., 1974. (This provides a general description of toxicity and carcinogenicity testing and also discusses some major problems in regulatory agencies.)

Epstein, S. S. *The Science of the Total Environment,* Vol. 4, pp. 1, 205, 1975. (This is a detailed review of the carcinogenicity data on aldrin and dieldrin.)

Fine, D., *et al., Science* (in progress), 1976.

Greenberg, D., *Washington Post,* January 19, 1975; *Science and Government Report,* April 1, 1975. (This provides a general discussion on N.C.I. priorities and environmental carcinogenesis.)

Innes, R., *et al., Journal of the National Cancer Institute,* Vol. 42, p. 1101, 1969.

McCann, J., *et al., Proceedings of the National Academy of Science,* Vol. 72, December, 1975.

Rattner, S., *New York Times,* December 28, 1975.

Tepper, L., *Hearings Before a Subcommittee of the House Committee on Appropriations,* p. 63, May 6, 1974.

6

Occupational Stress and Coronary Heart Disease: A Review and Theoretical Integration

James S. House

· ·

Empirical Evidence

Two kinds of evidence point to an important role for occupational stress in the etiology of heart disease. First, there are standard epidemiological studies comparing morbidity or mortality rates for different demographic categories such as race, sex, age, occupation, education, ethnicity, region, or place of residence. While an observed difference between demographic categories in incidence of disease is ambiguous with respect to the causal mechanisms that produce it, such data are useful in suggesting hypotheses about the impact of occupational stress on heart disease. Stress is only one of the possible causal mechanisms, and well-designed research should assess relevant competing causes, such as diet, exercise, smoking, or family history. But a second type of research is needed to establish adequately a relationship between occupational stress and heart disease: it must relate specific types of stress to heart disease and show that the differential distribution of stress across demographic categories accounts, at least in part, for observed differences in mortality or morbidity between groups.

This literature review considers both broad demographic comparisons and more focused studies of specific types of occupational stress in relation to heart disease. The more focused studies present the major evidence relating specific objective work conditions and/or subjective perceptions of stress to heart disease. The process by which individual and social situational characteristics condition relationships of objective work conditions and/or subjective perceptions thereof to heart disease is also considered briefly. Unfortunately, no good empirical evidence is available on the influence of response modes upon the relationship between occupational stress and heart disease. This is a problem needing future research.

Demographic Comparisons

Aside from its increase with age, perhaps the most striking fact about the distribution of coronary heart disease (CHD) in the American population of working age is the degree to which it afflicts young and middle-aged males and spares young and middle-aged white females. Throughout the period of peak occupational endeavor (ages 25 to 64 years), the mortality rate from CHD among white males is from 2.75 to 6.50 times greater than the white female rate, while non-white males die from CHD at a rate only 1.35 to 1.91 times greater than the non-white female rate. Among females, those who are black or of lower social status run a significantly greater risk of death from CHD, but there are no sizeable or consistent race or status differences among males (see mortality data for 1959–61 in Moriyama et al., 1971:58–64; also see Antonovsky, 1968; Marks, 1967).

Interestingly, few have speculated about the potential role of occupational stress in producing these sex differences. Moriyama et al. (1971) discount the possibility that the unique female hormonal make-up prior to menopause can account for the difference, since no noticeable increase in female death rates follows the age of menopause. But these same authors then suggest only that we look to differences in diet, physical activity, and smoking as explanations; they do not mention occupational or other social stress. If occupational stress contributes to the sex differences in CHD mortality, there should be evidence of a declining sex difference as female employment and equality increase. And, in fact, Moriyama et al. (1971) report that, between 1940 and the late 1950's, male CHD death rates steadily increased, while white female rates steadily declined; but since then the male rate seems to have levelled off, while the female rate (for ages 35 to 54 years) is rising.

The sizeable occupational differences in CHD morbidity and mortality also suggest the potential etiological importance of occupational stress (Guralnick, 1963). In a number of studies cited here, men in occupations involving "greater stress" showed higher susceptibility to heart disease. Yet, such occupational comparisons have generally produced few interpretable results since little effort has been made to specify types of stresses which might explain occupational differences. As Suchman (1967), Jenkins (1971), and others have suggested, identification of specific stresses and their differential distribution across occupations is *sine qua non* for establishing work-related stress as an explanation of occupational differences in heart disease. Demographic comparisons can suggest the potential relevance of occupational stress to CHD, but more focused studies must demonstrate that relevance.

Focused Studies

Studies of social psychological aspects of work in relation to CHD constitute the largest and most productive body of research relating occupational
stress to chronic diseases. The studies to be reviewed here use essentially
two measures of health: (1) actual disease entities such as heart attacks;
and (2) behavioral and physiological factors known to increase the risk of
such disease (high levels of cigarette smoking, obesity, blood sugar, blood
pressure, cholesterol, etc.). Studies using actual disease as the dependent
variable are of two types—retrospective and prospective. In a retrospective
study persons with heart disease are compared on measures of occupational stress with a control group of persons without this disease. A major
methodological flaw here is that differences between the heart disease and
control groups may be a result rather than a cause of heart disease. In a
prospective design asymptomatic persons are interviewed about their lives
and work and then followed until some develop heart disease. Here the
evidence is more convincing that the social psychological characteristics
differentiating those who do and do not incur the disease are, in fact,
causes of the disease.

Studies utilizing "risk factors" of heart disease as dependent variables
are usually cross-sectional, and occasionally prospective. In a cross-
sectional study, occupational stress and risk factors are measured at
about the same time and their associations determined. Although correlations cannot establish causality, it is usually more plausible to assume,
for example, that job satisfaction affected blood pressure rather than *vice
versa*. A number of longitudinal and/or experimental studies clearly demonstrate that changes in work-related variables cause changes in risk
factors. Despite the flaws in any single study, a rather convincing pattern
of results emerges from the studies considered below.

Job Satisfaction and Self-Esteem

A number of retrospective studies in the United States and other countries
found that persons with coronary disease were significantly more dissatisfied with their overall jobs or aspects thereof (e.g., tedious details, lack of
recognition, poor relations with co-workers, poor working conditions) and/
or had more work "problems" and difficulties (Jenkins, 1971). Three different samples of occupations (N's = 16, 12, and 36, respectively) studied by
Sales and House (1971) produced consistently negative and generally very
significant correlations across occupations between average levels of job
satisfaction and heart disease mortality rates. The relationships were strongest for intrinsic job satisfaction measures and in white collar, as opposed to
blue collar, occupations. Relationships between average levels of job dissatisfaction and mortality from a variety of other causes (tuberculosis, cancer,
diabetes, influenza, pneumonia, and accidents) were nonexistent. Con-

trolling for occupational status via partial correlation did not seriously diminish the relationship between satisfaction and CHD.

House (1972) reported correlations between a three-item index of job satisfaction and a variety of heart disease risk factors (e.g., smoking, obesity, cholesterol, blood pressure, and blood sugar) for a sample of 288 men representing the full range of occupations in a total community (the Tecumseh Community Health Study of the University of Michigan). Correlations across the total sample were near zero. However, further analyses revealed rather different correlations in specific age and occupational subgroups. As in the Sales and House study, correlations were in the expected negative direction more often among white-collar than among blue-collar workers. Interestingly, the expected relationships generally emerged for men 45 or more years of age, but a positive relationship was found for younger men. Among older men (i.e., 45+ years of age), correlations between satisfaction and a CHD risk summary measure were significantly negative for professionals and salaried managers ($r = -.31$) and for industrial foremen and workers ($r = -.25$).

These results highlight a persisting problem in the occupational stress and heart disease literature. The subject population for most studies is restricted to white-collar workers and/or specific organizations. Results from such homogeneous samples often do not replicate across the full range of more heterogeneous populations. The dangers in generalizing from quite limited samples to all employed males (much less females) cannot be overemphasized.

Self-esteem in work is closely related to job satisfaction. House (1972) found occupational self-esteem in work to be even more strongly and negatively associated with heart disease risk than was job satisfaction, again especially among middle-aged and older white-collar workers. However Kasl et al. (1968) and Kasl and Cobb (1970) longitudinally compared male blue-collar workers terminated by factory closings with a steadily employed control group. Self-esteem declined with job loss and rose with reemployment. Significant negative correlatons between self-esteem and CHD risk factors emerged both at any given point in time and over time.

In an earlier study, Kasl and French (1962) found that men whose occupational self-esteem was low frequented their company dispensaries much more often than those with higher self-esteem. Perhaps low work self-esteem predisposes men to a wider variety of illnesses than just heart disease. Men who felt their jobs were dull and boring also made more dispensary visits. In contrast, Caplan (1971) and French et al. (1965) found no clear relationships between self-esteem and heart disease risk among professional workers. Nevertheless, evidence is mounting to support a contention that low satisfaction and self-esteem in work predispose men to heart disease and perhaps to other diseases as well.

Job Pressures

The layman's conception of occupational "stress" is reflected best in studies about effects of high levels of work load, responsibility, and role conflict or ambiguity—what will here be termed job "pressures." A series of studies by French and his colleagues have found associations between feelings of work overload and elevated heart disease risk in a variety of populations. Work overload refers to feelings that job demands exceed one's capacities, given one's available time, resources, and abilities. Deadlines are a frequent source of overload. Among 104 university professors, men who felt overloaded had significantly higher cholesterol and significantly lower self-esteem (French et al., 1965). An unpublished study of 22 white-collar employees of the National Aeronautics and Space Administration (NASA) related feelings of overload to higher levels of heart rate and cholesterol (Caplan and French, 1968), but a later study of a large NASA sample failed to replicate that finding (Caplan, 1971). These studies also found significant positive correlations between subjective reports of work overload and more objective measures (ranging from wives' reports of the number of hours their husbands worked to direct observational measures of the demands made on men by others in the organization). These objective measures were also associated with elevated heart disease risk, but the results suggest that the effects of objective job conditions are mediated through the person's subjective experience of overload or "stress" (as has been assumed in the framework developed that is above).

These data are in line with earlier studies relating work load and job pressures to changes in heart disease risk factors. A seminal investigation found marked increases in serum cholesterol in tax accountants as the April 15 deadline for filing Federal income tax returns approached (Friedman et al., 1957). A number of studies have found significantly higher levels of cholesterol in medical students on the day before examinations as compared with times when they were not facing tests (see review by Sales, 1969b). It is plausible that these changes are attributable to increased work load under tax deadline or examination pressures. They also highlight what it is about work overload, as opposed to sheer work load, that makes it stressful—the feeling that one does not have enough time or ability and hence may fail (Pepitone, 1967).

Responsibility for the work of others has recently been implicated as a correlate of selected heart disease risk factors and possibly other illnesses. Caplan (1971) found the NASA managers, scientists, and engineers who spent a higher percentage of their time on such responsibilities smoked more cigarettes and had higher diastolic blood pressure. Studies showing high levels of CHD risk factors among executives (e.g., Montoye et al., 1967) might also support this responsibility hypothesis, although consistently positive relationships have not been found between managerial status and actual CHD (Hinkle, et al., 1968).

House's (1972) total community study produced further support for the role of job pressures in heart disease risk. A composite measure of job pressures (including work overload, responsibility, and role conflict) was associated with significantly greater heart disease risk in virtually the whole range of occupations. As with the findings on job satisfaction and self-esteem in this study, occupational stress effects were much more pronounced among men 45 to 65 years of age.

Several studies have also documented a relationship between occupational pressure or stress and actual coronary heart disease. Russek (1962) asked a number of practicing professionals to rank several categories of practice within the fields of medicine, dentistry, and law by the amount of "occupational stress" involved in each speciality. Regardless of the specific profession involved, individuals in the "high stress" categories reported higher incidences of coronary disease. A second Russek (1965) study compared 100 young coronary patients and 100 controls. Here Russek (1965:189) found that "prolonged emotional strain associated with job responsibility" preceded the heart attacks of 91 percent of the patients, while such strain was evident in only 20 percent of the control group. Further, this between-group difference exceeded those for family history of heart disease, diet, obesity, smoking, and physical exercise. In a similar study (Miles et al., 1954), 50 percent of heart disease patients, but only 12 percent of a control group, reported working long hours with few vacations prior to disease onset. Weiss et al. (1957) and Pearson and Joseph (1963) report similar conclusions.

Thus, there is rather consistent evidence that job pressures (measured both objectively and subjectively), such as work overload, responsibility and role conflict, significantly increase heart disease risk and actual coronary heart disease. Of all findings reviewed here, these have been replicated in the largest number of studies and across the widest range of populations. Further corroboration of these results appears in the data on personality and social situational factors influencing these relationships.

Incongruity and Change

A final set of factors seems increasingly important as sources of occupational stress leading to heart disease, though their exact social psychological meaning is unclear. A variety of evidence is accumulating that a life history of occupational mobility or rapid change in occupational environment predisposes men to heart disease. Caplan (1971), following Terreberry (1968), speaks of "complexification" of occupational environments (or rate at which things change or become increasingly complex) as a form of work overload taxing one's ability to adapt to new demands. Both occupationally or geographically mobile persons who expose themselves to change, complexity, and new demands and those whose environment changes rapidly seem to experience greater heart disease (cf. review by Smith, 1967) and perhaps greater illness of all kinds (e.g., Holmes and Rahe, 1967). The accumulating evidence that persons whose status is incongruent on two dimensions (e.g., men with low education in high status jobs) are more prone to heart disease may reflect effects of work overload (the job demands exceed their capacity) or prior occupational mobility rather than "status incongruity" *per se* (cf. reviews by Smith, 1967; Jenkins, 1971; see also Hinkle et al., 1968). The evidence on the relationship of status consistency to heart disease, however, must be subjected to rigorous methodological scrutiny that has recently been applied to this concept in sociology (see Hodge and Siegel, 1970). Attention must also be paid to the specification of intervening or conditioning variables (cf. House and Harkins, 1973).

Conditioning Variables

Conditioning Personal Characteristics

Thus far, direct relationships between objective aspects of work situations or subjective perceptions thereof and heart disease have been considered. Where the evidence is based on subjective reports of dissatisfaction or job pressures, these subjective reports are presumably the outcome of interactions between objective situational characteristics (role demands or expectations, the nature of the job, and its rewards) and individual characteristics (motives, needs, abilities, etc.). However, attempts to document this empirically are just beginning with at least modest success (e.g., Blood and Hulin, 1967; Caplan, 1971; French et al., in press; Turner and Lawrence, 1965).

More importantly, a large and growing body of literature indicates that men with a certain type of "behavior pattern" are more prone to coronary heart disease. This behavior pattern has been most extensively investigated by Friedman, Rosenman, and Jenkins, who labelled it the "Type A behavior-pattern," characterized by:

> . . . excessive drive, aggressiveness, ambition, involvement in competitve activities, frequent vocational deadlines, (and) an enhanced sense of time urgency. . . . The converse . . . pattern, called Type B is characterized by the relative absence of this *interplay of psychological traits and situational pressures* (Jenkins et al., 1967:371, emphasis added).

In a long series of studies (including an ongoing prospective study of 3,400 men now followed for over eight years) the Type A (relative to Type B) has been shown to be significantly higher on known heart disease risk factors and significantly more likely (by a factor of 1.4 to 6.5 in different analyses) to have an actual "heart attack" (see Jenkins, 1971; and Sales, 1969a, 1969b, for thorough reviews of these studies). The risk of recurrent and fatal heart attacks has also been shown to be higher for the Type A. Other investigators have found similar results, and in several studies, the Type A variable has been shown to have significant predictive power even when levels of a whole range of standard physiological risk factors are statistically controlled (Jenkins, 1971). The meaning of these results remains unclear however since the Type A pattern reflects "an interplay of psychological traits and situational pressures." To some extent these results may further demonstrate the importance of work overload and other "job pressures" reviewed above.

What role is played by psychological traits? Sales (1969a) suggested that the Type A person possesses personality traits (e.g., impatience, ambition, competitiveness, aggressiveness) causing self-selection into jobs involving greater "stress" (e.g., "time urgency," "frequent vocational deadlines," etc.), but no direct empirical test of this proposition has yet been made. Similarly, House (1972) suggested that a central psychological trait of the Type A is his "desire for social achievement" (reflected in ambition, competitiveness, aggressiveness, etc.), a trait apparently analogous to what others term "status-seeking" or extrinsic motivation for working (i.e., desire for money, status, recognition) as opposed to intrinsic motivation (i.e., desire for interesting, self-satisfying work). House predicted that persons with extrinsic motivations for working were more likely to choose jobs involving greater occupational stress and, hence, to experience heart disease, while intrinsically motivated persons would avoid highly stressful work and, hence, heart disease. Partial support for these hypotheses was found among white-collar workers, but, among lower blue-collar factory workers, intrinsic motivation was positively related to occupational stress and heart disease risk. These and other findings from that study indicate the difficulty of generalizing from the limited samples usually studied in this field (i.e., white collar, and often professional, workers) to all employed men.

Another approach to the meaning of the Type A behavior pattern asserts that under potentially stressful objective conditions Type A persons are more prone to perceive stress and manifest increases in heart disease or its risk factors. Caplan (1971) found support for this contention in research on NASA professionals. He proposes that the dramatic and consistent results derived from the Friedman et al. program of research may be due to the fact that the classification of a man as Type A indicates that he both possesses certain personality traits and experiences greater situational pressures. The role of personality in leading men into situations of stress and/or in accentuating the effects of such situations deserves further research.

Conditioning Social Characteristics

Just as personality factors may determine whether a person experiences stress and how he reacts to it, so may other characteristics of the work situation. As already noted, social and organizational change are likely to increase the stresses felt by individuals. Existing evidence indicates that individuals in positions involving great contact with external environments (and hence more varied and perhaps changing inputs) suffer greater emotional strain (Kahn et al., 1964) and heart disease risk (Caplan, 1971). Alternatively, the surrounding social environment may provide resources mitigating stress effects on individuals. Prescriptive theories of work organizations suggest that social support from peers, superiors, and subordinates improves the ability of men to cope with job stresses and, therefore, should enhance physical and mental health (e.g., Likert, 1967).

. . . .

Occupational Stress and Longevity

Given the accumulating evidence relating occupational stress to coronary heart disease and the significance of heart disease as a cause of death, occupational stress should also be a potent predictor of general mortality and, conversely, longevity. Evidence from demographic comparisons and from at least one focused study suggests that this is so.

Demographic Comparisons

In general, women, whites, and persons of higher educational or social status live longer and have lower age-adjusted mortality rates from many, though not all, diseases (cf. Palmore and Jeffers, 1971; Kitigawa and Hauser, 1968). Social status differentials are greater among women than men, and larger for communicable diseases than for such major chronic diseases as ulcer, stroke, arthritis, cancer, or heart disease (Kitigawa and Hauser, 1968; Lerner, 1969). Thus, social status and color differentials in general mortality probably stem more from poor living conditions and inadequate medical care or from social stress outside of work than from occupational stresses *per se.* There are, of course, occupational differences in most disease incidences, but in many cases the reasons for them remain unclear. However, the sex difference in longevity, just as that in heart disease mortality discussed above, again suggests a central role of work in the genesis of disease (cf. discussion in Palmore and Jeffers, 1971:284 ff).

Focused Studies

The best evidence that "stress" in life and work determines mortality and longevity comes from the Duke Longitudinal Study of Aging (Palmore, 1969a, 1969b; Palmore and Jeffers, 1971). This panel study has been carried out on 268 volunteers, ages 60 to 94 years (median age 70), at the time of their initial interview and physical examination. Although not a random sample, the distribution of the volunteers by sex, race, and occupation approximated that of the area from which they were drawn. The dependent variable was a Longevity Quotient—the number of years a person actually lived divided by the actuarially expected number of years remaining at the time of the initial examination.

For the total sample, *work satisfaction* was the strongest predictor of the Longevity Quotient (r=.26). It remained one of the three strongest predictors for all subgroups of the sample except for blacks, and was strongest (r=.38) among those (males, age 60 to 69 years) most likely to be working full-time. The second best longevity predictor (r=.26) in the total sample was the interviewing social worker's rating of the respondent's overall "happiness." These two social psychological measures (1) predicted longevity more accurately than either an overall physical functioning rating by the examining physician (r=.21) or a measure of the use of tobacco (r=.21); and (2) remained a strong predictor even when the aforementioned physical variables were controlled via multiple regression.

Conclusions

Traditional sociological and epidemiological research on social factors in heart disease has most often involved comparing disease rates across categories of standard demographic variables such as occupation, sex, race, or ethnicity. "Stress" is often presumed to be a mediating variable in such research, but the nature of the stress seldom is specified carefully and almost never measured independently. As noted above, such research can at best yield suggestive results. Only when all variables that mediate and/or condition the relationship between objective social conditions and health outcomes are explicitly conceptualized and measured can we have an adequate understanding of the effect of social stress on heart disease.

. . . There is considerable evidence that occupational stress plays a significant role in the etiology of coronary heart disease and probably other chronic diseases as well. Particularly noteworthy is the accumulation of studies documenting a relationship between stress and heart disease even when a variety of more medically recognized variables (e.g., heredity, diet, exercise, etc.) are controlled. However, we are just beginning to understand the complexities in the relationship between occupational stress and heart disease. . . .

Note

This paper is based in part on a report prepared for the Secretary's Committee on Work in America, Department of Health, Education and Welfare. I am grateful for the helpful comments and suggestions of the following people on earlier drafts of this paper: Sidney Cobb, John R. P. French, Jr., Elizabeth Bates Harkins, Wendy F. House, Berton Kaplan, George Maddox, Erdman Palmore, and Thomas Regan. Work on this paper has also been supported in part by a Biomedical Sciences Support Grant (5S05RR077007) from the National Institutes of Health and by Public Health Service Research Grant (HD0068) from NICHD.

References

Antonovsky, A. 1968. "Social class and the major cardiovascular diseases." Journal of Chronic Diseases 21 (May):65–108.

Appley, Mortimer H., and Richard Trumbull (eds.). 1967. Psychological Stress. New York: Appleton-Century-Crofts.

Blood, M. R., and C. L. Hulin. 1967. "Alienation, environmental characteristics and worker responses." Journal of Applied Psychology 51 (June):284–290.

Caplan, Robert. 1971. Organizational Stress and Individual Strain: A Social-Psychological Study of Risk Factors in Coronary Heart Disease among Administrators, Engineers, and Scientists. Unpublished Ph.D. thesis. Ann Arbor: University of Michigan.

Caplan, Robert, and John R. P. French, Jr. 1968. Final Report to NASA. Unpublished manuscript. Ann Arbor: University of Michigan.

Cobb, Sidney. 1972. A Report on the Health of Air Traffic Controllers Based on Aeromedical Examination Data. Unpublished report to the Federal Aviation Agency. Ann Arbor: University of Michigan.

Coelho, G. V., D. A. Hamburg and J. E. Adams (eds.). In press. Coping and Adaptation: Interdisciplinary Perspectives. New York: Basic Books.

Epstein, F. H. 1965. "The epidemiology of coronary heart disease: A review." Journal of Chronic Diseases 18 (August):735–774.

Felton, J. S., and R. Cole. 1963, "The high cost of heart disease." Circulation 27 (May): 957–962.

French, John R. P., Jr., C. John Tupper and Ernst Mueller. 1965. Workload of University Professors. Cooperative Research Project No. 2171, U.S. Office of Education. Ann Arbor: University of Michigan.

French, J. R. P., Jr., W. Rodgers and S. Cobb. In press. "Adjustment as person-environment fit." In G. V. Coelho, D. A. Hamburg and J. E. Adams (eds.),

Coping and Adaptation: Interdisciplinary Perspectives. New York: Basic Books.

Friedman, M., R. H. Rosenman and V. Carroll. 1957. "Changes in the serum cholesterol and blood clotting time of men subject to cyclic variation of occupational stress." Circulation 17 (May):852–961.

Graham, S., and L. G. Reeder. 1972. "Social factors in the chronic illness." Pp. 63–107 in Howard E. Freeman, Sol Levine and Leo G. Reeder (eds.), Handbook of Medical Sociology. Englewood Cliffs: Prentice-Hall.

Guralnick, Lillian. 1963. "Mortality by occupation and cause of death among men 20 to 64." National Center for Health Statistics. Vital Statistics Special Reports 53 (September): Number 3.

Hinkle, L. E., Jr. 1961. "Ecological observations on the relation of physical illness, mental illness, and the social environment." Psychosomatic Medicine 23 (July-August): 289–297.

Hinkle, L. E., Jr., L. H. Whitney, E. W. Lehman, J. Dunn, B. Benjamin, R. King, A. Platum and B. Flehinger. 1968. "Occupation, education, and coronary heart disease." Science 161 (July):238–246.

Hodge, R. W., and P. M. Siegel. 1970. "Nonvertical dimensions of social stratification." Pp. 512–520 in Edward O. Laumann, Paul M. Siegel, and Robert W. Hodge (eds.), The Logic of Social Hierarchies. Chicago: Markham.

Holmes, T. H., and R. H. Rahe. 1967. "The social readjustment rating scale." Journal of Psychosomatic Research 11 (August):213–225.

House, James S. 1972. The Relationship of Intrinsic and Extrinsic Work Motivations to Occupational Stress and Coronary Heart Disease Risk. Unpublished Ph.D. thesis. Ann Arbor: University of Michigan.

House, James S., and Elizabeth Bates Harkins. 1973. Why and When Is Status Inconsistency Stressful? Unpublished manuscript. Durham: Duke University.

Jenkins, C. D. 1971. "Psychologic and social precursors of coronary disease." New England Journal of Medicine 284 (February 4, February 11):244–255; 307–317.

Jenkins, C. D., R. H. Rosenman and M. Friedman. 1967. "Development of an objective psychological test for the determination of the coronary-prone behavior pattern." Journal of Chronic Diseases 20 (June):371–379.

Kahn, Robert L., Donald M. Wolfe, Robert P. Quinn, J. Dietrich Snoek and Robert A. Rosenthal. 1964. Organizational Stress: Studies in Role Conflict and Ambiguity. New York: John Wiley.

Kasl, S. V., and J. R. P. French, Jr. 1962. "The effects of occupational status on physical and mental health." Journal of Social Issues 18 (July):67–89.

Kasl, S.V., S. Cobb and G. Brooks. 1968. "Changes in serum uric acid and cholesterol levels in men undergoing job loss." Journal of the American Medical Association 206 (November):1500–1507.

Kasl, S. V., and S. Cobb. 1970. "Blood pressure changes in men undergoing job loss: A preliminary report." Psychosomatic Medicine 32 (January–February):19–38.

Kitigawa, Evelyn M., and P. M. Hauser. 1968. "Education differentials in mortality by cause of death: United States, 1960." Demography 5 (February):318–353.

Lazarus, Richard S. 1966. Psychological Stress and the Coping Process. New York: McGraw-Hill.

Lerner, M. 1969. "Social differences in physical health." Pp. 69–112 in John Kosa, Aaron Antonovsky and Irvin K. Zola (eds.), Poverty and Health: A Sociological Analysis. Cambridge: Harvard University Press.

Levine, Sol, and Norman Scotch. 1970. Social Stress. Chicago: Aldine.

Likert, Rensis. 1967. The Human Organization: Its Management and Value. New York: McGraw-Hill.

Marks, Renee. 1967. "Factors involving social and demographic characteristics: A review of empirical findings." Pp. 51–108 in S. Leonard Syme and Leo G. Reeder (eds.), Social Stress and Cardiovascular Disease. Milbank Memorial Fund Quarterly 45 (April): Part 2.

Matsumoto, Y. S. 1970. "Social stress and coronary heart disease in Japan: A hypothesis." Milbank Memorial Fund Quarterly 48 (January):9–13.

McGrath, Joseph E. (ed.). 1970. Social and Psychological Factors in Stress. New York: Holt, Rinehart and Winston.

Mechanic, David. 1962. Students Under Stress. New York: Free Press.

———. 1970. "Some problems in developing a social psychology of adaptation to stress." Pp. 104–123 in Joseph McGrath (ed.), Social and Psychological Factors in Stress. New York: Holt, Rinehart, and Winston.

Miles, H. H. W., S. Waldfogel, E. Barrabee and S. Cobb. 1954, "Psychosomatic study of 46 young men with coronary artery disease." Psychosomatic Medicine 16 (November–December):455–477.

Montoye, H. J., J. A. Faulkner, H. J. Dodge, W. M. Mikkelson, R. W. Willis, III and W. D. Block. 1967. "Serum uric acid concentration among business executives and observations on other coronary heart disease risk factors." Annals of Internal Medicine 66 (May):838–850.

Moriyama, Iwao M., Dean E. Krueger and Jeremiah Stamler. 1971. Cardiovascular Diseases in the United States. Cambridge: Harvard University Press.

Palmore, E. B. 1969a."Physical, mental, and social factors in predicting longevity." Gerontologist 9 (Summer):103–108.

———. 1969b. "Predicting longevity: A follow-up controlling for age." Gerontologist 9 (Winter):247–250.

Palmore, Erdman B., and Frances Jeffers (eds.). 1971. Prediction of Life Span. Boston: D. C. Heath-Lexington.

Pearson, H. E. S., and J. Joseph. 1963. "Stress and occlusive coronary-artery disease." The Lancet 1 (February): 415–418.

Pepitone, A. 1967. "Self, social environment, and stress." Pp. 182–199 in Mortimer H. Appley and Richard Trumbull (eds.). Psychological Stress. New York: Appleton-Century-Crofts.

Russek, H. I. 1962. "Emotional stress and coronary heart disease in American physicians, dentists, and lawyers." American Journal of Medical Science 243 (June):716–725.

———. 1965. "Stress, tobacco, and coronary heart disease in North American professional groups." Journal of the American Medical Association 192 (April):189–194.

Sales, S. M. 1969a. Differences Among Individuals in Affective, Behavioral, Biochemical, and Physiological Responses to Variations in Work Load. Unpublished Ph.D. thesis. Ann Arbor: University of Michigan.

————. 1969b. "Organizational roles as a risk factor in coronary heart disease." Administrative Science Quarterly 14 (September):325–336.

Sales, S. M., and J. House. 1971. "Job dissatisfaction as a possible risk factor in coronary heart disease." Journal of Chronic Diseases 23 (May):861–873.

Seashore, Stanley. 1954. Group Cohesiveness in the Industrial Work Group. Institute for Social Research. Ann Arbor: University of Michigan.

Selye, Hans. 1956. The Stress of Life. New York: McGraw-Hill.

Smith, Thomasina. 1967. "Sociocultural incongruity and change: A review of empirical findings." Pp. 17–46 in S. Leonard Syme and Leo G. Reeder (eds.), Social Stress and Cardiovascular Disease. Milbank Memorial Fund Quarterly 45 (April): Part 2.

Suchman, E. A. 1967. "Factors involving social and demographic characteristics: Appraisal and implications for theoretical development." Pp. 109–116 in S. Leonard Syme and Leo G. Reeder (eds.), Social Stress and Cardiovascular Disease. Milbank Memorial Fund Quarterly 45 (April):Part 2.

Syme, S. L. 1967. "Implications and future prospects." Pp. 175–181 in S. Leonard Syme and Leo G. Reeder (eds.), Social Stress and Cardiovascular Disease. Milbank Memorial Fund Quarterly 45 (April):Part 2.

Syme, S. Leonard and Leo G. Reeder (eds.) 1967. Social Stress and Cardiovascular Disease. Milbank Memorial Fund Quarterly 45 (April):Part 2.

Terreberry, S. 1968. The Organization of Environments. Unpublished Ph.D. thesis. Ann Arbor: University of Michigan.

Turner, A. N., and P. R. Lawrence. 1965. Industrial Jobs and the Worker: An Investigation of Response to Task Attributes. Harvard University Graduate School of Business Administration, Division of Research. Cambridge: Harvard University.

Weiss, E., B. Dlin, H. R. Rollin, H. K. Fischer and C. R. Bepler. 1957. "Emotional factors in coronary occlusion." Archives of Internal Medicine 99 (April):628–641.

7

Hypertension in American Society: An Introduction to Historical Materialist Epidemiology

Peter L. Schnall and Rochelle Kern

Introduction

The causes of essential hypertension—a disease that afflicts an estimated 50 million American adults—remains a medical mystery despite more than a hundred years of research efforts by scientists and physicians (Freis, 1976). Moreover, in the absence of an adequate medical understanding of the cause(s) of hypertension, millions of dollars are currently spent on extensive education and treatment programs (National HBP Education Program, 1978). This paper examines what medicine has learned about essential hypertension, how it has studied and explained the disease, and the limitations of its explanation and approach. We will describe a relatively new perspective on social epidemiology that is being developed and applied by a growing number of scholars and health providers: "historical materialist epidemiology" (HME). We will then use the perspective of HME to examine what is known about essential hypertension and to suggest new directions for research to understand and prevent this major health problem.

This paper is a preliminary analysis, provocative, we hope, in its questioning of the traditional medical perspective and in its use of the developing historical materialist epidemiology to suggest an alternative, more adequate approach to understanding not only essential hypertension but other health problems as well. HME gives us the beginnings of an explanatory perspective to identify and understand the connections among the organization of society, the nature and distribution of disease within society, and the available methods and dominant modes of treating and explaining diseases. While this is an enormous task, HME and the issues it raises provide a promising direction for future understanding of the relationship between disease and society.

The Problem of Hypertension

What Is Hypertension and Why Is It a Problem?

Hypertension, or chronic high blood pressure, has been defined by the medical profession as the presence of a sustained elevation of blood pressure in an individual greater than 140/90 (HDFP, 1979).[1] What this means is that when blood pressure is measured, the pressure of the blood against the walls of the arteries generated by the pumping of the heart in a normal, healthy adult should be no greater than 140 systolic (the highest pressure generated by the heart during the peak of its contraction) over 90 (the lowest pressure generated by the heart during its relaxation phase). Using this measurement of normal blood pressure, more than 50 million American adults have what is called "essential hypertension" and are seen by the medical profession as candidates for treatment (Relman, 1980). Essential hypertension is distinguished from secondary hypertension in that the latter is known to be caused by, or is secondary to, a particular organic problem, such as kidney disease; in the former, what we will refer to only as *hypertension* throughout the rest of this paper, the causes of the elevated blood pressure are unknown (or, in the medical view, are as yet "undiscovered") (Harrison, 1977: 1307).

Hypertension is a known health problem. Chronic elevation of blood pressure causes serious damage to the human body and may lead, if uncontrolled, to stroke, heart disease and heart attack, kidney disease and renal failure, and other organic problems. These serious consequences of untreated hypertension can be prevented or at least postponed if the blood pressure is lowered to normal. Unfortunately, people with hypertension often experience no symptoms of the disease, leading to its characterization in public service messages as "the silent killer." Nearly half of all deaths in this country are from cardiovascular disease, including coronary heart disease, hypertension-induced heart disease, and stroke (DHEW, 1980).

How Has Hypertension Been Studied by Medicine?

There is a great deal known about hypertension and the organic damage it causes. Medical science has utilized the "medical model" paradigm both to search for the causes of hypertension and to explain its consequences. That paradigm sees hypertension as an organic abnormality caused by some disturbances within the body that results in the physiological alteration of the circulatory system. By and large, as with other diseases, the medical model's perspective of hypertension sees it as *a* disease with one or more identifiable *organic* causes. Ironically, the inability of the medical model to explain the presence of hypertension in so much of the American population results in part from the extraordinary success of its doctrine of specific etiology (Dubos, 1959) for providing explanations for a range of diseases which plagued human populations during the nineteenth and early twentieth centuries. We will review briefly some of the landmark discoveries of medicine about blood pressure and hypertension.

There is a long tradition of laboratory research on the anatomical and physiological functioning of the human body. As early as 1658, John Jacob Reiter was performing autopsies in order to discover the cause of apoplexy (stroke) and learned that cerebral hemorrhages were caused by ruptured arteries. Throughout the nineteenth century, laboratory research into the physiology of blood circulation made remarkable progress with numerous discoveries about the nature of cardiovascular functioning, and the mechanisms by which the heart and nervous system maintain blood pressure in the arteries. By the end of the nineteenth century it was clinically established that a "hard" pulse and increased blood pressure could result in stroke (Ruskin, 1956).

Scientific technological inventions contributed to the growth of knowledge about hypertension. In the early nineteenth century, Jean Leonard Poisseule developed the mercury hemodyamometer which eventually led to the development of the modern blood pressure cuff, generally credited to Scipione Riva-Rocci in 1896 (Castiglione, 1947: 842). With the development of the blood pressure cuff (a mechanical device which allows a numerical measurement of blood pressure), there was a formative discovery about hypertension. It was generally believed that diseases of the kidneys were responsible for both high blood pressure and stroke until Theodore Janeway noted in 1906 that individuals could have increased blood pressure without evidence of kidney disease (Janeway, 1906).

Throughout the twentieth century, using the medical paradigm, physicians pursued the identification of the causes of increased blood pressure with some important successes. These successes included the identification of the causes of what we earlier distinguished as secondary hypertension. However, evidence soon emerged that a great percentage of the population had elevated blood pressure which could not be attributed to one of the identified causes of secondary hypertension. The realization of the prevalence and patterns of essential hypertension began to take form and give the picture of hypertension we have today. While the predominant scientific hypothesis of the medical model was that hypertension is a disease with a *specific etiology* and that, therefore, people with hypertension constitute a distinct and separable population from those without hypertension, medicine has failed to demonstrate the validity of this hypothesis.

As early as 1931 in a review of available studies, Wetherby (1932) found that the bulk of research on American population groups revealed that blood pressure tends to rise continuously with age, is higher in men than in women, until about the age of forty when women's blood pressure tends to exceed and then become significantly higher than men's by the age of about fifty. Other population studies have failed to discover a natural dividing line between those with high blood pressure and those without it (Pickering, 1961). Further evidence that those with hypertension don't constitute a population separate from those without hypertension is found in data from the Actuarial Society of America (1941) that shows mortality (death) rates increase with arterial pressure, and that the relationship is curvilinear, with there being *no point* below which blood pressure is unrelated to mortality.

In 1933 the federal government mandated the keeping of vital statistics for all states in the United States. Hypertension and its consequences such as stroke emerged as the third ranked cause of death for all Americans. The important association between hypertension and coronary heart disease (the nation's number one killer) began to attract scientific attention in the 1940s. At the beginning of that decade Davis and Klainer (1940) published an article noting an association for their patients under the age of fifty between the presence of hypertension and an increased incidence of coronary artery disease.

Following World War II medical research focused on trying to understand the cause of coronary heart disease. Prospective community studies, such as the famous Framingham Study, followed large groups of people over time and monitored their health in order to see what organic problems and behaviors (e.g., cigarette smoking) lead to coronary heart disease. These studies primarily focused on white, middle-class people and they conceptualized hypertension as an independent variable and coronary heart disease as a dependent variable (i.e., hypertension was seen as something that caused coronary heart disease). The results of these prospective community studies was to show that hypertension was a "risk factor" for the development of coronary heart disease (Kannel, 1969). A "risk factor" is one that, when present, increases the prevalence of the dependent variable, coronary heart disease, in a group by at least twofold as compared to its prevalence in a group in which no risk factor is present.

Medical Explanations of Hypertension

Unfortunately, no prospective study of essential hypertension as a dependent variable has been carried out in the United States. Medical explanations of the cause of hypertension have focused on three variables: (1)

aging, (2) genetically inherited susceptibility, and (3) increased salt intake. We will briefly review each of these as possible explanations as well as the data which examine the relationship of a fourth variable, stress, to hypertension.

(1) Some medical explanations posit that hypertension is the *natural* consequence of growing old, and that because people live longer, we're just seeing more of it now. There are two serious problems with this explanation. First, not everybody's blood pressure goes up with age, even within American society. Second, cross-cultural data shows that in other societies (e.g., primitive hunting and gathering societies), there is little or no increase in blood pressure with age. This is true even for some groups having racial and genetic inheritances identical with groups in the United States (Page, 1976).

(2) The genetic explanation of hypertension was given impetus by the finding that blacks have prevalence rates of hypertension two to three times higher than whites in the United States (e.g., DHEW, 1964). Genetic theories of increased susceptibility to hypertension were supported by results of twin studies (Thomas, 1973). As with all twin studies in which the twins are raised in the same household, however, these studies cannot control for the relative influence of the sharing of both genes and environment. In fact, some studies have found that familial influence and not genetic susceptibility accounts for hypertension in some children (Zinner, 1971).

Several other findings limit the power of genetic theories to explain hypertension. First, there is a rapid rise in the prevalence of high blood pressure in black populations when they migrate from their communities of origin to industrialized urban centers (Eyer, 1975; Page, 1976). Likewise, genetic explanations cannot account for why blacks have the same prevalence rate as whites up to about the age of twenty-four and why only then do black males show a rapid increase in their rates of hypertension compared to their white male counterparts (DHEW, 1978: 13). Inheritance perhaps plays a role via increased suspectibility in some people, but genetic explanations alone cannot account for the development and distribution of hypertension in the American population.

(3) Salt intake appears to be a prerequisite variable in the development of hypertension, but, like genetic variables, it alone cannot explain hypertension. There has been a linear increase in salt consumption in Western societies which parallels the increase in blood pressure in the population. On the other hand, there are a number of primitive communities that use salt in their diets but do not show increased blood pressure with age (Thomas, 1959). Further, those individuals in the United States whose blood pressure does not increase with age have the same salt intake as do those who do develop hypertension. Experimental attempts to induce (cause) hypertension in human subjects with normal blood pressure by

giving them salt were not "successful" (Dahl, 1960). Salt may play a contributory role in the development of hypertension, but only in combination with other variables.

In addition to looking at age, genetic susceptibility, and salt intake, a great deal of research has been conducted in the past twenty years to find a specific abnormality of a particular body organ to explain the cause of hypertension. No single abnormality of the body, however, has been identified which can account for the findings regarding the prevalance of hypertension in the United States (Freis, 1976). Before turning to a discussion of an alternative epidemiological perspective on high blood pressure and hypertension, we want to examine briefly a fourth variable which has been broadly identified as a correlate of elevated blood pressure: stress.

(4) There is a range of data that indicates that stress causes increases in human blood pressure. However, there is no adequate research on the relationship of sustained stress to the etiology of hypertension. We note as well that there is disagreement as to the exact definition of stress and how best to measure it. (See, for example, Brown, 1974; Dohrenwend, 1974; and Waldron, 1977.) Among the available evidence on stress and hypertension are studies which found elevated blood pressure in men who lost their jobs (Kasl and Cobb, 1970), in populations who live in "deprived neighborhoods (Harburg et al., 1970), in prisoners forced to live in crowded cells as compared to prisoners in private cells (D'Atri and Ostfeld, 1975), and among air traffic controllers compared to lower-ranking and less-stressed airmen (Cobb and Rose, 1973). Recent evidence indicates that people's blood pressure varies regularly—day by day and minute by minute, in response to environmental stimuli (Pickering, 1975). Blood pressure increases during arguments, sex, and exercise, and decreases in relaxation and sleep.

We will return to a discussion of the role of stress in hypertension, but we would like here to point out that there is evidence that stress influences blood pressure but the role of stress in hypertension is not one of the major concerns in the medical literature on hypertension. When data on stress and blood pressure have been incorporated into medical conceptualizations, it has been in terms of *individual* characteristics that correlate with elevated blood pressure—for example, personality types and individual susceptibility. (See, e.g., Shapiro, 1979.) In short, stress is treated in the medical model as an individual characteristic similar to the individual organic variables reviewed above.[2] It is this identification of environmental influences as "psychosocial" characteristics that leads to medical recommendations for individual behavioral adjustments to decreased blood pressure through, for example, bio-feedback and relaxation techniques.

To summarize, medicine conceptualizes the disease of hypertension as the consequence of some disturbance within the individual organism. The various explanations offered by medicine, including age, genetic susceptibility, salt intake, and psychosocial susceptibility to stress all locate both the cause and potential cure of hypertension within the individual. While each of these variables has been studied within this model of individual correlates to elevations in blood pressure, none has provided an adequate explanation for either the cause of hypertension or its distribution.

Historical Materialist Epidemiology

The Context of the Emergence of HME

The serious limitations of scientific medicine's ability to explain or treat chronic diseases has contributed to a growing disenchantment with medicine and a reassessment of the medical paradigm which for so long has dominated American medical care. It has become increasingly clear through careful historical analyses of the decline of mortality over the past hundred years that the elimination of infectious diseases as major causes of mortality was tied to a number of social changes, including improvements in sanitation and nutrition, rather than to the specific treatments of medicine (Dubos, 1959; McKeown, 1971; Powles, 1973; Knowles, 1977). Likewise, it is becoming equally clear that chronic diseases also have a relationship to the organization of society, and in particular, to the physical and social environments in which people live and work (Epstein, 1976; House, 1974).

These recognitions of the social components of disease and the limitations of scientific medicine did not develop in a vacuum, but were fueled and made popular in part by a number of social and political struggles that took place over the past twenty-five years. In this context there emerged a strong leftist health movement in the United States, composed of people who were by and large current or future medical care workers. Through organizations such as The Medical Committee for Human Rights, these progressive health workers contributed to an analysis of the way American society creates and sustains ill health in certain segments of the population, and fails to provide equitable, accessible and adequate medical care to all. (See, for example, Bodenheimer et. al., 1972; Ehrenreich and Ehrenreich, 1970; and all of Health/PAC.) As part of the growing understanding of the relationship of health and medical care to the priorities of American society, the reemergence of Marxism within the newly politicized colleges and universities of the 1960s and 1970s provided the intellectual resources for the development of an examination of the basic societal causes of disease and ill health and the relationship of these causes to the political economy of capitalism in particular. These intellectual and social developments provided the historical context in which HME developed and within which it must be examined and appraised.

The Marxist Analysis of Capitalism and the Health of Citizens

There is a long tradition of scholarship documenting the consequences of capitalist production on the health of both its paid labor force and the rest of its citizens. The most explicit analysis of this relationship, and a central work for the historical development of historical materialist epidemiology, is Friedrich Engle's (1845) analysis of the conflict of workers and owners in Great Britain in the nineteenth century. In *The Conditions of the Working Class in England,* Engels examined the social conditions produced by early capitalism and their consequences for the health of the working class. Under early (or primitive) capitalism, an industrial working class, a proletariat, was created for the first time in history with no means of subsistence other than the sale of its labor. Early capitalism mechanized the farm and used land for the grazing of animals, giving rise to enclosures, which meant, ultimately, the creation of a surplus of workers forced to migrate from their farms to urban centers to find work (Engels, 1958 [1845]). The need to accumulate capital (property and money) led businesses to minimize the cost of labor power by providing only the cheapest of shelter, food and working conditions (including wages) for its workers. This process resulted in the rise of the great slums of Britain in the nineteenth century and a range of diseases endemic to those particular living conditions—for example, tuberculosis (which still exists in American slums), typhoid, and other infectious epidemics. These diseases, argued Engels, were the social and physical products of early capitalism.

Capitalism has undergone enormous transformation from its early primitive stages to its current stage of what has been termed advanced monopoly capitalism (O'Conner, 1973; Sweezy, 1968). In the process, the nature of work and social life has been altered in the past 150 years, and these changes have been accompanied by a great improvement in the standard of living for the majority of Americans. With this improved standard of living, early deaths from infectious diseases decreased, but the resultant increase in life expectancy has been accompanied by the rise of chronic diseases, including coronary heart disease, cancer, and hypertension and stroke.

By the economic laws of capitalism and capitalist accumulation, it is necessary for businesses to constantly expand their markets, compete with each other, grow ever-larger or, failing that, be swallowed up by even larger businesses. Twentieth-century capitalism is characterized by enormous corporations—firms like General Motors, IBM, AT&T, and Exxon—which dominate the American economy (Baran and Sweezy, 1966). Declining competition created by increasing control by fewer and fewer firms within an economic sector increases the power of corporations and the dependence of workers. So, modern capitalism is characterized by efforts to increase "worker productivity"—that is, the amount of goods or services produced by workers in a given period of time for a given wage. This can be accomplished by introducing technologies to automate portions of the work process and thus eliminate workers and the wages they earn, by getting workers to work harder and thereby produce more in the same time period for the same wage, or by decreasing wages and benefits for workers. As a result, a continuous struggle emerges in the workplace between the owners' need to increase surplus value and the workers' attempts to keep their wages up with the cost of living and to limit the degree of their exploitation in the job market. This struggle between workers and owners—between the working class and the capitalist class—is seen by Marxists as a central struggle within capitalist society with significant consequences on the health of workers and their families.

During the past six years a number of politically active, progressive health workers and scholars have utilized the philosophy, economic theory, and methodology of Marxism in conjunction with the findings and methods of social epidemiology to study the nature of health and illness in modern society. By conceptualizing historical materialist epidemiology, they have produced a theoretical perspective that differs from that of traditional social epidemiology in its attempts to relate the patterns of disease in society to the economic and social relations which are the historical underpinnings of that society:

> [Historical] Materialist Epidemiology maintains that the history of a particular human disease is a unique nonrepetitive process, which obeys discoverable laws and results from discoverable relationships. These relationships are essentially social in nature. It is the same social environment which forms the context within which we live that also forms the context within which disease arises. The physics and chemistry of diseases may recur again and again. But the causes of these phenomena and the reason for their spread are socially rooted and historical in nature. (Gaynor et al., 1976)[3]

How then does a Marxist perspective inform the study of epidemiology? First, a Marxist perspective alerts us to the important sociological role of economic relations in society. The organization of work and the work process, the distribution of economic wealth and power, and the creation of particular forms of stratification all emerge from a capitalist political economy.[4] Among the particular features of American capitalism are racism, sexism, the chronic unemployment of large segments of the population, significant movement of the population due to the demands for a mobile labor force, crowded and decaying urban centers, and the stratification of society by social class. While not all of these inequalities are unique to American capitalism, they are all *integral* to it and need to be understood as part of the larger social organization of a capitalist economy. Second, a Marxist perspective gives us empirical and theoretical categories by which to locate significant social variations in the health of citizens—categories which emerge from an understanding of the particular inequalities of capitalism as well as the stresses and conflicts produced by a capitalist mode of production. Marxism gives us not only the categories of analysis, but a theory and methodology by which to understand those social, economic, and psychological categories.[5] That scholarship encourages an historical perspective and an understanding of the conflicts and contradictions which characterize the ongoing process of capitalism (Waitzkin, 1978).

In one example of the use of HME to understand disease patterns, Eyer and Sterling (1977) examined the consequences of unavoidable swings in a capitalist economy. They were concerned with the continuous social disruptions engendered by the American economy with its requirements of mobility and a competitive striving for success. They present evidence that disease and death vary among the population according to the predictable patterns of social mobility, urban living, and swings in the economy, including unemployment and periods of industrial expansion. In another article, Eyer (1977b) looked specifically at the effect of the swings in the American economy—the so-called booms and falls—on the mortality rate. He found that booms in the economy, those periods of increased productivity and increased pressures on workers to produce, were characterized by increased death rates:

> The causes of death involved in this variation range from infectious diseases through accidents to heart disease, cancer and cirrhosis of the liver, and include the great majority of all causes of death. Less than 2% of the death rate—that for suicide and homicide—varies directly with unemployment . . . the role of social stress is probably predominant. Overwork and the fragmentation of community through migration are two important sources of stress which rise with the boom, and they are demonstrably related to the causes of death which show this variation. (Eyer, 1977b:125.)

While there is continuing debate about whether these economic swings indeed cause the patterns of death that Eyer claims (Brenner, 1977; Eyer, 1977a), there is no doubt that in order to develop a fully articulated analysis of the relationship of society and disease, we need to examine and understand the particular consequences of changes in the economy on people's health. We cannot present here all the work done within the perspective of HME[6] but we can note a range of health issues that have been examined from and informed by this perspective, including suicide (Hopper and Guttmacher, 1979), violence against women (Stark, Flitcraft, and Frazier, 1979), the epidemic (Stark, 1977b), and occupational health (Turshen, 1977; Gaynor, 1977; Stark, 1977a; HMO Packet #5, 1979; Sterling, 1978). In addition, there is a range of works which utilizes a Marxist paradigm to analyze the features of the medical care system as it relates to the political economy. (See, for example, HMO Packet #6, 1979; Salmon, 1977; Navarro, 1977 and 1978; and Rodberg and Stevenson, 1977.)

An important study of the social origins of hypertension—and a work that did much to stimulate the development of HME—was an early work by Joseph Eyer on "Hypertension as a disease of modern society." In that study, Eyer identifies two features of modern society as being critical to the development of hypertension in the population: (1) the disruption of social communities, and (2) the rise of hierarchically controlled, time-pressured work. For Eyer the central feature of modernization is the

> ... wresting of control over social resources ... from the village communities and craft organizations ... and placing this control in the hands of a new ruling class, either private or state capitalists ... [This] transfer of power entails the destruction of the settled rural kin-based extended family and village community ... delegating socialization and work training to an extra communal educational system (Eyer, 1975: 547).

Eyer concludes that people who are uprooted from stable communities, thrust into hostile, competitive urban environments experience great elevations in their blood pressure. Of equal importance is the continual development of new technology and work organization that characterizes modern society.

> Combined with the accompanying specialization and hierarchical division of labor, this development necessitates multiple work role adjustments during the life-span, and this in turn means that a higher proportion of people experience a lack of fit between their skills and preparation and the work position they find themselves in. (Eyer, 1975: 548)

While Eyer attempts to relate these changes in modern society to the social relations of capitalism, his analysis is limited by his puzzling conclusion that there "... is no relation between the economic level of the population and rates of death from hypertension or between family income and blood pressure ..." (Eyer, 1975: 548–549). For Eyer, all residents of modern society experience elevations in blood pressure. As we will see, however, specific features of capitalist society (e.g., differentials in income) *are* correlated with differences in both prevalence of hypertension and subsequent morbidity from this disease.

Utilizing Historical Materialist Epidemiology to Understand Hypertension

Drawing on the perspective of historical materialist epidemiology, we would hypothesize that there is an identifiable relationship between the patterns of hypertension in American society and the (historically changing) political economic organization of society. We know that capitalism generates particular inequalities, divisions, conflicts, and stresses among its citizens, although understanding the relationship between these particular social forms and disease patterns is an enormous task. Likewise, it is important to remember that not everybody who is oppressed, stressed, or underpaid develops hypertension (or even gets sick). As social scientists, however, we are interested in trends in the population rather than the "exception to the rule," and so we begin by looking at patterned differences. Ultimately we would need to know a lot more about the details of the effects of both physical and social differences (including the role of personality) before we could develop a fully adequate understanding of the causes of hypertension. We suggest that by examining the variations in the distribution of hypertension in American society according to the social and physical categories suggested by HME, we can begin to develop this understanding.

This is not an easy task, in part because existing data are usually gathered by researchers who utilize the medical model to design their studies, collect their data, and analyze their findings. These limitations affect the types of analyses we can generate from available research. We present the following as a preliminary evaluation of what HME can tell us about hypertension, an evaluation based on available epidemiological data, with all its limitations. With this in mind, then, we turn to five categories suggested by the HME perspective as relevant social categories for the study of disease: (1) social class, (2) occupation, (3) race/ethnicity, (4) gender, and (5) age.

Social Class and Hypertension

The fact that poverty is associated with increased prevalence rates of all diseases has been well documented (Kitagawa and Hauser, 1973). Interestingly, there is limited information on the relationship of income to hypertension. Social class, by which Marxists mean people's relationship to the economy, is often referred to as "socioeconomic status" and is measured only indirectly in many studies by occupation, level of education, or income.[7] HME leads us to hypothesize that those people with the least economic benefit from work, or those unable to support themselves and their families (i.e., the poor and working class) would show more evidence of hypertension than wealthier populations. To test this hypothesis on available data, however, we will have to look at both income and education as indicators of social class.

> Mean systolic blood pressure levels in the U.S. population are found to be inversely related to the size of the family income. As family income increases from less than $3000 to $10,000 or more per year, the mean systolic pressure of the population age 7–74 decreases [as well] . . . (DHEW, 1977: 15–16.)[8]

Utilizing education as an indicator of socioeconomic status (i.e., higher levels of education represent higher social class), a similar relationship to income is found: "blood pressure shows a significant inverse relationship to education level..." (DHEW, 1977: 16). This finding is replicated in another study where "prevalence of hypertension was [found to be] inversely related to level of education among both blacks and whites, i.e., the greater the number of school years completed, the lower the prevalence of hypertension..." (HDFP, 1977: 354). The differences between the extremes of education are also quite marked:

> Those completing college had approximately 40 percent lower prevalence rates of hypertension than did those completing less than ten years of school (36.9 percent lower in black college graduates and 41.6 percent lower in white college graduates). (HDFP, 1977: 354.)

This relationship between level of education and prevalence of hypertension holds up in all age groups, although it is more marked in the younger populations and is a "considerably more striking" relationship among blacks than whites. So, for example, among the black population between 30–39 years of age, those with a college education were found to have a hypertension prevalence rate almost 50 percent *lower* than those blacks with less than ten years of formal education (HDFP, 1977: 354).

When income has been studied directly, the strongest relationship between income and prevalence of hypertension was found for the age group 35–49, where the prevalence of hypertension is three times higher in the group whose annual income is less than $5,000 than the group with an annual income of $15,000 or more (Harris, 1973). Interestingly, no large-scale studies of the prevalence of hypertension among the upper class have been carried out. In fact, the National Health Survey (a major source of national health information) lumps together all those who earn more than $14,000 into one group. In addition, no research has carefully analyzed available data on income, education, *and* occupation simultaneously in one analysis. So, the exact relationship of social class to hypertension can only be approximated, although it is clear that there is a relationship between income and prevalence of hypertension.

Occupation and Hypertension

An association between certain occupations and an increased prevalence of hypertension has been demonstrated. However, little can be learned about the national distribution of hypertension by occupational category as there are practically no national data available by occupation. The National Health Survey for 1960–1962 gathered data on hypertension and occupation and found that certain occupations had higher prevalence rates than others. However, no follow-up or long-term prospective study was done to identify the characteristics of the occupations correlated with elevations in blood pressure. In fact, the National Health Survey did not collect data on hypertension again until 1970–1972, but at this time did not collect data on occupation.

In a review of several smaller studies on occupation and hypertension, Mustacchi examines the possible physical causes of hypertension within the workplace. Among the physical characteristics of work associated with high blood pressure are continuous exposure to noise, physical vibrations, extremes of heat and cold, and a range of chemicals and toxins (Mustacchi, 1977).

Recently, Karasek and his co-workers have been developing a more adequate understanding of the relationship among work, stress, and hypertension through a detailed examination of particular features of occupations and rates of hypertension (Karasek et al., 1978). Among the variables they found associated with hypertension are time-pressured work, a lack of freedom over work and the conditions of work, and working under close supervision. Assuming the replicability of these findings, questions arise as to the specific features of occupations which are responsible for elevations in blood pressure. We might ask, for example, whether it is the repetitive nature of certain jobs that causes hypertension, or the lack of worker control over the worksite (as when assembly lines are speeded up by management or work breaks limited to increase worker productivity)? Perhaps it is the workers' lack of control over the future of their jobs which contributes to hypertension (plants may close with little or no notice to workers, moving whole companies to areas or other countries where lower wages can be paid to poorer workers). These issues are raised by utilizing the perspective of HME and by some of the initial findings of correlations between occupation and rates of hypertension, although as yet they have not been specifically investigated. This suggests to the sociologist that there are "natural" experiments possible which might permit a better understanding of what it is about work that contributes to hypertension. For example, by comparing factories or plants organized traditionally (in which workers have little or no control over their work or the work process) with more innovative settings (in which workers collectively own and manage whole plants or have more control than under the traditional work organizations), we might be able to identify and document what we can only hypothesize to be differences in stress and consequent rates of hypertension in different occupational situations.

Race/Ethnicity and Hypertension

As was discussed earlier, the discovery of higher rates of hypertension among American blacks was interpreted (and still is by many medical scientists) as evidence of a genetic etiology of hypertension, at least among blacks. This perspective was initially weakened by data collected in cross-cultural anthropological studies which demonstrated that groups of blacks living in Africa in their original tribal conditions, and with genetic inheritance identical with that of American blacks, did not demonstrate progressive increases in blood pressure with age (Page, 1976). Migration studies as well demonstrate that during the process of adjustment to modern, industralized societies, these groups evidence increases in their levels of blood pressure.

Before looking at variations among blacks, let us look at the data on the difference between hypertension in blacks and whites. There is a systematic difference in the patterns and prevalence of hypertension among whites and blacks in the United States. Without controlling for age or social class (or anything else), one study found that among males, the hypertension prevalence ratio of blacks to whites was 1.9 and for females was a higher 2.2. In comparing the patterns of age and blood pressure elevations for blacks and whites, studies have found that black and white males have similar levels of blood pressure up until about the age of twenty-four, whereupon the population of black men has progressively greater elevations of blood pressure with increasing age than white men. (HDFP, 1977; DHEW, 1977). A similar pattern for females shows an increase in prevalence of hypertension in black women compared to white women after about the age of twenty-five (DHEW, 1977).

During the past fifteen years a number of researchers have studied patterns of hypertension among blacks while controlling for other variables, including age, social class, and community disruption. By comparing poor blacks with poor whites living under similar social circumstances (e.g., in communities with significant amounts of social stress as measured by high crime and juvenile delinquency rates, high rates of other violence, and high rates of divorce), these researchers have sought to identify the specific influence of race versus other social characteristics on patterns of hypertension. In all these studies, when both socioeconomic status and levels of social or community disruption were controlled for, the differences in prevalence rates between blacks and whites dropped significantly (Harburg, 1973; James and Kleinbaum, 1976; Keil et al., 1977).

The fact that a small but significant difference still persists between blacks and whites even when controlling for social class and community disruption points to the possibility that institutionalized racism with its damaging psychological and social consequences may contribute independently to the stress experienced by blacks, and therefore to the etiology of hypertension. (This would parallel the finding that Reed [1981] reports on the consequences of institutionalized racism on infant mortality in the United States.) Alternatively, the data may be interpreted to mean genetic inheritance does play a small role in the etiology of hypertension among blacks.

Given the pattern of increased hypertension among blacks (i.e., that the difference between whites and blacks increases with age), we might hypothesize that somewhere in their mid-twenties, black people are forced to recognize the reality of their social situation—a reality in this country characterized by high unemployment, poor paying jobs with little prospect for advancement, and persistent patterns of social discrimination based on race. In his study of blacks and whites in Detroit, Harburg found a significantly increased amount of repressed anger in those blacks with elevated blood pressure compared to those blacks with normal levels of blood pressure. Perhaps, Harburg theorized, blacks faced with a bleak future internalize their anger because of their socialization and the fear of the consequences of expressing their rage, resulting in the patterns of hypertension he found (Harburg, 1973).

Hypertension and Gender

For both women and men in the United States, average blood pressure increases with age, but from twenty-five years on, the rate is substantially higher in women than in men (DHEW, 1977). Up until about the age of forty-five, men's (as a population) blood pressure is greater than women's. After that, for both blacks and whites, women's blood pressure surpasses and remains higher than men's (HDFP, 1977; DHEW, 1977; Kannel et al., 1969). While this patterned difference between women and men's rates of hypertension has been known and replicated for years, little is known beyond this about the differences in blood pressure by gender. In fact, little is known about women's health patterns in general (Olesen, 1977). Much more about variations among different groups of women needs to be learned. However, limitations in the epidemiological data collected about women often prevent such intra-gender comparisons.

In one recently published study of coronary heart disease among women, comparisons between women who worked outside the home with housewives revealed important differences among working women, as well as among women with different numbers of children. Although somewhat limited and not directly a study of hypertension, we can see in this study the potential for important differentiations among groups of women suggested by the findings that numbers of children and type of job correlated more with coronary heart disease than whether or not a woman worked outside the home *per se* (Haynes and Feinleib, 1980). Without an adequate understanding of the details of women's lives, including their domestic and family arrangements, we cannot really illuminate variations in women's health patterns (Kanter, 1977; Verbrugge, 1979).

One explanation for the pattern of female hypertension has to do with acknowledging the decreasing social and cultural value of women in our society as they age (Stannard, 1971). There is evidence, for example, that when women devote their younger years exclusively to unpaid domestic work, including the raising of children, they are more likely to become ill after their children are grown and leave home (Bart, 1970). For many

Table 1
Prevalence per 100 of Hypertension by Race and Age: United States, 1974

Age	All persons 17 years and over	White	Black
All ages over 17 years	16.8	16.0	24.1
17–24 years	4.2	4.1	5.3
25–44 years	9.5	8.6	17.9
45–64 years	24.2	22.7	39.1
65 years and over	36.3	35.3	47.2

Source: DHEW, 1978. "Characteristics of persons with hypertension: United States, 1974." Edited by Abigail J. Moss. Vital and Health Statistics, Data from National Health Survey. DHEW Publication No. (PHS) 79–1549 [series 10, no. 121], p. 4.

women, aging means the loss of identity along with the loss of a socially valued role. This would possibly explain the pattern of increased hypertension in middle class women, but since many working class women don't really shift their work patterns with age, such an explanation may be inapplicable to them. Without better data on variations in women's domestic lives, differences by social class between women's patterns of work and health, and more information on women's health patterns in general, any possible explanation of women's patterns of hypertension remain speculative (Lipman-Bluman, 1977).

Age and Hypertension

As mentioned earlier, a consistent finding in studies of prevalence patterns of hypertension is that hypertension increases with the age of the population (DHEW, 1977; Kannel et al., 1969; DHEW, 1978). As seen in Table 1, the prevalence of hypertension increases for both blacks and whites with each age increment.

Although we earlier noted that cross-cultural evidence does not support the hypothesis that increased blood pressure is part of the "natural" process of aging, we can hypothesize that the increasing prevalence of hypertension with age in the United States has a social and economic basis. We suggest there are two interrelated processes that account for the findings concerning age and hypertension. First, stress has a cumulative effect over the course of any particular person's lifetime, so that we see a gradual but constant increase in blood pressure with increased age among most Americans. Second, being old in our society is itself a negative experience for many, with its own particular sets of stresses and difficulties. Many old people must live on fixed incomes from inadequate Social Security or retirement benefits; many are forced to live in nursing homes for lack of alternatives; and the elderly are enormously overrepresented among the poor in this country. No longer able to be of "economic value" unless they are wealthy, the elderly find themselves without social or cultural value in a society that honors wealth and gives privilege only to those who can afford to buy it. The point for this discussion is that age, like gender and race, is not simply a physical characteristic (although it is often conceptualized so by medical research), but is a social and psychological one as well. It is in understanding the social nature of aging that we can begin to get some insight into the stresses and problems that the elderly have which can lead to sustained elevations in blood pressure and perhaps explain the American patterns of hypertension by age.

Summary and Conclusions

We have seen that certain groups of people in American society are more likely to have hypertension than others. Hypertension varies with social class (being more prevalent among those with less income and less education), race (being more prevalent among blacks than whites), age (it varies directly with age), occupation (certain occupations, and particular features of work situations are correlated with higher rates of hypertension), and gender (women have lower prevalence rates than men until their mid-forties when they surpass and exceed men's rates, and after the age of twenty-five, women's rates of hypertension increase more rapidly than do men's).

While a great deal of information has been collected relating these various social categories to prevalence rates of hypertension, each of these correlations treats the social variables as if they were independent of one another. The studies reviewed presented these variables as if they were characteristics of individuals rather than reflections of patterns of society. HME would suggest alternatively that we examine these correlations and categories *simultaneously* in order to identify the broad social and physical context in which hypertension occurs. Social class, occupation, race, age, and gender are interrelated in the organization of society. The political economy of capitalism (with its particular social and cultural characteristics) gives rise to both the organization of American society and the distribution and patterns of disease within it.

Historical materialist epidemiology makes those connections through a social analysis informed by a Marxist perspective. That perspective gives priority to the economic relations in society generated by the organization of production (work) and the distribution of material resources.

Before drawing any further conclusions, we want to reiterate the preliminary nature of HME, point out what we regard as some serious limitations in its perspective, and offer some suggestions for its future direction. Among its limitations are: (1) the overemphasis on wage labor, (2) the need for a feminist perspective and an understanding of the domestic sphere, and (3) the need for original, prospective empirical research.

(1) Traditional Marxist approaches, including HME,[9] focus on the importance of paid (wage) labor and the social relations of production as the crucial processes of society. While it is certainly the case that the organization of work under capitalism produces a range of stressful work conditions as well as an unequal distribution of wealth and power in society, we need to go beyond the organization of paid labor in order to understand all of the patterns of hypertension we find. The widespread existence of hypertension among the chronically unemployed as well as those who perform unpaid labor in the home (most women in our society) are two patterns which, while related to the political economy of capitalism, represent different sorts of stresses than those found within the factory. Perhaps the perception that one lacks control over one's life (true for both the employed and unemployed) is a central factor in the development of hypertension. Likewise, the small but significant percentage of hypertension among blacks that is not explained by their economic situation requires a fuller understanding of the social, psychological, and physical consequences of racism. We suggest that an adequate HME perspective will need to expand the range of social situations examined beyond those most directly related to paid labor in order to develop a full understanding of the processes involved in the development of hypertension in our society.

(2) There is a growing feminist literature that points to the limitations of Marxism to account for either the particular experiences of women in society (including their patterns of morbidity and mortality) or the relationships of men and women. (See, for example, Eisenstein, 1979; Kuhn and Wolpe, 1978; Mitchell, 1971; Firestone, 1970.) A major point of this feminist critique is the serious limitations in the Marxist understanding of the family and the domestic sphere. (See, for example, Poster, 1978; Zaretsky, 1976.) In order to account for the particular patterns of hypertension among women, and the variations among groups of women, we need to expand HME to understand the related but separate effects of the "sex/gender system" (institutionalized male dominance) and capitalism on both women and men (Rubin, 1975).

(3) The last problem reflects the available epidemiological research on chronic disease, so much of which utilizes a traditional medical model to gather and analyze its data. We suggest the critical need for original empirical research that is prospective and incorporates the theoretical and empirical categories of HME (as expanded to include unpaid labor, nonwork social and psychological variables, and an adequate understanding of the consequences of sexism, the lives of women, and the role of the domestic sphere). Such research would be able to provide the sort of data we currently lack in order to test the hypothesized relationships between the organization of American society and the patterns of disease among its citizens. While HME helps us to identify possible and significant correlations (e.g., between social class and hypertension), without better data we cannot identify the causal processes that are involved in the etiology of

hypertension (or any other chronic disease). Although no perspective can provide the total explanation for a chronic disease, research examining HME's hypotheses will enlighten our understanding of the social production of disease in a new way.

While this article cannot begin to address the complex social and political reasons why medicine has failed to explore the social basis of hypertension, it is easily demonstrable by examining the available medical literature that medicine continues to rely on a paradigm that does not (and cannot) incorporate social structural variables into the explanation and prevention of chronic disease. HME has as an explicit part of its theory the corollary possibility of the prevention of disease by changing those social and political conditions that contribute to its development. So, we would conclude from our examination of hypertension that we need to identify and understand better the social bases of stress as well as the relevant physical conditions which contribute to chronic elevations in blood pressure, and work to eliminate them in order to prevent the continued epidemic of hypertension in our society. This stance unfortunately is exactly the opposite of that of the current campaign of organized medicine, the National Heart, Blood and Lung Institute (part of the Department of Health, Education and Welfare), and the American pharmaceutical industry, which have joined forces to attempt to "cure" hypertension by placing 50 million (or more!) American adults on medications for even mild elevations in blood pressure (Relman, 1980). Indeed, this campaign has taken the direction of seeking increasingly sophisticated methods of ensuring patient "compliance" with medication regimens in order to guarantee the "success" of treatment.

We are certainly not opposed to those with severe hypertension being given the option of taking medications to lower their blood pressure: indeed, they should take such medications. However, in the long run, the most logical and safe approach to eliminating hypertension is to prevent it. This means, of course, identifying and eliminating those sources of both physical and social stress that are causing so many people to be plagued by this chronic and serious disease. Only through an analysis such as HME can we develop an integrated understanding of the relationship between society and disease, and thereby begin to develop insights and recommendations to eliminate hypertension through its prevention.

Notes

We thank Peter Conrad and Kim Hopper for their extensive conceptual and editorial suggestions, and Gail Garbowski for her background research contributions. We take full responsibility for the ideas presented here. (The order of author listing was determined by the flip of a coin.)

1. Until about five years ago, the higher cutoff of 160/95 was used within medicine as the measurement of "normal" blood presure. (See, for example, Inter-Society Commission for Heart Disease Resources, 1970.)
2. An early effort to develop a socio-medical analysis of hypertension was by Stahl et al. (1975) and suggested a model in which cognition (or perception) mediates between social structure and the development of hypertension (and other diseases). However, the ultimate suggestion that physicians become involved in the "manipulation of perception" is not only questionable, but relies once again on an individualistic conceptualization of disease and cure.
3. See also Schnall (1977) for an early introduction to the conceptualization of HME.
4. While non-capitalist societies also have chronic disease (including hypertension), the major focus of HME has been on the particular disease patterns prevalent under capitalism. Certainly, comparative and cross-cultural work needs to be done in order to isolate the particular products of American capitalism from those of other forms of political economic organization. One problem is the increasingly international influence of capitalism through multinational corporations, so that any analysis of "underdeveloped" Third World countries would necessarily have to address their relationship to capitalist economies.
5. At this point we note that there are limitations in the Marxist perspective, and in HME, and these will be discussed in the last section of this paper.
6. Two valuable published resources of work are: *The Review of Radical Political Economics* (Special Issue on "The Political Economy of Health"), Vol. 9, No. 1, Spring, 1977, available through URPE, 41 Union Square West, Room 901, New York, NY 10003, and *The International Journal of Health Services* (published quarterly and to be found in most university libraries).
7. In one major study of hypertension, the researchers actually gathered data on family income as well as the occupation of the "head of household," but chose to use only education as a measure of socioeconomic status. Their failure to use family income and occupation, as well as their failure to develop more adequate measures of social class, remains a serious limitation in their study (HDFP, 1977).
8. This citation refers to the findings of the United States National Health Survey.
9. There is variation within the writings of those who see their work as contributing to an historical materialist epidemiology. In particular, some have tried to expand the traditional Marxist emphasis on paid labor and the social relations of production, although this emphasis does dominate the bulk of HME writings. One notable exception is Hopper and Guttmacher (1979).

References

Actuarial Society of America and The Association of Life Insurance Medical Directors. 1941. "Supplement to 'Blood Pressure Study.'" New York: Actuarial Society of America and The Association of Life Insurance Medical Directors.

Baran, Paul, and Paul Sweezy. 1966. Monopoly Capital. New York: Monthly Review Press.

Bart, Pauline. 1970. "Portnoy's mother's complaint." Trans-action (November-December).

Bodenheimer, Thomas, Steve Cummings and Elizabeth Harding. 1972. Billions for Bandaids. San Francisco: Medical Committee for Human Rights.

Brenner, Harvey. 1977. "Health costs and benefits of economic policy." International Journal of Health Services 7, 4: 581–623.

Brown, George. 1974. "Meaning, measurement, and stress of life events." Pp. 217–244 in Barbara S. Dohrenwend and Bruce P. Dohrenwend (ed.), Stressful Life Events: Their Nature and Effects. New York: John Wiley and Sons.

Castiglione, Arturo. 1947. A History of Medicine. New York: Alfred A. Knopf.

Cobb, S., and R. M. Rose. 1973. "Hypertension, peptic ulcer, and diabetes in air traffic controllers." The Journal of The American Medical Association 224: 489–492.

Dahl, L. 1960. "Possible role of salt intake in the development of essential hypertension." Pp. 53ff in K. Bock and P. Cottier (eds.), Essential Hypertension. Berlin: Springer-Verlag.

D'Atri, D. A., and A. M. Ostfeld. 1975. "Crowding: Its effects on the elevation of blood pressure in a prison setting." Preventive Medicine 4: 550–566.

Davis, David, and Max Klainer. 1940. "Studies in hypertensive heart disease I. The incidence of coronary atherosclerosis in cases of essential hypertension." American Heart Journal 19: 185–192.

DHEW. 1964. "Hypertension and hypertensive heart disease, United States, 1960–1962." Vital and Health Statistics from the National Center for Health Statistics, Data from National Health Survey. DHEW [series 11, no. 13].

DHEW. 1977. "Blood pressure levels of persons 6–74 years, United States, 1971–1974." Edited by Jean Roberts. Department of Health, Education and Welfare. DHEW No. (HRA) 78–1648 [series 11, number 203].

DHEW. 1978. "Characteristics of persons with hypertension: United States, 1974." Edited by Abigail J. Moss. Vital and Health Statistics, Data from National Health Survey. DHEW Publication No. (PHS) 79–1549 [series 10, no. 121].

DHEW. 1980 "Births, marriages, divorces, and deaths for 1979." Monthly Vital Statistics Report, Provisional Statistics from the National Center for Health Statistics. Department of Health, Education and Welfare. DHEW Publication No. (PHS) 80–1120 [vol. 28, no. 12] (March 14).

Dohrenwend, Bruce P. 1974. "Problems in defining and sampling the relevant populations of stressful life events." Pp. 275–312 in Barbara S. Dohrenwend and Bruce P. Dohrenwend (eds.), Stressful Life Events. New York: John Wiley and Sons.

Dubos, René. 1959. Mirage of Health. New York: Harper and Row.

Ehrenreich, Barbara, and John Ehrenreich. 1970. The American Health Empire: Power, Profits and Politics. New York: Random House.

Eisenstein, Zillah R. (ed.). 1979. Capitalist Patriarchy and the Case for Socialist Feminism. New York: Monthly Review Press.

Engels, Friedrich. 1958. [1845] The Condition of the Working Class in England. Stanford, California: Stanford University Press.

Epstein, Samuel. 1976. "The political and economic basis of cancer." Technology Review 78: 1–7.

Eyer, Joseph. 1975. "Hypertension as a disease of modern society." International Journal of Health Services 5, 4: 539–558.

Eyer, Joseph. 1977a. "Does unemployment cause the death rate peak in each business cycle? A multifactor model of death rate change." International Journal of Health Services 7, 4: 625–662.

Eyer, Joseph. 1977b. "Prosperity as a cause of death." International Journal of Health Services 7, 1: 125–150.

Eyer, Joseph, and P. Sterling. 1977. "Stress-related mortality and social organization." The Review of Radical Political Economics 9, 1 (Spring): 1–44.

Firestone, Shulamith. 1970. The Dialectic of Sex. New York: William Morrow and Co., Inc.

Freis, Edward. 1976. "Salt, volume and the prevention of hypertension." Circulation 53, 4: 589–595.

Gaynor, David, et al. 1976. "Materialist epidemiology." HMO Packet #1: ME/1.

Gaynor, David. 1977. "Materialist epidemiology applied to occupational health and safety." HMO Packet #2: The Social Etiology of Disease (Part I): 23–28.

Harburg, E.W., J. Schull, J. C. Erfurt, and M. A. Schork. 1970. "A family-set method for estimating heredity and stress I. A pilot survey of blood pressure among Negroes in high and low stress areas, Detroit, 1966–1967." Journal of Chronic Disease 23: 69–81.

Harburg, E. W. 1973. "Socio-ecological stress, suppressed hostility, skin color, and black-white male blood pressure." Psychosomatic Medicine 35, 4.

Harris, L. 1973. "The public and high blood pressure." A Survey Conducted for the National Heart and Lung Institute. Department of Health, Education and Welfare 74–356.

Harrison, T. R. 1977. Harrison's Principles of Internal Medicine, Eighth Edition. Edited by George W. Thorn, et al. New York: McGraw-Hill Book Company.

Haynes, Suzanne, and Manning Feinleib. 1980. "Women, work and coronary heart disease: Prospective findings from the Framingham heart study." American Journal of Public Health 70, 2 (February): 133–141.

Health/PAC, 17 Murray Street, New York NY 10007.

HMO Packet #5. 1979. "Work and Health." Unpublished collection of papers available from: Dean Baker, 207 W. 106th Street, New York, NY 10025.

HMO Packet #6. 1979. "Imperialism, Dependency and Health. The Political and Economic Determinants of Health and Nutrition. Case Studies in Latin America." Unpublished collection of papers available from: Sally Guttmacher, Columbia University School of Public Health, Division of Sociomedical Sciences, 600 W. 168th Street, New York, NY 10032.

Hopper, Kim, and Sally Guttmacher. 1979. "Rethinking suicide: Notes toward a critical epidemiology." International Journal of Health Services 9, 3: 417–438.

House, James. 1974. "Occupational stress and coronary heart disease: A review and theoretical integration." Journal of Health and Social Behavior 15 (March): 17–27.

Hypertension Detection and Follow-up Cooperative Group [HDFP]. 1977. "Race, education and prevalence of hypertension: Hypertension Detection and Follow-up Program Cooperative Group." American Journal of Epidemiology 106, 5 (November): 351–361.

Hypertension Detection and Follow-up Cooperative Group [HDFP]. 1979. "Five-year findings of the Hypertension Detection and Follow-up Program I, Reduction in mortality of persons with HBP, including mild hypertension." and "Five-year findings of the Hypertension Detection and Follow-up Program II, Mortality by race-sex to age." Journal of the American Medical Association [JAMA] 242, 23: 2562–2577.

Inter-Society Commission for Heart Disease Resources. 1970. "Primary prevention of the atherosclerotic diseases." Circulation 43: A55.

James, Sherman, and David Kleinbaum. 1976. "Socioecologic stress and hypertension related mortality rates in North Carolina." American Journal of Public Health 66, 4 (April).

Janeway, Theodore. 1906. "The diagnostic significance of persistent high arterial pressure." American Journal of Medical Sciences 131: 772–779.

Kannel, William, et al. 1969. "Blood pressure and risk of coronary heart disease: The Framingham study." Diseases of the Chest 56: 43–52.

Kanter, Rosabeth Moss. 1977. Work and Family in the United States: A Critical Review and Agenda for Research and Policy. New York: Russell Sage.

Karasek, Robert, et al. 1978. "Job decision latitude, job demands and coronary heart disease, A cross-sectional and prospective study of Swedish men." Unpublished paper quoted with author's permission (December).

Kasl, S.V., and S. Cobb. 1970. "Blood pressure changes in men undergoing job loss: A preliminary report." Psychosomatic Medicine 2: 19–38.

Keil, Julian, et al. 1977. "Hypertension: Effects of social class and racial admixture." American Journal of Public Health 67, 7 (July): 634–639.

Kitagawa, E. M., and P. Hauser. 1973. Differential Mortality in the United States: A Study in Socioeconomic Epidemiology. Cambridge, Mass: Harvard University Press.

Knowles, John. 1977. "The responsibility of the individual." Daedalus (Winter).

Kuhn, Annette, and Ann Marie Wolpe (eds.). 1978. Feminism and Materialism, Women and Modes of Production. London: Routledge and Kegan Paul.

Lipman-Bluman, Jean. 1977. "Demographic trends and issues in women's health." Pp. 11–22 in V. Olesen (ed.), Women and Their Health: Research Implications for a New Era. Proceedings of a Conference Held at San Francisco, California, August 1–2, 1975. National Center for Health Services Research.

McKeown, Thomas. 1971. "A historical appraisal of the medical task." In G. McLachlan and T. McKeown (eds.), Medical History and Medical Care: A Symposium of Perspectives. New York: Oxford University Press.

Mitchell, Juliet. 1971. Woman's Estate. New York: Random House.

Mustacchi, Piero. 1977. "The interface of the work environment and hypertension." Medical Clinics of North America 61, 3 (May): 531–545.

National High Blood Pressure Education Program. 1978. "Info-memo." National Heart, Lung and Blood Institute 13 (May).

Navarro, Vicente. 1977. "Political power, the state, and their implications in medicine." The Review of Radical Political Economics 9, 1 (Spring): 61–80.

Navarro, Vicente. 1978. "The crisis of the western system of medicine in contemporary capitalism." International Journal of Health Services 8, 2: 179–211.

O'Connor, James. 1973. The Fiscal Crisis of the State. New York: St. Martin's Press.

Olesen, Virginia (ed.). 1977. Women and Their Health: Research Implications for a New Era. Proceedings of a Conference Held at San Francisco, California, August 1–2, 1975. National Center for Health Services Research.

Page, Lot. 1976. "Epidemiological evidence on the etiology of human hypertension and its possible prevention." American Heart Journal 91, 4 (April): 527–534.

Pickering, George W. 1961. The Nature of Essential Hypertension. New York: Grune and Stratton, Inc.

Pickering, George. 1975. "Hypertension: Natural histories and consequences." In J. H. Laragh (ed.), Hypertension Manual: Mechanisms, Methods, Management. New York: Dun-Donnelly Publishing Corporation.

Poster, Mark. 1978. Critical Theory of the Family. New York: Seabury Press.

Powles, John. 1973. "On the limitations of modern medicine." Science, Medicine and Man 1: 1–30.

Reed, Wornie. 1981. "Suffer the children: Some effects of racism on the health of black infants." In Part Two of this volume.

Relman, Arnold S. 1980. "Mild hypertension: No more benign neglect." New England Journal of Medicine 302, 5 (January 31): 293–294.

Rodberg, Leonard, and Gelvin Stevenson. 1977. "The health care industry in advanced capitalism." The Review of Radical Political Economics 9, 1 (Spring): 104–115.

Rubin, Gayle. 1975. "The traffic in women: Notes on the 'political economy' of sex." Pp. 157–210 in Rayna Reiter (ed.), Toward an Anthropology of Women. New York: Monthly Review Press.

Ruskin, Arthur. 1956. Classics in Arterial Hypertension. Charles C. Thomas Publishers.

Salmon, J. Warren. 1977. "Monopoly capital and the reorganization of the health sector." The Review of Radical Political Economics 9, 1 (Spring): 125–133.

Schnall, Peter L. 1977. "An introduction to Historical Materialist Epidemiology." HMO Packet #2, The Social Etiology of Disease (Part I): 1–9.

Shapiro, Alvin (ed.). 1979. "The role of stress in hypertension—A symposium." The Journal of Human Stress 4, 2 (June): 7–26.

Stahl, Sidney M., et al. 1975. "A model for the social sciences and medicine: The case for hypertension." Social Science and Medicine 9: 31–38.

Stannard, Una. 1971. "The mask of beauty." Pp. 187–203 in Vivian Gornick and Barbara K. Moran (eds.), Woman in Sexist Society. New York: Basic Books.

Stark, Evan. 1977a. "The cutting edge in occupational health." HMO Packet #3: The Social Etiology of Disease (Part II), Implications and Applications of HME: 52–62.

Stark, Evan. 1977b. "The epidemic as a social event." International Journal of Health Services 7, 4: 681–705.

Stark, Evan, Anne Flitcraft and William Frazier. 1979. "Medicine and patriarchal violence: The social construction of a 'private' event." International Journal of Health Services 9, 3: 461–493.

Sterling, T. D. 1978. "Does smoking kill workers or working kill smokers? Or the mutual relationship between smoking, occupation, and respiratory disease." International Journal of Health Services 8, 3: 437–452.

Sweezy, Paul. 1968. The Theory of Capitalist Development. New York: Monthly Review Press.

Thomas, C. B. 1973. "Genetic patterns of hypertension in man." In G. Onesti, K. E. Kim, and J. H. Moyer (eds.), Hypertension Mechanism and Management. New York: Grune and Stratton, Inc.

Thomas, E. 1959. The Harmless People. New York: Vintage.

Turshen, Meredeth. 1977. "Worker safety and health." HMO Packet #3: The Social Etiology of Disease (Part II), Implications and Applications of HME: 41–51.

Verbrugge, Lois. 1979. "Marital status and health." Journal of Marriage and Family (May): 267–285.

Waitzkin, Howard. 1978. "A Marxist view of medical care." Annals of Internal Medicine 89: 264–278.

Waldron, Ingrid. 1977. "Society, 'stress' and illness." HMO Packet #2: The Social Etiology of Disease (Part I): 105–107.

Wetherby, Macnider. 1932. "A comparison of blood pressure in men and women." Annals of Internal Medicine 6: 754–770.

Zaretsky, Eli. 1976. Capitalism, the Family and Personal Life. New York: Harper Colophon.

Zinner, S. H., P. S. Levy and E. H. Kass. 1971. "Familial aggregation of blood pressure in childhood." New England Journal of Medicine 284:401–404.

The Experience of Illness

DISEASE NOT ONLY INVOLVES the body. It also affects people's social relationships, self-image, and behavior. The social psychological aspects of illness are related in part to the biophysiological manifestations of disease, but are also independent of them. The very act of defining something as an illness has consequences that are independent of any effects of biophysiology.

> When a veterinarian diagnoses a cow's condition as an illness, he does not merely by diagnosis change the cow's behavior; to the cow, illness [disease] remains an experienced biophysiological state, no more. But when a physician diagnoses a human's condition as an illness, he changes the man's behavior by diagnosis: a social state is added to a biophysiological state by assigning the meaning of illness to disease. (Freidson, 1970: 223.)

Much of the sociological study of illness has centered on the *sick role* and *illness behavior.* Talcott Parsons (1951) argued that in order to prevent the potentially disruptive consequences of illness on a group or society, there exists a set of shared cultural rules (norms) called the "sick role." The sick role legitimates the deviations caused by illness and channels the sick into the reintegrating physician-patient relationship. According to Parsons the sick role has four components: (1) the sick person is exempted from normal social responsibilities, at least to the extent it is necessary to get well; (2) the individual is not held responsible for his or her condition and cannot be expected to recover by an act of will; (3) the person must recognize that being ill is undesirable and must want to recover; and (4) the sick person is obligated to seek and cooperate with "expert" advice, generally that of a physician. Sick people are not blamed for their illness, but must work toward recovery. There have been numerous critiques and modifications of the concept of the sick role, such as its inapplicability to chronic illness and disability, but it remains a central sociological way of seeing illness experience (Segall, 1976).

Illness behavior is essentially how people act when they develop symptoms of disease. As one sociologist notes, it includes ". . . the ways in which given symptoms may be differentially perceived, evaluated, and acted (or not acted) upon by different kinds of persons . . . whether by reason of early experience with illness, differential training in respect to symptoms, or whatever" (Mechanic, 1962). Reaction to symptoms, use of social networks in locating help, and compliance with medical advice are some of the activities characterized as illness behavior.

Illness behavior and the sick role, as well as the related concept of *illness career* (Suchman, 1965), are all more or less based on a perspective that all (proper) roads lead to medical care. They tend to create a "doctor-centered" picture by making the receipt of medical care the centerpiece of sociological attention. Such concepts are essentially "outsider" perspectives on the experience of illness. While these viewpoints may be useful in their own right, none of them has the actual subjective experience of illness as a central concern. They don't analyze illness from the sufferer's (or patient's) viewpoint. A few sociologists (e.g., Strauss and Glaser, 1975) have attempted to develop more subjective "insider" accounts of what it is like to be sick. These accounts focus more on individuals' perceptions of illness, interactions with others, the effects of illness on identity, and people's strategies for managing illness symptoms than do the abstract notions of illness careers or sick roles.

The two articles in this section illuminate the subjective side of illness. Mark Zborowski's classic article, "Cultural Components in Response to Pain," combines outsider and insider viewpoints in offering a cultural analysis of the experience of pain. As he shows, pain may be physiological in cause but it is affected by social variables. Pain is often the first sign of illness but its perception varies by culture. Indeed, as Zola (1966) and others have demonstrated, cultural factors profoundly influence symptoms, how we behave when we get sick, and what we do about it. To ignore the cultural realm is to misunderstand the illness experience. In "Chronic Illness," Anselm Strauss depicts the experience of chronic illness in the social worlds in which people live. Most of the problems of people with chronic illness are apart from medical care. Strauss shows, from the patient's viewpoint, how family interaction, handling medical regimens, and finding ways to "get by" are central in the personal managing of illness and the "disease trajectory."

When we understand and treat illness as a subjective as well as objective experience we no longer treat patients as diseases but as people who are sick. This is an important dimension of human health care.

References

Freidson, Eliot. 1970. Profession of Medicine. New York: Dodd, Mead.

Mechanic, David. 1962. "The concept of illness behavior." Journal of Chronic Diseases. 15: 189–94.

Parsons, Talcott. 1951. The Social System. New York: Free Press.

Segall, Alexander. 1976. "The sick role concept: Understanding illness behavior." Journal of Health and Social Behavior. 17 (June): 163–70.

Suchman, Edward. 1965. "Stages of illness and medical care." Journal of Health and Social Behavior. 6: 114–28.

Strauss, Anselm, and Barney Glaser. 1975. Chronic Illness and the Quality of Life. St. Louis: C. V. Mosby.

Zola, Irving Kenneth. 1966. "Culture and symptoms." American Sociological Review. 31: 615–30.

8

Cultural Components in Responses to Pain

Mark Zborowski

This paper reports on one aspect of a larger study: that concerned with discovering the role of cultural patterns in attitudes toward and reactions to pain which is caused by disease and injury—in other words, responses to spontaneous pain (1).

Some Basic Distinctions

In human societies biological processes vital for man's survival acquire social and cultural significance. Intake of food, sexual intercourse or elimination—physiological phenomena which are universal for the entire living world—become institutions regulated by cultural and social norms, thus fulfilling not only biological functions but social and cultural ones as well. Metabolic and endocrinal changes in the human organism may provoke hunger and sexual desire, but culture and society dictate to man the kind of food he may eat, the social setting for eating or the adequate partner for mating.

Moreover, the role of cultural and social patterns in human physiological activities is so great that they may in specific situations act against the direct biological needs of the individual, even to the point of endangering his survival. Only a human being may prefer starvation to the breaking of a religious dietary law or may abstain from sexual intercourse because of specific incest regulations. Voluntary fasting and celibacy exist only where food and sex fulfill more than strictly physiological functions.

Thus, the understanding of the significance and role of social and cultural patterns in human physiology is necessary to clarify those aspects of human experience which remain puzzling if studied only within the physiological frame of reference.

Pain is basically a physiological phenomenon and as such has been studied by physiologists and neurologists such as Harold Wolff, James Hardy, Helen Goodell, C. S. Lewis, W. K. Livingston and others. By using the most ingenious methods of investigation they have succeeded in clarifying complex problems of the physiology of pain. Many aspects of perception and reaction to pain were studied in experimental situations involving the most careful preparation and complicated equipment. These investigators have come to the conclusion that "from the physiological point of view pain qualifies as a sensation of importance to the self-preservation of the individual" (2). The biological function of pain is to provoke special reactive patterns directed toward avoidance of the noxious stimulus which presents a threat to the individual. In this respect the function of pain is basically the same for man as for the rest of the animal world.

However, the physiology of pain and the understanding of the biological function of pain do not explain other aspects of what Wolff, Hardy and Goodell call the *pain experience,* which includes not only certain "associated feeling states" (3). It would not explain, for example, the acceptance of intense pain in torture which is part of the initiation rites of many primitive societies, nor will it explain the strong emotional reactions of certain individuals to the slight sting of the hypodermic needle.

In human society pain, like so many other physiological phenomena, acquires specific social and cultural significance, and accordingly, certain reactions to pain can be understood in the light of this significance. As Drs. Hardy, Wolff and Goodell state in their recent book, ". . . the culture in which a man finds himself becomes the conditioning influence in the formation of the individual reaction patterns to pain . . . A knowledge of group attitudes toward pain is extremely important to an understanding of the individual reaction" (4).

In analyzing pain, it is useful to distinguish between self-inflicted, other-inflicted and spontaneous pain. Self-inflicted pain is defined as deliberately self-inflicted. It is experienced as a result of injuries performed voluntarily upon oneself, e.g., self-mutilation. Usually these injuries have a culturally defined purpose, such as achieving a special status in the society. It can be observed not only in primitive cultures but also in contemporary societies on a higher level of civilization. In Germany, for instance, members of certain student or military organizations would cut their faces with a razor in order to acquire scars which would identify them as members of a distinctive social group. By other-inflicted pain is meant pain inflicted upon the individual in the process of culturally accepted and expected activities (regardless of whether approved or disapproved), such as sports, fights, war, etc. To this category belongs also pain inflicted by the physician in the process of medical treatment. Spontaneous pain usually denotes the pain sensation which results from disease or injury. This term also covers pain of psychogenic nature.

Members of differnt cultures may assume differing attitudes towards these various types of pain. Two of these attitudes may be described as pain expectancy and pain acceptance. Pain expectancy is anticipation of pain as being unavoidable in a given situation, for instance, in childbirth, in sports activities or in battle. Pain acceptance is characterized by a willingness to experience pain. This attitude is manifested mostly as an inevitable component of culturally accepted experiences, for instance, as part of initiation rites or part of medical treatment. The following example will help to clarify the differences between pain expectancy and pain acceptance. Labor pain is expected as part of childbirth, but while in one culture, such as in the United States, it is not accepted and therefore various means are used to alleviate it, in some other cultures, for instance in Poland, it is not only expected but also accepted, and consequently nothing or little is done to relieve it. Similarly, cultures which emphasize military achievements expect and accept battle wounds, while cultures which emphasize pacifistic values may expect them but will not accept them.

In the process of investigating cultural attitudes toward pain it is also important to distinguish between pain apprehension and pain anxiety. Pain apprehension reflects the tendency to avoid the pain sensation as such, regardless of whether the pain is spontaneous or inflicted, whether it is accepted or not. Pain anxiety, on the other hand, is a state of anxiety provoked by the pain experience, focused upon various aspects of the causes of pain, the meaning of pain or its significance for the welfare of the individual.

Moreover, members of various cultures may react differently in terms of their manifest behavior toward various pain experiences, and this behavior is often dictated by the culture which provides specific norms according to the age, sex and social position of the individual.

The fact that other elements as well as cultural factors are involved in the response to a spontaneous pain should be taken into consideration. These other factors are the pathological aspect of pain, the specific physiological characteristics of the pain experience, such as the intensity, the duration and the quality of the pain sensation, and finally, the personality of the individual. Nevertheless, it was felt that in the process of a careful investigation it would be possible to detect the role of the cultural components in the pain experience.

The Research Setting

In setting up the research we were interested not only in the purely theoretical aspects of the findings in terms of possible contribution to the understanding of the pain experience in general; we also had in mind the practical goal of a contribution to the field of medicine. In the relationship between the doctor and his patient the respective attitudes toward pain may play a crucial role, especially when the doctor feels that the patient exaggerates his pain while the patient feels that the doctor minimizes his suffering. The same may be true, for instance, in a hospital where the members of the medical and nursing staff may have attitudes toward pain different from those held by the patient, or when they expect a certain pattern of behavior according to their cultural background while the patient may manifest a behavior pattern which is acceptable in his culture. These differences may play an important part in the evaluation of the individual pain experience, in dealing with pain at home and in the hospital, in administration of analgesics, etc. Moreover, we expected that this study of pain would offer opportunities to gain insight into related attitudes toward health, disease, medication, hospitalization, medicine in general, etc.

With these aims in mind the project was set up at the Kingsbridge Veterans Hospital, Bronx, New York (5), where four ethno-cultural groups were selected for an intensive study. These groups included patients of Jewish, Italian, Irish and "Old American" stock. Three groups—Jews, Italian, and Irish—were selected because they were described by medical people as manifesting striking differences in their reaction to pain. Italians and Jews were described as tending to "exaggerate" their pain, while the Irish were often depicted as stoical individuals who were able to take a great deal of pain. The fourth group, the "Old Americans," were chosen because the values and attitudes of this group dominate in this country and are held by many members of the medical profession and by many descendants of the immigrants who, in the process of Americanization, tend to adopt American patterns of behavior. The members of this group can be defined as White, native-born individuals, usually Protestant, whose grandparents, at least, were born in the United States and who do not identify themselves with any foreign group, either nationally, socially or culturally.

The Kingsbridge Veterans Hospital was chosen because its population represents roughly the ethnic composition of New York City, thus offering access to a fair sample of the four selected groups, and also because various age groups were represented among the hospitalized veterans of World War I, World War II and the Korean War. In one major respect this hospital was not adequate, namely, in not offering the opportunity to investigate sex differences in attitude toward pain. This aspect of research will be carried out in a hospital with a large female population.

In setting up this project we were mainly interested in discovering certain regularities in reactions and attitudes toward pain characteristic of the four groups. Therefore, the study has a qualitative character, and the efforts of the researchers were not directed toward a collection of material suitable for quantitative analysis. The main techniques used in the collection of the material were interviews with patients of the selected groups, observation of their behavior when in pain and discussion of the individual case with doctors, nurses and other people directly or indirectly involved in the pain experience of the individual. In addition to the interviews with patients, "healthy" members of the respective groups were interviewed on their attitudes toward pain, because in terms of the original hypothesis those attitudes and reactions which are displayed by the patients of the given cultural groups are held by all members of the group regardless of whether or not they are in pain although in pain these attitudes may come more sharply into focus. In certain cases the researchers have interviewed a member of the patient's immediate family in order to check the report of the patient on his pain experience and in order to find out what are the attitudes and reactions of the family toward the patient's experience.

These interviews, based on a series of open-ended questions, were focused upon the past and present pain experiences of the interviewee. However, many other areas were considered important for the understanding of this experience. For instance, it was felt that complaints of pain may play an important role in manipulating relationships in the family and the larger social environment. It was also felt that in order to understand the specific reactive patterns in controlling pain it is important to know certain aspects of child-rearing in the culture, relationships between parents and children, the role of infliction of pain in punishment, the attitudes of various members of the family toward specific expected, accepted pain experiences, and so on. The interviews were recorded on wire and transcribed verbatim for an ultimate detailed analysis. The interviews usually lasted for approximately two hours, the time being limited by the condition of the interviewee and by the amount and quality of his answers. When it was considered necessary an interview was repeated. In most of the cases the study of the interviewee was followed by informal conversations and by observation of his behavior in the hospital.

The information gathered from the interviews was discussed with members of the medical staff, especially in the areas related to the medical aspects of the problem, in order to get their evaluation of the pain experience of the patient. Information as to the personality of the patient was checked against results of psychological testing by members of the psychological staff of the hospital when these were available.

The discussion of the material presented in this paper is based on interviews with 103 respondents, including 87 hospital patients in pain and 16 healthy subjects. According to their ethno-cultural background the respondents are distributed as follows: "Old Americans," 26; Italians, 24; Jews, 31; Irish, 11; and others, 11 (6). In addition, there were the collateral interviews and conversations noted above with family members, doctors, nurses and other members of the hospital staff.

With regard to the pathological causes of pain the majority of the interviewees fall into the group of patients suffering from neurological diseases, mainly herniated discs and spinal lesions. The focusing upon a group of patients suffering from a similar pathology offered the opportunity to investigate reactions and attitudes toward spontaneous pain which is symptomatic of one group of diseases. Nevertheless, a number of patients suffering from other diseases were also interviewed.

This paper is based upon the material collected during the first stage of study. The generalizations are to a great extent tentative formulations on a descriptive level. There has been no attempt as yet to integrate the results with the value system and the cultural pattern of the group, though here and there will be indications to the effect that they are part of the culture pattern. The discussions will be limited to main regularities within three groups, namely, the Italians, the Jews and the "Old Americans." Factors related to variations within each group will be discussed after the main prevailing patterns have been presented.

Pain Among Patients of Jewish and Italian Origin

As already mentioned, the Jews and Italians were selected mainly because interviews with medical experts suggested that they display similar reactions to pain. The investigation of this similarity provided the opportunity to check a rather popular assumption that similar reactions reflect similar attitudes. The differences between the Italian and Jewish culture are great enough to suggest that if the attitudes are related to cultural pattern they will also be different despite the apparent similarity in manifest behavior.

Members of both groups were described as being very emotional in their responses to pain. They were described as tending to exaggerate their pain experience and being very sensitive to pain. Some of the doctors stated that in their opinion Jews and Italians have a lower threshold of pain than members of other ethnic groups, especially members of the so-called Nordic group. This statement seems to indicate a certain confusion as to the concept of the threshold of pain. According to people who have studied the problem of the threshold of pain, for instance Harold Wolff and his associates, the threshold of pain is more or less the same for all human beings regardless of nationality, sex or age.

In the course of the investigation the general impressions of doctors were confirmed to a great extent by the interview material and by the observation of the patients' behavior. However, even a superficial study of the interviews has revealed that though reactions to pain appear to be similar the underlying atitudes toward pain are different in the two groups. While the Italian patients seemed to be mainly concerned with the immediacy of the pain experience and were disturbed by the actual pain sensation which they experienced in a given situation, the concern of patients of Jewish origin was focused mainly upon the symptomatic meaning of pain and upon the significance of pain in relation to their health, welfare, and eventually, for the welfare of the families. The Italian patient expressed in his behavior and in his complaints the discomfort caused by pain as such, and he manifested his emotions with regard to the effects of this pain experience upon his immediate situation in terms of occupation, economic situation and so on; the Jewish patient expressed primarily his worries and anxieties as to the extent to which the pain indicated a threat to his health. In this connection it is worth mentioning that one of the Jewish words to describe strong pain is *yessurim,* a word which is also used to describe worries and anxieties.

Attitudes of Italian and Jewish patients toward pain-relieving drugs can serve an an indication of their attitude toward pain. When in pain the Italian calls for pain relief and is mainly concerned with the analgesic effects of the drugs which are administered to him. Once the pain is relieved the Italian patient easily forgets his sufferings and manifests a happy and joyful disposition. The Jewish patient, however, often is reluctant to accept the drug, and he explains this reluctance in terms of concern about the effects of the drug upon his health in general. He is apprehensive about the habit-forming aspects of the analgesic. Moreover, he feels that the drug relieves his pain only temporarily and does not cure him of the disease which may cause the pain. Nurses and doctors have reported cases in which patients would hide the pill which was given to them to relieve their pain and would prefer to suffer. These reports were confirmed in the interviews with the patients. It was also observed that many Jewish patients after being relieved from pain often continued to display the same depressed and worried behavior because they felt that though the pain was currently absent it may recur as long as the disease was not cured completely. From these observations it appears that when one deals with a Jewish and Italian patient in pain, in the first case it is more important to relieve the anxieties with regard to the sources of pain, while in the second it is more important to relieve the actual pain.

Another indication as to the significance of pain for Jewish and Italian patients is their respective attitudes toward the doctor. The Italian patient seems to display a most confident attitude toward the doctor which is usually reinforced after the doctor has succeeded in relieving pain, whereas the Jewish patient manifests a skeptical attitude, feeling that the fact that the doctor has relieved his pain by some drug does not mean at all that he is skillful enough to take care of the basic illness. Consequently, even when the pain is relieved, he tends to check the diagnosis and the treatment of one doctor against the opinions of other specialists in the field. Summarizing the difference between the Italian and Jewish attitudes, one can say that the Italian attitude is characterized by a present-oriented apprehension with regard to the actual sensation of pain, and the Jew tends to manifest a future-oriented anxiety as to the symptomatic and general meaning of the pain experience.

It has been stated that the Italians and Jews tend to manifest similar behavior in terms of their reactions to pain. As both cultures allow for free expression of feelings and emotions by words, sounds and gestures, both the Italians and Jews feel free to talk about their pain, complain about it and manifest their sufferings by groaning, moaning, crying, etc. They are not ashamed of this expression. They admit willingly that when they are in pain they do complain a great deal, call for help and expect sympathy and assistance from other members of their immediate social environment, especially from members of their family. When in pain they are reluctant to be alone and prefer the presence and attention of other people. This behavior, which is expected, accepted and approved by the Italian and Jewish cultures often conflicts with the patterns of behavior expected from a patient by American or Americanized medical people. Thus they tend to describe the behavior of the Italian and Jewish patient as exaggerated and over-emotional. The material suggests that they do tend to minimize the actual pain experiences of the Italian and Jewish patient regardless of whether they have the objective criteria for evaluating the actual amount of pain which the patient experiences. It seems that the uninhibited display of reaction to pain as manifested by the Jewish and Italian patient provokes distrust in American culture instead of provoking sympathy.

Despite the close similarity between the manifest reactions among Jews and Italians, there seem to be differences in emphasis especially with regard to what the patient achieves by these reactions and as to the specific manifestations of these reactions in the various social settings. For instance, they differ in their behavior at home and in the hospital. The Italian husband, who is aware of his role as an adult male, tends to avoid verbal complaining at home, leaving this type of behavior to the women. In the hospital, where he is less concerned with his role as a male, he tends to be more verbal and more emotional. The Jewish patient, on the contrary, seems to be more calm in the hospital than at home. Traditionally the Jewish male does not emphasize his masculinity through such traits as stoicism, and he does not equate verbal complaints with weakness. Moreover, the Jewish culture allows the patient to be demanding and complaining. Therefore, he tends more to use his pain in order to control interpersonal relationships within the family. Though similar use of pain to manipulate the relationships between members of the family may be present also in some other cultures it seems that in the Jewish culture this is not disapproved, while in others it is. In the hospital one can also distinguish variations in the reactive patterns among Jews and Italians. Upon his admission to the hospital and in the presence of the doctor the Jewish patient tends to complain, ask for help, be emotional even to the point of crying. However, as soon as he feels that adequate care is given to him he becomes more restrained. This suggests that the display of pain reaction serves less as an indication of the amount of pain experienced than as a means to create an atmosphere and setting in which the pathological cause of pain will be best taken care of. The Italian patient, on the other hand, seems to be less concerned with setting up a favorable situation for treatment. He takes for granted that adequate care will be given to him, and in the presence of the doctor he seems to be somewhat calmer than the Jewish patient. The mere presence of the doctor reassures the Italian patient, while the skepticism of the Jewish patient limits the reassuring role of the physician.

To summarize the description of the reactive patterns of the Jewish and Italian patients, the material suggests that on a semi-conscious level the Jewish patient tends to provoke worry and concern in his social environment as to the state of his health and the symptomatic character of his pain, while the Italian tends to provoke sympathy toward his suffering. In one case the function of the pain reaction will be the mobilization of the efforts of the family and the doctors toward a complete cure, while in the second case the function of the reaction will be focused upon the mobilization of effort toward relieving the pain sensation.

On the basis of the discussion of the Jewish and Italian material two generalizations can be made: (1) *Similar reactions to pain manifested by members of different ethno-cultural groups do not necessarily reflect similar attitudes to pain.* (2) *Reactive patterns similar in terms of their manifestations may have different functions and serve different purposes in various cultures.*

Pain Among Patients of "Old American" Origin

There is little emphasis on emotional complaining among "Old American" patients. Their complaints about pain can best be described as reporting on pain. In describing pain, the "Old American" patient tries to find the most appropriate ways of defining the quality of pain, its localization, duration, etc. When examined by the doctor he gives the impression of trying to assume the detached role of an unemotional observer who gives the most efficient description of his state for a correct diagnosis and treatment. The interviewees repeatedly state that there is no point in complaining and groaning and moaning, etc., because "it won't help anybody." However, they readily admit that when pain is unbearable they may react strongly, even to the point of crying, but they tend to do it when they are alone. Withdrawal from society seems to be a frequent reaction to strong pain.

There seem to be different patterns in reacting to pain depending on the situation. One pattern, manifested in the presence of members of the family, friends, etc., consists of attempts to minimize pain, to avoid complaining and provoking pity; when pain becomes too strong there is a tendency to withdraw and express freely such reactions as groaning, moaning, etc. A different pattern is manifested in the presence of people who, on account of their profession, should know the character of the pain experience because they are expected to make the appropriate diagnosis, advise the proper cure and give the adequate help. This tendency to avoid deviation from certain expected patterns of behavior plays an important role in the reaction to pain. This is also controlled by the desire to seek approval on the part of the social environment, especially in the hospital, where the "Old American" patient tries to avoid being a "nuisance" on the ward. He seems to be, more than any other patient, aware of an ideal pattern of behavior which is identified as "American," and he tends to conform to it. This was characteristically expressed by a patient who answered the question how he reacts to pain by saying, "I react like a good American."

An important element in controlling the pain reaction is the wish of the patient to cooperate with those who are expected to take care of him. The situation is often viewed as a team composed of the patient, the doctor, the nurse, the attendant, etc., and in this team everybody has a function and is supposed to do his share in order to achieve the most successful result. Emotionality is seen as a purposeless and hindering factor in a situation which calls for knowledge, skill, training and efficiency. It is important to note that this behavior is also expected by American or Americanized members of the medical or nursing staff, and the patients who do not fall into this pattern are viewed as deviants, hypochondriacs and neurotics.

As in the case of the Jewish patients, the American attitude toward pain can be best defined as a future-oriented anxiety. The "Old American" patient is also concerned with the symptomatic significance of pain which is correlated with a pronounced health-consciousness. It seems that the "Old American" is conscious of various threats to his health which are present in his environment and therefore feels vulnerable and is prone to interpret his pain sensation as a warning signal indicating that something is wrong with his health and therefore must be reported to the physician. With some exceptions, pain is considered bad and unnecessary and therefore must be immediately taken care of. In those situations where pain is expected and accepted, such as in the process of medical treatment or as a result of sports activities, there is less concern with the pain sensation. In general, however, there is a feeling that suffering pain is unnecessary when there are means of relieving it.

Though the attitudes of the Jewish and "Old American" patients can be defined as pain anxiety they differ greatly. The future-oriented anxiety of the Jewish interviewee is characterized by pessimism or, at best, by skepticism, while the "Old American" patient is rather optimistic in his future-orientation. This attitude is fostered by the mechanistic approach to the body and its functions and by the confidence in the skill of the expert which are so frequent in the American, in that the body is often viewed as a machine which has to be well taken care of, be periodically checked for dysfunctioning and eventually, when out of order, be taken to an expert who will "fix" the defect. In the case of pain the expert is the medical man who has the "know-how" because of his training and experience and therefore is entitled to full confidence. An important element in the optimistic outlook is faith in the progress of science. Patients with intractable pain often stated that though at the present moment the doctors do not have the "drug" they will eventually discover it, and they will give the examples of sulfa, penicillin, etc.

The anxieties of a pain-experiencing "Old American" patient are greatly relieved when he feels that something is being done about it in terms of specific activities involved in the treatment. It seems that his security and confidence increase in direct proportion to the number of tests, X-rays, examinations, injections, etc., that are given to him. Accordingly, "Old American" patients seem to have a positive attitude toward hospitalization, because the hospital is the adequate institution which is equipped for the necessary treatment. While a Jewish and an Italian patient seem to be disturbed by the impersonal character of the hospital and by the necessity of being treated there instead of at home, the "Old American" patient, on the contrary, prefers the hospital treatment to the home treatment, and neither he nor his family seems to be disturbed by hospitalization.

To summarize the attitude of the "Old American" toward pain, he is disturbed by the symptomatic aspect of pain and is concerned with its incapacitating aspects, but he tends to view the future in rather optimistic colors, having confidence in the science and skill of the professional people who treat his condition.

Some Sources of Intra-Group Variation

In the description of the reactive patterns and attitudes toward pain among patients of Jewish and "Old American" origin certain regularities have been observed for each particular group regardless of individual differences and variations. This does not mean that each individual in each group manifests the same reactions and attitudes. Individual variations are often due to specific aspects of pain experience, to the character of the disease which causes the pain or to elements of the personality of the patient. However, there are also other factors that are instrumental in provoking these differences and which can still be traced back to the cultural backgrounds of the individual patients. Such variables as the degree of Americanization of the patient, his socio-economic background, education and religiosity may play an important role in shaping individual variations in the reactive patterns. For instance, it was found that the patterns described are manifested most consistently among immigrants, while their descendants tend to differ in terms of adopting American forms of behavior and American attitudes toward the role of the medical expert, medical institutions and equipment in controlling pain. It is safe to say that the further the individual is from the immigrant generation the more

American is his behavior. This is less true for the attitudes toward pain, which seem to persist to a great extent even among members of the third generation and even though the reactive patterns are radically changed. A Jewish or Italian patient born in this country of American-born parents tends to *behave* like an "Old American" but often expresses *attitudes* similar to those which are expressed by the Jewish or Italian people. They try to appear unemotional and efficient in situations where the immigrant would be excited and disturbed. However, in the process of the interview, if a patient is of Jewish origin he is likely to express attitudes of anxiety as to the meaning of his pain, and if he is an Italian he is likely to be rather unconcerned about the significance of his pain for the future.

The occupational factor plays an important role when pain affects a specific area of the body. For instance, manual workers with herniated discs are more disturbed by their pain than are professional or business people with a similar disease because of the immediate significance of this particular pain for their respective abilities to earn a living. It was also observed that headaches cause more concern among intellectuals than among manual workers.

The educational background of the patient also plays an important role in his attitude with regard to the symptomatic meaning of a pain sensation. The more educated patients are more health-conscious and more aware of pain as a possible symptom of a dangerous disease. However, this factor plays a less important role than might be expected. The less educated "Old American" or Jewish patient is still more health-conscious than the more educated Italian. On the other hand, the less educated Jew is as much worried about the significance of pain as the more educated one. The education of the patient seems to be an important factor in fostering specific reactive patterns. The more educated patient, who may have more anxiety with regard to illness, may be more reserved in specific reactions to pain than an unsophisticated individual, who feels free to express his feelings and emotions.

· ·

The analysis of cultural factors in responses to pain is tentative and incomplete. It is based upon only one year of research which has been devoted exclusively to collection of raw material and formulation of working hypotheses. A detailed analysis of the interviews may call for revisions and reformulations of certain observations described in this paper. Nevertheless, the first objectives of our research have been attained in establishing the importance of the role of cultural factors in an area relatively little explored by the social sciences. We hope that in the course of further research we shall be able to expand our investigation into other areas of the pain problem, such as sex differences in attitudes toward pain, the role of age differences and the role of religious beliefs in the pain experience. We hope also that the final findings of the study will contribute to the growing field of collaboration between the social sciences and medicine for the better understanding of human problems.

Notes and References

1. This paper is based upon material collected as part of the study "Cultural Components in Attitudes toward Pain," under a grant of the U. S. Public Health Service.
2. James D. Hardy, Harold G. Wolff and Helen Goodell, *Pain Sensations and Reactions,* Williams and Wilkins Company, 1952, p. 23.
3. Ibid., p. 204.
4. Ibid., p. 262.
5. I should like to take the opportunity to express my appreciation to Dr. Harold G. Wolff, Professor of Neurology, Cornell University Medical College, Dr. Hiland Flowers, Chief of Neuropsychiatric Service, Dr. Robert Morrow, Chief of Clinical Psychology Section, Dr. Louis Berlin, Chief of Neurology Section, and the Management of the hospital for their cooperation in the setting up of the research at the Kingsbridge Veterans Hospital.
6. Italian respondents are mainly of South Italian origin; the Jewish respondents, with one exception, are all of East European origin. Whenever the Jews are mentioned they are spoken of in terms of the culture they represent and not in terms of their religion.

9

Chronic Illness

Anselm Strauss

Smallpox, diphtheria, polio, measles—conquered through immunization. Tuberculosis, leprosy, plague, yellow fever, malaria—defeated or checked by sanitation, improved living conditions and effective treatment.

In the old days, people who died from diseases contracted them quickly, reached crisis shortly thereafter, and either died or pulled through.

Modern medical researchers have changed this dramatic pattern by taming many once-devastating ailments. Improved conditions of living, along with effective medical skills and technology, have altered the nature of illness in scientifically advanced societies. While patients suffering from communicable diseases once filled most hospitals, treatment centers now serve mainly those afflicted with chronic ailments.

Many who would have died soon after contracting a disease now live and endure their affliction. Today most illnesses are chronic diseases—slow-acting, long-term killers that can be treated but not cured. A 1964 survey by the Department of Health, Education and Welfare indicates that about 40 percent of all Americans suffer from one or more chronic diseases; one out of every four so afflicted have lost some days at work because of disabling symptoms.

A large and growing body of medical literature presents detailed discussions of etiology, symptomatology, treatments and regimens. This outpouring of information, however, generally ignores a basic aspect of chronic illness—how to deal with such ailments in terms that are *social*—not simply medical. How can patients and professionals cope with health-related problems of family disruption, marital stress, role destruction and adjustment, stigmatization and even loss of body mobility?

Each chronic condition brings with it multiple problems of living. Among the most pressing are preventing and managing medical crises (that go even to death), managing regimens, controlling symptoms, organizing one's time efficiently, preventing or living with social isolation, adjusting to changes in the disease trajectory, and normalizing interaction and life, despite the disease. To handle those problems, people develop basic strategies which call for an organization of effort (including that of kinsmen, neighbors and health professionals). To establish and maintain this organization requires certain resources (financial, medical, familial and so forth), as well as interactional and social skills in order to make the necessary arrangements.

Medicine and the health professionals are very much included in this scheme but are neither at the scheme's focal point nor even constitute its primary elements. What is primary is simply the question of living: the difference between chronic sufferers and "normal people" merely being that the former must live with their diseases, their symptoms and often with their regimens. Medicine may contribute, but it is secondary to "carrying on."

Coping with Crises

Some chronic diseases carry a constant threat of grave medical crises. Diabetics may fall into insulin coma and die; epileptics can go into convulsions (which of themselves are not lethal) and be killed in a fall or a traffic accident. In order to prevent crises, minimize their effects, get the critically ill person into the hands of a physician or a hospital staff—and if need be actually save him—the person himself and possibly his kinsmen must be organized and prepared to handle all contingencies.

Relevant to the question of crises is how far they can go (to, or short of, death), how fast they appear, the clarity of advance warning signals to laymen or even to health professionals, the probability of recurrence, the predictability of their appearance, the complexity of the saving operations, and the speed and completeness of recovery from them.

The ability to read signs that portend a crisis is the first important step in managing chronic illness. Thus, diabetics or the parents of diabetic children learn how to recognize the signs of oncoming sugar shortage or insulin shock and what to do in case of actual crisis. Likewise, epileptics and sickle cell disease sufferers, if they are fortunate enough to have warning signs before their crises, learn to prepare themselves: if they are in public they get themselves to a place of safety and sit or lie down. Diabetics may carry instructions with them and may also carry those materials, like sugar or candy or insulin, which counteract the crisis; and epileptics may stuff handkerchiefs between their teeth just before convulsions.

When signs aren't properly read, are read too slowly or are interpreted as meaning something else, then people die or come close to dying. This may happen the first time a cardiac patient experiences severe chest pains and doesn't yet know their cause or treatment. (After the first sequence the patient may put his doctor's name close to the telephone for emergency use.) Even physicians may misread signs and so precipitate a crisis—even death. If an unconscious sickle cell anemia sufferer is brought bleeding to a hospital he may die if the natural immediate effort is made to stop his bleeding. Patients who carry instructions with them can sometimes avoid difficulties. Whenever an unconscious individual is brought into the emergency room of the nearest hospital, physicians there understandably may treat him for the wrong disease. Inexperienced patients who are on kidney dialysis machinery may not realize that their machinery is working incorrectly and that their bodies are nearing crisis. The complexity of the human body can cause even experienced persons to misread important signs.

Any breakdown or disruption of the crisis-preventing or crisis-coping organization can be disastrous. Family strain can lead to the abandonment of or lessening control over regimens, and temporary absence of "protective agents" or of "control agents" (such as mothers of diabetic children who are prone to eat too much candy) can also be traumatic. A divorce or separation that leaves an assisting agent (a mother helping her cystic-fibrosis child with absolutely necessary exercises) alone, unrelieved with her task, can gradually or quickly lead to a crisis. (One divorced couple arranged matters so that the father relieved the mother on weekends and some evenings.) Even an agent's illness can lead to the relaxation of regimens or the elimination of activities that might otherwise prevent crisis.

There is also a post-crisis period, in relation to the organization of effort. Some failure of organization right in the hospital can be seen when the staff begins to pull away from a cardiac patient, recently saved from a heart attack, but now judged "less critical" than other patients. Back home, of course, such patients require plenty of family organization to prevent additional attacks. What is not so evident is that the patient and his family may read signs of improvement where few exist, or that contingencies may arise which render faulty the organization for crisis prevention and crisis management. Relevant variables here are the length and rapidity of recovery—since both of these may vary for different disease conditions.

During an extended period of crisis the family may need to make special arrangements about their time (for visiting the hospital, for nursing the patient at home) and their living space (having the bed downstairs rather than upstairs, living near the hospital during the peak of the crisis). They may have to juggle the family's finances or spell each other in nursing the patient during his crisis. Even the patient himself—in trying to get better rather than giving up—may have to contribute to the necessary organization of effort to bring the family through the crisis period.

Unless the physician is absolutely helpless in the face of a given chronic disease, he will suggest or command some kind of regimen. Adhering to regimens, though, is a very complex matter, for regimens can sometimes set problems so difficult that they may present more hardships than the symptoms themselves.

Patients do not adhere to regimens automatically. Those who accept and maintain a regimen must have abiding trust in the physician, evidence that the requirements work without producing distressing or frightening side-effects (or that the side-effects are outweighed by symptom relief or fear of the disease itself), and the guarantee that important daily activities, either of the patient or of the people around him, can continue relatively uninterrupted.

In addition to the time it takes and the discomfort it causes, an important property of a given regimen is whether it is visible to other people, and what visibility may mean to the patient. If the regimen means that a stigmatized disease can be suspected or discovered, the person is unlikely to carry it out in public. (Tuberculosis patients sometimes have this problem.) If the visible regimen is no more than slightly embarrassing or is fully explainable, then its visibility is much less likely to prevent its maintenance in public or private.

Another property is also important: if the regimen appears to work for the patient, then that *may* convince him that he should continue with it. But continuance is problematic, not only because the other properties noted above may counteract his best intentions or his good sense, but because once a regimen has brought symptom relief, the patient may forego the routine—no matter what the physician says. This is exactly what happens when tuberculosis patients see their symptoms disappear, and figure that now they can cut out—partially or totally—their uncomfortable regimen.

The very properties of the regimen, then, constitute contributing conditions for adhering, relaxing or even rejecting the prescribed activities. Thus, if the patient simply denies that he has the disease (as with tuberculosis, where many patients experience no symptoms), he may not carry out his regimen. Instructions for a treatment routine may leave him confused or baffled: cardiac patients told to "rest" or "find their own limits" can be frustrated because they don't really know what "sufficient rest" means.

Patients and kinsmen inevitably enter into negotiations with each other, and sometimes with the physician, over relaxing or otherwise changing (substituting one drug for another, one activity for another) the regimen. They are negotiating not only over such matters as the elimination of discomfort and side-effects, but also the possibility of making the management of ordinary life easier or even possible. Physicians, of course, recognize much of this bargaining, but they may not realize just how high the stakes can be for the patient and his family. If a doctor ignores those factors, his patient may go shopping for another physician or, at the least, he may quietly alter his regimen or substitute part of it with something recommended by an amateur—pharmacist, friend or relative.

Symptom Management

The control of symptoms is obviously linked with adherence to effective regimens. Like adherence to regimen, symptom control is not merely a matter of medical management. Most of the time, the patient is far from medical facilities, so he and his family must rely upon their own judgment, wisdom and ingenuity in controlling symptoms—quite aside from faithfully following the prescribed regimens. Some physicians—probably not many—recognize that need for judgment.

Whatever the sophisticated technical references may be, the person who has symptoms will be concerned primarily with whether he hurts, faints, trembles visibly, has had his mobility or his speech impaired, or is evidencing some kind of disfigurement. How much they interfere with his life and social relationships depends on whether they are permanent or temporary, predictable or unpredictable, publicly visible or invisible; also on their degree (as of pain), their meaning to bystanders (as of disfigurement), the nature of the regimen called for to control the symptom, and of course on the kinds of lifestyle and social relations which the sufferer has been accustomed to.

Even minor, occasional symptoms may lead to some changing of habits, and major symptoms may call for the redesigning or reshaping of important aspects of a patient's life-style. Thus, someone who begins to suffer from minor back pains is likely to learn to avoid certain kinds of chairs and even discover to his dismay that a favorite sitting position is precisely the one he must forego. Major adjustments could include moving to a one-story house, buying clothes that cloak disfigurement, getting the boss to assign jobs that require less strength, using crutches or other aides to mobility. In one case a mailman suffering from colitis lived "on a leash" having arranged never to be very far from that necessary toilet. Emphysema patients learn to have "puffing stations" where they can recoup from lack of breath while looking like they have stopped normally.

Ideas for redesigning activities may come from others, too. A community nurse taught an emphysema patient how to rest while doing household chores; a sister taught a patient afflicted with brittle bones (because of a destructive drug) how to get up from the toilet, minus a back brace, without breaking bones in her back. Another woman figured out how her cardiac-arthritic grandfather could continue his beloved walks on his farm, by placing wooden stumps at short distances so that he could rest as he reached each one. Unfortunately, kinsmen and health professionals can function in just the opposite fashion: for instance, a woman with multiple sclerosis had carefully arranged her one-room apartment so that every object she needed was literally within arm's reach: but the public health nurse who visited her regarded the place as in a terrible shambles and proceeded to tidy things up herself.

Perhaps inventiveness, just as much as finances or material resources, is what makes the difference between reaching and not reaching some relatively satisfying redesign of life. The cancer patient with lessened energy who can ingeniously juggle her friends' visits and telephone calls can maintain a relatively unimpaired social life. Arthritic farm women who can get neighbors to bring in groceries can live on their farms during the summer although they must move to town for the winter months. One multiple sclerosis patient who is a student not only has rearranged her apartment but persuaded various people to help her manage despite her increasingly restricted mobility. A veritable army of people have come to her aid: the university architect redesigned certain of the public toilets for her wheelchair and also put in some ramps; the handy men around the university help her up and down stairs, by appointment; they also have rebuilt her cupboards so that she can reach them from her wheelchair; and so on.

Lack of imagination about useful redesigning makes symptom control harder. This lack of imaginative forethought can be seen in many homes for the elderly where stiff-jointed or low-energy people must struggle to rise from sitting positions on low sofas and chairs, or must painstakingly pick their way along highly polished corridors—minus handrails.

The reshaping of activities pertains also to the crucial issue of "interaction." A variety of judicious or clever maneuvers can keep one's symptoms as inobtrusive as possible. Sometimes the tactics are very simple: a college teacher with bronchitis, whose peak load of coughing up sputum is in the morning, arranges his teaching schedule so that he can stay at home, or at least in his office, until after lunchtime. Another person who tends continually to have a runny allergic nose always carries tissue in her hand when in public. Another with a tendency to cough carries cough drops with him—especially important when he attends concerts. An epileptic may have to persuade acquaintances that his epileptic fits are not communicable! Emphysema sufferers learn to sit down or lean against buildings in such a fashion that they are not mistaken for drunks or loiterers.

Agents of various kinds can also be useful—wives who scout out the terrain at a public meeting to find the least obtrusive spot, and then pass on the information to their husbands in wheelchairs or on crutches. Spouses may have prearranged signals to warn each other when a chronic symptom (for example, runny nose) starts appearing. In a more dramatic instance a couple was attending a party when the husband noticed his wife's temporarily slurred speech—a sign of her tiredness and pain from cancer. Since they did not want to have their friends know of her illness, he acted quickly to divert the others' attention and soon afterward manufactured an excuse so that they could leave the party.

When visible symptoms cannot easily be disguised, misleading explanations may be offered—fainting, for instance, is explained away by someone "in the know" as a temporary weakness due to flu or to some other reasonable cause. When a symptom cannot be minimized, then a wife may attempt to prepare others for the distressing sight or sound of her husband's affliction. The sufferer himself may do this, as when a cancer patient who had lost much weight warned friends, over the phone, that when they visited they would find her not looking like herself at all. Each friend who visits is very likely, in turn, to warn other friends what to expect.

Various chronic diseases lead to such disruption that they call for some temporal re-ordering. One all-too-familiar problem is too much time. It may only be temporary, as with persons who are waiting out a post-crisis period, but, for the disabled elderly or victims of multiple sclerosis, it may be a permanent condition. Among the consequences are boredom, decreased social skills, family strains, negative impact on identity and even physical deterioration.

Just as common is not enough time. Not only is time sopped up by regimens and by symptom control, but those who assist the patient may expend many hours on their particular tasks. Not to be totally engulfed, they in turn may need to get assistants (babysitters, housecleaners, cooks) or redistribute the family workload. Occasionally the regimens require so much time, or crises come so frequently (some sickle cell anemia sufferers have been hospitalized up to 100 times), that life simply gets organized around those events; there is not enough time for much of anything else. Even just handling one's symptoms or the consequences of having symptoms may require so much time that life is taken up mainly with handling them. Thus, a very serious dermatological condition forced one woman to spend hour after hour salving her skin; otherwise she would have suffered unbearably. Unfortunately, the people who suffer cannot leave their bodies. Kinsmen and other assisting agents, however, may abandon their charges out of desperation for what the temporal engulfment is doing to their own lives. Abandonment, here, may mean shifting the burdens to a nursing home or other custodial institution, such as a state mental institution.

The term "dying trajectory" means the course of dying as defined by various participants in it. Analogously, one can also think of the course of the chronic disease (downward in most instances). Like the dying trajectory, that course can be conceived as having two properties. First, it takes place over time: it has duration. Specific trajectories can vary greatly in duration. Some start earlier, some end later. Second, a trajectory has shape. It may plunge straight down; it may move slowly but steadily downward; it may vacillate slowly, moving slightly up and down before diving downward radically; it may move slowly down at first, then hit a long plateau, then plunge abruptly even to death. Neither the duration nor shape of a dying trajectory is a purely objective physiological property. Both are perceived properties; their dimensions depend on when the perceiver initially defines someone as diseased and on his expectations of how the disease course will proceed. (We can add further that the dying trajectory consists merely of the last phases of some chronic disease trajectories.) Each type of disease (multiple sclerosis, diabetes and so forth) or subtype (different kinds of arthritis) may have a range of variation in trajectory, but they certainly tend to be patterned in accordance with duration and shape.

It would be much too simplistic to assert that specific trajectories determine what happens to a sense of identity; but certainly they do contribute, and quite possibly in *patterned* ways. Identity responses to a severe heart attack may be varied, but awareness that death can be but a moment away—every day—probably cannot but have a different impact on identity than trajectories expected to result in slow death, or in leaving one a "vegetable" or perfectly alive but a hopeless cripple.

We have alluded to the loss of social contact, even extending to great social isolation, that may be a consequence of chronic disease and its management. This loss is understandable given the accompanying symptoms, crises, regimens and often difficult phasing of trajectories.

It is not difficult to trace some of the impact on social contact of varying symptoms, in accordance with their chief properties. The disfigurement associated with leprosy leads many to stay in leper colonies; they prefer the social ease and normal relationships that are possible there. Diseases which are (or which the sufferer thinks are) stigmatizing are kept as secret as possible. But talking about his illness with friends who may understand can be comforting. Some may find new friends (even spouses) among fellow sufferers, especially through clinic visits or special clubs formed around the illness or disability (such as those formed by kidney failure victims and people who have had ileostomies). Some virtually make careers of doing voluntary work for those clubs or associations. People can also leave circles of friends whom they feel might now be unresponsive, frightened or critical and move to more sympathetic social terrain. An epileptic who has used a warning tactic and has moved to a supportive terrain said:

> I'm lucky, I still have friends. Most people who have epilepsy are put to the side. But I'm lucky that way. I tell them that I have epilepsy and that they shouldn't get scared if I fall out. I go to things at the church—it's the church people that are my friends. I just tell them and then it is okay. They just laugh about it and don't get upset.

Some people may choose to allow their diseases to advance rather than put up with their regimens. One cardiac patient, for instance, simply refused to give up his weekly evening playing cards with "the boys"—replete with smoking, beer drinking and late hours—despite his understanding that this could lead to further heart attacks. Another cardiac patient avoided coffee breaks at work because everyone smoked then. He stayed away from many social functions for the same reasons. He felt that people probably thought him "unsociable," but he was not able to think of any other way to stop himself from smoking. Perhaps the extreme escape from—not minimization or prevention of—social isolation was exhibited by one woman with kidney disease who chose to go off dialysis (she had no possibility of getting a transplant), opting for a speedy death because she saw an endless time ahead, dependence on others, inability to hold down a job, increasing social isolation and a purposeless life. Her physicians accepted her right to make this choice.

Those who cannot face physically altered friends may avoid or even abandon them. One individual who was losing weight because of cancer remarked bitterly that a colleague of his had ducked down the street, across campus, to avoid meeting him. Spouses who have known great intimacy together can draw apart because of an illness: a cardiac husband may fear having sex or may be afraid of dying but cannot tell his wife for fear of increasing *her* anxiety. The awkwardness that others feel about discussing death and fear of it isolates many chronically ill people from their friends— even from their spouses. During the last phases of a disease trajectory, an unbridgeable gap may open up between previously intimate spouses.

Even aside from the question of death fears, friends may draw apart because the patient is physically isolated from the mainstream of life. One stroke patient who temporarily lost the ability to speak described what happened between himself and his friends: "I felt unguarded and my colleagues—who pretty soon found their conversation drying up in the lack of anything from me—felt bored, or at any rate I thought they were. My wife, who was ususally present, saved the conversation from dying—she was never at loss for a word." A cardiac patient hospitalized away from his home town at first received numerous cards and telephone calls, but once his friends had reached across the distance they chose to leave him alone, doubtless for a variety of reasons. He and his wife began to feel slightly abandoned. Later, when he had returned to part-time work, he found that his fellow executives left him relatively alone at first, knowing that he was far from recuperated. Despite his conscious knowledge that his colleagues were trying to help, he still felt out of things.

Friends and relatives may withdraw from patients who are making excessive demands or who have undergone personality changes caused by a crisis or the progress of a disease. Abandonment may be the final result. Husbands desert, spouses separate and adult children place their elderly parents in nursing homes. In some kinds of chronic diseases, especially stigmatic (leprosy) or terribly demanding (mental illness), friends and relatives and even physicians advise the spouse or kinsmen quite literally to abandon the sick person: "It's time to put her in the hospital." "Think of the children." "Think of yourself—it makes no sense." "It's better for her, and you are only keeping her at home because of your own guilt." These are just some of the abandonment rationales that are offered, or which the person offers himself. Of course, the sick person, aware of having become virtually an intolerable burden, may offer those rationales also—though not necessarily alleviating his own sense of estrangement.

The chief business of a chronically ill person is not just to stay alive or to keep his symptoms under control, but to live as normally as possible despite his symptoms and his disease. In the case of chronically ill children, parents work very hard at creating some semblance of a normal life for their offspring. "Closed awareness" or secrecy is the ruling principle of family life. No one tells the child he is dying. Parents of children with leukemia, for example, have a very difficult time. For much of the time, the child actually may look quite well and live a normal life—but his parents have to work very hard at *acting* normal unless they can keep the impending death well at the back of their minds. The parents with children with longer life expectancies need not work so hard to maintain a normal atmosphere in their homes, except insofar as the child may rebel against aspects of a restrictive regimen which he feels makes *his* life abnormal. Some of the difficulties which chronic sufferers experience in maintaining normal interaction are reflected in the common complaint that blind and physically handicapped people make—that people assume they cannot walk and work like ordinary mortals, but rush up to help them do what they are quite capable of doing as anyone else. The non-sick, especially strangers, tend to overemphasize the sick person's visible symptoms, so that they come to dominate the interaction. The sick person fights back by using various tactics to disavow his deviant status: he hides the intrusive symptom—covers it with clothes, puts the trembling hand under the table—or if it can't be hidden, then minimizes its impact by taking attention away from it—like a dying woman who has lost a great deal of weight but who forces visitors to ignore her condition by talking cheerfully and normally about their mutual interests.

Artful Striving

In setting guidelines for "acting normal" there is much room for disagreement between the ill person and those near to him about just how ill he is. The sick person may choose more invalidism than his condition really warrants. After a crisis or a peak period of symptoms, the sick person may find himself rushed by others—including his helping agents—who either misjudge his return to better health—or simply forget how sick he might still be since he does not show more obvious signs of his current condition. All patients who have partial-recovery trajectories necessarily run that hazard. ("Act sicker than you look or they will quickly forget you were so ill" was the advice given to one cardiac patient who was about to return to his executive job.)

The more frequent reverse phenomenon is when the sick person believes his condition is more normal than others believe. His friends and relatives tell him, "Take it easy, don't rush things." His physician warns him that he will harm himself, even kill himself, if he doesn't act in accordance with the facts of his case. But it sometimes happens that the person really has a very accurate notion of just how he feels. One man who had had a kidney transplant found himself having to prove to his fellow workers that he was not handicapped—doing extra work to demonstrate his normality. A slightly different case is the ill person who may know just how ill he is but wishes others to regard him as less ill and allow him to act accordingly. One dying man who was trying to live as normally as possible right down through his last days found himself rejecting those friends, however well intentioned, who regarded him as "dying now" rather than as "living fully to the end."

As the trajectory of the ill person's health continues downward, he may have to come to terms with a lessened degree of normality. We can see this very clearly with those who are slowly dying, when both they and their friends or kinsmen are quite willing to settle for "something less" at each phase of the downward trajectory, thankful at least for small things. It is precisely when the chronically ill cannot settle for lower levels of functioning that they opt out of this life. When their friends and relatives cannot settle for less, or have settled for as much as they can stand, then they too opt out of his life: by separation, divorce or abandonment. Those who are chronically ill from diseases like multiple sclerosis or other severe forms of neurological illness (or mental illness, for that matter) are likely to have to face this kind of abandonment by others. The chronically ill themselves, as well as many of their spouses, kinsmen and friends, are remarkably able to accommodate themselves to increasingly lower levels of normal interaction and style; they can do this either because of immense closeness to each other or because they are grateful even for what little life and relationship remain. They strive manfully—and artfully—to "keep things normal" at whatever level that has come to mean.

We must not forget, either, that symptoms and trajectories may stabilize for long periods of time, or in fact not change for the worst at all: then the persons so afflicted simply come to accept, on a long-term basis, whatever restrictions are placed on their lives. Like Franklin D. Roosevelt, they live perfectly normal (even super-normal!) lives in all respects except for whatever handicaps may derive from their symptoms or their medical regimens. To keep interaction normal, they need only develop the requisite skills to make others ignore or de-emphasize their disabilities.

Helping those afflicted with chronic diseases means far more than simply displaying compassion or having medical competence. Only through knowledge of and sensitivity to the *social* aspects of symptom control, regimen management, crisis prevention, handling dying and death itself, can one develop truly beneficial strategies and tactics for dealing with specific diseases and chronic illness in general.

The Social Organization of Medical Care

In Part Two we turn from the production of disease and illness to the social organizations created to treat it. Here we begin to examine the institutional aspects of health and illness—the medical care system. We look at the social organization of medical care historically, structurally, and, finally, interactionally. We seek to understand how this complex system operates and how its particular characteristics have contributed to the current health care crisis.

The Professionalization of Medicine: Creating a Monopoly

PHYSICIANS HAVE A PROFESSIONAL MONOPOLY of medical practice in America. They have an exclusive state-supported right, manifested in the "licensing" of physicians, to medical practice. With their licenses, physicians can legally do what no one else can, including cutting into the human body and prescribing drugs.

Until the latter part of the nineteenth century various groups and individuals (homeopaths, midwives, botanical doctors, etc.) competed for the "medical turf." By the second decade of this century virtually only M.D. physicians had the legal right to practice medicine in this country. One might suggest that physicians achieved their exclusive rights to the nation's medical territory because of their superior scientific and clinical achievements, a line of reasoning which suggests that physicians demonstrated superior healing and curative skills and the government therefore supported their rights against less effective healers and quacks. But this seems not to have been the case. As we noted earlier, most of the improvement in the health status of the population resulted from social changes, including better nutrition, sanitation, and a rising standard of living rather than from the interventions of clinical medicine. Medical techniques were in fact rather limited, often even dangerous, until the early twentieth century. As L. J. Henderson observed, " . . . somewhere between 1910 and 1912 in this country, a random patient, with a random disease, consulting a doctor chosen at random, had, for the first time in the history of mankind, a better than fifty-fifty chance of profiting from the encounter" (quoted in Blumgart, 1964).

The success of the American Medical Association (AMA) in consolidating medical power in its own organizational hands was central to the securing of a monopoly for M.D. physicians. Although the AMA has lost some power recently to the "corporate rationalizers" in medicine (e.g., health insurance industry, hospital organizations [Alford, 1972]), its monopoly over professional practice remains intact. (The creation and maintenance of this medical monopoly has been more of a political than a scientific achievement.) By virtue of their monopoly of medical practice, physicians have been able to gain dominance over the entire field of medicine, including the right to define what constitutes disease and how to treat it. As Freidson (1970a:251) has observed, "The medical profession has first claim to jurisdiction over the label illness and *anything* to which it may be attached, irrespective of its capacity to deal with it effectively."

Physicians also gained "professional dominance" over the organization of medical services in the United States (Freidson: 1970b). This monopoly gave the medical profession functional autonomy and a structural insulation from outside evaluations of medical practice. In addition, professional dominance includes not only the exclusive right to treat disease, but also the right to limit and evaluate the performance of most other medical-care workers. Finally, the particular vision of medicine that became institutionalized included a "clinical mentality" (Freidson, 1970a) which focused on medical responsibility to *individual* patients rather than to the community or public.

In the first essay in this section, "Professionalization, Monopoly, and the Structure of Medical Practice," Peter Conrad and Joseph W. Schneider present a brief review of the historical development of this medical monopoly. They examine the case of abortion in the nineteenth century to highlight how specific medical interests were served by a physician-led crusade against abortion. By successfully outlawing abortion and institutionalizing their own professional ethics, "regular" physicians were able to eliminate effectively some of their competitors and secure greater control of the medical market.

Richard W. Wertz and Dorothy C. Wertz expand on this theme of monopolization and professional dominance in "Notes on the Decline of Midwives and the Rise of Medical Obstetricians." They investigate the medicalization of childbirth historically and the subsequent decline of midwifery in this country. Female midwifery, which continues to be practiced in most industrialized and developing countries, has been virtually eliminated in the United States. Wertz and Wertz show that it was not merely professional imperialism that led to the exclusion of midwives (although this played an important role), but also a subtle and profound sexism within and outside the medical profession. They postulate that the physicians' monopolization of childbirth resulted from a combination of a change in middle-class women's views of birthing, physicians' economic interests, and the development of sexist notions which suggested that women weren't suitable for attending births. Physicians became increasingly interventionist in their childbirth practice partly due to their training (they felt they had to "do" something) and their desire to use instruments "to establish superior status" and treat childbirth as an illness rather than a natural event. In recent years we have seen the re-emergence of nurse midwives, but their work is usually limited to hospitals under medical dominance (Rothman, 1979). Also, there are presently a small number of "lay" midwives whose practice is confined to quasi-illegal situations outside of medical control (See Arms, 1975).

In the final article in this section, "Professional Dominance and the Ordering of Health Services," Eliot Freidson analyzes some of the consequences of professional monopolization. He first describes medicine as having an "organized autonomy" and then shows how it also has a professional dominance over the medical division of labor. He describes how professional practice, rather than bureaucratic organization, contributes to the discomfort and dissatisfaction patients experience in medical encounters. Freidson notes that the jurisdiction of medicine is widening and that the profession exerts an unwarranted influence on the planning and financing of services in the health field.

References

Alford, Robert. 1972. "The political economy of health care: Dynamics without change." Politics and Society. 2: 127–164.

Arms, Suzanne. 1975. Immaculate Deception. Boston: Houghton Mifflin Company.

Blumgart, H. L. 1964. "Caring for the patient." New England Journal of Medicine. 270:449–56.

Freidson, Eliot. 1970a. Profession of Medicine. New York: Dodd, Mead.

———. 1970b. Professional Dominance. Chicago: Aldine.

Rothman, Barbara Katz. 1979. Two Models of Maternity Care: Defining and Negotiating Reality. Unpublished Ph.D. Dissertation, New York University.

10

Professionalization, Monopoly, and the Structure of Medical Practice

Peter Conrad and Joseph W. Schneider

· ·

Medicine has not always been the powerful, prestigious, successful, lucrative, and dominant profession we know today. The status of the medical profession is a product of medical politicking as well as therapeutic expertise. This discussion presents a brief overview of the development of the medical profession and its rise to dominance.

Emergence of the Medical Profession: up to 1850

In ancient societies, disease was given supernatural explanations, and "medicine" was the province of priests or shamans. It was in classical Greece that medicine began to emerge as a separate occupation and develop its own theories, distinct from philosophy or theology. Hippocrates, the great Greek physician who refused to accept supernatural explanations or treatments for disease, developed a theory of the "natural" causes of disease and systematized all available medical knowledge. He laid a basis for the development of medicine as a separate body of knowledge. Early Christianity depicted sickness as punishment for sin, engendering new theological explanations and treatments. Christ and his disciples believed in the supernatural causes and cures of disease. This view became institutionalized in the Middle Ages, when the Church dogma dominated theories and practice of medicine and priests were physicians. The Renaissance in Europe brought a renewed interest in ancient Greek medical knowledge. This marked the beginning of a drift toward natural explanations of disease and the emergence of medicine as an occupation separate from the Church (Cartwright, 1977).

But European medicine developed slowly. The "humoral theory" of disease developed by Hippocrates dominated medical theory and practice until well into the 19th century. Medical diagnosis was impressionistic and often inaccurate, depicting conditions in such general terms as "fevers" and "fluxes." In the 17th century, physicians relied mainly on three techniques to determine the nature of illness: what the patient said about symptoms; the physician's own observations of signs of illness and the patient's appearance and behavior; and more rarely, a manual examination of the body (Reiser, 1978, p. 1). Medicine was by no means scientific, and "medical thought involved unverified doctrines and resulting controversies" (Shryock, 1960, p. 52). Medical practice was a "bedside medicine" that was patient oriented and did not distinguish the illness from the "sick man" (Jewson, 1976). It was not until Thomas Sydenham's astute observations in the late 17th century that physicians could begin to distinguish between the patient and the disease. Physicians possessed few treatments that worked regularly, and many of their treatments actually worsened the sufferer's condition. Medicine in colonial America inherited this European stock of medical knowledge.

Colonial American medicine was less developed than its European counterpart. There were no medical schools and few physicians, and because of the vast frontier and sparse population, much medical care was in effect self-help. Most American physicians were educated and trained by apprenticeship; few were university trained. With the exception of surgeons, most were undifferentiated practitioners. Medical practices were limited. Prior to the revolution, physicians did not commonly attend births; midwives, who were not seen as part of the medical establishment, routinely attended birthings (Wertz and Wertz, 1977). William Rothstein (1972) notes that "American colonial medical practice, like European practice of the period, was characterized by the lack of any substantial body of usable scientific knowledge" (p. 27). Physicians, both educated and otherwise, tended to treat their patients pragmatically, for medical theory had little to offer. Most colonial physicians practiced medicine only part-time, earning their livelihoods as clergymen, teachers, farmers, or in other occupations. Only in the early 19th century did medicine become a full-time vocation (Rothstein, 1972).

The first half of the 19th century saw important changes in the organization of the medical profession. About 1800, "regular," or educated, physicians convinced state legislatures to pass laws limiting the practice of medicine to practitioners of a certain training and class (prior to this nearly anyone could claim the title "doctor" and practice medicine). These state licensing laws were not particularly effective, largely because of the colonial tradition of medical self-help. They were repealed in most states during the Jacksonian period (1828-1836) because they were thought to be elitist, and the temper of the times called for a more "democratic" medicine.

The repeal of the licensing laws and the fact that most "regular" (i.e., regularly educated) physicians shared and used "a distinctive set of medically invalid therapies, known as 'heroic' therapy," created fertile conditons for the emergence of *medical sects* in the first half of the 19th century (Rothstein, 1972, p. 21). Physicians of the time practiced a "heroic" and invasive form of medicine consisting primarily of such treatments as bloodletting, vomiting, blistering, and purging. This highly interventionist, and sometimes dangerous, form of medicine engendered considerable public opposition and resistance. In this context a number of medical sects emerged, the most important of which were the homeopathic and botanical physicians. These "irregular" medical practitioners practiced less invasive, less dangerous forms of medicine. They each developed a considerable following, since their therapies were probably no less effective than those of regulars practicing heroic medicine. The regulars attempted to exclude them from practice; so the various sects set up their own medical schools and professional societies. This sectarian medicine created a highly *competitive* situation for the regulars (Rothstein, 1972). Medical sectarianism, heroic therapies, and ineffective treatment contributed to the low status and lack of prestige of early 19th-century medicine. At this time, medicine was neither a prestigious occupation nor an important economic activity in American society (Starr, 1977).

The regular physicians were concerned about this situation. Large numbers of regularly trained physicians sought to earn a livelihood by practicing medicine (Rothstein, 1972, p. 3). They were troubled by the poor image of medicine and lack of standards in medical training and practice. No doubt they were also concerned about the competition of the irregular sectarian physicians. A group of regular physicians founded the American Medical Association (AMA) in 1847 "to promote the science and art of medicine and the betterment of public health" (quoted in Coe, 1978, p. 204). The AMA also was to set and enforce standards and ethics of "regular" medical practice and strive for exclusive professional and economic rights to the medical turf.

The AMA was the crux of the regulars' attempt to "professionalize" medicine. As Magali Sarfatti Larson (1977) points out, professions organize to create and control *markets*. Organized professions attempt to regulate and limit the competition, usually by controlling professional education and by limiting licensing. Professionalization is, in this view, "the process by which producers of special services sought to constitute *and control* the market for their expertise" (Larson, 1977, p. xvi). The regular physicians and the AMA set out to consolidate and control the market for medical services. As we shall see in the next two sections, the regulars were successful in professionalization, eliminating competition and creating a medical monopoly.

Crusading, Deviance, and Medical Monopoly: The Case of Abortion

The medical profession after the middle of the 19th century was frequently involved in various activities that could be termed social reform. Some of these reforms were directly related to health and illness and medical work; others were peripheral to the manifest medical calling of preventing illness and healing the sick. In these reform movements, physicians became medical crusaders, attempting to influence public morality and behavior. This medical crusading often led physicians squarely into the moral sphere, making them advocates for moral positions that had only peripheral relations to medical practice. Not infrequently these reformers sought to change people's values or to impose a set of particular values on others. . . . We now examine one of the more revealing examples of medical crusading: the criminalization of abortion in American society.[1]

Most people are under the impression that abortion was always defined as deviant and illegal in America prior to the Supreme Court's landmark decision in 1973. This, however, is not the case. American abortion policy, and the attendant defining of abortion as deviant, were specific products of medical crusading. Prior to the Civil War, abortion was a common and largely legal medical procedure performed by various types of physicians and midwives. A pregnancy was not considered confirmed until the occurrence of a phenomenon called "quickening," the first perception of fetal movement. Common law did not recognize the fetus before quickening in criminal cases, and an unquickened fetus was deemed to have no living soul. Thus most people did not consider termination of pregnancy before quickening to be an especially serious matter, much less murder. Abortion before quickening created no moral or medical problems. Public opinion was indifferent, and for the time it was probably a relatively safe medical procedure. Thus, for all intents and purposes, American women were free to terminate their pregnancies before quickening in the early 19th century. Moreover, it was a procedure relatively free of the moral stigma that was attached to abortion in this century.

After 1840 abortion came increasingly into public view. Abortion clinics were vigorously and openly advertised in newspapers and magazines. The advertisements offered euphemistically couched services for "women's complaints," "menstrual blockage," and "obstructed menses." Most contemporary observers suggested that more and more women were using these services. Prior to 1840 most abortions were performed on the unmarried and desperate of the "poor and unfortunate classes." However, beginning about this time, significantly increasing numbers of middle- and upper-class white, Protestant, native-born women began to use these services. It is likely they either wished to delay childbearing or thought they already had all the children they wanted (Mohr, 1978, pp. 46-47). By

1870 approximately one abortion was performed for every five live births (Mohr, 1978, pp. 79–80).

Beginning in the 1850s, a number of physicians, especially moral crusader Dr. Horatio Robinson Storer, began writing in medical and popular journals and lobbying in state legislatures about the danger and immorality of abortion. They opposed abortion before and after quickening and under Dr. Storer's leadership organized an aggressive national campaign. In 1859 these crusaders convinced the AMA to pass a resolution condemning abortion. Some newspapers, particularly *The New York Times,* joined the antiabortion crusade. Feminists supported the crusade, since they saw abortion as a threat to women's health and part of the oppression of women. Religious leaders, however, by and large avoided the issue of abortion; either they didn't consider it in their province or found it too sticky an issue to discuss. It was the physicians who were the guiding force in the antiabortion crusade. They were instrumental in convincing legislatures to pass state laws, especially between 1866 and 1877, that made abortion a criminal offense.

Why did physicians take the lead in the antiabortion crusade and work so directly to have abortion defined as deviant and illegal? Undoubtedly they believed in the moral "rightness" of their cause. But social historian James Mohr (1978) presents two more subtle and important reasons for the physicians' antiabortion crusading. First, concern was growing among medical people and even among some legislators about the significant drop in birthrates. Many claimed that abortion among married women of the "better classes" was a major contributor to the declining birthrate. These middle- and upper-class men (the physicians and legislators) were aware of the waves of immigrants arriving with large families and were anxious about the decline in production of native American babies. They were deeply afraid they were being betrayed by their own women (Mohr, 1978, p. 169). Implicitly the antiabortion stance was classist and racist; the anxiety was simply that there would not be enough strong, native-born, Protestant stock to save America. This was a persuasive argument in convincing legislators of the need of antiabortion laws.

The second and more direct reason spurring the physicians in the antiabortion crusade was to aid their own nascent professionalization and create a monopoly for regular physicians. . . . the regulars had formed the AMA in 1847 to promote scientific and ethical medicine and combat what they saw as medical quackery. There were, however, no licensing laws to speak of, and many claimed the title "doctor" (e.g., homeopaths, botanical doctors, eclectic physicians). The regular physicians adopted the Hippocratic oath and code of ethics as their standard. Among other things, this oath forbids abortion. Regulars usually did not perform abortions; however, many practitioners of medical sects performed abortions regularly, and some had lucrative practices. Thus for the regular AMA physicians the limitation of abortion became one way of asserting their own professional domination over other medical practitioners. In their crusading these physicians had translated the social goals of cultural and professional dominance into moral and medical language. They lobbied long and hard to convince legislators of the danger and immorality of abortion. By passage of laws making abortion criminal any time during gestation, regular physicians were able to legislate their code of ethics and get the state to employ sanctions against their competitors. This limited these competitors' markets and was a major step toward the regulars' achieving a monopolization of medical practice.

In a relatively short period the antiabortion crusade succeeded in passing legislation that made abortion criminal in every state. A by-product of this was a shift in American public opinion from an indifference to and tolerance of abortion to a hardening of attitudes against what had until then been a fairly common practice. The irony was that abortion as a medical procedure probably was safer at the turn of the 20th century than a century before, but it was defined and seen as more dangerous. By 1900 abortion was not only illegal but deviant and immoral. The physicians' moral crusade had successfully defined abortion as a deviant activity. This definition remained largely unchanged until the 1973 Supreme Court decision, which essentially returned the abortion situation to its pre-1850 condition.

. . . .

Growth of Medical Expertise and Professional Dominance

Although the general public's dissatisfaction with heroic medicine remained, the image of medicine and what it could accomplish was improving by the middle of the 19th century. There had been a considerable reduction in the incidence and mortality of certain dread diseases. The plague and leprosy had nearly disappeared. Smallpox, malaria, and cholera were less devastating than ever before. These improvements in health engendered optimism and increased people's faith in medical practice. Yet these dramatic "conquests of disease" were by and large *not* the result of new medical knowledge or improved clinical medical practice. Rather, they resulted from changes in social conditions: a rising standard of living, better nutrition and housing, and public health innovations like sanitation. With the lone exception of vaccination for smallpox, the decline of these diseases had nearly nothing to do with clinical medicine (Dubos, 1959; McKeown, 1971). But despite lack of effective treatments, medicine was the beneficiary of much popular credit for improved health.

The regular physicians' image was improved well before they demonstrated any unique effectiveness of practice. The AMA's attacks on irregular medical practice continued. In the 1870s the regulars convinced legislatures to outlaw abortion and in some states to restore licensing laws to restrict medical practice. The AMA was becoming an increasingly powerful and authoritative voice representing regular medical practice.

But the last three decades of the century saw significant "breakthroughs" in medical knowledge and treatment. The scientific medicine of the regular physicians was making new medical advances. Anesthesia and antisepsis made possible great strides in surgical medicine and improvements in hospital care. The bacteriological research of Koch and Pasteur developed the "germ theory of disease," which had important applications in medical practice. It was the accomplishments of surgery and bacteriology that put medicine on a scientific basis (Freidson, 1970a, p. 16). The rise of scientific medicine marked a death knell for medical sectarianism (e.g., the homeopathic physicians eventually joined the regulars). The new laboratory sciences provided a way of testing the theories and practices of various sects, which ultimately led to a single model of medical practice. The well-organized regulars were able to legitimate their form of medical practice and support it with "scientific" evidence.

With the emergence of scientific medicine, a unified paradigm, or model, of medical practice developed. It was based, most fundamentally, on viewing the body as a machine (e.g., organ malfunctioning) and on the germ theory of disease (Kelman, 1977). The "doctrine of specific etiology" became predominant: each disease was caused by a specific germ or agent. Medicine focused solely on the internal environment (the body), largely ignoring the external environment (society) (Dubos, 1959). This paradigm proved fruitful in ensuing years. It is the essence of the "medical model". . . .

The development of scientific medicine accorded regular medicine a convincing advantage in medical practice. It set the stage for the achievement of a medical monopoly by the AMA regulars. As Larson (1977) notes, "Once scientific medicine offered sufficient guarantees of its superior effectiveness in dealing with disease, the state willingly contributed to the creation of a monopoly by means of registration and licensing" (p. 23). The new licensing laws created regular medicine as a *legally enforced monopoly of practice* (Freidson, 1970b, p. 83). They virtually eliminated medical competition.

The medical monopoly was enhanced further by the Flexner Report on medical education in 1910. Under the auspices of the Carnegie Foundation, medical educator Abraham Flexner visited nearly all 160 existing medical schools in the United States. He found the level of medical education poor and recommended the closing of most schools. Flexner urged stricter state laws, rigid standards for medical education, and more rigorous examinations for certification to practice. The enactment of Flexner's recommendations effectively made all nonscientific types of medicine illegal. It created a near total AMA monopoly of medical education in America.

In securing a monopoly, the AMA regulars achieved a unique professional state. Medicine not only monopolized the market for medical services and the training of physicians, it developed an unparalleled "professional dominance." The medical profession was *functionally autonomous* (Freidson, 1970b). Physicians were insulated from external evaluation and were by and large free to regulate their own performance. Medicine could define its own territory and set its own standards. Thus, Eliot Freidson (1970b) notes, "while the profession may not everywhere be free to control the *terms* of its work, it is free to control the *content* of its work" (p. 84).

The domain of medicine has expanded in the past century. This is due partially to the prestige medicine has accrued and its place as the steward of the "sacred" value of life. Medicine has sometimes been called on to repeat its "miracles" and successful treatments on problems that are not biomedical in nature. Yet in other instances the expansion is due to explicit medical crusading or entrepreneurship. This expansion of medicine, especially into the realm of social problems and human behavior, frequently has taken medicine beyond its proven technical competence (Freidson, 1970b). . . .

The organization of medicine has also expanded and become more complex in this century. In the next section we briefly describe the structure of medical practice in the United States.

Structure of Medical Practice

Before we leave our discussion of the medical profession, it is worthwhile to outline some general features of the structure of medical practice that have contributed to the expansion of medical jurisdiction.

The medical sector of society has grown enormously in the 20th century. It has become the second largest industry in America. There are about 350,000 physicians and over 5 million people employed in the medical field. The "medical industries," including the pharmaceutical, medical technology, and health insurance industries, are among the most profitable in our economy. Yearly drug sales alone are over $4.5 billion. There are more than 7000 hospitals in the United States with 1.5 million beds and 33 million inpatient and 200 million outpatient visits a year (McKinlay, 1976).

The organization of medical practice has changed. Whereas the single physician in "solo practice" was typical in 1900, today physicians are engaged increasingly in large corporate practices or employed by hospitals or other bureaucratic organizations. Medicine in modern society is becoming bureaucratized (Mechanic, 1976). The power in medicine has become diffused, especially since World War II, from the AMA, which represented the individual physician, to include the organizations that represent bureaucratic medicine: the health insurance industry, the medical schools, and the American Hospital Association (Ehrenreich and Ehrenreich, 1970). Using Robert Alford's (1972) conceptualizations, corporate rationalizers have taken much of the power in medicine from the professional monopolists.

Medicine has become both more specialized and more dependent on technology. In 1929 only 25 percent of American physicians were fulltime specialists; by 1969 the proportion had grown to 75 percent (Reiser, 1978). Great advances were made in medicine, and many were directly related to technology: miracle medicines like penicillin, a myriad of psychoactive drugs, heart and brain surgery, the electrocardiograph, CAT scanners, fetal monitors, kidney dialysis machines, artificial organs, and transplant surgery, to name but a few. The hospital has become the primary medical workshop, a center for technological medicine.

Medicine has made a significant economic expansion. In 1940, medicine claimed about 4 percent of the American gross national product (GNP); today it claims about 9 percent, which amounts to more than $150 billion. The causes for this growth are too complex to describe here, but a few factors should be noted. American medicine has always operated on a "fee-for-service" basis, that is, each service rendered is charged and paid for separately. Simply put, in a capitalist medical system, the more services provided, the more fees collected. This not only creates an incentive to provide more services but also to expand these medical services to new markets. The fee-for-service system may encourage unnecessary medical care. There is some evidence, for example, that American medicine performs a considerable amount of "excess" surgery (McCleery and Keelty, 1971); this may also be true for other services. Medicine is one of the few occupations that can create its own demand. Patients may come to physicians, but physicians tell them what procedures they need. The availability of medical technique may also create a demand for itself.

The method by which medical care is paid for has changed greatly in the past half-century. In 1920 nearly all health care was paid for directly by the patient-consumer. Since the 1930s an increasing amount of medical care has been paid for through "third-party" payments, mainly through health insurance and the government. About 75 percent of the American population is covered by some form of medical insurance (often only for hospital care). Since 1966 the government has been involved directly in financing medical care through Medicare and Medicaid. The availability of a large amount of federal money, with nearly no cost controls or regulation of medical practice, has been a major factor fueling our current medical "cost crisis." But the ascendancy of third-party payments has effected the expansion of medicine in another way: more and more human problems become defined as "medical problems" (sickness) because that is the only way insurance programs will "cover" the costs of services. . . . .

In sum, the regular physicians developed control of medical practice and a professional dominance with nearly total functional autonomy. Through professionalization and persuasion concerning the superiority of their form of medicine, the medical profession (represented by the AMA) achieved a legally supported monopoly of practice. In short, it cornered the medical market. The medical profession has succeeded in both therapeutic and economic expansion. It has won the almost exclusive right to reign over the kingdom of health and illness, no matter where it may extend.

Note

We rely on James C. Mohr's (1978) fine historical account of the origins and evolution of American abortion policy for data and much of the interpretation in this section.

References

Alford, R. The political economy of health care: dynamics without change. *Politics and Society* 1972 2 (2), 127–64.

Cartwright, F. F. *A Social History of Medicine*. New York: Longman, 1977.

Coe, R. *The Sociology of Medicine*. Second edition. New York: McGraw-Hill, 1978.

Dubos, R. *Mirage of Health*. New York: Harper and Row, 1959.

Ehrenreich, B., and Ehrenreich, J. *The American Health Empire*. New York: Random House, 1970.

Freidson, E. *Profession of Medicine*. New York: Dodd, Mead, 1970a.

Freidson, E. *Professional Dominance*. Chicago: Aldine, 1970b.

Jewson, N. D. The disappearance of the sick-man from medical cosmology, 1770–1870. *Sociology*, 1976, 10, 225–44.

Kelman, S. The social nature of the definition of health. In V. Navarro, *Health and Medical Care in the U.S.* Farmingdale, N.Y.: Baywood, 1977.

Larson, M. S. *The Rise of Professionalism*. Berkeley: California, 1977.

McCleery, R. S., and Keelty, L. T. *One Life-One Physician: An Inquiry into the Medical Profession's Performance in Self-regulation*. Washington, D.C.: Public Affairs Press, 1971.

McKeown, T. A historical appraisal of the medical task. In G. McLachlan and T. McKeown (eds.), *Medical History and Medical Care: A Symposium of Perspectives*. New York: Oxford, 1971.

McKinlay, J. B. The changing political and economic context of the physician-patient encounter. In E. B. Gallagher (ed.), *The Doctor-Patient Relationship in the Changing Health Scene*. Washington, D.C.: U.S. Government Printing Office, 1976.

Mechanic, D. *The Growth of Bureaucratic Medicine*. New York: Wiley, 1976.

Mohr, J. C. *Abortion in America*. New York: Oxford, 1978.

Reiser, S. J. *Medicine and the Reign of Technology*. New York: Cambridge, 1978.

Rothstein, W. G. *American Physicians in the Nineteenth Century: From Sects to Science*. Baltimore: Johns Hopkins, 1972.

Shryock, R. H. *Medicine and Society in America: 1660–1860*. Ithaca, N.Y.: Cornell, 1960.

Starr, P. Medicine, economy and society in nineteenth-century America. *Journal of Social History*, 1977, 10, 588–607.

Wertz, R., and Wertz, D. *Lying-In: A History of Childbirth in America*. New York: Free Press, 1977.

11

Notes on the Decline of Midwives and the Rise of Medical Obstetricians

Richard W. Wertz and Dorothy C. Wertz

. . . .

The Americans who were studying medicine in Great Britain [in the late eighteenth century] discovered that men could bring the benefits of the new midwifery to birth and thereby gain income and status. In regard to the unresolved question of what medical arts were appropriate, the Americans took the view of the English physicians, who instructed them that nature was usually adequate and intervention often dangerous. From that perspective they developed a model of the new midwifery suitable for the American situation.

From 1750 to approximately 1810 American doctors conceived of the new midwifery as an enterprise to be shared between themselves and trained midwives. Since doctors during most of that period were few in number, their plan was reasonable and humanitarian and also reflected their belief that, in most cases, natural processes were adequate and the need for skilled intervention limited, though important. Doctors therefore envisaged an arrangement whereby trained midwives would attend normal deliveries and doctors would be called to difficult ones. To implement this plan, Dr. Valentine Seaman established a short course for midwives in the New York (City) Almshouse in 1799, and Dr. William Shippen began a course on anatomy and midwifery, including clinical observation of birth, in Philadelphia. Few women came as students, however, but men did, so the doctors trained the men to be man-midwives, perhaps believing, as Smellie had contended, that the sex of the practitioner was less important than the command of new knowledge and skill.[1]

As late as 1817, Dr. Thomas Ewell of Washington, D.C., a regular physician, proposed to establish a school for midwives, connected with a hospital, similar to the schools that had existed for centuries in the great cities of Europe. Ewell sought federal funding for his enterprise, but it was not forthcoming, and the school was never founded. Herein lay a fundamental difference between European and American development of the midwife. European governments provided financial support for medical education, including the training of midwives. The U.S. government provided no support for medical education in the nineteenth century, and not enough of the women who might have aspired to become midwives could afford the fees to support a school. Those who founded schools turned instead to the potentially lucrative business of training the many men who sought to become doctors.[2]

Doctors also sought to increase the supply of doctors educated in America in the new midwifery and thus saw to it that from the outset of American medical schools midwifery became a specialty field, one all doctors could practice.

The plans of doctors for a shared enterprise with women never developed in America. Doctors were unable to attract women for training, perhaps because women were uninterested in studying what they thought they already knew and, moreover, studying it under the tutelage of men. The restraints of traditional modesty and the tradition of female sufficiency for the management of birth were apparently stronger than the appeal of a rationalized system for a more scientific and, presumably, safer midwifery system.

Not only could doctors not attract women for training in the new science and arts, but they could not even organize midwives already in practice. These women had never been organized among themselves. They thought of themselves as being loyal not primarily to an abstract medical science but to local groups of women and their needs. They reflected the tradition of local self-help empiricism that continued to be very strong in America. Americans had never had a medical profession or medical institutions, so they must have found it hard to understand why the European-trained doctors wished to organize a shared, though hierarchical, midwifery enterprise. How hard it was would be shown later, when doctors sought to organize themselves around the new science of midwifery, in which they had some institutional training. Their practice of midwifery would be governed less by science and professional behavior than by empirical practice and economic opportunity.

In the years after 1810, in fact, the practice of midwifery in American towns took on the same unregulated, open-market character it had in England. Both men and women of various degrees of experience and training competed to attend births. Some trained midwives from England immigrated to America, where they advertised their ability in local newspapers.[3] But these women confronted doctors trained abroad or in the new American medical schools. They also confronted medical empirics who presented themselves as "intrepid" man-midwives after having imbibed the instrumental philosophy from Smellie's books. American women therefore confronted a wide array of talents and skills for aiding their deliveries.

Childbirth in America would not have any neat logic during the nineteenth century, but one feature that distinguished it from childbirth abroad was the gradual disappearance of women from the practice of midwifery. There were many reasons for that unusual development. Most obvious was the severe competition that the new educated doctors and empirics brought to the event of birth, an event that often served as entrance for the medical person to a sustained practice. In addition, doctors lost their allegiance to a conservative view of the science and arts of midwifery under the exigencies of practice; they came to adopt a view endorsing more extensive interventions in birth and less reliance upon the adequacy of nature. This view led to the conviction that a certain mastery was needed, which women were assumed to be unable to achieve.

Women ceased to be midwives also because of a change in the cultural attitudes about the proper place and activity for women in society. It came to be regarded as unthinkable to confront women with the facts of medicine or to mix men and women in training, even for such an event as birth. As a still largely unscientific enterprise, medicine took on the cultural attributes necessary for it to survive, and the Victorian culture found certain roles unsuitable for women. Midwives also disappeared because they had not been organized and had never developed any leadership. Medicine in America may have had minimal scientific authority, but it was beginning to develop social and professional organization and leadership; unorganized midwives were an easy competitive target for medicine. Finally, midwives lost out to doctors and empirics because of the changing tastes among middle- and upper-class women; for these women, the new midwifery came to have the promise of more safety and even more respectability.[4]

Midwives therefore largely ceased to attend the middle classes in America during the nineteenth century. Except among ethnic immigrants, among poor, isolated whites, and among blacks, there is little significant evidence of midwifery. This is not to say that there were no such women or that in instances on the frontier or even in cities when doctors were unavailable women did not undertake to attend other women. But educated doctors and empirics penetrated American settlements quickly and extensively, eager to gain patients and always ready to attend birth. The very dynamics of American mobility contributed to the break-up of those communities that had sustained the midwives' practices.

Because of continued ethnic immigration, however, by 1900 in many urban areas half of the women were still being delivered by immigrant midwives. The fact that ethnic groups existed largely outside the development of American medicine during the nineteenth century would pose a serious problem in the twentieth century.

Native-born educated women sought to become doctors, not midwives, during the nineteenth century. They did not want to play a role in birth that was regarded as inferior and largely nonmedical—the midwife's role—but wished to assume the same medical role allowed to men.

It is important to emphasize, however, that the disappearance of midwives at middle- and upper-class births was not the result of a conspiracy between male doctors and husbands. The choice of medical attendants was the responsibility of women, upon whom devolved the care of their families' health. Women were free to choose whom they wished. A few did seek out unorthodox practitioners, although most did not. But as the number of midwives diminished, women of course found fewer respectable, trained women of their own class whom they might choose to help in their deliveries.

In order to understand the new midwifery [i.e. medical obstetrics], it is necessary to consider who doctors were and how they entered the medical profession. The doctors who assumed control over middle-class births in America were very differently educated and organized from their counterparts in France or England. The fact that their profession remained loosely organized and ill-defined throughout most of the nineteenth century helps to explain their desire to exclude women from midwifery, for often women were the only category of people that they could effectively exclude. Doctors with some formal education had always faced competition from the medical empirics—men, women, and even freed slaves—who declared themselves able to treat all manner of illnesses and often publicly advertised their successes. These empirics, called quacks by the orthodox educated doctors, offered herbal remedies or psychological comfort to patients. Orthodox physicians objected that the empirics prescribed on an individual, trial-and-error basis without reference to any academic theories about the origins and treatment of disease. Usually the educated physician also treated his patients empirically, for medical theory had little to offer that was practically superior to empiricism until the development of bacteriology in the 1870s. Before then there was no convincing, authoritative, scientific nucleus for medicine, and doctors often had difficulty translating what knowledge they did have into practical treatment. The fundamental objection of regular doctors was to competition from uneducated practitioners. Most regular doctors also practiced largely ineffective therapies, but they were convinced that their therapies were better than those of the empirics because they were educated men. The uneducated empirics enjoyed considerable popular support during the first half of the nineteenth century because their therapies were as often successful as the therapies of the regulars, and sometimes less strenuous. Like the empirics, educated doctors treated patients rather than diseases and looked for different symptoms in different social classes. Because a doctor's reputation stemmed from the social standing of his patients, there was considerable competition for the patronage of the more respectable families.

The educated, or "regular," doctors around 1800 were of the upper and middle classes, as were the state legislators. The doctors convinced the legislators that medicine, like other gentlemen's professions, should be restricted to those who held diplomas or who had apprenticed with practitioners of the appropriate social class and training. State licensure laws were passed, in response to the Federalist belief that social deference was due to professional men. The early laws were ineffectual because they did not take into account the popular tradition of self-help. People continued to patronize empirics. During the Jacksonian Era even the nonenforced licensing laws were repealed by most states as elitist; popular belief held that the practice of medicine should be "democratic" and open to all, or at least to all men.[5]

In the absence of legal control, several varieties of "doctors" practiced in the nineteenth century. In addition to the empirics and the "regular" doctors there were the sectarians, who included the Thomsonian Botanists, the Homeopaths, the Eclectics, and a number of minor sects of which the most important for obstetrics were the Hydrotherapists.

The regular doctors can be roughly divided into two groups: the elite, who had attended the better medical schools and who wrote the textbooks urging "conservative" practice in midwifery; and the great number of poorly educated men who had spent a few months at a proprietary medical school from which they were graduated with no practical or clinical knowledge. (Proprietary medical schools were profit-making schools owned by several local doctors who also taught there. Usually such schools had no equipment or resources for teaching.) In the eighteenth century the elite had had to travel to London, or more often Edinburgh, for training. In 1765, however, the Medical College of Philadelphia was founded, followed by King's College (later Columbia) Medical School in 1767 and Harvard in 1782. Obstetrics, or "midwifery," as it was then called, was the first medical specialty in those schools, preceding even surgery, for it was assumed that midwifery was the keystone to medical practice, something that every student would do after graduation as part of his practice. Every medical school founded thereafter had a special "Professor of Midwifery." Among the first such professors were Drs. William Shippen at Philadelphia, Samuel Bard at King's College, and Walter Channing at Harvard. In the better schools early medical courses lasted two years; in the latter half of the nineteenth century some schools began to increase this to three, but many two-year medical graduates were still practicing in 1900.

A prestigious medical education did not guarantee that a new graduate was prepared to deal with patients. Dr. James Marion Sims, a famous nineteenth-century surgeon, stated that his education at Philadelphia's Jefferson Medical College, considered one of the best in the country in 1835, left him fitted for nothing and without the slightest notion of how to treat his first cases.[6] In 1850 a graduate of the University of Buffalo described his total ignorance on approaching his first obstetrical case:

> I was left alone with a poor Irish woman and one crony, to deliver her child . . . and I thought it necessary to call before me every circumstance I had learned from books—I must examine, and I did—But whether it was head or breech, hand or foot, man or monkey, that was defended from my uninstructed finger by the distended membranes, I was as uncomfortably ignorant, with all my learning, as the foetus itself that was making all this fuss.[7]

Fortunately the baby arrived naturally, the doctor was given great praise for his part in the event, and he wrote that he was glad "to have escaped the commission of murder."

If graduates of the better medical schools made such complaints, those who attended the smaller schools could only have been more ignorant. In 1818 Dr. John Stearns, President of the New York Medical Society, complained, "With a few honorable exceptions in each city, the practitioners are ignorant, degraded, and contemptible."[8] The American Medical Association later estimated that between 1765 and 1905 more than eight hundred medical schools were founded, most of them proprietary, money-making schools, and many were short-lived. In 1905 some 160 were still in operation. Neither the profession nor the states effectively regulated those schools until the appearance of the Flexner Report, a professional self-study published in 1910. The report led to tougher state laws and the setting of standards for medical education. Throughout much of the nineteenth century a doctor could obtain a diploma and begin practice with as little as four months' attendance at a school that might have no laboratories, no dissections, and no clinical training. Not only was it easy to become a doctor, but the profession, with the exception of the elite who attended elite patients, had low standing in the eyes of most people.[9]

Nineteenth-century women could choose among a variety of therapies and practitioners. Their choice was usually dictated by social class. An upper-class woman in an Eastern city would see either an elite regular physician or a homeopath; if she were daring, she might visit a hydropathic establishment. A poor woman in the Midwest might turn to an empiric, a poorly-educated regular doctor, or a Thomsonian botanist. This variety of choice distressed regular doctors, who were fighting for professional and economic exclusivity. As long as doctors were organized only on a local basis, it was impossible to exclude irregulars from practice or even to set enforceable standards for regular practice. The American Medical Association was founded in 1848 for those purposes. Not until the end of the century, however, was organized medicine able to re-establish licensing laws. The effort succeeded only because the regulars finally accepted the homeopaths, who were of the same social class, in order to form a sufficient majority to convince state legislators that licensing was desirable.

Having finally won control of the market, doctors were able to turn to self-regulation, an ideal adopted by the American Medical Association in 1860 but not put into effective practice until after 1900. Although there had been progress in medical science and in the education of the elite and the specialists during the nineteenth century, the average doctor was still woefully undereducated. The Flexner Report in 1910 revealed that 90 percent of doctors were then without a college education and that most had attended substandard medical schools.[10] Only after its publication did the profession impose educational requirements on the bulk of medical practitioners and take steps to accredit medical schools and close down diploma mills. Until then the average doctor had little sense of what his limits were or to whom he was responsible, for there was often no defined community of professionals and usually no community of patients.

Because of the ill-defined nature of the medical profession in the nineteenth century and the poor quality of medical education, doctors' insistence on the exclusion of women as economically dangerous competitors is quite understandable. As a group, nineteenth-century doctors were not affluent, and even their staunchest critics admitted that they could have made more money in business. Midwifery itself paid less than other types of practice, for many doctors spent long hours in attending laboring women and later had trouble collecting their fees. Yet midwifery was a guaranteed income, even if small, and it opened the way to family practice and sometimes to consultations involving many doctors and shared fees. The family and female friends who had seen a doctor "perform" successfully were likely to call him again. Doctors worried that, if midwives were allowed to deliver the upper classes, women would turn to them for treatment of other illnesses and male doctors would lose half their clientele. As a prominent Boston doctor wrote in 1820, "If female midwifery is again introduced among the rich and influential, it will become fashionable and it will be considered indelicate to employ a physician."[11] Doctors had to eliminate midwives in order to protect the gateway to their whole practice.

They had to mount an attack on midwives, because midwives had their defenders, who argued that women were safer and more modest than the new man-midwives. For example, the *Virginia Gazette* in 1772 carried a "LETTER on the present State of MIDWIFERY," emphasizing the old idea that "Labour is Nature's Work" and needs no more art than women's experience teaches, and that it was safer when women alone attended births.

> It is a notorious fact that more Children have been lost since Women were so scandalously indecent as to employ Men than for Ages before that Practice became so general. . . . [Women midwives] never dream of having recourse to Force; the barbarous, bloody Crochet, never stained their Hands with Murder. . . . A long unimpassioned Practice, early commenced, and calmly pursued is absolutely requisite to give Men by Art, what Women attain by Nature.

The writer concluded with the statement that men-midwives also took liberties with pregnant and laboring women that were "sufficient to taint the Purity, and sully the Chastity, of any Woman breathing." The final flourish, "True Modesty is incompatible with the Idea of employing a MAN-MIDWIFE," would echo for decades, causing great distress for female patients with male attendants. Defenders of midwives made similar statements throughout the first half of the nineteenth century. Most were sectarian doctors or laymen with an interest in women's modesty.[12] No midwives came forward to defend themselves in print.

The doctors' answer to midwives' defenders was expressed not in terms of pecuniary motives but in terms of safety and the proper place of women. After 1800 doctors' writings implied that women who presumed to supervise births had overreached their proper position in life. One of the earliest American birth manuals, the *Married Lady's Companion and Poor Man's Friend* (1808), denounced the ignorance of midwives and urged them to "submit to their station."[13]

Two new convictions about women were at the heart of the doctors' opposition to midwives: that women were unsafe to attend deliveries and that no "true" woman would want to gain the knowledge and skills necessary to do so. An anonymous pamphlet, published in 1820 in Boston, set forth these convictions along with other reasons for excluding midwives from practice. The author, thought to have been either Dr. Walter Channing or Dr. Henry Ware, another leading obstetrician, granted that women had more "passive fortitude" than men in enduring and witnessing suffering but asserted that women lacked the power to act that was essential to being a birth attendant:

> They have not that power of action, or that active power of mind, which is essential to the practice of a surgeon. They have less power of restraining and governing the natural tendencies to sympathy and are more disposed to yield to the expressions of acute sensibility . . . where they become the principal agents, the feelings of sympathy are too powerful for the cool exercise of judgment.[14]

The author believed only men capable of the attitude of detached concern needed to concentrate on the techniques required in birth. It is not surprising to find the author stressing the importance of interventions, but his undervaluing of sympathy, which in most normal deliveries was the only symptomatic treatment necessary, is rather startling. Clearly, he hoped to exaggerate the need for coolness in order to discountenance the belief of many women and doctors that midwives could safely attend normal deliveries.

The author possibly had something more delicate in mind that he found hard to express. He perhaps meant to imply that women were unsuited because there were certain times when they were "disposed to yield to the expressions of acute sensibility." Doctors quite commonly believed that during menstruation women's limited bodily energy was diverted from the brain, rendering them, as doctors phrased it, idiotic. In later years another Boston doctor, Horatio Storer, explained why he thought women unfit to become surgeons. He granted that exceptional women had the necessary courage, tact, ability, money, education, and patience for the career but argued that, because the "periodical infirmity of their sex . . . in every case . . . unfits them for any responsible effort of mind," he had to oppose them. During their "condition," he said, "neither life nor limb submitted to them would be as safe as at other times," for the condition was a "temporary insanity," a time when women were "more prone than men to commit any unusual or outrageous act."[15]

The author of the anonymous pamphlet declared that a female would find herself at times (i.e., during menstruation) totally unable to manage birth emergencies, such as hemorrhages, convulsions, manual extraction of the placenta, or inversion of the womb, when the newly delivered organ externally turned itself inside out and extruded from the body, sometimes hanging to the knees. In fact, an English midwife, Sarah Stone, had described in 1737 how she personally had handled each of these emergencies successfully. But the author's readers did not know that, and the author himself could have dismissed Stone's skill as fortuitous, exercised in times of mental clarity.[16]

The anonymous author was also convinced that no woman could be trained in the knowledge and skill of midwifery without losing her standing as a lady. In the dissecting room and in the hospital a woman would forfeit her "delicate feelings" and "refined sensibility"; she would see things that would taint her moral character. Such a woman would "unsex" herself, by which the doctors meant not only that she would lose her standing as a "lady" but also, literally, that she would be subject to physical exertions and nervous excitements that would damage her female organs irreparably and prevent her from fulfilling her social role as wife and mother.[17]

. . . .

The exclusion of women from obstetrical cooperation with men had important effects upon the "new practice" that was to become the dominant tradition in American medical schools. American obstetric education differed significantly from training given in France, where the principal maternity hospitals trained doctors clinically alongside student midwives. Often the hospital's midwives, who supervised all normal births, trained the doctors in normal deliveries. French doctors never lost touch with the conservative tradition that said "Dame Nature is the best midwife." In America, where midwives were not trained at all and medical education was sexually segregated, medicine turned away from the conservative tradition and became more interventionist.

Around 1810 the new midwifery in America appears to have entered a new phase, one that shaped its character and problems throughout the century. Doctors continued to regard birth as a fundamentally natural process, usually sufficient by itself to effect delivery without artful assistance, and understandable mechanistically. But this view conflicted with the exigencies of their medical practice, which called upon them to demonstrate skills. Gradually, more births seemed to require aid.

Young doctors rarely had any clinical training in what the theory of birth meant in practice. Many arrived at a birth with only lectures and book learning to guide them. If they (and the laboring patient) were fortunate, they had an older, experienced doctor or attending woman to explain what was natural and what was not. Many young men were less lucky and were embarrassed, confused, and frightened by the appearances of labor and birth. Lacking clinical training, each had to develop his own sense of what each birth required, if anything, in the way of artful assistance; each had to learn the consequence of misdirected aids.[18]

If the doctor was in a hurry to reach another patient, he might be tempted to hasten the process along by using instruments or other expedients. If the laboring woman or her female attendants urged him to assist labor, he might feel compelled to use his tools and skills even though he knew that nature was adequate but slow. He had to use his arts because he was expected to "perform." Walter Channing, Professor of Midwifery at Harvard Medical School in the early nineteenth century, remarked about the doctor, in the context of discussing a case in which forceps were used unnecessarily, that he "must do something. He cannot remain a spectator merely, where there are too many witnesses and where interest in what is going on is too deep to allow of his inaction." Channing was saying that, even though well-educated physicians recognized that natural processes were sufficient and that instruments could be dangerous, in their practice they also had to appear to *do* something for their patient's symptoms, whether that entailed giving a drug to alleviate pain or shortening labor by using the forceps. The doctor could not appear to be indifferent or inattentive or useless. He had to establish his identity by doing something, preferably something to make the patient feel better. And if witnesses were present there was perhaps even more reason to "perform." Channing concluded: "Let him be collected and calm, and he will probably do little he will afterwards look upon and regret."[19]

If educated physicians found it difficult in practice to appeal before their patients to the reliability of nature and the dangers of instruments, one can imagine what less confident and less competent doctors did with instruments in order to appear useful. A number of horror stories from the early decades of the century have been retailed by men and women who believed that doctors used their instruments unfairly and incompetently to drive midwives from practice.[20] Whatever the truth may be about the harm done, it is easy to believe that instruments were used regularly by doctors to establish their superior status.

If doctors believed that they had to perform in order to appear useful and to win approval, it is very likely that women, on the other hand, began to expect that more might go wrong with birth processes than they had previously believed. In the context of social childbirth, which . . . meant that women friends and kin were present at delivery, the appearance of forceps in one birth established the possibility of their being used in subsequent births. In short, women may have come to anticipate difficult births whether or not doctors urged that possibility as a means of selling themselves. Having seen the "best," perhaps each woman wanted the "best" for her delivery, whether she needed it or not.

Strange as it may sound, women may in fact have been choosing male attendants because they wanted a guaranteed performance, in the sense of both guaranteed safety and guaranteed fashionableness. Choosing the best medical care is itself a kind of fashion. But in addition women may have wanted a guaranteed audience, the male attendant, for quite specific purposes; namely, they may have wanted a representative male to see their pain and suffering in order that their femininity might be established and their pain verified before men. Women, then, could have had a range of important reasons for choosing male doctors to perform: for themselves, safety; for the company of women, fashion; for the world of men, femininity.

So a curious inconsistency arose between the principle of noninterference in nature and the exigencies of professional practice. Teachers of midwifery continued to stress the adequacy of nature and the danger of instruments. Samuel Bard, Dean of King's College Medical School, wrote a text on midwifery in 1807 in which he refused even to discuss forceps because he believed that interventions by unskilled men, usually inspired by Smellie's writings, were more dangerous than the most desperate case left to nature. Bard's successors made the same points in the 1830s and 1840s. Dr. Chandler Gilman, Professor of Obstetrics at the College of Physicians and Surgeons in New York from 1841 to 1865, taught his students that "Dame Nature is the best midwife in the world. . . . Meddlesome midwifery is fraught with evil. . . . The less done generally the better, Non-interference is the cornerstone of midwifery."[21] This instruction often went unheeded, however, because young doctors often resorted to instruments in haste or in confusion, or because they were poorly trained and unsupervised in practice, but also, as we have indicated, because physicians, whatever their state of knowledge, were expected to do something.

What they could do—the number of techniques to aid and control natural processes—gradually increased. In 1808, for example, Dr. John Stearns of upper New York State learned from an immigrant German midwife of a new means to effect the mechanics of birth. This was ergot, a powerful natural drug that stimulates uterine muscles when given orally. Ergot is a fungus that grows on rye and other stored grains. It causes powerful and unremitting contractions. Stearns stressed its value in saving the doctor's time and in relieving the distress and agony of long labor. Ergot also quickens the expulsion of the placenta and stems hemorrhage by compelling the uterus to contract. Stearns claimed that ergot had no ill effects but warned that it should be given only after the fetus was positioned for easy delivery, for it induced an incessant action that left no time to turn a child in the birth canal or uterus.

There was in fact no antidote to ergot's rapid and uncontrollable effects until anesthesia became available in later decades. So if the fetus did not move as expected, the drug could cause the uterus to mold itself around the child, rupturing the uterus and killing the child. Ergot, like most new medical arts for birth, was a mix of danger and benefit. Critics of meddlesome doctors said that they often used it simply to save time. However true that was, ergot certainly fitted the mechanistic view of birth, posed a dilemma to doctors about wise use, and enlarged the doctors' range of arts for controlling birth. Doctors eventually determined that using ergot to induce labor without an antidote was too dangerous and limited its use to expelling the placenta or stopping hemorrhage.[22]

Despite the theory of the naturalness of birth and the danger of intervention, the movement in midwifery was in the opposite direction, to less reliance on nature and more reliance on artful intervention. The shift appeared during the 1820s in discussions as to what doctors should call themselves when they practiced the new midwifery. "Male-midwife," "midman," "man-midwife," "physician man-midwife," and even "andro-boethogynist" were terms too clumsy, too reminiscent of the female title, or too unreflective of the new science and skill. "Accoucheur" sounded better but was French. The doctors of course ignored Elizabeth Nihell's earlier, acid suggestion that they call themselves "pudendists" after the area of the body that so interested them. Then an English doctor suggested in 1828 that "obstetrician" was as appropriate a term as any. Coming from the Latin meaning "to stand before," it had the advantage of sounding like other honorable professions, such as "electrician" or "geometrician," in which men variously understood and dominated nature.[23]

The renaming of the practice of midwifery symbolized doctors' new sense of themselves as professional actors. In fact, the movement toward greater dominance over birth's natural processes cannot be understood unless midwifery is seen in the context of general medical practice. In that perspective, several relations between midwifery and general practice become clearly important. In the first place, midwifery continued during the first half of the nineteenth century to be one of the few areas of general practice where doctors had a scientific understanding and useful medical arts. That meant that practicing midwifery was central to doctors' attempts to build a practice, earn fees, and achieve some status, for birth was one physical condition they were confident they knew how to treat. And they were successful in the great majority of cases because birth itself was usually successful. Treating birth was without the risk of treating many other conditions, but doctors got the credit nonetheless.

In the second place, however, birth was simply one condition among many that doctors treated, and the therapeutic approach they took to other conditions tended to spill over into their treatment of birth. For most physical conditions of illness doctors did not know what processes of nature were at work. They tended therefore to treat the patient and the patient's symptoms rather than the processes of disease, which they did not see and were usually not looking for. By treating his or her symptoms the doctors did something for the patient and thereby gained approbation. The doctors' status came from pleasing the patients rather than from curing diseases. That was a risky endeavor, for sometimes patients judged the treatment offered to relieve symptoms to be worthless or even more disabling than the symptoms themselves. But patients expected doctors to do something for them, an expectation that carried into birth also. So neither doctors nor patients were inclined to allow the natural processes of birth to suffice.

There is no need to try to explain this contradiction by saying that doctors were ignorant, greedy, clumsy, hasty, or salacious in using medical arts unnecessarily (although some may have been), for the contradiction reflects primarily the kind of therapy that was dominant in prescientific medicine.

The relations between midwifery and general medical practice become clearer if one considers what doctors did when they confronted a birth that did not conform to their understanding of birth's natural processes. Their mechanistic view could not explain such symptoms as convulsions or high fevers, occasionally associated with birth. Yet doctors did not walk away from such conditions as being mysterious or untreatable, for they were committed to the mastery of birth. Rather, they treated the strange symptoms with general therapies just as they might treat regular symptoms of birth with medical arts such as forceps and ergot.

Bloodletting was a popular therapy for many symptoms, and doctors often applied it to births that seemed unusual to them. If a pregnant woman seemed to be florid or perspiring, the doctor might place her in a chair, open a vein in her arm, and allow her to bleed until she fainted. Some doctors bled women to unconsciousness to counter delivery pains. A doctor in 1851 opened the temporal arteries of a woman who was having convulsions during birth, "determined to bleed her until the convulsion ceased or as long as the blood would flow." He found it impossible to catch the blood thrown about during her convulsions, but the woman eventually completed her delivery successfully and survived. Bloodletting was also intitiated when a woman developed high fever after delivery. Salmon P. Chase, Lincoln's Secretary of the Treasury and later Chief Justice, told in his diary how a group of doctors took 50 ounces of blood from his wife to relieve her fever. The doctors gave careful attention to the strength and frequency of her pulse, debating and deliberating upon the meaning of the symptom, until finally Mrs. Chase died.[24]

For localized pain, doctors applied leeches to draw out blood from the affected region. A distended abdomen after delivery might merit the application of twelve leeches; a headache, six on the temple; vaginal pain also merited several.[25]

Another popular therapy was calomel, a chloride of mercury that irritated the intestine and purged it. A woman suffering puerperal fever might be given extended doses to reduce swelling by purging her bodily contents. If the calomel acted too violently, the doctors could retard it by administering opium. Doctors often gave emetics to induce vomiting when expectant women had convulsions, for they speculated that emetics might be specifics for hysteria or other nervous diseases causing convulsions.

An expectant or laboring woman showing unusual symptoms might be subjected to a battery of such agents as doctors sought to restore her symptoms to a normal balance. In a famous case in Boston in 1833 a woman had convulsions a month before her expected delivery. The doctors bled her of 8 ounces and gave her a purgative. The next day she again had convulsions, and they took 22 ounces of blood. After 90 minutes she had a headache, and the doctors took 18 more ounces of blood, gave emetics to cause vomiting, and put ice on her head and mustard plasters on her feet. Nearly four hours later she had another convulsion, and they took 12 ounces, and soon after, 6 more. By then she had lapsed into a deep coma, so the doctors doused her with cold water but could not revive her. Soon her cervix began to dilate, so the doctors gave ergot to induce labor. Shortly before delivery she convulsed again, and they applied ice and mustard plasters again and also gave a vomiting agent and calomel to purge her bowels. In six hours she delivered a stillborn child. After two days she regained consciousness and recovered. The doctors considered this a conservative treatment, even though they had removed two-fifths of her blood in a two-day period, for they had not artificially dilated her womb or used instruments to expedite delivery.[26]

Symptomatic treatment was intended not simply to make the patient feel better—often the treatment was quite violent, or "heroic"—but to restore some balance of healthy appearances. Nor were the therapies given to ailing women more intrusive or different from therapies given to suffering men. The therapies were not, in most instances, forced upon the patients without their foreknowledge or consent. People were often eager to be made healthy and willing to endure strenuous therapies to this end. Doctors did believe, however, that some groups of people were more susceptible to illness than others and that different groups also required, or deserved, different treatments.

These views reflected in large part the doctors' awareness of cultural classifications of people; in other words, the culture's position on the relative social worth of different social classes influenced doctors' views about whose health was likely to be endangered, how their endangered health affected the whole society, and what treatments, if any, were suitable. For birth this meant, for example, that doctors believed it more important for them to attend the delivery of children by middle- and upper-class women than the delivery of children by the poor. It meant that doctors expected "fashionable" women to suffer more difficult deliveries because their tight clothing, rich diet and lack of exercise were unhealthy and because they were believed to be more susceptible to nervous strain. It also meant that doctors thought it fitting for unmarried and otherwise disreputable mothers not to receive charitable care along with other poor but respectable women.

There is abundant evidence that doctors came to believe in time that middle- and upper-class women typically had more difficult deliveries than, for example, farm women. One cannot find an objective measure of the accuracy of their perception, nor, unfortunately and more to the point, can one find whether their perception that some women were having more difficult deliveries led doctors consistently to use more intervention in attending them than in attending poorer women with normal deliveries. Doctors' perception of the relative difficulty of deliveries was part of their tendency to associate different kinds of sickness with different social classes. They expected to find the symptoms of certain illnesses in certain groups of people, and therefore looked for those particular symptoms or conditions. In the nineteenth century upper-class urban women were generally expected to be sensitive and delicate, while farm women were expected to be robust. Some doctors even believed that the evolutionary result of education was to produce smaller pelves in women and larger heads in babies, leading to more difficult births among civilized women. There is no evidence that these beliefs were medically accurate. Whether a doctor considered a patient "sick" or "healthy" depended in part upon class-related standards of health and illness rather than on objective scientific standards of sickness.

Treatment probably varied according to the doctor's perception of a woman's class and individual character. At some times and places the treatment given probably reflected the patient's class as much as her symptoms. Thus some doctors may have withheld the use of instruments from their upper-class patients in the belief that they were too fragile to undergo instrumental delivery. The same doctors may have used instruments needlessly on poor patients, who were considered healthy enough to stand anything, in order to save the doctor's time and permit him to rush off to the bedside of a wealthier patient. On the other hand, some doctors may have used instruments on the upper-class women in order to shorten labor, believing that they could not endure prolonged pain or were too weak to bring forth children unassisted, and also in order to justify higher fees. The same doctors may have withheld forceps from poor women whom they considered healthy enough to stand several days of labor. Unfortunately, there is no way of knowing exactly how treatments differed according to class, for very few doctors kept records of their private patients. The records now extant are for the small number of people, perhaps 5 percent of the population, who were treated in hospitals in the nineteenth century. Only poor women, most unmarried, delivered in hospitals, so the records do not cover a cross-section of classes. These hospital records do indicate a large number of instrumental deliveries and sometimes give the reasons as the patient's own "laziness" or "stupidity" in being unable to finish a birth. It is likely that doctors' expectations of lower-class performance are reflected here. Hospital records also reflect the use of poor patients for training or experimentation, another reason for a high incidence of instrumental deliveries.

The fact that doctors' tendency to classify patients according to susceptibility did not lead to consistent differences in treatment is an important indication that they were not merely slavish adherents to a mechanistic view of nature or to cultural and class interests. Doctors were still treating individual women, not machines and not social types. The possibility of stereotypical classification and treatment, however, remained a lively threat to more subtle discernments of individual symptoms and to truly artful applications of treatment in birth.

At the same time, it was possible that patients would find even unbiased treatments offensively painful, ineffective, and expensive, or would doubt that the doctor had a scientific reason for giving them. Such persons could seek other treatments, often administered by laypeople or by themselves. Yet those treatments, including treatments for birth, were also directed toward symptoms. At a time when diseases were unrecognized and their causes unknown, the test of therapy was the patient's whole response, not the curing of disease. So patients who resented treatments as painful, ineffective, or officious rejected the doctor and the treatments. A woman who gave birth in Ohio in 1846 recalled that the doctor bled her and then gave her ergot even though the birth was proceeding, in her view, quite normally. She thought he was simply drunk and in a hurry and angrily judged him a "bad man."[27]

The takeover of birth by male doctors in America was an unusual phenomenon in comparison to France and England, where traditional midwifery continued as a much more significant part of birth. Practice developed differently in America because the society itself expanded more rapidly and the medical profession grew more quickly to doctor in ever new communities. American mobility left fewer stable communities than in France or England, and thus networks of women to support midwives were more often broken. The standards of the American medical profession were not so high or so strictly enforced as standards in other countries, and thus there were both more "educated" doctors and more self-proclaimed doctors in America to compete with midwives. So American midwives disappeared from view because they had less support from stable communities of women and more competition from male doctors.

The exclusion of women from midwifery and obstetrics had profound effects upon practice. Most obviously, it gave obstetrics a sexist bias; maleness became a necessary attribute of safety, and femaleness became a conditon in need of male medical control. Within this skewed view of ability and need, doctors found it nearly impossible to gain an objective view of what nature could do and what art should do, for one was identified with being a woman and the other with being a man.

The bias identified functions, attributes, and prerogatives, which unfortunately could become compulsions, so that doctors as men may have often felt that they had to impose their form upon the processes of nature in birth. Obstetrics acquired a basic distortion in its orientation toward nature, a confusion of the need to be masterful and even male with the need for intervention.

Samuel Bard, one of the few doctors to oppose the trend, remarked that the young doctor, too often lacking the ability to discriminate about natural processes, often became alarmed for his patient's safety and his own reputation, leading him to seek a speedy instrumental delivery for both. A tragedy could follow, compounded because the doctor might not even recognize that he had erred and might not, therefore, learn to correct his practice. But doctors may also have found the "indications" for intervention in their professional work—to hurry, to impress, to win approval, and to show why men rather than women should attend births.

The thrust for male control of birth probably expressed psychosexual needs of men, although there is no basis for discussing this historically. The doctor appears to history more as a ritualistic figure, a representative man, identifying and enforcing sexual roles in critical life experiences. He also provided, as a representative scientist, important rationalizations for these roles, particularly why women should be content to be wives and mothers, and, as a representative of dominant cultural morality, determined the classifications of women who deserved various kinds of treatment. Thus the doctor could bring to the event of birth many prerogatives that had little to do with aiding natural processes, but which he believed were essential to a healthy and safe birth.

Expectant and laboring women lost a great deal from the exclusion of educated female birth attendants, although, of course, they would not have chosen men if they had not believed men had more to offer, at least in the beginning decades of the century. Eventually there were only men to choose. Although no doubt doctors were often sympathetic, they could never have the same point of view as a woman who had herself borne a child and who might be more patient and discerning about birth processes. And female attendants would not, of course, have laid on the male prerogatives of physical and moral control of birth.

. . . .

References

1. Valentine Seaman, *The Midwives' Monitor and Mother's Mirror* (New York, 1800); Lewis Scheffey, "The Early History and the Transition Period of Obstetrics and Gynecology in Philadelphia," *Annals of Medical History,* Third Series, 2 (May, 1940), 215–224.
2. John B. Blake, "Women and Medicine in Ante-Bellum America," *Bulletin of the History of Medicine* 34, No. 2 (March-April 1965):108–109; see also Dr. Thomas Ewell, *Letters to Ladies* (Philadelphia, 1817) pp. 21–31.
3. Julia C. Spruill, *Women's Life and Work in the Southern Colonies* (New York: Norton, 1972), pp. 272–274; Jane Bauer Donegan, "Midwifery in America, 1760–1860: A Study in Medicine and Morality." Unpublished Ph.D. dissertation, Syracuse University, 1972, pp. 50–52.
4. Alice Morse Earle (ed.), *Diary of Anna Green Winslow, a Boston Schoolgirl of 1771* (Detroit: Singing Tree Press, 1970), p. 12 and n. 24.
5. William G. Rothstein, *American Physicians in the Nineteenth Century: From Sects to Science* (Baltimore: Johns Hokpkins Press, 1970), pp. 47–49.

6. J. Marion Sims, *The Story of My Life* (New York, 1888), pp. 138–146.

7. *Buffalo Medical Journal* 6 (September, 1850):250–251.

8. John Stearns, "Presidential Address," *Transactions of the New York State Medical Society* 1:139.

9. Sims, *Story of My Life*, pp. 115–116.

10. Abraham Flexner, *Medical Education in the United States and Canada: A Report to the Carnegie Foundation for the Advancement of Teaching* (New York, 1910).

11. Anonymous, *Remarks on the Employment of Females as Practitioners in Midwifery*, 1820, pp. 4–6. See also Samuel Gregory, *Man-Midwifery Exposed and Corrected* (Boston, 1848) pp. 13, 49; Donegan, "Midwifery in America," pp. 73–74, 240; Thomas Hersey, *The Midwife's Practical Directory; or, Woman's Confidential Friend* (Baltimore, 1836), p. 221; Charles Rosenberg, "The Practice of Medicine in New York a Century Ago," *Bulletin of the History of Medicine* 41 (1967):223–253.

12. Spruill, *Women's Life and Work*, p. 275; Gregory, *Man-Midwifery Exposed*, pp. 13, 28, 36.

13. Samuel K. Jennings, *The Married Lady's Companion and Poor Man's Friend* (New York, 1808), p. 105.

14. Anonymous, *Remarks*, p.12.

15. Horatio Storer, M.D., *Criminal Abortion* (Boston, 1868), pp. 100–101n.

16. Sarah Stone, *A Complete Practice of Midwifery* (London, 1737).

17. Anonymous, *Remarks*, p. 7.

18. Harold Speert, M.D., *The Sloane Hospital Chronicle* (Philadelphia: Davis, 1963), pp. 17–19; Donegan, "Midwifery in America," p. 218.

19. Walter Channing, M.D., *A Treatise on Etherization in Childbirth, Illustrated by 581 Cases* (Boston, 1848), p. 229.

20. Gregory, *Man-Midwifery Exposed*, pp. 13, 28, 36; Hersey, *Midwife's Practical Directory*, p. 220; Wooster Beach, *An Improved System of Midwifery Adapted to the Reformed Practice of Medicine . . .* (New York, 1851), p. 115.

21. Speert, *Sloane Hospital Chronicle*, pp. 31–33, 77–78.

22. Palmer Findlay, *Priests of Lucina: The Story of Obstetrics* (Boston, 1939), pp. 220–221.

23. Elizabeth Nihell, *A Treatise on Art of Midwifery: Setting Forth Various Abuses Therein, Especially as to the Practice with Instruments* (London, 1760), p. 325; Nicholson J. Eastmen and Louis M. Hellman, *Williams Obstetrics*, 13th Ed. (New York: Appleton-Century-Crofts, 1966), p. 1.

24. Rothstein, *American Physicians*, pp. 47–49.

25. *Loc. cit.*

26. Frederick C. Irving, *Safe Deliverance* (Boston, 1942), pp. 221-225.

27. Harriet Connor Brown, *Grandmother Brown's Hundred Years, 1827–1927* (Boston, 1929), p. 93.

12

Professional Dominance and the Ordering of Health Services: Some Consequences

Eliot Freidson

A great many words have been spoken in discussions of what a profession is, or rather, what the best definition of "profession" is. Unfortunately, discussion has been so fixed on the question of definition that not much analysis has been made of the significance and consequences of some of the elements common to most definitions. The most critical of such under-examined elements are organizational in character and are related to the organization of practice and the division of labor. Such elements are critical because they deal with facets of professional occupations that are independent of individual motivation or intention, and that may, as Carlin has suggested for law,[1] minimize the importance to behavior of the personal qualities of intelligence, ethicality, and trained skill imputed to professionals by most definitions. The key to such institutional elements of professions, I believe, lies in the commonly invoked word "autonomy." Autonomy means "the quality or state of being independent, free, and self-directing."[2] In the case of professions, autonomy apparently refers most of all to control over the content and the terms of work. That is, the professional is self-directing in his work.

From the single condition of self-direction or autonomy I believe we can deduce or derive virtually all the other institutional elements that are included in most definitions of professions. For example, an occupational group is more likely to be self-directing in its work when it has obtained a legal or political position of privilege that protects it from encroachment by other occupations. This is one of the functions of licensure, which provides an occupation with a legal monopoly over the performance of some strategic aspect of its work and effectively prevents free competition from other occupations. In the United States, for example, the physician is virtually the only one who can legally prescribe drugs and cut into the body. Competitors are left with being able to talk to patients and to lay hands *on* the body, but they may not penetrate the body chemically or physically.

Second, an occupational group is not likely to be able to be self-directing if it cannot control the production and particularly the application of knowledge and skill in the work it performs. This is to say, if the substance of its knowledge and skill is known to and performed by others, the occupation cannot be completely autonomous because those others can legitimately criticize and otherwise evaluate the way it carries out its work. The extended period of education controlled by the profession in an exclusively segregated professional school rather than in a variegated liberal arts school and a curriculum that includes some *special* theoretical content (whether scientifically proven or not) may represent a declaration that there is a body of special knowledge and skill necessary for the occupation that is not represented in colleges of arts and sciences or their specialized departments. The existence of such self-sufficient schools in itself rules out as *legitimate* arbiters of the occupation's work those with specialized training in the same area who received their training from some other kind of school. The professional school and its curriculum, of course, also constitute convenient institutional criteria for licensure, registration, or other exclusionary legal devices.

Third, a code of ethics or some other publicly waved banner of good intentions may be seen as a formal method of declaring to all that the occupation can be trusted, and so of persuading society to grant the special status of autonomy. The very existence of such a code implies that individual members of the occupation have the personal qualities of professionalism, the imputation of which is also useful for obtaining autonomy. Thus, most of the commonly cited attributes of professions may be seen either as consequences of their autonomy or as conditions useful for persuading the public and the body politic to grant such autonomy.

Autonomy and Dominance in the Division of Labor

Clearly, however, autonomy is not a simple criterion. One can think of many occupations that are autonomous merely by virtue of the esoteric character of their craft or the circumstances in which they work. Nightclub magicians and circus acrobats, for example, form autonomous occupations by virtue of their intensive specialization in an area of work that is itself narrowly specialized without at the same time constituting part of an interdependent division of labor. Other occupations, like cab drivers or lighthouse keepers, are fairly autonomous because their work takes place in a mobile or physically segregated context that prevents others from observing, and therefore evaluating and controlling, performance. In all these cases we have *autonomy by default*. An occupation is left wholly to its own devices because there is no strong public concern with its work, because it works independently of any functional division of labor, and because its work (in complexity, specialization, or observability) precludes easy evaluation and control by others. Where we find autonomy by default, we find no formal institutions in existence that serve to protect the occupation from competition, intervention, evaluation, and direction by others. Should interest in such an autonomous occupation be aroused among other workers or in society, its autonomy would prove to be fragile indeed without the introduction of such institutions. In short, *organized autonomy* is most stable and relevant to professions.

When we look at occupations engaged in such a complex division of labor as is found in the field of health, however, we find that with the exception of dentistry the only occupation that is truly autonomous is medicine itself.[3] It has the authority to direct and evaluate the work of others without in turn being subject to formal direction and evaluation by them. Paradoxically, its autonomy is sustained by the *dominance* of its expertise in the division of labor. It is true that some of the occupations it dominates—nursing for example—claim to be professions, as do other groups that lack either organized autonomy or dominance, such as school-teachers and social workers. But surely there is a critically significant difference between dominant professions and those others that claim the name but do not possess the status. While the members of all may be committed to their work, may be dedicated to service, and may be specially educated, the dominant profession stands in an entirely different structural relationship to the division of labor than does the subordinate profession. To ignore that difference is to ignore something major. One might call many occupations "professions" if one so chooses, but there is a difference between the dominant profession and the others. In essence the difference reflects the existence of a *hierarchy of institutionalized expertise*. That hierarchy of expertise, which is almost as definite as the hierarchy of office to be found in rational-legal monocratic bureaucracies,[4] can have the same effect on the experience of the client as bureaucracy is said to have. Let me briefly indicate how.

The Client in the Health Organization

Unlike education, where most services are given within complex organizations, most personal services in the field of health have been given in settings that are, organizationally, analogous to small shops. For a number of reasons, however, the proportion of personal health services given in complex organizations like hospitals seems to be increasing. It is the service in these complex organizations that has been most criticized for dehumanizing care, but is it bureaucratic office or institutionalized expertise that produces the client experience underlying that criticism?

Some complaints, like the cost of hospitalization, reflect the method of financing medical care in the United States rather than organization as such. Other complaints—such as those about poor food, noise, and general amenities—reflect the economic foundation and capital plant of the institution rather than its organization. For our present question, two sets of complaints seem most important—those related to the physical treatment for sickness and those related to the discomforts of being in a patient role in medical organizations.

Clearly, many complaints about the depersonalization of the client in the medical organization concern what some technical, ostensibly therapeutic, procedures do to people.[5] Simply to be strapped on a rolling table and wheeled down corridors, into and out of elevators, and, finally, into an operating room for the scrutiny of all is to be treated like an object, not a person. To be anesthetized is to become literally an object without the consciousness of a person. And to be palpated, poked, dosed, purged, cut into, probed, and sewed is to find oneself an object. In such cases, it is the technical work of the profession, not bureaucracy, that is responsible for some of the unpleasantness the client experiences in health organizations. That unpleasantness is partly analogous to what the industrial worker suffers when the machine he works on requires him to make limited, repetitive motions at some mechanically paced speed. It is directly analogous to what is suffered by the raw materials shaped by worker and machine in industry.

Such discomfort may easily be excused by the outcome—that is, improvement or cure is generally thought to be a product well worth the discomfort of being treated like an object. The problem, though, is to determine exactly how much of that treatment has any necessary bearing at all on the technical outcome. There is no doubt that some of the management of the patient has little or no bearing on the purely technical requirements for treatment.[6] Some practices bear on the bureaucratic problem of administering services to a number of individuals in a manner that is fair, precise, predictable, and economical. Other practices bear on the convenience of the staff, medical or otherwise, and while they may be justified by reference to staff needs as workers, such justification has no bearing on staff expertise as such. Without denying the role of formal bureaucratic organization in creating some of the problem, it is the role of the professional worker himself I wish to examine more closely, if only because, in medical and other organizations, the professional worker is specifically antibureaucratic, insisting on controlling the management of treatment himself. The question is, how do professional practices contribute to the unhappy experience of the patient?

The best way of beginning to answer this question lies in recalling the distinction I made between an object and a person. An object does not possess the capacity for understanding, and its behavior cannot be influenced by its understanding. When a person is treated *as if* he were an object, he will nonetheless behave on the basis of his understanding of that treatment. Naturally, his understanding is formed in part by what he brings with him into the treatment setting. It is also formed by the sense he himself can make of what is happening to him in the treatment setting. Since the treatment setting is presumably dominated by specialized, expert procedures, however, the most critical source of his information and understanding lies in the staff and its ability and inclination to communicate with the patient. If the staff does not communicate to the patient the meaning of and justification for what is done to him, it in essence refuses him the status of a responsible adult or of a person in the full sense of the word.

The extent to which the staff withholds information from the patient and avoids communicative interaction with him has been a common criticism of the operation of such medical organizations as hospitals.[7] The complaint is that no one tells the client what is going to be done to him, why, and when. And after he has been treated no one tells him why he feels the way he does, what can be expected subsequently, and whether or not he will live or die. The charge is that so little information is provided him that the patient cannot evaluate why he is being treated in a certain manner. Experience is mysteriously meaningless when it includes long waits for something unknown to happen or for something that does not happen, being awakened for an apparently trivial reason, being examined by taciturn strangers who enter the room unintroduced, perceiving lapses in such routines as medication and feeding without knowing whether error or intent is at issue. Surely this experience is little different from that of Kafka's antibureaucratic hero of *The Castle*.

Explanation by the staff constitutes acknowledgment of the client's status as a responsible adult capable of intelligent choice and self-control. In commercial organizations such acknowledgment does occur, however superficially, by "personalized" forms. Why does it not occur in hospitals? Part of the reason may stem from the necessity to treat clients in batches standardized by their technical status and by the services required. Some reason may also be found in understaffing and overwork, which excuses the minimization of interaction with some in order to maximize it with those with more "serious" problems. But these reasons do not explain why *bureaucratic* solutions to the problem of communication are not adopted—for example, distributing brochures explaining and justifying hospital routines, describing the experience of "typical" cholycystectomies, mastectomies, or heart patients from the first day through convalescence, and including answers to "commonly asked questions." The prime reason for the failure to communicate with the patient does not, I believe, lie in underfinancing, understaffing, or bureaucratization. Rather, it lies in the professional organization of the hospital and in the professional's conception of his relation to his clients.

Professional Control of Information

In the medical organization the medical profession is dominant. This means that all the work done by other occupations and related to the service of the patient is subject to the order of the physician.[8] The profession alone is held competent to diagnose illness, treat or direct the treatment of illness, and evaluate the service. Without medical authorization little can be done for the patient by paraprofessional workers. The client's medication, diet, excretion, and recreation are all subject to medical orders. So is the information given to the patient. By and large, without medical authorization paramedical workers are not supposed to communicate anything of significance to the patient about what his illness is, how it will be treated, and what the chances are for improvement. The physician himself is inclined to be rather jealous of the prerogative and is not inclined to authorize other workers to communicate information to the patient. Consequently, the paraprofessional worker who is asked for information by a patient is inclined to pass the buck like any bureaucrat. "You'll have to ask your doctor," the patient is told.

The dominant professional, then, is jealous of his prerogative to diagnose and forecast illness, holding it tightly to himself. But while he does not want anyone else to give information to the patient, neither is he himself inclined to do so. A number of reasons are advanced for this disinclination—the difficulty of being sure about diagnosis and precise about prognosis being perhaps the most neutral and technical of them all. Another reason is the physician's own busy schedule; he does not have the time to talk with the patient, and more serious cases need his attention. But the reasons of uncertainty and time-pressure are rather too superficial to dwell on. In the former case, the fact of uncertainty can constitute communication, though as Davis has shown[9] it can be asserted to avoid communication; in the latter case, surely the task can be delegated if time is lacking the doctor. For our present purposes, the most revealing argument against communication is based on characteristically professional assumptions about the nature of their clients. The argument, which goes back at least as far as Hippias' defensive remarks in the Hippocratic Corpus, asserts that, lacking professional training, the client is too ignorant to be able to comprehend what information he gets and that he is, in any case, too upset at being ill to be able to use the information he does get in a manner that is rational and responsible.[10] From this it follows that giving information to the patient does not help him, but rather upsets him and creates additional "management problems" for the physician. Thus, the patient should not be treated like an adult, but rather like a child, given reassurance but not information. To do otherwise would only lead to the patient being upset and making unnecessary trouble for the staff. Characteristically, the professional does not view the client as an adult, responsible person.

In addition, it is worth pointing out the implications of the professional insistence on faith or trust rather than persuasion. The client, lacking professional training, is thought to be unequipped for intelligent evaluation or informed cooperation with his consultant. Essentially, he is expected either to have faith in his consultant and do what he is told without searching question or else to choose another consultant in whom he does have faith. To question one's doctor is to show lack of faith and is justifiable grounds for the doctor to threaten to withdraw his services. Such insistence on faith, I believe, rests on more than the purely functional demands of an effective therapeutic or service relationship. It also neutralizes threat to status. The very special social position of institutionalized privilege that is the profession's is threatened as well as demeaned by the demand that advice and action be explained and justified to a layman. If he must justify himself to a layman, the professional must use grounds of evidence and logic common to both professional and layman and cannot use esoteric grounds known and subscribed to by the profession alone. Insistence on faith constitutes insistence that the client give up his role as an independent adult and, by so neutralizing him, protect the esoteric foundation of the profession's insitutionalized authority.[11]

Other Workers in the Professional Organization

Thus far I have pointed out that in medical organizations, the source of a client's alienation is professional rather than bureaucratic authority.[12] Some alienating characteristics of professional authority may lead to practices with a curiously bureaucractic look to them, including such notorious practices as passing the buck and such a notorious problem as (in the form of requiring doctors' orders) red tape. In this organization the client's position is similar to his position in civil service bureaucracies—he is handled like an object, given little information or opportunity for choice, and made to feel less than a responsible adult. And what of the subordinate worker in this setting dominated by a profession?

. . . many writers have felt that the worker as well as the client suffers from the bureaucratization of production by a monocratic administration. Lacking identification with the prime goals of the organization, lacking an important voice in setting the formal level and direction of work, and performing work that has been so rationalized as to become mechanical and meaningless, a minute segment of an intricate mosaic of specialized activities that he is in no position to perceive or understand, the worker is alienated. In contrast to the bureaucratized worker, however, the professional is said to be committed to and identified with his work so that it retains meaning for him, becoming in fact a central life interest. This may be true for dominant professions, but what of the other occupations working in the organization that the professional dominates? Are they not prone to alienation?

By and large, this question has not been asked in past studies, for the emphasis has been more on the positive response of "professionalism" than on the negative responses of alienation. What evidence there is, however, indicates that there are serious problems of worker morale in professional settings. Available studies are fairly clear about the existence of hierarchy in the professional health organization and about a decrease of participation in decision making the farther down the hierarchy one goes. Neither the ends nor the means of their work seem to be a matter for legitimate determination by lower-level workers, though, of course, they do sometimes have a very strong informal influence on such determination. Furthermore, even in situations where the stated official expectation is free participation by all workers in conferences about the running of such units as wards, participation has been observed to be quite unequal.[13]

The paraprofessional worker is, then, like the industrial worker, subordinated to the authority of others. He is not, however, subordinated solely to the authority of bureaucratic office, but also to the putatively superior knowledge and judgment of professional experts. In some studies this authority is characterized as a kind of stratification,[14] in others as a function of status.[15] In very few, if any, studies is that status or stratification said to be of administrative or bureaucratic origin. It is instead largely of professional origin. In a few studies the notion of alienation has been specifically cited.[16] Clearly, while there is no comparative evidence to allow us to determine whether more or fewer workers are alienated from professional than from bureaucratic organizations, neither hierarchical nor authoritarian tendencies are missing in the professional organization of the division of labor, nor are alienation, absenteeism, low morale, and high turnover insignificant problems. It is as true for the worker as for the patient that the professionally organized division of labor has pathologies similar to those stemming from bureaucracy.

Substantive Bias in Client Services

Thus far I have compared the influence of professional authority with the influence of bureaucratic authority on the experience of both client and worker in the physically limited corporate body we usually call an organization. However, because interorganizational relations may themselves be seen as organization and since the production of particular goods and services is rarely limited to the confines of a single corporate body requiring a variety of functions from outside "the" organization, it seems useful to continue my comparison in the rather broader context of planning and coordinating service as such. I have already noted that the common assumption is that expert authority has a neutral, functional foundation rather than, like bureaucratic authority, the foundation of arbitrary office. If this is so, we should expect the influence of expert authority on the support and planning of services to be highly functional, lacking arbitrary bias from the special vantage of bureaucratic office. Our expectation is not met in health services. There, the dominant profession exercises great influence on the disposition of resources that makes services available for clients. The character of that influence does stem from professional views of the purely functional considerations of what service is needed to accomplish some desired end, but *those views have been distorted by the lenses of a special occupational perspective.*

To understand how resources get distributed to the varied health services sought or required by the client, we must keep in mind the fact that the *medical* division of labor is not functionally complete. It is composed solely of those occupations and services controlled by the dominant profession. Outside it are some performing work that is functionally and substantively related to the profession but not subject to the profession's authority. In matters of health in the United States, such occupations as dentistry, optometry, chiropracty, and clinical psychology exemplify by their independent existence the functional incompleteness of the medically ordered division of labor. Furthermore, there are occupational groups whose work is often at least partly related to health problems but which are not recognized medical occupations; schoolteachers, specialized training and guidance personnel, social workers, and even ministers may be cited here. These are not part of the medically ordered division of labor either. Thus, while the profession stands as the supreme authority in the medical division of labor, the medical division of labor does not encompass all health-related activities of the larger health-related division of labor. Nonetheless, the distribution of support and resources tends to move disproportionately through the medical division of labor.

I have argued for the distinction of a type of profession that has ultimate authority over its work in such a way that it is self-directing or autonomous and dominant in a division of labor. In the case of medicine, a strategic facet of its authority is its delineation of pathology, the definitions of health and illness that guide the application of knowledge to human ills. The physician is the ultimate expert on what is health and what illness and on how to attain the former and cure the latter. Indeed, his perspective leads him to see the world in terms of health and illness, and the world is presently inclined to turn to him for advice on all matters related to health and illness regardless of his competence. Given the highly visible miracles medicine has worked over the past century, the public has even been inclined to ask the profession to deal with problems that are not of the biophysical character for which success was gained from past efforts. What were once recognized as economic, religious, and personal problems have been redefined as illness and have therefore become medical problems.[17] This widening of medical jurisdiction has had important consequences for the allocation of resources to client services.

No philanthropies today seem to be able to attract more financial support than those devoting themselves to illness, particularly those of children. If the label of illness can be attached to a problem it receives extensive support and also becomes dominated by medical institutions even when there is no evidence that medical institutions have any especially efficacious way of dealing with the problem. By virtue of controlling the notions of illness and health, medicine has in fact become a giant umbrella under which a disparate variety of workers (including sociologists) can be both financed and protected from overly close outside scrutiny merely through their semantic connection with health. But those who do not or cannot choose to huddle under the umbrella, even though their work is health-related, tend to find it difficult to obtain support.

One rather obvious consequence is the uneven distribution of resources to health-related activities. For example, it was pointed out recently that heavy financing has been given to medical research into mental deficiency, only a small amount of which is biologically or genetically caused, while *educational* facilities for the training and teaching of mental deficients have been sorely underfinanced.[18] Less obvious and more important to public welfare is the extent to which this uneven distribution of resources emphasizes some hypotheses and investigatory and therapeutic models at the expense of others equally plausible. For example, it was recently noted that work in rehabilitation has come under medical supervision, resulting in an inappropriate emphasis on the traditional authoritarian therapeutic relationship of medicine that I have already discussed.[19] It has also been noted that the disease model has dominated the approach to mental illness.[20] By and large, within the well-financed division of labor dominated by the profession and under its protective umbrella, most work is limited to that which conforms to the special perspective and substantive style of the profession—a perspective that emphasizes the individual over the social environment, the treatment of rare and interesting over common and uninteresting disorders, the cure rather than the prevention of illness, and preventive medicine rather than what might be called "preventive welfare"—social services and resources that improve the diet, housing, way of life, and motivation of the people without their having to undertake clinical consultation with a practitioner. In short, I suggest that by virtue of its position in the public esteem and in its own division of labor, the dominant profession of the field of health exerts a special and biased influence on planning and financing services of the general field within which it is located. The prime criterion for determining that emphasis is not necessarily functional in character, but social and structural—whether or not the services can be dominated by or be put under the umbrella of the dominant profession. The consequence for the client is an array of differentially supported services that may not be adequate for his needs and interests.

Finally, I might point out that given this array of health-related services differentially developed and supported by functional and other considerations, still further qualification of the kind of service a client is likely to get is exercised by the dominant profession. In general, I wish to suggest that when some of the relevant services lie outside the medical division of labor and some inside, serious problems of access to care and of the rational coordination of care are created by the barriers that the profession erects between that segment of the division of labor it does dominate and that segment it does not.[21]

Perhaps the simplest way of discussing these barriers is to examine the process by which clients move through the division of labor. They move in part by their own choice and selection of consultants and in part by their consultants' choice of and referral to other consultants or technicians. To the extent that the client moves through the division of labor by his own volition, he is responsible for his own care and his consultants are dependent on him for relevant information about his problem. But to the extent to which the client is being guided by consultants, the character of his experience and care is dependent on the substantive direction of his consultants' referrals and on the exchange of information bearing on treatment among them. Here is where the professionally created barrier is found. Within the general health division of labor, the referral of clients tends to go in only one direction—into the smaller medical division of labor, without also going from the medical into the larger system. This is also generally true of the transmission of information about the client. To put it more bluntly, teachers, social workers, ministers, and others outside the medical division of labor refer to physicians and communicate information about the client to them, but physicians are not likely either to refer clients to them or to provide them with the results of medical investigation.[22]

By the same token, physicians do not routinely refer to clinical psychologists, optometrists, chiropractors, and others outside the medical division of labor but clearly within the health division of labor. They are likely to refer only when they are sure that the limited services they may order—psychological testing rather than psychotherapy, spectacle fitting and sales rather than refractions, and minor manipulations for medically untreatable muscular-skeletal complaints rather than for other complaints—will be performed, and no more. They are also, wittingly or not, likely to discourage such workers' referrals to them by reciprocating neither referrals nor information about their findings. And from at least one study there is evidence that medically oriented workers are prone to reject the patient if he comes to them from the wrong source.[23]

By and large, physicians refer to and communicate extensively with only those who, within the medical division of labor, are subject to their prescription, order, or direction. Indeed, physicians are likely to be very poorly informed about any institutional and occupational resources that lie outside their own jurisdiction. And, as is quite natural for people who have developed commitment to their work, they are likely to be suspicious of the value of all that lies outside their domain, including the competence and ethicality of those working outside. Their commitment leads them to deprecate the importance of extramedical services, and their position as professionals encourages them to restrict their activities to the medical system they control. So long as this is all their clients need or want, no harm is done save for the possibility that the professional's response to outside services may encourage those outside to avoid or delay in referring clients to the physician. Even when outside services are necessary for the client's well-being, referral to them may be delayed or never undertaken and the client's interests left unprotected.

Notes

1. Jerome Carlin, *Lawyers' Ethics* (New York: Russell Sage Foundation, 1966). It should be noted that Carlin's findings also were that a stable individual attribute of ethicality influenced behavior independently of the setting. A recent study of college students found the same thing. See William J. Bowers, "Normative Constraints on Deviant Behavior in the College Context," *Sociometry,* *31* (December, 1968), 370–385.
2. *Webster's Third New International Dictionary* (Springfield, Mass.: C. & C. Merriam Co., 1967), p.148.
3. See Eliot Freidson, "Paramedical Personnel," in *International Encyclopedia of the Social Sciences* (New York: Macmillan and Free Press, 1968), Vol. 10, pp. 114–120, for more discussion on the medical division of labor.
4. A recent article argues persuasively against the value of using the idea of formal bureaucratic organization to analyze settings in which professionals work, pointing out that even in industrial settings the idea does not faithfully reflect observed behavior. See Rue Bucher and Joan Stelling, "Characteristics of Professional Organization," *Journal of Health and Social Behavior,* 10 (1969), 3–15. The same point may be made for the division of labor I describe. However, formal bureaucratic organization and formal occupational jurisdiction and authority do provide limits of a fairly definite nature; just as a

stenographer cannot negotiate with her employer over who will chair a policy making meeting, so a nurse cannot negotiate with a surgeon over who will perform an operation.

5. Important in this context is Erving Goffman's "The Medical Model and Mental Hospitalization," in Erving Goffman, *Asylums* (Garden City, N.Y.: Doubleday, 1961), pp. 321–386.

6. For an extended analysis of the substance of expertise which tries to indicate what is genuine and what spurious in medical work, see Eliot Freidson, *Profession of Medicine: A Study of the Sociology of Applied Knowledge* (New York: Dodd-Mead, 1970), Chapter 15.

7. For example, see the following: Julius A. Roth, "The Treatment of Tuberculosis as a Bargaining Process," in A. M. Rose, ed., *Human Behavior and Social Processes* (Boston: Houghton Mifflin, 1962), pp. 575–588; Jeanne C. Quint, "Institutionalized Practices of Information Control," *Psychiatry,* 28 (1965), 119–132.

8. For example, see Albert F. Wessen, "Hospital Ideology and Communication Between Ward Personnel" in E. G. Jaco, ed., *Patients, Physicians, and Illness* (New York: Free Press, 1958), pp. 448–468.

9. Fred Davis, "Uncertainty in Medical Prognosis, Clinical and Functional," *American Journal of Sociology,* 66 (1960), 41–47.

10. See, for example, the material in Barney G. Glaser and Anselm L. Strauss, *Awareness of Dying* (Chicago: Aldine, 1965).

11. For a more extensive discussion of the professional ideology see Freidson, *Profession of Medicine,* Chapter 8.

12. For a rare study of patients using a measure of alienation, see John W. Evans, "Stratification, Alienation, and the Hospital Setting," *Engineering Experiment Station Bulletin* No. 184, Ohio State University, 1960.

13. For example, see the findings in William Caudill, *The Psychiatric Hospital as a Small Society* (Cambridge, Mass.: Harvard University Press, 1958), and William A. Rushing, *The Psychiatric Professions* (Chapel Hill: University of North Carolina Press, 1964), pp. 258–259.

14. See M. Seeman and J. W. Evans, "Stratification and Hospital Care," *American Sociological Review,* 26 (1961), 67–80, 193–204, and Ivar Oxaal, "Social Stratification and Personnel Turnover in the Hospital," *Engineering Experiment Station Monograph* No. 3, Ohio State University, 1960.

15. See E. G. Mishler and A. Tropp, "Status and Interaction in a Psychiatric Hospital," *Human Relations,* 9 (1956), 187–205, and William R. Rosengren, "Status Stress and Role Contradictions: Emergent Professionalization in Psychiatric Hospitals," *Mental Hygiene,* 45 (1961), 28–39.

16. See Rose L. Coser, "Alienation and the Social Structure: Case Study of a Hospital," in E. Freidson, ed., *Hospital in Modern Society* (New York: Free Press, 1963), pp. 231–265, and L. I. Pearlin, "Alienation from Work: A Study of Nursing Personnel," *American Sociological Review,* 27 (1962), 314–326.

17. For an extended discussion of the relative place of notions of health and illness in modern society, see Freidson, *Profession of Medicine,* Chapter 12.

18. George W. Albee, "Needed—A Revolution in Caring for the Retarded," *Trans-action,* 5 (1968), 37–42.

19. Albert F. Wessen, "The Apparatus of Rehabilitation: An Organizational Analysis," in Marvin B. Sussman, ed., *Sociology and Rehabilitation* (Washington, D. C.: American Sociological Association, 1966), pp. 148–178.
20. See Marline Taber et al., "Disease Ideology and Mental Health Research," *Social Problems, 16* (1969), 349–357, for a recent statement.
21. See the discussion in William L. Kissick, "Health Manpower in Transition," *The Milbank Memorial Fund Quarterly, 46* (January 1968), Part 2, pp. 53–91, for this and many other relevant points.
22. For work bearing on these statements see Elaine Cumming et al., *Systems of Social Regulation* (New York: Atherton, 1968), and Eugene B. Piedmont, "Referrals and Reciprocity: Psychiatrists, General Practitioners, and Clergymen," *Journal of Health and Social Behavior, 9* (1968), 29–41.
23. See David Schroder and Danuta Ehrlich, "Rejection by Mental Health Professionals: A Possible Consequence for Not Seeking Appropriate Help for Emotional Disorders," *Journal of Health and Social Behavior, 9* (1968), 222–232.

The Social Organization of Medical Care Workers and Services

MEDICAL CARE IN THE UNITED STATES is an enormous and complex industry, involving thousands of organizations, the expenditure of billions of dollars each year, and the employment of millions of workers. There are discernible patterns in the types and distribution of medical services available in any society. These patterns reflect and reinforce the socio-cultural context in which they are found, including the political, economic, and cultural priorities of a society (Waitzkin and Waterman, 1974: 8). The composition of the labor force in most sectors of society reflects that society's distribution of power and privilege. This section examines (1) the organization and distribution of medical care services; and (2) the nature of the medical care labor force in this country.

(1) Our medical care system has been described as ". . . acute, curative, [and] hospital-based . . ." (Knowles, 1977: 2). That is, we have a *medical* care system (as distinguished from a *health* care system)[1] organized around the cure and/or control of serious diseases and the repairing of physical injuries rather than the "caring" for the sick or prevention of disease. The American medical care system is highly technological, specialized and, increasingly, centralized. More and more medical care is delivered in large bureaucratic institutions, many of them hospitals. And these organizations now employ more than 75 percent of all medical care workers (DHEW, 1978: 336). Our medical care system is becoming increasingly hospital-centered.

Since 1900 there has been a gradual increase in the number of hospitals in the United States to the current total of over 7,000. In fact, as of 1976, there were 7,274 long- and short-term hospitals, 20,185 nursing homes (long-term residential institutions for the old and very sick), and an additional 6,280 "inpatient health facilities" (unspecified) (DHEW, 1978: 349). Until about the mid-1960s there was also a sharply increasing number of hospital beds; since then the number has dropped back down to about 350 beds per 1,000 people, the level found in the mid-1950s (The University of Michigan: 1976). These figures are averages, of course, and do not tell us about the distribution of the beds or their availability to people. Approximately 50 percent of all hospitals in 1976 were owned by nonprofit organizations, with another 36 percent owned by either federal, state, or local governments. The remaining 14 percent were owned by profit-making organizations; however, 75 percent of all nursing homes at that time were profit-making institutions (DHEW, 1978: 349).

The first article in this section, "Health Care and Medical Care in the United States," by Victor W. Sidel and Ruth Sidel addresses the issue of how and why medical care services are organized and distributed the way they are in the United States. The authors find a serious maldistribution of medical services, coupled with a set of economic and political priorities that has produced a medical care system unresponsive to the health needs of many of its citizens. Why this should be so in a country that invests so much money in medical care—more than any other country in the world—remains a central question in their article and throughout this book.

(2) The growth and expansion of medical care institutions has engendered a rapid expansion of the medical labor force. The number of people employed between 1970 and 1977 in the medical care industry in the United States expanded 50 percent—from 4.2 million to 6.3 million.[2] Medical care workers constitute about 7 percent of the total American labor force. Approximately 58 percent of all medical care workers are employed by hospitals, 15 percent by convalescent institutions (nursing homes), 11 percent in doctors' offices, 5 percent in dentists' offices, and the remainder in offices of other health practitioners and at other medical service sites. Some of these workers are physicians, but the vast majority are not. In fact, physicians make up *less than 6 percent* of the entire medical labor force (DHEW, 1978: 333–337).

Approximately half of the total medical labor force provides nursing-related services. Only about 4 percent of the hospital workforce are physicians. As Caress (1976: 178) notes, "There are about the same number of physicians as there are maintenance men in American hospitals." Among hospital workers there is an enormous range in the level of education and skill required to carry out their jobs.

Of all hospital employees 43.5 percent are either RN's [registered nurses] (16.2 percent), LPN's [licensed practical nurses] and LVN's [licensed vocational nurses] (7.4 percent) or aides, orderlies and attendants (19.9 percent). The remainder of hospital workers are in clinical technology (3.2 percent), pharmacy (0.8 percent), administration (0.6 percent), dentistry (0.6 percent) and even smaller representations in other categories. (Caress, 1976: 178.)

Medical care workers include some of the highest paid employees in our nation (physicians) and some of the lowest paid (until the early 1970s many hospital workers were not even covered by minimum wage laws). More than 75 percent of all medical workers are women, although more than 85 percent of all physicians are men. Many of these women are members of Third World and minority groups, and most come from working-class and lower-middle class backgrounds. Almost all physicians are white and upper middle class. In short, the structure of the medical workforce reflects the inequalities of American society in general.

This medical care workforce structure can be pictured as a broad-based triangle, with a small number of highly paid physicians and administrators at the very top. These men (and they are mostly men) by and large control the administration of medical care services *within* institutions. As one moves toward the bottom of the triangle, there are increasing numbers of significantly lower-paid female workers with little or no authority in the medical delivery organization. This triangle is layered with a growing number of licensed occupational categories of workers, a number currently close to 300 different medical occupations (Caress, 1976: 168). There is practically no movement of workers from one category to another, since each requires its own specialized training and qualifications, requirements which are largely controlled through licensing procedures authorized by the American Medical Association's Committee on Education. Professional dominance, as discussed in the previous section, is highly evident throughout the division and organization of medical labor.

The development of this rigidly layered or *stratified* medical labor force is the result of a complex historical process, deeply connected to the development of the hospital as a central site of American medical care delivery. Susan Reverby explores this connection in the second article in this section, "Re-forming the Hospital Nurse: The Management of American Nursing." She traces the relationship of the development of the division of labor within nursing, the efforts of nursing to gain professional power, and the changing organizational needs of the hospital administrators.

In the final article, "The Influence of Social Class Structure on the American Health Sector," Vicente Navarro examines the relationship of society's structure to the medical care system in particular. Concerned with what he sees as the overly narrow focus of so much medical and social sciences research, Navarro contends that if we are to understand the nature of the division of labor within medical care, we must understand its relationship to the division of labor in our society in general. Navarro argues that the medical labor force mirrors the social class divisions that exist under the particular political economy of the United States. He points out, as have others, that while medical care workers may hope to better themselves economically and socially through education and training, these mechanisms have *not* produced significant change in the class composition of the medical labor force. Rather, as another writer puts it, the workers are competing with each other for "smaller pieces" of a "bigger pie" (Caress, 1976: 168). This had led to the extreme fragmentation of both the medical labor force and the services they provide. This situation implicitly raises the issue of the consequences of the current distribution of power and privilege within the medical labor force on the quality of medical care, and the issue of options available to medical workers to effect changes in the current system.

Notes

1. The distinction between "medical" and "health" care is one made by Sidel and Sidel in their article in this section.
2. Inclusion of those people who work in health related occupations but were not employed in the health care industry *as defined* by the Bureau of the Census—e.g., school nurses, medical school faculty—adds another 560,000 medical care workers to the 1977 total (DHEW, 1978: 333).

References

Caress, Barbara. 1976. "The health workforce: Bigger pie, smaller pieces." Pp. 163–170 in David Kotelchuck, Prognosis Negative. New York: Vintage Books. [Reprinted from Health/PAC Bulletin, January/February, 1975.]

Department of Health, Education and Welfare. 1978. Health United States 1978. DHEW Publication No. (PHS) 76-1232: December. Ratio of physicians computed from data in Table 119 using the 1977 total of health service employees [6,328,000] and the average number of total active physicians from the totals listed for 1975 and projected for 1980 in Table 121 [400,000].

Knowles, John. 1977. "Introduction." John Knowles (ed.), Doing Better and Feeling Worse: Health in the United States. Daedalus. 106, 1: Winter.

The University of Michigan. 1976. School of Public Health, Department of Medical Care Organization. Medical Care Chart Book, Sixth Edition. Revised, September.

Waitzkin, Howard, and Barbara Waterman. 1974. The Exploitation of Illness in Capitalist Society. Indianapolis: The Bobbs-Merrill Co., Inc.

13

Health Care and Medical Care in the United States

Victor W. Sidel and Ruth Sidel

. . . .

Although in one sense the U.S. medical-care system is highly structured—for the benefit of those who control it and of some of those who work in it—in another sense it is so fragmented, the responsibilities so diffuse, the levels of control so manifold, the communication and coordination between its parts so haphazard, that—except for the euphemisms "pluralistic" and "pragmatic"—the system almost defies brief description.

One type of analysis, analogous in some ways to the classifications of levels of prevention, is the definition of various levels of care as "primary," "secondary" and "tertiary" according to the severity of the illness and the nature of the medical response that is required.

At the first level, the patient with relatively minor symptoms or who is worried about his health may seek reassurance or care in a number of different ways. Self-care, often with medications available without prescription ("over the counter"), is the most frequent response to common symptoms or anxiety which an individual feels on a given day. Such an individual may turn to members of his family for advice and care, or to nonprofessional people within his community. Teachers or fellow workers are often consulted on various types of health problems. In some cultures spiritualists, herbalists or other well-defined individuals within the culture are consulted at times of minor illness, or even illness of greater severity.

The first contact with the professional medical system is often with a professional other than a physician. Pharmacists, for example, play an important role in first-contact professional care. If a physician is to be consulted as the point of first-contact professional care, the choice of the type of physician to be contacted is quite different from country to country. In most countries the physician of first contact will be a "primary-care physician," which, as we define the term, signifies a physician based in the community rather than in a hospital; a physician people first turn to, who does not regularly see referrals from other physicians; who provides continuing care rather than episodic care; and who serves the function of integrating the work of referral specialists and other community resources in relation to the patient's care.

In this sequence, "secondary care" is that which is provided by specialists, either on an ambulatory basis or in the hospital, and "tertiary care" is that which is provided in specialized hospitals by highly specialized or subspecialized personnel. In the United States, however, first-contact primary care is often provided by specialists, by emergency rooms and by hospital outpatient departments—resources which in other societies are largely reserved for secondary or even tertiary care.

Beyond these three levels of medical care is that of long-term care for the chronically ill or disabled. In the United States, long-term care is often provided in chronic hospitals or in nursing homes for those whose illnesses are so severe that function outside of an institution is impossible or, in an increasing number of instances, for those who have no alternative place with either family or friends in which they can be given the care they need while continuing to function within the society.

Another framework for analysis is based on the nature of the controlling institution. These institutions are usually divided into three basic groups, one conventionally defined as "public" (meaning governmental) and two defined as "private," although the distinctions increasingly have less and less meaning.

Let us begin with the elements of the system in the "public" sector. All levels of government play a role in health care and in medical care, with a complex mix of direct operating responsibility for some elements, funding for others, and regulation for yet others. The federal government directly *operates* medical-care delivery programs for military personnel and their families, for veterans and for native Americans on reservations. It *finances* medical care for the aged and for a limited group of other disabled people through Medicare and indirectly pays a major part of the cost of medical care for the poor through Medicaid; it is the major funding agency for the construction of medical facilities and for medical research; and it provides a large part of the funding for medical education directly to medical schools and indirectly through scholarships and loan funds for medical students. Finally, the federal government has important *regulatory* authority over health and medical affairs involving "interstate commerce," such as food and drugs, occupational health and safety, and environmental pollution. Overall, federal money accounts for nearly 30 percent of all U.S. health expenditures. These include about 25 percent of all funds spent on personal health and medical-care services, 65 percent of the investment in biomedical research and development, and over 45 percent of the revenues of the nation's medical schools.

State governments provide medical care directly for many of the mentally ill and, until recently, those with tuberculosis; they administer and contribute to the financing of health care for the poor through Medicaid;

they conduct statewide public health programs; they operate medical schools, usually through a state university, and contribute to the financing of others; and they license hospitals and a wide range of health workers.

Local governments, at the county and municipal levels, often provide inpatient and ambulatory-care services directly for the poor. They also carry out a wide variety of public health functions, including the collecting of vital statistics and statistics on reportable illnesses; controlling communicable diseases, including tuberculosis and venereal diseases; monitoring environmental sanitation, including water quality and supervision of foods and eating places; providing maternal and child health services, including school health services; and conducting programs of health education.

In short, almost all "public health services" in the United States and many personal medical-care services are directly provided by government agencies, and many other personal medical-care services are financed by government.

The two parts of the "private" sector are defined as "profit-making" (sometimes called, for historical reasons, "proprietary" or, for public-relations reasons, "investor-owned") and "nonprofit-making" (sometimes termed "voluntary" or "eleemosynary").

Examples of parts of the system almost entirely in the profit-making sector are nursing homes; pharmaceutical research, manufacture, distribution and sale; and commercial health-insurance companies. For the United States as a whole, most ambulatory medical and dental care is in the profit-making part of the private sector, although the situation is different in the centers of some of our largest cities where many of these services are provided by government or by voluntary hospitals. Only a small fraction of U.S. hospital beds lie in profit-making hospitals, many of which are owned by groups of physicians.

The "nonprofit" sector includes the voluntary hospitals, which contain over 60 percent of the country's acute-general-care beds; many of the nation's medical schools, including some of its most prestigious ones; and insurance organizations in each state affiliated with each other under the name of Blue Cross and Blue Shield, providing insurance respectively for hospitalization costs and for doctors' fees.

In sum, a large part of the U.S. medical-care system—as contrasted with its health-care system—is controlled by the private sector, even though, as we have seen, large amounts of it are financed publicly. Furthermore, the fact that medical care is largely controlled by the private sector and that health care is largely controlled by the public sector is surely one of the major reasons for the overwhelmingly greater investment in treatment rather than in prevention. This is especially true for ambulatory care. Of the 1.1 billion patient visits made annually in the United States (an average of five visits per person per year), two-thirds are made to private medical practitioners and private group practices, almost all on a fee-for-service basis. Another 18 percent of the visits nationwide—though a far higher percent in the inner cities—are made to hospital outpatient departments and emergency rooms, many of them also in the "private" (albeit "nonprofit") sector.

The situation shifts markedly when one looks at inpatient hospital care. Mainly because of the large number of long-stay beds in mental hospitals owned by state and local governments, and to a lesser extent the number of beds in the federal government's Veterans Administration, Armed Services, and Public Health Service hospitals, approximately half the U.S. hospital beds are in government-owned and -operated hospitals. Only 5 percent of the beds are in proprietary hospitals, owned and operated for profit. The remaining 45 percent are in voluntary hospitals, operated on a nonprofit basis by churches, other organized groups, or by self-elected and self-perpetuated boards of trustees.

It is of interest that since 1946 the ratio of hospital beds of all kinds to population has decreased, from one bed for every 100 people to one for every 130 people. The decrease has occurred largely in federal hospitals and in psychiatric, tuberculosis and other long-term hospitals. At the same time, however, there has been an increase in the bed/population ratio for short-term general hospitals. There are now approximately 4.5 short-term general medical and surgical beds per 1000 population (one for every 225 people); of these, in contrast to the situation for long-stay beds, only about one-third are operated by government. There has also been a trend over this period to larger hospitals, with a reduction in the number of hospitals having less than 100 beds. Despite the fact that hospitals have increased in size in the name of efficiency and despite the net movement of people from rural areas to metropolitan areas where hospitals are larger, the level of bed occupancy has changed almost not at all from 1946 (75 percent) to 1975 (76 percent).

The training and practice of the health workers in the system are also fragmented and there is little accountability to the public. Patterns for education of physicians are largely set by nongovernmental bodies, such as the Association of American Medical Colleges, and by the medical schools themselves. Although there is an increasing attempt at coordination of criteria for licensure and the use of a standardized national examination, licensure standards are set on a state-by-state basis, almost in every case by physician-dominated boards with little public accountability. Except for the internal standards set by hospitals and other medical institutions, which vary widely and are often unenforced, any physician, whatever his or her training, can legally do anything in medical practice: perform neurosurgery, counsel people with marital problems or read X rays. For physicians who practice largely outside institutions, fear of malpractice suits is almost the only deterrent—other than conscience—to undertaking procedures in which they have had only minimal training or experience.

Figure 1. *Distribution of Physicians by Specialization Status in the United States, 1949–1972*

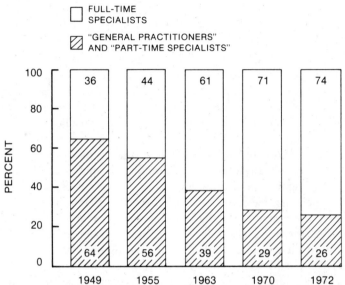

Modified by the authors from a figure prepared by the University of Michigan School of Public Health from data published by the U.S. Public Health Service (before 1970) and the National Center for Health Statistics (1970 and 1972). The data include only M.D.s in private practice.

Of the approximately 375,000 active physicians in the United States (one for every 550 people), almost 8 percent are employed by the federal government and approximately 20 percent are in salaried hospital practice; some of the former and most of the latter are in training programs, usually as interns and residents. Approximately another 10 percent are employed in teaching, administration, research and other activities not directly related to patient care. The remaining 60 percent of active doctors are employed in "office-based" patient care; most of them practicing on a fee-for-service basis.

Physicians are largely free to choose their own form of postgraduate training and their own form of practice. As a result over the past quarter-century there has been a major shift away from primary care—first-contact, continuing integrated care for the patient—and a major shift toward specialist practice, as shown in Figure 1. Even if one includes doctors who say they "limit their practice" to internal medicine and pediatrics, the supply of primary-care doctors in the United States has fallen sharply from 1930, when there was approximately one for every 1000 people, to 1970, when there was one for every 2000.

There has been somewhat of a reversal in the 1970s, due in part to the efforts of the federal and state governments, but the number of specialist physicians still far exceeds the number of primary-care physicians. In fact, the United States probably exceeds all other countries in the world in the extent to which medical care is given by physicians who consider themselves specialists rather than generalists or even, as is the increasing trend in the United States, as "specialists" in "family practice."

The result, of course, of this specialization and of the benefit coverage of most health-insurance policies, which cover hospital care but rarely ambulatory care and even more rarely continuing and preventive care, is a medical-care system devoted largely to technological diagnosis and treatment for serious acute illness and relatively little to care for less serious acute illness and to care for chronic illness and disability.

Similar kinds of analyses can be applied to nurses and other health workers. Among the major differences is that most nurses, for example, are salaried rather than fee-for-service entrepreneurs, that a far higher percentage of them are women, and that their incomes are far lower than those of doctors. But there are also vast similarities: a fragmentation of training patterns with little public control, an increasing emphasis in training (the "university-trained" nurse) and in practice (the "nurse-clinician") on technology rather than care, and gross geographic and social maldistribution.

The gross maldistribution of health workers in the United States can be seen by a regional, a state-by-state, or a community-by-community analysis. In 1973 there was, for example, one doctor for every 1343 people in South Dakota, compared to one for every 432 people in New York . . . The differences among states are not simply a result of differences in population density; Vermont and Iowa, for example, have approximately the same population density, but there is one physician for every 565 people in Vermont compared to one for every 999 in Iowa. The wealth of the state, and its desirability to physicians as a place to live and work, appear to be the major attractions.

The same is true for other types of health workers. There is one registered nurse, for example, for every 400 to 500 persons in the South Central states while in the New England states there is one nurse for every 150 to 200 people; an average person in the South, in other words, has available less than half the number of nurses than does his counterpart in the Northeast.

Not only is there gross maldistribution among regions and among states, but there is similar maldistribution within states and within cities. In a study performed in the Appalachian states in 1967, the ratio of physicians to population in counties with a median disposable income of more than $5000 per family was, with the exception of one state, consistently higher than the ratio in counties with an income of $5000 or less per family . . . In Maryland, Tennessee and Alabama, for example, there were almost three times as many doctors per capita in the rich counties as in the poor counties, and in Virginia, West Virginia and North Carolina, there were about twice as many per capita for the wealthy counties as for the poor.

Individual small, relatively isolated communities often have severe difficulty in recruiting or in keeping a physician. The National Health Service Corps estimated in 1976 that there were 748 U.S. communities that lacked a physician. These doctorless communities were located in 46 states; every one of the United States, with the exception of Hawaii, Massachusetts, New Jersey and Rhode Island, had at least one town needing a doctor.

Inside the large cities the maldistribution of physicians is equally severe, but it is harder to demonstrate statistically because many of the teaching hospitals, with their large numbers of doctors, are located in the midst of what have become the poorest urban areas. However, because they limit their practice to specialties or subspecialties or because they are in training for these specialties, most of these hospital-based doctors are unavailable to meet the general medical-care needs of the poor who surround them. A study performed in Boston, for example, showed that the number of general-care physicians per capita was twice as high in affluent areas studied as in poor ones.

Even when general-care doctors are available—often grudgingly—in outpatient departments and in the emergency rooms of the hospitals (and, because of the inaccessibility of general medical care elsewhere, the emergency room is becoming the place in which much primary medical care is currently being given), there are great barriers to access by the poor. Members of the New York City Department of Health in the mid-1960s described some of the remaining barriers, even when those imposed by cost of care are removed, which keep poor people from equitable access to medical care. These include inadequate transportation, complex and imposing institutions, difficulty in taking time off from work or in finding someone to take care of the children, and the fragmentation and repeated visits common in such care.

Medicaid, which was intended to ameliorate some of the inequity of access, has indeed brought physicians into the urban ghetto, but the nature of the financial incentives which brought them in have led to other forms of abuse. One is the promotion of brief and unnecessarily frequent visits, with the "ping-ponging" of patients from one physician to another, often in a shared facility known as a "Medicaid mill." This is done so that each physician may charge a separate fee for the partial service rendered. For the same reason—receipt of extra fees—the number of lab tests and number of prescriptions seem far in excess of the number needed. There are exceptions, of course, both among some principled and therefore in fact self-sacrificing individual doctors operating in fee-for-service practice and in those few instances where Medicaid has been used to support forms of practice different from fee-for-service care.

Paradoxically, programs like Medicaid themselves produce limited access to care, due to their reimbursement levels and their bureaucratic structure. Patients in New York State are required to reregister for Medicaid monthly, no matter how sick or how poor they are. Delays of up to six months or longer in payments to providers of care are common, and limitations on reimbursement often have little or no relationship to actual costs, causing many physicians, pharmacists and other providers to refuse to accept Medicaid patients.

. . . .

Interestingly, the distribution of hospital beds in the United States is much more equitable than that of physicians. In 1948 some states had as few as two general medical and surgical hospital beds per 1000 population. Since that year, however, the Hill-Burton program, a federal hospital-construction program, has spent more than $12 billion, in addition to even greater amounts of local funds, for hospital construction and modernization. As a result of these vast expenditures the distribution of hospital beds throughout the country has become much more balanced. States such as Mississippi, Alabama, Georgia and Tennessee, which had the lowest bed/ population ratios in 1948, are now at the national average or above it. Some of the states with particularly high bed/population ratios in 1948 have experienced a decrease, and within states there is also evidence of a more equitable distribution of hospital facilities between rich and poor areas. In some ways hospital-bed distribution is used to "make up for" shortages of physicians; states, like South Dakota, which have low physician-to-population ratios, have relatively high hospital bed/population ratios. While part of the object of the Hill-Burton program was to "lure" physicians into rural areas by building hospitals there, the strategy has largely been a failure.

There is indeed gross maldistribution and social misuse of hospital resources, but it takes a different form than that of physicians and other health workers. The maldistribution and misuse occur in the competition among hospitals, particularly in urban areas, for prestige-enhancing equipment and for patients to keep the beds full.

Examples of needless and dangerous duplication of expensive equipment are ubiquitous. It was estimated in 1971, for example, that the number of teletherapy units (containing X-ray equipment used for treating certain kinds of cancer) concentrated on Chicago's near-South Side could, if properly distributed, take care of the needs of the entire state of Illinois. There were teletherapy units in Chicago that had never even been used since their installation because no one knew how to operate the equipment. Furthermore, the Chicago Regional Hospital Study estimated that a more rational distribution of teletherapy and coronary-care units might cut the operating costs of Chicago hospitals by as much as 10 percent.

The most commonly cited examples of expensive and hazardous duplication of services lie in the field of open-heart surgery, in which complex and costly heart-lung machines are used to maintain the patient's blood flow while surgeons repair or replace valves or other parts of the heart. The duplication of such units is so extensive that, despite intense competition for patients, many hospitals manage to attract only a few candidates for such surgery and thus perform extremely few such operations. The Inter-Society Commission for Heart Disease Resources reported that in 1969, 360 U.S. hospitals were equipped to do open-heart surgery. Of these, 220 average 50 operations or less a year—less than one per week. The commission, composed of experts in heart disease, advises that an open-heart surgery unit can maintain its skills and function efficiently only if it does a minimum of 200 operations a year, a minimum of 4 on the average per week. Of the 360 U.S. hospitals with units, only 15 actually performed 200 or more in 1969.

. . . .

The most recent rush to duplicate facilities has been for computed tomographic (CT) scanners which can diagnose conditions that previously could only be found by exploratory surgery or other invasive techniques. The machines cost an average of $500,000 to purchase and install and $100,000 annually to run. In mid-1976 there were over 300 CT scanners in operation in the United States and over 500 more approved for installation. The hospital portion of the private sector is now under some control by federally mandated Health Systems Agencies and other hospital planning bodies, so the hospital competition is somewhat constrained. Private offices and group practices are not so constrained and there is some evidence that an extraordinarily expensive piece of technology will move into areas of use in which there is even less quality and utilization control than in hospitals; almost 20 percent of CT installations are already in private offices.

In short, the fragmentation and the lack of accountability of the U.S. medical-care system have led to severe inequities, inefficiency and danger. In all areas of medical care, with the possible exception of hospitalization, the poor and nonwhite, who by almost every measure have far greater needs for care than do the more affluent, have less than equitable access to medical care. And the duplications and overlapping areas of high technology in medicine vastly increase the cost of care and undermine the competence in its use.

. . . .

Health care is not only a huge industry when measured by the amount of money and technology poured into it, it is also huge in terms of the

Figure 2. *Number of Health Workers in the United States, 1900–1974*

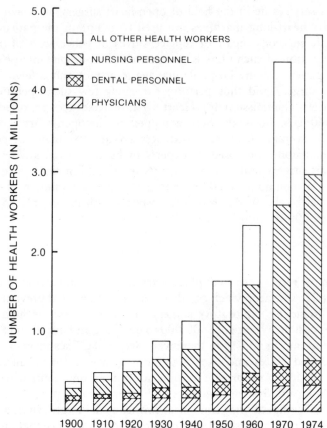

Prepared by the authors from data published by the National Center for Health Statistics.

number of people employed in it. As shown in Figure 2, almost five million people work in health care—some 5 percent of the employed population of the United States.

Of these health workers, approximately one-half—some two and a half million—are employed in providing what are called "nursing services," including registered nurses, licensed practical nurses, nurses' aides, order-lies and home health aides. About 375,000 (8 percent) are physicians, most with the M.D. degree, but also including a much smaller number with the degree of doctor of osteopathy, who in all states are licensed to do anything that a physician with an M.D. degree can do. The remainder are employed in approximately 100 other skilled and unskilled occupa-tions, including such varied roles as ambulance attendants, laboratory technicians, pharmacists, receptionists, radiologic technicians, dieticians, secretaries, dental assistants and research scientists.

Over the panoply of facilities and people that is the U.S. medical-care system, the physician has reigned supreme. His or (rarely, but increasingly) her dominance over the U.S. health system has been derived, at least in part, from his authority over and dominance of his patients, a phenomenon which has existed since prehistoric times when the practice of medicine originated in magic and was a priestly art.

There are, of course, still elements of the priesthood in the physician's role, in how he sees himself and how he is viewed by patients and co-workers alike. The authority of the physician today is still based both on the "authority of office" (that is, on the fact that he is a member of the guild), on the "authority of knowledge" (that is, on the assumption that he has special technical competence) and on the "authority of class" (that is, on the often vast social-class difference between him and other health workers or patients). Because the technical competence is more complex and more powerful than ever before, and because the income and prestige differences are huge and increasing, today more than ever his authority takes precedence over all others in the health field.

The physician guards the powers conferred on him, in part by controlling the information made available to patients and to the general public, a control as rigid in its technological form as was the ancient guarding of priestly rituals. A fictionalized account of one physician's internship vividly conveys this withholding of information and its function:

> I didn't show her the X-rays; none of us ever showed parents the studies themselves. It was a kind of informal tradition that you were to interpret what the lab results revealed, not show the tests. The idea was not to make the parents nervous with technical details they were not prepared to understand. That it could also be a device to keep control, to keep the mystery—and patient respect—alive and working, had not occurred to me then.

But there are even larger issues at stake than the mystification of the individual patient and family. The physician is now in a position to control vast resources—resources for medical-care services, for medical education and for research. In an age when billions of dollars are spent at the bidding of technologists and technocrats and when the vast majority of the people in every society possesses insufficient knowledge and information (as opposed to intelligence and judgment) on which to base sound decisions, physicians and other technocrats of medicine become extraordinarily powerful in the technological decision-making process.

Furthermore, the process itself becomes self-perpetuating, the technology becomes an end in itself, and the only ones who can discuss the technology with adequate understanding (who have the tools to deal with the issues) are those who control it. What should be a political decision, in its original sense—made with the good of the polity in view—often becomes a narrow technical decision made by those whose judgment must at least in part be colored by their view of what's in it for them.

Between the macrocosm of social policy and the microcosm of the doctor's office, the modern U.S. hospital has come more and more to resemble a modern industrial plant with its elaborate division of labor and the increasing alienation of the hospital worker. Most hospital workers remain at their entry-level jobs unless they acquire more formal training or other credentials even though they often learn skills on the job and perform tasks at a higher level.

The result is a rigid occupational hierarchy with an elaborate system of rank identifications such as uniforms and titles and an equally rigid social-class system. In 1970, 98 percent of U.S. physicians were white, 91 percent were male and predominantly from middle- and upper-middle-class families; while 92 percent of nurses were white, 98 percent were female and from predominantly middle- and lower-middle-class families. Of the total enrolled in training programs administered by hospitals in 1973–74, 86 percent of practical-nurse trainees were white and 96 percent were female; while 64 percent of nurse's-aide trainees were white and 87 percent were female, and 64 percent of orderly-trainees were white and 14 percent were female.

Thus it is clear that in general as income and power drop, the domination by white males ends and medical professions become overwhelmingly female and increasingly nonwhite. As one practical nurse described the hierarchy in the hospital where she worked, "You have to see this place as a giant bureaucracy. I'm at the bottom of it, or maybe the patients are, and there's not a lot an individual can do."

The physician is of course at the top of the medical-care structure, earns the most money . . . and has the most power. . . . The income differentials between those at the top and those at the bottom have markedly increased over the past two decades.

The nurse is typically subordinate to both the physician and the hospital, and early in her training learns to play what one observer has called the "doctor-nurse game," the object of which is that the nurse "be bold, have initiative and be responsible for making significant recommendations, while at the same time [appearing] passive." She must "make her recommendations appear to be initiated by the physicians," taking care not to disturb the physician's narcissism or feelings of omnipotence.

The doctor's role vis-à-vis other health professionals and paraprofessionals is even more distant and authoritarian. In hospital settings those persons who are in continuous and intimate contact with patients are workers with the lowest status and least power in the institution. Eliot Freidson's description of the alienated industrial worker seems to fit the medical paraprofessional as well:

Lacking identification with the prime goals of the organization, lacking an important voice in setting the formal level and direction of work, and performing work that has been so rationalized as to become mechanical and meaningless, a minute segment of an intricate mosaic of specialized activities that he is in no position to perceive or understand, the worker is alienated.

In spite of this alienation, more and more of the caring functions of medicine are left to the nurse's aides, the LPNs, the orderlies. Furthermore, since workers in the primarily female caring professions of nursing and social work have been awakened to their low status by the women's movement, members of these professions have in significant numbers attempted to "move up" into traditionally male and therefore higher-status teaching or administrative roles, leaving the caring function increasingly to powerless paraprofessionals with still lower status.

Thus we may view the typical structure of a large medical institution as a pyramid with the usually white, male physician on top, his orders carried out by middle-level professionals who are generally women, and with the patients and the "dirty work" left to low-paid, frequently alienated, largely black female paraprofessionals at the bottom of the pyramid.

Although acceptance into medical school has shifted somewhat in recent years toward the female (24 percent of the entering class in 1975 compared to 6 percent 20 years earlier) and toward "minority" students (8 percent of the entering class in 1975), the more pronounced trend has been toward higher and higher intellectual requirements; the percentage of students with A averages in medical school has increased from 13 percent in 1965 to 44 percent in 1975. This, together with the rapid increase in medical school (and college) tuition—in one medical school now over $10,000 per year for four years—discriminates more and more against the socially and educationally disadvantaged. Yet, there is absolutely no evidence that intellectual attainment beyond a given level is necessary for technical proficiency or that intellectual attainment at any level is correlated with skill in providing humane medical care. Furthermore, the emphasis on grades, particularly in science courses, and the intense competition for the limited number of medical school places, has led to enormous anxieties among premedical students and a profound distortion of the undergraduate learning experiences.

Furthermore, once in medical school, the educational pattern is largely irrelevant—and actually seems to be inimical—to the practice of medicine, particularly of primary medical care. Much of the work in the preclinical sciences is based on the needs and desires of a "science" faculty and has little use meeting patients' needs. A very large percentage of the clinical work is done on (the word "on" is usually more appropriate than "with") hospitalized patients in large teaching hospitals. In most medical schools well over 50 percent of the teaching is done on "horizontal" rather than "vertical" patients. As Jack Geiger has commented, "It's like teaching forestry in a lumber yard." Moreover, while studies of how patients actually need and use medical care indicate that patients' needs lie largely outside the hospital, the teaching nevertheless concentrates on the small fraction of care that takes place not only in a hospital, but in the university medical center tertiary-care hospital.

Inappropriate intellectualization and academization of training occurs among other health workers as well. A recent report by the secretary of education of Massachusetts states that he finds absolutely no evidence that registered nurses who hold bachelor's degrees are any more competent in patient care than are those who have graduated from hospital-based schools, yet diploma nurses find it difficult to get jobs at comparable pay to baccalaureate nurses. Registered nurses with diplomas, the report stated, find themselves "squeezed" between the registered nurses with bachelor's degrees, on one hand, and the licensed practical nurses, who have lesser levels of technical skills and thus command far less salary, on the other. At all of these levels, nurses, like other health workers, are judged more by how academic their training was and by their degrees and licenses than by what they can actually do for the patient.

New categories of personnel are constantly being added to the system, both in response to the demands of technology and to the demands of patient care. One response over the past ten years to the shortage and inappropriate use of health personnel has been the development of physician's assistant programs. The effort has been highly publicized, but the number of new workers trained is still quite small.

The term "physician's assistant" includes a range of health workers—variously called physician's associates, MEDEX (for "medical extenders"), clinical associates, child-health associates and others. "Assistant to the primary-care physician," for example, is a generic term used for an assistant who performs certain specified tasks under the direction and supervision of a physician in a number of settings, from a physician's office to a hospital. The assistant has a wide range of duties which include taking patients' case histories, performing physical examinations, drawing blood samples, giving intravenous injections and infusions, providing immunizations, suturing and caring for wounds, and other specific tasks usually performed by doctors.

Programs to train PAs (the abbreviation is in part a way of avoiding the problem of whether they should be called "assistants" or "associates") were begun in the mid-1960s at a time when the Vietnam War was annually producing thousands of military medical corpsmen whose knowledge and experience were being lost to the civilian world after their discharge. Because the PA concept was originally seen as a way to utilize those trained in the military medical corps and at the same time provide needed medical manpower, the new medical professionals were expected to be predominantly male. The nursing profession, not unreasonably, saw the development as yet another device of the medical establishment to under-cut the predominantly female nursing profession, and in response the new professional role of "nurse practitioner" has been developed.

Since the first PA program at Duke University in 1965, some 4000 students have graduated from the roughly 60 training programs now ac-credited by the AMA. The programs, which now graduate about 1300 PAs a year, vary enormously in their requirements and even in the length of the program. Some 40 states have enacted legislation governing the use of PAs.

Severe problems have developed. There are conflicts between PA and nurse-practitioner programs in determining status, hierarchy and which training programs will receive how much money from the federal govern-ment. Although most PAs are trained in primary care, some are already reflecting the specialization of the medical profession; they are being trained in such diverse medical specialties as anesthesiology, pathology, surgery, obstetrics and orthopedics, and in these roles the PAs are adding to the specialization within medicine rather than providing additional pri-mary care.

And, of course, for the PA, as for the nurse practitioner, the nurse, the nurse's aide and other health workers, there is usually almost no chance to become a physician. The only pathway to advancement is through admin-istration, supervision and teaching, with the result that the most skilled health workers either feel trapped and frustrated in their subsidiary roles or are forced to move further and further away from direct patient care.

Another, perhaps even more basic, criticism is that PAs and nurse practitioners may become the physicians for the poor while the rich are able to purchase and demand care by "real" doctors. While this criticism is still for the most part more theoretical than real, the danger in an unregu-lated, fee-for-service system certainly exists. The issue is how the medical-care system chooses to use these new workers—as part of an effort to bring greater equity to the system, or to further stratify the already highly stratified provision of health care.

Up to this point PAs are not changing the nature of American medicine but rather shoring up its current organization and priorities. Nationally, 77 percent of PA graduates are absorbed into private practices. The physi-cians who add PAs to their practice often charge their regular fees for a visit conducted entirely or largely by a PA, and pocket the difference between the PA's salary (from $7500 to $22,500 a year, relatively modest compared to a doctor's income) and the fee charged.

In short, these new health roles act to further the physician's control of the health-care system.

There are some areas, however, in which the physician's dominance of the medical-care system is being effectively threatened. The increasing size, complexity and corporate structure of the hospital give its professional managers new power over the workshop in which a large share of the physician's income is generated. The increasing cost of medical care and its major financing through insurance companies and tax levy funds give regulators and claims examiners new power over the physician's income and therefore over his pattern of practice.

The response of many physicians is to join together in what they view as—and sometimes call—"physician's unions." Strikes have been threatened, and over some issues, such as malpractice insurance rates, have even been partially carried out in some areas. While some physicians question the "ethics" of such actions—which, to be effective, will leave patients without a source of continuing or even emergency care—it seems likely that when the provocation is seen as large enough a significant percentage of physicians will be willing to use methods traditionally identified with the working class.

Some critics see unionization of physicians as a step forward, a breaking down of some of the elitist pretensions of the physician, even as a "proletarianization" of physicians. One major difference, of course, is that the threat to withhold services is often the only significant leverage available to workers wishing to improve their wages or working conditions, while most doctors already have other powerful resources and methods for control and change at their disposal. Another is that most workers are economically damaged by even a short strike, while most doctors can afford to strike for a prolonged period either because of their accumulated wealth or their expectation of future large incomes.

Others therefore fear that the elitist attitudes will not change but simply be further expressed through the power of organized deprivation of services, a deprivation which will become the ultimate weapon in the hands of an already powerful group.

Notes

A recent detailed and comprehensive description of the United States health-care and medical-care system, with an extensive bibliography, may be found in Steven Jonas and others, *Health Care Delivery in the United States* (New York: Springer Publishing Co., 1977). Detailed data on distribution of hospitals and health workers, on physicians' visits and on health problems may be found in *Health United States 1975*, DHEW Publication no. (HRA) 76-1232. Detailed data on the geographic distribution of doctors, nurses and other health workers are presented in *Health Resources Statistics*, issued annually by the National Center for Health Statistics; the most recent volume, for 1975, is DHEW Publication no. (HRA) 76-1509.

An analysis of barriers to health care for the poor was made by L. Bergner and A. S. Yerby, "Low Income and Barriers to Use of Health Services," *New England*

Journal of Medicine 278 (March 7, 1968): 541–6. The study of teletherapy units in the city of Chicago and the report of the Inter-Society Commission were discussed by Spencer Klaw in *The Great American Medicine Show*, (New York: Viking Press, 1975).

Data on the current numbers of health workers in the United States may be found in the annual editions of *Health Resources Statistics*, cited above. Distribution of health workers in 1970 and projections to 1990 were presented in *The Supply of Health Manpower*, DHEW Publication no. (HRA) 75–38. An analysis of the authority of the physician has been presented by Eliot Freidson in *Professional Dominance: The Social Structure of Medical Care* (New York: Atherton Press, 1970), pp. 108–9.

The quotation on the withholding of information is from Ronald J. Glasser, *Ward 402* (New York: Pocket Books, 1974), p. 69.

A discussion of characteristics and roles of health workers can be found in Barbara Ehrenreich and John H. Ehrenreich, "Hospital Workers: Class Conflicts in the Making," and in Carol A. Brown, "Women Workers in the Health Service Industry," published, respectively, in the *International Journal of Health Services* 5, no. 1 (1975): 43–51; no. 2 (1975): 173–84; and in Vicente Navarro, "Women in Health Care," *New England Journal of Medicine* 292 (February 20, 1975): 398–402. A series of articles describing nurse-doctor relationships is presented in Bonnie Bullough and Vern Bullough, eds., *New Directions for Nurses* (New York: Springer Publishing Co., 1971), particularly Leonard I. Stein, "The Doctor-Nurse Game," pp. 129–37. Further analysis of these relationships can be found in Shirley A. Smoyak, "Problems in Interprofessional Relations," *Bulletin of the New York Academy of Medicine* 53 (January–February 1977): 51–9. The quotation describing the alienated worker is taken from Freidson's *Professional Dominance*, p. 144.

Data on the characteristics of U.S. medical students are published regularly in the *Journal of Medical Education* and annually in the medical-education issue of the *Journal of the American Medical Association;* the December 27, 1976, issue gives data for the classes entering and graduating in 1975.

Further material on the development of the "intermediate" categories of health personnel and the issues surrounding their training can be found in the following sources: Donald M. Pitcairn and Daniel Flahault, eds., *The Medical Assistant: An Intermediate Level of Health Care Personnel*, Public Health Paper no. 60 (Geneva: World Health Organization, 1974); Alfred M. Sadler, Jr., Blair L. Sadler, and Ann A. Bliss, *The Physician's Assistant: Today and Tomorrow* (Cambridge, Mass.: Ballinger Publishing Co., 1975); Susan Reverby, "The Sorcerer's Apprentice," in Kotelchuck, ed., *Prognosis Negative* (New York: Vintage, 1976): 215–229; Margaret E. Mahoney, "The Future Role of Physician's Assistants and Nurse Practitioners," in John Z. Bowers and Elizabeth Purcell, eds., *National Health Services: Their Impact on Medical Education and Their Role in Prevention* (New York: Josiah Macy, Jr., Foundation, 1973), pp. 124–42; and Anthony Robbins, "Allied Health Manpower—Solution or Problem?" *New England Journal of Medicine* 286 (April 27, 1972): 918–23. Examples of studies on their effectiveness and acceptance include Charles E. Lewis and others, "Activities, Events and Outcomes in Ambulatory Patient Care," *New England Journal of Medicine* 280 (March 20, 1969): 645–9; Evan Charney and Harriet Kitzman, "The Child-Health Nurse

(Pediatric Nurse Practitioner) in Private Practice: A Controlled Trial," *New England Journal of Medicine* 285 (December 9, 1971): 1353–8. Eugene C. Nelson, Arthur R. Jacobs, and Kenneth G. Johnson, "Patients' Acceptance of Physicians' Assistants," *Journal of the American Medical Association* 228 (April 1, 1974): 63–7; and Lawrence S. Linn, "Patient Acceptance of the Family Nurse Practitioner," *Medical Care* 14 (April 1976): 357–64. Marianne G. Dekker documents "First Doctor Opposition to Physician's Assistants" in *Medical Economics*, September 6, 1976. Warnings that the use of nonphysician personnel to provide primary care is likely to further the two-class nature of medical care in the United States, with the poor cared for by those with less training, were sounded by Milton Terris, "False Starts and Lesser Alternatives," *Bulletin of the New York Academy of Medicine* 53 (January–February 1977): 129–40, and Milton I. Roemer, "Primary Care and Physician Extenders in Affluent Countries," *International Journal of Health Services* 7 (Fall 1977): 545–55.

The decrease in home visits, demonstrated by the National Health Interview Survey, was summarized in *Forward Plan for Health FY 1978–82.*

14

Re-forming the Hospital Nurse: The Management of American Nursing

Susan Reverby

The labyrinthine hospital, filled with multitudes of personnel in a rainbow assortment of uniforms, is the norm for the contemporary medical institution in the United States. But the hospital has not always been a huge specialized acute care institution with a complex staffing pattern. For most of its history, the institution was run by relatively few people and served a generalized social welfare function. As the hospital's purpose and function have changed, so has its division of labor. This article is a brief overview of this transformation as it has affected and was effected by the largest segment of the hospital workforce: the nurses. It explores the impact of the confluence of the professional aspirations of nursing and the managerial thrusts of the hospital administrations.[1]

Until the early twentieth century, most people, even when acutely ill, were cared for not in the hospital, but at home by relatives, friends or a neighborhood nurse. The hospital was more an institution primarily for the very poor or transients in need of food and shelter as much as medical and surgical attention. Conditions in many hospitals, as in the most disreputable nursing homes of today, were often abominable: dirty, unkempt, understaffed, places of little hope and much despair. Alcohol, considered an important medicine, was dispensed as frequently to the staff as to the patients.

Many of the women who provided what nursing care there was were either patients themselves, inmates of an adjacent prison or almshouse, or women hired almost off the streets. Strength, in particular a strong back, and a somewhat pleasing disposition, were the major job requirements. Thus, for example, the matron of a Boston hospital placed this ad in the newspaper in 1874: "Wanted, a nurse for the Boston Lying-In Hospital, Experience not required."[2] When she couldn't find someone to take the job (she reported the applicants weren't prepossessing enough), she had one of the recuperating patients become the hospital laundress, and she moved the laundress up to nurse. Similarly, in 1913, a survey of New York hospitals noted that "... in the absence of other institutions where the periodic and semi-respectable drunks can live and work, they can, to the best advantage to themselves and to the City, be supported as workers in the City's hospitals."[3]

But not all the nurses, even in the worst of hospitals, were the immoral and inexperienced semi-alcoholics so bitingly satirized by Dickens in Sairey Gamp and Betsy Prig in his novel *Martin Chuzzlewitt*. Many women (and much of the hospital workforce was women) became permanent employees and stayed at their jobs for many years. They learned and accumulated some skills on the job and gained what one historian has called an "ad hoc" professionalism.[4] These women often did everything in the institution: washing dishes, mending the linen, cleaning hoppers and bedpans, but also careful watching, skilled bandaging, bathing, and assisting in operations and deliveries.

The hospital's major decisions were made primarily by the administrator, called a superintendent, and the board of trustees. As medical care was less important in the hospital, the medical staff's power over decisions was not as large as it is today.[5] But in a hospital world in which stays were measured in weeks and months, not days, many of the patients were more convalescent than acutely ill, and doctor and trustee visits more rituals than daily occurrences. Thus a strong hospital culture developed which linked the patients and workers together in a web of both class and circumstance. Frequent clashes between the rules of the institution and its daily life were common.[6]

Beginning in 1873, as part of general reform effort in social welfare and the necessity for finding more respectable work for the daughters of the lower middle classes, several nurses' training schools, attached to hospitals, were founded in this country. Several of the early schools were independent institutions with their own funds and boards, but by the 1880s, most schools were organized and controlled by the hospitals, which realized the "students" could be used as a source of more docile, "non-wage" labor. The early schools, despite the efforts of nursing reformers, were primarily hiring halls for the hospitals in which student drop-outs were replaced on an individual basis whenever the necessity arose, with no concern for organized classes or a graded curriculum.[7]

Student nurses became the key nursing workers in the hospitals and made possible the rapid expansion in the number of hospitals in the late nineteenth and early twentieth centuries. Graduate nurses were sometimes used in supervisory positions, but it was more common to find such positions filled by a senior nursing student. The hospital administrations were quick to realize that the nursing students were not only cheaper, but as employees were preferable to either untrained attendants or graduate nurses for several reasons.

First, students could be trained into the exact routine of the hospital and would not bring the knowledge of different routines from other hospitals with them. Second, since training lasted for two to three years, the students became a relatively permanent workforce who could be depended upon to stay longer than other employees, if they did not die or break down from the overwork. Any time lost to illness, however, had to be made up before the student received her diploma. Third, management could exert more discipline and control over students than it could over employees who, not seeing the work as something to be endured until graduation, might quit more readily. The nursing leadership, anxious to develop the proper "character" in their charges and to shed the image of the nurse as an intemperate lowlife, saw the necessity for strict disciplining. Their emphasis on the hierarchy and military-like obedience, however, in the face of their lack of control over the schools, left the students easily open ideologically and in practice to exploitation by the hospitals. Lavinia Dock, one of the early leaders of American nursing, stated succinctly: "Discipline and strict subordination of the school makes it possible for the hospital to exact from [the nursing students] an amount of work it would be quite impossible to exact from women over whom it had no special hold. . . ."[8]

Since the nursing students were pushed onto the wards with almost no training and were expected to do everything, strict supervision of these unskilled women was necessary if any degree of quality care was to be obtained. Nursing leaders rightly believed that good supervision would help with the on-the-job training of the nursing students. The system was far from flawless. An Iowa physician lamented: "We are entirely too careless in the operating rooms, and too many pupil nurses are put into operating rooms who are too stupid ever to learn operating technic, too many who are too careless, and who have not been long enough in the school to have acquired the proper mental attitude toward the profession of nursing."[9]

Since the hospital was also a school, control over the nurses was sanctioned by the ideology of *in loco parentis* as well. Adherence to such strict control over work meant that the hospitals could admit virtually any warm body to the nursing school knowing that the supervision and teaching of strict routines would largely make up for the deficit in knowledge and training. Consequently, the public often viewed the hospital nursing school as " . . . a sort of respectable reform school where its mental or disciplinary cases can be sent," as a 1928 nursing reform report noted.[10]

For the graduate nurse conditions of labor were quite different. After graduation, most nurses left the hospital to become private duty nurses. They were hired by patients and worked individually in the home. Hiring took place either by word of mouth or through registries established in the major cities by the nursing alumnae associations, commercial businesses, the hospitals, and medical societies. For a small fee, nurses could register, give their prices and their preferences for work.[11]

In private duty nursing, the only real supervision was that given by doctors, and this was at best haphazard and uneven. Nurses were still expected to kowtow and cover for the physicians and their mistakes. Dr. William L. Richardson, for example, told the graduating class at the Boston Training School for Nurses on June 18, 1886 to "always be loyal to the physician." He warned them not to be "tempted" to impress the doctor with their knowledge because "what error can be more stupid?"[12] Although the private duty nurse was technically working "independently," she was in fact dependent on the physicians for her reputation and often for her actual case loads. The difference in the situation for nurses and physicians was clearly reflected in the language used to describe their respective positions: a doctor out on his own was in private *practice*, the nurse was working on private *duty*.

Graduate nurses increasingly in the 1920s worked in hospitals as private duty or special nurses for the paying patients in their private rooms. Hospitals usually kept registries, mostly of their own graduates, but patients could obtain private duty nurses anywhere they pleased. The presence of the private duty nurse was a constant problem for both the nursing supervisors and the hospital administrators. She was independent of the rules, discipline and supervision of the hospital and its nursing hierarchy. Often her patients were not considered to be "that sick" and the fact that she worked less diligently than the other nurses was deeply resented.[13] Moreover, she was not responsible for anything but the care of her one patient. Because she was usually older than the students and out of school, she often used older or different techniques, a practice which clearly disturbed nursing supervisors bent on teaching the students their own particular or more modern ways of doing things.[14]

Hospital administrators were even more concerned about the behavior of private duty nurses who could tell their patients about failings in the hospitals. Since their patients were usually well-to-do people in the community, the hospitals could ill afford to have their problems or limitations revealed to them.[15] Where they could, hospitals retaliated against these nurses, limiting their registry lists and using these as blacklists to keep out particularly troublesome nurses. Nurses frequently complained about discrimination on the part of the hospitals.[16]

The outbreak of World War I and the flu pandemic of 1918 were critical events which helped shape personnel relations within the hospitals. Both made the hospitals more acutely aware of shortages, the cost of labor turnover, and the need for better trained workers. Problems of quality and the division of labor intensified in the 1920s.

This new concern for quality in the workforce was closely related to the change in the nature of patients using the hospital. As the institutions expanded and the scientific and sanitary basis for care improved, more middle and upper class patients began to use the hospital. By 1931, the income from private, paying patients, rather than public funds or private donations, was the most important source of hospital income.

Because of the difference in the kind of patient hospitals served and their importance to hospital income, administrators began increasingly to worry about the quality of the workforce and the impressions they made on the patients. Thus during the 1920s and 1930s the hospital managers moved both to downgrade the scope of authority of their workers through increasing the division of labor and to upgrade their quality through better selection and standardization of training and through the provision of better ancillary benefits. In direct patient care areas, in particular, nursing, the changes were made in training and the types of workers.

The administrators' first line of attack was upon the stratum in the hospital which would be equivalent to lower middle management or foremen in industry: the head nurses and matrons in charge of the housekeeping departments. As administrators tried to chart lines of authority and make concrete rules about procedures, these "foremen" quickly sensed a threat to their authority. They clearly understood that the development of bureaucratic rules and the clear demarcation of authority would limit their control over their work.

Henry Hurd, one of the editors of *The Modern Hospital,* editorialized that matrons and nurses sometimes had "the impulse" or an "overwhelming desire" to organize or supervise the work in departments that were not their own. He was particularly concerned that these women did not want to give up the power of purchasing to a central authority. "The result of all this," he pointed out, "is a confusion of duty, a mingling of responsibilities, and a loss of efficiency, costly to the institution, all of which are most unwise." Such plans led to increased departmental dependence on centralized planning and control of the administrators.[17]

The nurses and matrons realized this and fought as best they could. Counseling and cajoling on the part of the administrators did not always result in cooperation. When department heads refused to give up their broader decision-making powers, *The Modern Hospital* counseled firings, and letters to the journals make it clear that dismissals were common.[18] At the same time the administrators moved to increase the division of labor. The extent to which this division of labor and increasing substitution of lower-skilled workers occurred varied depending upon both the hospital's size and funding source.[19] Regardless of the speed of substitution, however, increasing division of labor in the direct patient care areas resulted from the convergence and delicate balance of professional pressures and scientific management principles. The establishment of nurse's aides illustrates this tension.

During the shortages of the First World War and the flu pandemic many hospitals briefly introduced nurse's aide programs. Toward the end of the period 1910–1919, the expansion of these programs and other quick nursing courses produced an oversupply rather than a shortage of nurses.[20] With funding from the Rockefeller Foundation, a commission was established in 1918 to study nursing and nursing education.[21] When the report, known as the Goldmark Report after its principle investigator, Josephine Goldmark, was issued in 1922, it established two principles which were to become more generally accepted in subsequent years: (1) subsidiary grades of nurses serving patients with mild cases and serving as nurses' assistants in the hospitals should be licensed, and (2) such workers should be trained in the hospitals, apart from regular nursing students. The report also recommended that nurses increasingly be trained in universities and transformed into hospital foremen.[22]

The Goldmark report was not greeted with hosannas from most physicians and administrators. They were unwilling to give up the cheaper nursing students or to upgrade to any higher professional status the "uppity nurses."[23] Other doctors, notably Charles Mayo of the Mayo Clinic, went as far as to accuse the nursing profession of being the most "autocratic closed shop" in the country and to suggest that professional nurses could be done away with completely and "100,000 country girls could be trained as subnurses."[24] With such powerful opposition, while numerous hospitals began setting up training programs for aides in the 1920s and 1930s, widespread use of aides did not occur until the shortages of World War II.

Most of the hospitals in the 1920s and 1930s were, however, more concerned about the nature of their nursing staff than they were with the question of aides. Long debates ensued during these years over who the nursing worker should be, how she should be trained and who should control her work. Decisions about the kind of nursing worker necessary were based in part upon attempts to determine a nurse's productivity and how many patients she could care for in an hour. How to "scientifically" ascertain this number was and still is a question which is extremely difficult to answer.

A survey of nurses in the New York City hospitals in 1913, concluded: " . . . no recognized standards of the numbers of nurses that should be employed to a given number of beds and admissions existed."[25] The problem was based in part on the fact that, while the hospitals could regularize the number of beds they had, the occupancy rate of those beds always was variable. It was difficult for hospitals to know their staffing needs from day to day.

Among nursing's more educated leadership, there was a real willingness to experiment with different forms of work organization. This leadership also hoped that better training and planning could upgrade the nurse's status and dignity. Many of the early leaders worked with the scientific management movement in an attempt to apply its principles to nursing. Minnie Goodnow, a nursing superintendent and nurse historian, informed the 1914 annual hospital convention that nurses were training students "as Mr. Gilbreth does his bricklayers, and as all the efficiency engineers are doing in factories and business offices."[26] M. Adelaide Nutting, the first full professor of nursing at Columbia University, became interested in scientific management and efficiency schemes through her work in the American Home Economics Association.[27] By the 1920s, the National League for Nursing Education introduced some of the first time-and-motion studies of nursing work.[28]

The 1932 report of a study conducted by the League had important implications for the changes in nursing in the 1930s. The study documented the variability in both patient census and nursing load which made it necessary to shift nurses from one service to another. When these nurses were students, however, their education and ultimately the quality of nursing care suffered. The researchers concluded that nursing students could not provide enough quality care and that "a supplementary general duty graduate nursing staff . . . [was] essential."[29] The study also found that one-third of the nurses' time was spent in "extratreatment activities or non-nursing duties." This finding laid the basis for further consideration of the introduction of ward clerks and nurse's aides to take over these functions.

The move toward the employment of graduate nurses was encouraged by the work of yet another major nursing study which issued several reports between 1928 and 1934.[30] The first report urged the closing of some nursing schools and the upgrading of training in those that remained. The national nursing groups began to reconsider their focus on private duty and to look increasingly at the hospital as a place to work.

It was not time and motion studies or the actions of the American Nurses' Association, however, which determined the gradual introduction of the graduate nurse to the hospital.[31] The expansion of nursing in the early 1920s had led to an oversupply; by 1928 the depression had already begun in nursing.[32] The plight of private duty nurses became even more acute as the Depression wore on and patients began to cut back on use of their services. The American Nurses' Association moved exceedingly slowly in assisting their members through pressure for shorter hours or relief.[33] By 1932, the national nursing groups reluctantly drafted an appeal letter to the trustees of American hospitals asking them to remember nurses in their hour of need and to begin to employ graduate nurses. The letter also noted that the dilemma for nursing was not just the result of the Depression but was due " . . . to a weakness of a system of accepting students primarily as workers in the hospital. . . ."[34]

Hospitals were at first reluctant to employ more graduate nurses. A 1927 questionnaire sent to five hundred supervisors questioning them on which type of worker they preferred showed that 76 percent wanted students; only 24 percent wanted graduate nurses.[35] The nursing supervisors were fearful of employing women used to working independently because " . . . they find even kindly direction irksome," as one nursing supervisor explained.[36]

Hospitals had been convinced by economics and by earlier demands of the nursing profession to use trained nursing students. They now seemed reluctant to give up their free labor in exchange for the graduate nurse, even if the Depression made her cheaper and more available. The 1928 nursing report remarked: "It is an extraordinary thing, but it seems to be a fact that hospitals regard the suggestion that they pay for their own nursing service as unreasonable . . . the student nurse is seen as an inalienable right. . . ."[37]

As the Depression wore on, however, more and more small hospitals were forced to close their nursing schools. The number of schools dropped from 1,885 in 1929 to 1,311 in 1940. Studies began to appear in the journals to show that nursing students were not cheaper, because of their high maintenance and supervision costs.[38] By 1934 a new study of nursing superintendents concluded that their position on the use of graduate nurses had shifted positively.[39]

Some hospitals at first experimented with a form of private group nursing, which allowed a group of private duty nurses to care for several private patients at once. The nursing associations, finally coming to understand that this meant allowing the graduate nurse to become the general floor duty nurse, attacked the group nursing plans as " . . . merely another attempt on the part of the hospital to saddle the patient with nursing costs the hospital itself should meet, if this is not merely one more attempt to bolster up an inadequate nursing service."[40]

By the end of the 1930s it became clear that graduate nurses could provide better quality nursing service, could function as supervisors for auxiliary personnel, and, if they were not cheaper than students, neither were they that much more expensive. The hospital nurse became more common than private duty or public health nurse by 1937 and the number of graduate nurses within hospitals climbed from 4,000 in 1929 to 28,000 in 1937.[41]

The nurses also slowly began to accept the idea of nurses' aides in the hospital, as long as the training programs followed the dictates of the Goldmark Report, limiting the training of aides and constantly reminding them " . . . that they are not and will not be nurses."[42] The attempt to develop a subsidiary nursing worker who was cheaper but could provide quality care caught the hospitals in a contradiction which they have yet to resolve. If aides were to be given less responsibility and pay than the nurses, then their duties had to be different and more narrowly circumscribed. Yet because they were going to be handling sick patients, not machine parts, they had to be taught to understand basic procedures and to cope with many different kinds of emergencies. It is therefore understandable that they would want to improve their skills and to grow into more responsible positions. Yet the credentialing barrier established by the nursing profession in its quest for status and control prevented this happening through a job ladder in the hospital.[43]

A report on a nurse's aide program from Cleveland City Hospital makes this point candidly from the perspective of the administration: " . . . There is keen resentment on the part of several students because they feel that there is too much class distinction in the hospital. Probably it is inevitable that in so large a group a few would lose perspective regarding their place. On the other hand, perhaps, we, in our enthusiasm for the experiment, painted too glowing a picture of the joys of domestic work on our wards. After all, there is not much glamour to cleaning and bed making, even if they are an expression of devotion. Undoubtedly the continuance of their interest will be one of our perplexing situations. . . ."[44]

Hospitals met this dilemma in several ways. First, the training programs emphasized again and again the limited role of the aide. She had to be socialized " . . . to continue to try and perfect herself in the skills that her assignments permit rather than to forge ahead to new accomplishment."[45] Second, nurses were shifted to paperwork and supervisory tasks and nurse's aides and practical or vocational nurses were left to do much of the direct patient care.[46] Since neither of these solutions really solved the "perplexing situation" for the hospitals, the aides responded in classic ways—shirking greater responsibilities, fighting with other workers, or quitting.[47]

Thus by the 1920s, turnover in hospitals relying heavily on aides first surfaced as a major issue. This dilemma was and continues to be unsolved by the hospital management. On the one hand, high turnover controlled the resentment of the workers, allowed the hospitals to continue to pay low wages and yet keep an unskilled workforce. On the other hand, such high turnover meant that new workers had to be constantly taught the routines and integrated into the hospitals, making the workforce less efficient—the goal the administrators were trying so hard to achieve.

As the hospital became the center of the health system, scientific medicine necessitated a skilled as well as a controlled labor force; more than this, hospitals needed employees who were socially acceptable to paying patients upon whom they were becoming increasingly dependent. Poor men and women from almshouses were neither skilled nor acceptable. Students, although at first socially compatible, were expensive to maintain and inadequate to the tasks. While graduate nurses meet the two former objections, they presented a threat to the institutional integrity of the hospital.

The graduate nurses, therefore, had to be incorporated into the hospital hierarchy. First, they were separated from their potential source of power—the paying patient. A new level of workers, aides, was introduced to take over many of the traditional nursing chores. Aides could be employed in nursing without risk to the administration. They had no collective memory of control over patient care, and were more easily contained because of differences in training, class and race from graduate nurses. Additionally, they were cheaper to employ.

Second, nurses were further removed from the bedside by being made supervisors. This served two purposes: it made clear to the aides that there was more to nursing than bedside care, and it seemingly elevated the RN by making her someone else's boss. Once incorporated into the administration of the hospital, nurses quickly gained a stake in its smooth functioning. Advancement in nursing consisted of climbing up the hospital hierarchy and meant implicit acceptance of the institution's terms.

In the face of institutionalization, however, nurses were not merely passive recipients of bureaucratic whims. Often they saw the dangers inherent in their situation. Unfortunately, many of their responses were inadequate to meet the challenge and ironically played into the hands of the very forces they needed to combat. Imitating the earlier, successful thrust of doctors for professional status, nurses called upon their own unique abilities to cope with the nursing demands of scientific medicine, inadvertently conferring their stamp of approval on the ideology of high technology medicine. Thus, the more professional the nurse, the further removed she became from the patients and the more vulnerable she became to administrator's control. Like the insect in the spider's web, the more the nurses fought, the more entwined they became.

Prior to World War II, the transformation of nursing from direct patient care to a variety of specialized roles, including administration, was accomplished with few changes in technology. Rather, it was effected by the division of nursing into subsections with the imposition of a multi-leveled hierarchy. For graduate nurses, it meant an end to the possibility of being autonomous practitioners who set their own work rules and controlled their own time. Unlike doctors, nurses became employees of institutions and were dependent upon and subject to those institutions' needs.

Thus, RN journals today are filled with articles about the threat to the existence of nursing coming from technicians below and doctors' assistants above. This pincer-like grip on the nursing profession is most frequently attributed to the technological proliferation within some aspects of nursing care and the complexity of hospital administration. Thus on the one hand, nurses are being replaced by lesser paid, lesser skilled people operating machines, and on the other, by clerical workers and computers. It is also becoming clearer that nurses cannot succeed in making demands on the institutions if they do it alone. In 1976 the nurses went on strike in Seattle, Washington. During the strike, the hospitals were able to replace them: aides, lpn's, pharmacy mates, supervisors took over their jobs. At the end of the strike, the hospitals were able to replace them with more lower level workers; nurses were clearly not indispensable.[48]

The nurses' responses are often to either recite the catalog of nurses' skills or to insist upon some mystical healing quality inherent in the nurse's touch. But, as the history of nursing demonstrates, the extinction of the profession, if it happens, will result from the increasing division of labor mystified and speeded up by high technology medicine. It can only be resisted and reversed through a critique of the "science" of medicine and nursing and the "science" of management. They go hand in hand.

References

For a more detailed and analytic study of the historical development of nursing, see my dissertation, "Apprenticeship to Duty: Nursing and Hospital Reform in the United States, 1860–1940" (Boston University, 1981). The research for this article was originally done under a grant from the Milbank Memorial Fund.

1. The history of the American hospital is just beginning to be written. See, for recent examples, Morris J. Vogel, *The Invention of the Modern Hospital, Boston 1870–1930* (Chicago: University of Chicago Press, 1980); David Karl Rosner, "A Once Charitable Enterprise: Health Care in Brooklyn, 1890–1914" (Unpublished dissertation, Harvard University, 1978); Charles E. Rosenberg, "And Heal the Sick: The Hospital and the Patient in 19th Century America," *Journal of Social History,* 1977, 10: 428–448, and "Inward Vision & Outward Glance: The Shaping of the American Hospital, 1880–1914," *Bulletin of the History of Medicine,* 1979, 53: 346–391.
2. "Diary of Eliza Higgins," Matron of Boston Lying-In Hospital, Volume I, June 1, 1874, Boston Hospital for Women, Public Relations Office.

3. Henry C. Wright, *Report of the Committee on Inquiry into the Departments of Health, Charities, and Bellevue and Allied Hospitals in the City of New York* (New York: Board of Estimate and Apportionment, 1913), p. 78.

4. Rosenberg, "And Heal the Sick . . . ," p. 434; and G. L. Sturtevant, "Personal Recollections of Hospital Life," *The Trained Nurse and Hospital Review,* 1917, 58: 129–131.

5. See Rosenberg, "Inward Vision & Outward Glance . . . ," passim.

6. See Rosenberg, "And Heal the Sick . . . ," *op. cit.* passim; and chapter two of my dissertation.

7. JoAnn Ashley, *Hospitals, Paternalism and the Role of the Nurse* (New York: Teachers' College Press, 1976).

8. Lavinia Dock, "The Relation of Training Schools to Hospitals," *Nursing of the Sick, 1893,* ed. Isabel Hampton (New York: McGraw Hill, 1949), p. 20; and Bonnie and Vern Bullough, *The Emergence of Modern Nursing* (New York: Macmillan, 1964), p. 144.

9. Iowa physician, "Pupil Nurses a Hazard to Patients," Letter in *Modern Hospital,* Vol. 3, No. 5, November, 1914, p. 314.

10. May Ayres Burgess, *Nurses, Patients and Pocketbooks* (New York: Committee on Grading of Nursing Schools, 1928), p. 347.

11. See Susan Reverby, " 'Neither for the Drawing Room Nor for the Kitchen,' Private Duty Nursing 1880–1914." Paper presented at the Organization of American Historians Meetings, April 15, 1978.

12. "Address on the Duties and Conduct of Nurses in Private Nursing" (Boston: Press of George H. Ellis, 1886), p. 22 (Box 8, Folder 3, Boston University Nursing Archives).

13. H. B. J., "The Special Nurse," Letter in *The Trained Nurse and Hospital Review,* Vol. 54, No. 2, February, 1915, p. 107.

14. *Ibid.*

15. John A. Hornsby and Richard E. Schmidt, *The Modern Hospital: Its Inspiration; Its Architecture; Its Equipment; Its Operation* (Philadelphia and London: W. B. Saunders and Company, 1913), passim.

16. Janet Geister, "Hearsay and Facts in Private Duty," *American Journal of Nursing,* Vol. 26, No. 7, July, 1926, pp. 515–528; Burgess, *op. cit.* pp. 80–93.

17. "Another Source of Friction in Hospital Administration," *Modern Hospital,* Vol. 6, No. 2, February, 1916, p. 112.

18. "Team Work in the Hospital," *Modern Hospital,* Vol. 4, No. 3, March, 1915, p. 220; "The Usual Duties of a Matron," *Modern Hospital,* Vol. 6, No. 6, June 1916, pp. 460–61.

19. Norman Metzger and Dennis Pointer, *Labor-Management Relations in the Health Services Industry: Theory and Practice* (Washington, D.C.: Science and Health Publications, Inc., 1972), p. 13.

20. Kathleen Canning and William Lazonick, "The Development of the Nursing Workforce in the United States: A Basic Analysis," *International Journal of Health Services,* November, 1975, p. 21.

21. Committee for the Study of Nursing Education, *Nursing and Nursing Education in the United States* (New York: Macmillan, 1923).

22. *Ibid.,* pp. 16, 26, 28.

23. Richard O. Beard, "The Report of the Rockefeller Foundation on Nursing Education, A Review and Critique," *American Journal of Nursing*, Vol. 23, No. 5, February, 1923, pp. 358–365; No. 6, March, 1923, pp. 460–466; No. 7, April, 1923, pp. 550–554; Canning and Lazonick, *op. cit.*, p. 23.
24. "Are Nurses Self-Seeking?" *American Journal of Nursing*, Vol. 21, No. 2, November, 1921, pp. 73–74.
25. Wright, "Report . . . ," *op. cit.*, p. 407.
26. "Efficiency in the Care of the Patient," *Transactions of the American Hospital Association*, 16th Annual Conference, 1914, p. 210.
27. Helen E. Marshall, *Mary Adelaide Nutting, Pioneer of Modern Nursing* (Baltimore: Johns Hopkins University Press, 1972), p. 158.
28. Elizabeth Greener, "A Study of Hospital Nursing Service," *Modern Hospital* 16 (January 1921): 99–102; A. Owens et al., "Some Times Studies," *American Journal of Nursing* 27 (February 1927): 99–101; Blanche Pfefferkorn and Marion Rottman, *Clinical Education in Nursing* (New York: Macmillan, 1932); for a review of the more contemporary literature on this, see Myrtle Aydelotte, *Nurse Staffing Methodology, A Review and Critique of Selected Literature* (Washington D.C.: Government Printing Office, 1970).
29. Pfefferkorn and Rottman, *op. cit.*, p. 59.
30. May Ayres Burgess' *Nurses, Patients and Pocketbooks,* published in 1928, was the first report in this research study. The final report was published as *Nursing Schools: Today and Tomorrow, The Final Report of the Committee on the Grading of Nursing Schools* (New York: Committee on the Grading of Nursing Schools, 1934).
31. *Ibid.*, p. 24.
32. Burgess, *op. cit.*, p. 83.
33. Canning and Lazonick, *op. cit.*, pp. 24–25; Bullough and Bullough, *op. cit.*, Chap. 5.
34. "National Nursing Groups Appeal to Hospital Trustees," *Modern Hospital,* Vol. 34, No. 1, July, 1932, p. 108.
35. Burgess, *op. cit.*, p. 290.
36. *Ibid.*, p. 531.
37. *Ibid.*, p. 434.
38. Malcolm MacEachern, "Which Shall We Choose—Graduate or Student Service?" *Modern Hospital*, Vol. 38, No. 6, June, 1932, pp. 94–104; Anna Wolf, "Is the Use of Graduate Nurses for Floor Duty Justified?" *Modern Hospital*, Vol. 33, No. 5, November, 1929, pp. 140–142; "How Many Students Can a Graduate Nurse Replace?" *Modern Hospital*, Vol. 41, No. 2, August, 1933, p. 86; J. C. Geiger, "An Important Change in Policy," *American Journal of Nursing*, Vol. 32, No. 2, February, 1932, p. 180; R. B. Brisbane, "Should the Small Hospital Employ Graduate or Student Nurses?," *Modern Hospital*, Vol. 28, No. 6, June, 1927, pp. 142–144.
39. *Nursing Schools: Today and Tomorrow, op. cit.*, p. 117.
40. Shirley Titus, "The Significance of General Duty Nursing to Our Profession," *American Journal of Nursing*, Vol. 31, No. 2, February, 1931, pp. 197–207, and "Group Nursing and How It Affects the Welfare of Patients," *Modern Hospital*, Vol. 35, No. 6, December, 1930, pp. 120–128.

41. Canning and Lazonick, *op. cit.*, p. 26.
42. A. C. Jensen, "Training Nursing Attendants," *Modern Hospital,* Vol. 51, No. 5, November, 1938, p. 68.
43. Emily Spieler, "Division of Laborers," *Health/PAC BULLETIN,* No. 45, November, 1972, pp. 3–17; and Susan Reverby, "From Aide to Organizer, the Oral History of Lillian Roberts," in Carol Berkin and Mary Beth Norton, eds., *Women of America, A History* (Boston: Houghton-Mifflin, 1979) pp. 289–317.
44. Winifred Shepler et al., "Standardized Training Course for Ward Aids," *Modern Hospital,* Vol. 51, No. 6, December, 1938, pp. 68–69.
45. *Ibid.*, p. 70; A. K. Haywood, "The Status of the Nursing Attendant," *Modern Hospital,* Vol. 19, No. 3, September, 1922, pp. 226–227.
46. Everett Hughes et al., *20,000 Nurses Tell Their Story* (Philadelphia: J. B. Lippincott, 1948), pp. 131–146.
47. M., "The Attendant, Her Place and Work," Letter in *American Journal of Nursing,* Vol. 20, No. 2, November, 1919, pp. 154–155.
48. Margaret Levi, "Functional Redundancy and the Process of Professionalization: The Case of Registered Nurses in the United States," paper presented to the 1978 International Sociological Association Meetings in Uppsala, Sweden, July 1978.

15

The Influence of Social Class Structure on the American Health Sector

Vicente Navarro

By Way of Introduction

In trying to understand the present composition, nature, and functions of the health sector in the United States, one is hampered by a great scarcity of literature, both in the sociological and the medical care fields, that would explain how the shape and form of the health sector—the tree—is determined by the same economic and political forces shaping the political and economic system of the United States—the forest. In fact, health services literature reveals what C. W. Mills (1), Birnbaum (2), and others (3, 4) have found in other areas of social research: a predominance of empiricism, leading to dominance of experts on trees who neither analyze nor question the forest but accept it as given.

Health services research, like most social research, has become more and more compartmentalized, with its practitioners turning into narrower and narrower specialists, superbly trained in their own fields, but with less and less comprehension of the total. And yet, the Hegelian dictum that "the truth is the whole" continues with its undiminished validity. Let me underline that I am not belittling empirical studies, i.e. the analysis of detail. Actually, the reader will see that I borrow heavily from the findings of empirical studies. But, as Baran and Sweezy (5) have indicated, "Just as the whole is always more than the sum of the parts, so the amassing of small truths about the various parts and aspects of society can never yield the big truths about the social order itself." There is, indeed, a need for explanation of how the parts are related to each other, and it is in meeting this need that our empiricists have fallen short and, for the most part, have remained silent. It is to break this deafening silence that this article has been written. Although admittedly full of assumptions, perceptions, and values, it will try to show that the composition and distribution of health resources are determined by the same forces that determine the distribution of economic and political power in our society. Indeed, I would postulate that the former cannot be understood without an understanding of the latter.

. . . .

The Class Structure of the United States, Outside and Within the Health Sector

In attempting to explain and understand the composition, functions, and nature of the health sector, one must look outside the health sector and first address a key question in any society, i.e. who owns and who controls the income and wealth of that society?[1] Thus, I have to revive a forgotten paradigm in social analysis in the United States: that of social class structure. In so doing, I am going against the mainstream of our sociological research, which assumes that this category has been transcended by the present reality of the United States, where it is considered that most of our population is middle class. Actually, it is assumed in most of the press and in most of academia that the contemporary United States, and the rest of the Western democracies for that matter, are being recast in a mold of middle-class conditions and styles of life.[2] Moreover, this situation is considered to be the result of social fluidity and mobility that are believed to falsify past characterizations of the United States as a class society. This conclusion, however, seems to confuse class consciousness with class interests. Indeed, the social reality that establishes the level of social aspiration of the American population as the consumption pattern of the middle class, and the assumed concomitant absence of class consciousness, do not deny the existence of social classes. In fact, as C.W. Mills (9) pointed out,

> ... the fact that men are not "class conscious" at all times and in all places does not mean that "there are no classes" or that "in America everybody is middle class." The economic and social facts are one thing. Psychological feelings may or may not be associated with them in rationally expected ways. Both are important, and if psychological feelings and political outlooks do not correspond to economic or occupational class, we must try to find out why, rather than throw out the economic baby with the psychological bath, and so fail to understand how either fits into the national tub.

Actually, there is not even convincing evidence that class consciousness or awareness do not exist. According to a study conducted in 1964, 56 percent of all Americans said that they thought of themselves as "working class," some 39 percent considered themselves "middle class," and 1 percent said they were "upper class." Only 2 percent rejected the whole idea of class (10).

An analysis of the social structure of the United States shows that there are indeed social classes in this country. . . . In such an analysis, we find at the top of our society the upper or corporate class which, by virtue of its ownership of a disproportionate share of the personal wealth and/or its control over that wealth, commands the most important sectors of our society. At the other extreme of the social spectrum, we find the majority of our population—the working class—composed primarily of industrial or blue-collar workers as well as farm workers and workers in the services sector, and representing 80 percent of the labor force. In between these two polar classes, there is the middle class, divided into upper and lower groupings and comprised of (a) professionals, (b) the business middle-class, (c) self-employed shopkeepers and craftsmen, and (d) office and sales workers. While aware of the simplifications that such a categorization implies, for reasons of brevity I shall refer to groups (a) and (b) as the upper-middle class, and groups (c) and (d) as the lower-middle class.

And the distribution of wealth and income closely follow these class lines, with the highest possession of both at the top and the lowest possession at the bottom, with a large gap in between. Using one of his excellent graphic analogies, Samuelson makes this skewed distribution quite clear. He states, in the eighth edition of *Economics,* "If we made today an income pyramid out of a child's blocks, with each layer portraying $1,000 of income, the peak would be far higher than the Eiffel Tower, but almost all of us would be within a yard of the ground" (11, p. 110). Moreover, these distribution patterns of wealth and income have remained remarkably constant over time. In the last retrospective study of the distribution of income, published in the 1974 annual *Economic Report of the President* (12) and widely reported in the press, it was found that "the bottom 20 percent of all families had 5.1 percent of the nation's income in 1947 and had almost the same amount (5.4 percent) in 1972. At the top, there was a similar absence of significant change. The richest 20 percent had 43.3 percent of the income in 1947 and 41.4 percent in 1972" (13).

This class structure in our society is also reflected in the composition of the different elements that participate in the health sector, either as owners, controllers, or producers of services. Indeed, considering just the health sector, and analyzing the owners, controllers, and producers of services in health institutions, we find that members of the upper class and, to a lesser degree, the upper-middle class (groups a and b of the middle class in the previous categorization), predominate in the decision-making bodies of our health institutions, i.e. the boards of trustees of foundations, teaching hospital institutions, medical schools, and hospitals. For the producers and the members of the labor force in the health sector we can see the distribution shown in Figure 1. At the top we find the physicians, who are mainly of upper-middle-class backgrounds and who had in 1970 a median annual net income of $40,000, which places them in the top 5 percent of our society. I should add that the majority of persons in this group are white and male, besides being upper-middle class. They represent 7.3 percent of the whole labor force in the health sector.

Below, very much below the upper class of the health sector, we find the level called paraprofessional. This could be defined as equivalent to the lower-middle-class category of office worker of the previous categorization (group d), i.e. nurses, therapists, technologists, and technicians, whose annual median income was approximately $6,000 in 1970. They represent 28.5 percent of the labor force in the health sector. This group is primarily female and is part of the lower-income group. Nine percent is black.

Below this group we find the working class per se of the health sector, the auxiliary, ancillary, and service personnel, representing 54.2 percent of the labor force, who are predominantly women (84.1 percent) and who include an overrepresentation of blacks (30 percent). This group's median income was $4,000 in 1970.

If we look at income distribution in the health sector, as we did for society in general, we find a similar structure, although here again, we find

Figure 1 *Persons employed in the delivery of health services in the United States, by sex, in 1970*

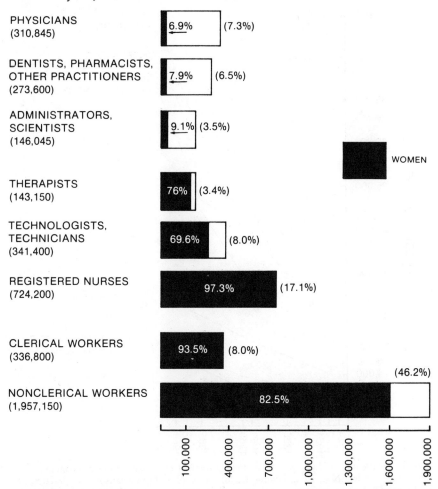

Source: For numbers of persons employed in the health services, Health Services and Mental Health Administration, *Health Resources Statistics: Health Manpower and Health Facilities, 1971,* U.S. Government Printing Office, Washington, D.C., 1972. Source for percentage of women physicians, M.Y. Pennell and J.E. Renshaw, Distribution of women physicians, 1970, *Journal of the American Medical Women's Association* 27(4): 197–203, 1972. Source for other categories, U.S. Bureau of the Census, 1970.

a great scarcity of information and a great absence of empirical data. Figure 2, however, shows the trend in the differentials of median income among the different groups of producers in the health sector from 1949 to 1970. Here we can see that there has been a very dramatic increase in the income differential between the top and bottom income groups of the health industry.

Figure 2. *The rise in income of selected personnel in the delivery of health services in the United States, 1949–1970*

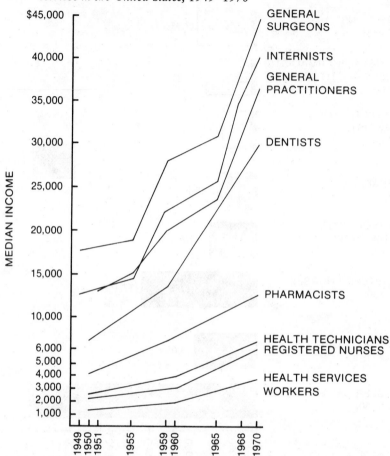

Source: For income of physicians, Continuing Survey of Physicians, Medical Economics Company, Oradell, N.J., 1972. Figures are for self-employed physicians in solo practice, under age 65. Source for income of dentists, Continuing Survey of Dentists, *Journal of the American Dental Association,* various years. Source for income of other wage groups, U.S. Bureau of the Census, *Statistical Abstract of the United States,* U.S. Government Printing Office, Washington, D.C., 1950, 1960, and 1970.

The Determinants of Income Differentials

Much has been written about the reasons for these income differentials. According to the orthodox economic paradigm, "every agent of production receives the amount of wealth that agent creates" and "every man receives all that he creates." Thus, workers' incomes depend on their productivity, i.e. "on the amount of capital available, on the one hand, and on workers' skills and education, on the other."[3] According to this interpretation, the conditions for social mobility are (a) increased education, to improve the workers' position in the market for their skills, and (b) equal opportunity for each worker in the competitive labor market. The strategy, then, is to increase educational opportunities and to break with the race and sex discrimination which prevents the proper functioning of the market forces. This paradigm is shared, incidentally, by the majority of people in the black and women's liberation movements within and outside the health sector. However, absent in this analysis is the concept of property and class. Actually, one of the widely accepted theoretical works on social inequality in today's United States, Rawls' *A Theory of Justice* (15), does not even mention the value of property as a source of social cleavage. Indeed, following the Weberian interpretation of status, Rawls and most of the exponents of what Barry (16) calls the liberal paradigm, maintain that social stratification is multidimensional, depending on a variety of factors such as education, income, occupation, religion, ethnicity, and so on (17).

Empirical evidence, however, seems to question the main assumptions of the liberal paradigm. Regarding the social mobility that is supposed to be the result of the widening of opportunities and of the free flow of labor market forces, and that is supposed to have caused the withering away of the social classes, Westergaard (18) and others have recently shown that although there has been some mobility among the different social groups or strata within each social class, there has been practically no mobility among social classes.

And the primary objective of education, instead of being the transmission of skills to aid upward mobility, seems to have been the perpetuation of social roles within the predefined social classes. Indeed, Bowles and Gintis (19), among others, have indicated how education, labor markets, and industrial structures interact to produce distinctive social strata *within* each class. A similar situation prevails in the health sector, where Simpson (20) and Robson (21) in England, and Kleinback (22) in the United States have shown how (a) the social class background of the main groups within the health labor force has not changed during the last 25 years, and how (b) education fixes and perpetuates those social backgrounds and replicates social roles. Actually, let me point out here that Flexner himself saw that as a function of medical education when he wrote that a primary aim of medical education was to separate the gentlemen (the upper class) from the quacks (the lower class).

Education, as a perpetuation of social roles, remains the same today as in Flexner's time. Simpson (20, p. 39), for instance, mentions that, within the five-scale grouping of classes in Britain, the offspring of social classes 1 and 2 (equivalent to our upper and upper-middle classes, as defined before) predominate in medicine:

In 1961 more than a third were from class 2, rather less than a third from class 3, and only 3 percent from classes 4 and 5 together. By 1966, social class 1 was contributing nearly 40 percent. The proportion of children of classes 1 and 2 in universities generally, derived from the Robbins Report, is about 59 percent. Individual medical schools vary between 69 and 73 percent. It is hard to believe that the small number of medical students selected from families of low average income exhausts the potentially good students contained in this large part of the population.

That this situation may even follow a predefined policy is indicated in the following statement from the Royal College of Surgeons (23):

... there has always been a nucleus in medical schools of students from cultured homes. ... This nucleus has been responsible for the continued high social prestige of the profession as a whole and for the maintenance of medicine as a learned profession. Medicine would lose immeasurably if the proportion of such students in the future were to be reduced in favour of the precocious children who qualify for subsidies from the Local Authorities and State purely on examination results.

A similar situation occurs in the United States, where Lyden, Geiger, and Peterson (24) reported in 1968 that only 17 percent of physicians were the children of craftsmen or skilled and unskilled laborers (who represented 57 percent of the whole labor force), while over 31 percent of physicians were children of professionals (representing 4.9 percent of the labor force). ... It is quite interesting and, I would add, not surprising, to note that while the underrepresentation of women and blacks among new entrants to the medical schools slowly, but steadily, diminished over the last decade, the underrepresentation of entrants with working-class and lower-middle-class backgrounds remained remarkably constant during the same period (25). Indeed, women, who represent 51 percent of the U.S. population, made up 6 percent of all medical students in 1961 and 17 percent in 1973, while blacks, representing 12 percent of the overall U.S. population, went during the same period from 3 to 9 percent of all medical students. During these years the percentage of medical students who came from families earning the median family income or below, representing approximately one-half of the population, remained at 12 percent. This percentage, incidentally, has remained the same since 1920.

These accumulated bits of evidence would seem to indicate that there is not an automatic trend toward diminishing class differences or bringing about social class mobility within and outside the health sector of the present United States, and, I would postulate, in that of most Western European societies. As in the past, experience seems to show that, as Harold Laski used to say, "the careful selection of one's own parents" remains among the most important variables explaining one's own power, wealth, income, and opportunities. The importance of this selection, moreover, seems to be particularly vital at the top. As C.W. Mills (26) said, "It is very difficult to climb to the top . . . it is much easier and much safer to be born there."

It would seem, then, that the liberal paradigm does not sufficiently explain the composition of the labor force and its class and income structure. Indeed, I would postulate that a better explanation of that structure would be that the inequalities of income, wealth, and . . . economic and political power, are functionally related to the way in which the means of production and reproduction of goods, commodities, and services, and the organs of legitimization in the United States, are owned, controlled, influenced, and directed. According to this interpretation, property and control of, and/or influence on, those means of production, reproduction, and legitimization are not just marginal factors in explaining class structure and income differentials, as the liberal paradigm would suggest, but key explanatory ones. Thus, in this alternative explanation, the overall distribution of wealth and income depends on who owns, controls, influences, and directs the means of production, reproduction, and legitimization in the different sectors of the U.S. economy. Overall income differentials among social classes, then, do not have so much to do with the free operation of the labor market forces, but more with the patterns of ownership and control of the main means of income-producing wealth and of the organs of legitimization, i.e. communication, education, and the agencies of the state. And according to this alternate explanation, education and other means of socialization are not the means of creating upward mobility among social classes, but actually are means of perpetuating patterns of control and ownership.

In summary, it can be postulated that social classes and income differentials come about because of the different degrees of ownership, control, and influence that different social classes have over the means of production and consumption and over the organs of legitimization, including the media, communications, education, and even the organs of state. Moreover, it can further be postulated that . . . these class influences determine not only the nature of the economic sectors in the United States today but also of the social sectors, including that of the health services.

. . . .

Notes

1. Simply stated, income is money coming from different sources, either as wages and salaries, dividends and profits, or as rent. Wealth is the value of people's possessions and property.
2. An example of a recent newspaper article exhibiting this belief is that by Kumpa (6). The most influential of the large body of sociological literature that negates the existence of classes in the United States is Bell (7). For a critique of this literature, see reference 8.

3. All these quotations are from Clark (14), the first work to enunciate the marginal productivity of income distribution. The most important contemporary work in this area is Samuelson (11).

References

1. Mills, C.W. *The Sociological Imagination.* Grove Press, New York, 1959.
2. Birnbaum, N. *Toward a Critical Sociology.* Oxford University Press, New York, 1971.
3. Dreitzel, H.P. *On the Social Basis of Politics.* Macmillan Company, New York, 1969.
4. Coulson, M.A., and Riddell, C. *Approaching Sociology: A Critical Introduction.* Routledge and Kegan Paul, London, 1973.
5. Baran, P., and Sweezy, P. *Monopoly Capital,* pp. 2–3. Monthly Review Press, New York, 1968.
6. Kumpa, P.J. Hail to the middle class! *Baltimore Sun* pp. K1 and K3, March 10, 1974.
7. Bell, D. *End of Ideology: On the Exhaustion of Political Ideas in the Fifties.* Free Press, New York, 1960.
8. Parker, R. *The Myth of the Middle Class: Notes on Affluence and Equality.* Liveright, New York, 1972.
9. Horowitz, I.L., editor. *Power, Politics and People: The Collected Essays of C. Wright Mills,* p. 317. Oxford University Press, New York, 1962. (Quoted in R. Miliband, *The State in Capitalist Society: An Analysis of the Western System of Power,* p. 20. Weidenfeld and Nicolson, London, 1969.)
10. Irish, M., and Prothro, J. *The Politics of American Democracy,* p. 38. Prentice-Hall, Englewood Cliffs, N.J., 1965. (Quoted in E.K. Hunt and H.J. Sherman, *Economics: An Introduction to Traditional and Radical Views,* p. 284. Harper and Row, New York, 1972.)
11. Samuelson, P. *Economics,* Ed. 8, p. 110. McGraw-Hill Book Company, New York, 1972.
12. United States Congress. *Economic Report of the President, 1974.* U.S. Government Printing Office, Washington, D.C., 1974.
13. Shanahan, E. Income distribution found unchanged. *New York Times* p. 10, February 2, 1974.
14. Clark, J.B. *The Distribution of Wealth.* Macmillan Company, New York, 1924. (Quoted in B. Silverman and M. Yanowitch, Radical and liberal perspectives on the working class. *Social Policy* 4(4):40–50, 1974.)
15. Rawls, J.A. *Theory of Justice.* Harvard University Press, Cambridge, Mass., 1971.
16. Barry B. *The Liberal Theory of Justice: A Critical Examination of the Principal Doctrines in "A Theory of Justice" by John Rawls.* Clarendon Press, Oxford, 1972.
17. Silverman, B., and Yanowitch, M. Radical and liberal perspectives on the working class. *Social Policy* 4(4):40–50, 1974.

18. Westergaard, J.H. Sociology: The myth of classlessness. In *Ideology in Social Science,* edited by R. Blackburn, pp. 199–163. Fontana, New York, 1972.
19. Bowles, S., and Gintis, H. IQ in the U.S. class structure. *Social Policy* 3(4 and 5): 65–96, 1973.
20. Simpson, M.A. *Medical Education: A Critical Approach.* Butterworths, London, 1972.
21. Robson, J. The NHS Company, Inc.? The social consequence of the professional dominance in the National Health Service. *Int. J. Health Serv.* 3(3):413–426, 1973.
22. Kleinbach, G. Social structure and the education of health personnel. *Int. J. Health Serv.* 4(2):297–317, 1974.
23. *Evidence of the Royal College of Surgeons to the Royal Commission on Doctors and Dentists Remuneration.* Her Majesty's Stationery Office, London, 1958. (Quoted in J. Robson, The NHS Company, Inc.? The social consequence of the professional dominance in the National Health Service. *Int. J. Health Serv.* 3(3):413–426, 1973.)
24. Lyden, F.J., Geiger, H.J., and Peterson, O. *The Training of Good Physicians.* Harvard University Press, Cambridge, Mass., 1968. (Cited in M.A. Simpson, *Medical Education: A Critical Approach,* p. 35. Butterworths, London, 1972.)
25. Kleinbach, G. Social Class and Medical Education. Department of Education, Harvard University, Cambridge, Mass., 1974.
26. Mills, C.W. *The Power Elite,* p. 39. Oxford University Press, New York, 1956.

Medical Industries

THE TWENTIETH CENTURY HAS SEEN the development of a part of
the corporate sector we can best call "medical industries." Medical
industries are corporate enterprises that market goods or services
in the health field. Although the "patent medicine" industry was
already well established in the nineteenth century (Young, 1961),
the expansion of medical industries in the past fifty years has been
remarkable. The pharmaceutical, health insurance, and medical
technology industries, on the one hand, and the proprietary hospital and nursing home industries, on the other, have experienced
phenomenal growth.

The expansion of medical industries is evidence of the profitability of medicine in American society. The pharmaceutical industry, the most developed medical industry, is the second most profitable industry in the country (Silverman and Lee, 1974). Nearly
three billion prescriptions were filled in 1979. Since prescription
drugs must be marketed through prescriptions written by physicians, the drug companies spend over $1 billion yearly on advertis-
ing and promotion to physicians (Nelson, 1976). This is more than
the teaching budgets of all medical schools combined (Schrag,
1978: 122). The total spent on advertising and promotion by the
pharmaceuticals amounts to about 25 percent of all their revenues,
as compared with 6 percent that goes into research.

The most widely prescribed, or "best selling," drugs today are
psychoactive medications, especially minor tranquilizers. In 1979,
160 million prescriptions were written for tranquilizers, over 60
million for Valium alone. Sixty to 80 percent of these drugs were
prescribed for women (Nellis, 1980). While the "pill for every ill"
ideology of the pharmaceutical industry reaps high profits, Valium
addiction is widespread and Valium abuse has been cited as the
most common drug problem seen in hospital emergency rooms.
The drug industry resists external controls, a resistance that has
led to serious consequences, such as deaths caused by the Dalkon
Shield (Johnston and Dowie, 1977).

The pharmaceutical industry is regulated in the United States by the Food and Drug Administration (FDA). Although this regulation is by no means completely effective (Sheskin, 1978), it places restrictions on the marketing of pharmaceuticals and, occasionally, on the type of drug that can be sold in this country. A major problem with the regulatory effectiveness of the FDA is that it is understaffed and therefore relies primarily on research data gathered by the pharmaceutical companies themselves. Furthermore, the FDA has no jurisdiction outside the United States. The pharmaceutical industry includes multinational corporations that depend on creating new markets to increase profits. It has taken to expanding its markets into Third World countries and there promoting (sometimes called "dumping") drugs for uses for which they are not approved in the United States and without the "warning" materials mandated for American markets. This kind of corporate colonialism has been called "the corporate crime of the century" by the investigative-reporting magazine *Mother Jones*.

The medical industries have "commodified" health in other ways—that is, they have turned certain goods and services into products or commodities that can be marketed to meet "health needs" that are created by the industry itself. An early instance of "commodification" was the promotion of Listerine to cure the "disease" of "halitosis." In recent years, a wide range of products have been marketed to meet "commodified health needs," such as products designed to alleviate feminine hygiene "problems" and instant-milk formulas to meet the "problem" of feeding infants.

Medicine itself is today industrialized. In less than a century it has grown from an occupation typified by a solo practitioner making the rounds by house calls into the second largest industry in America. Part of this growth is due to the expansion of hospitals and medical schools, which were weak and underdeveloped in 1900, but are at the core of medicine today. This is part of a shift in power of medicine from the "professional monopolists" (AMA physicians) to the "corporate rationalizers" (Alford, 1972).

Some medical schools and hospitals have been inclined to "colonize" certain medical publics as their own. Medical schools have been particularly adept at building "medical empires" which are likely to serve their teaching needs more than the health needs of the community (Ehrenreich and Ehrenreich, 1970). Many of these medical empires become small industries in themselves, creating a concentration of local medical power in elite medical-educational institutions more dedicated to management prerogatives than the public's health needs.

The two articles in this section examine different medical industries. James L. Goddard, a former commissioner of the FDA, describes the breadth of "The Medical Business" and the limits of the FDA's jurisdiction. He notes how the pharmaceutical industry has been able to maintain its high profit margins in spite of external pressures. How will the rapidly developing medical technology industry, which recently has given medicine CAT scanners, fetal monitoring units, and other high cost technology, affect the practice of medicine and the costs of medical care? Dorothy Nelkin and David J. Edelman present a case study in the development of a medical empire in "Centralizing Health Care." They show how the regionalization of medical care, protentially a beneficial change, can become a rationalization for medical empire building. The organizational needs of large university hospitals become priorities with little regard for the real health needs of the surrounding community.

Examination of medical industries raises the general question of the role of profitability in medicine, and whether corporations should so freely be able to capitalize on illness. The basic question is whether the medical care sector of society should have a profit-making corporate structure or a structure that is service oriented.

References

Alford, Robert L. 1972. "The political economy of health care: Dynamics without change." Politics and Society (Winter): 127–164.

Ehrenreich, John, and Barbara Ehrenreich. 1970. The American Health Empire. New York: Vintage.

Johnston, Tracy, and Mark Dowie. 1977. "A case of corporate malpractice." Reprinted in Claudia Dreifus (Ed.) Seizing Our Bodies. New York: Vintage.

Nellis, Muriel. 1980. "Hooked, women and prescription drugs." Boston Globe Magazine. (January 13): 10–12.

Nelson, Gaylord. 1976. "Advertising and the national health." Journal of Drug Issues. 6 (1): 28–33.

Schrag, Peter. 1978. Mind Control. New York: Pantheon.

Sheskin, Arlene. 1978. "Dangerous and unhealthy alliances: The pharmaceutical industry and the Food and Drug Administration." In John Conrad (Ed.) The Evolution of Criminal Justice. Beverly Hills, Calif.: Sage Publications.

Silverman, Milton, and Philip R. Lee. 1974. Pills, Profits and Politics. Berkeley: University of California Press.

Young, James H. 1971. The Toadstool Millionaires. Princeton: Princeton University Press.

16

The Medical Business

James L. Goddard

The biggest item in the average American's budget after food, shelter, clothing and transportation is medical care. It is also the fastest-rising major component. Between 1950 and 1972, while the four leading items were increasing about 200 percent, the cost of medical care was increasing more than 400 percent. In 1950 medical care absorbed only 4.6 percent of the average budget; 22 years later it accounted for 7.5 percent. The nation's total health bill in 1972 was $70 billion, or $350 per capita. In this article I shall be concerned with the substantial fraction of the total medical-care bill that supports the "medical business": the $11 billion expended for drugs, medical supplies and equipment. To put the $11 billion in perspective, it is roughly a third of what Americans spent in 1972 on new automobiles.

In the field of ethical pharmaceuticals—drugs sold only on prescription—there are some 22,000 trade-name products in the marketplace. In the field of devices, medical equipment and supplies there is no reliable estimate of the number of products manufactured but it almost certainly exceeds 20,000. They range from cotton balls, sutures and tongue depressors to $100,000 blood-analysis machines that can measure 12 components in a blood sample at the rate of 60 samples per hour. There are more differences than similarities between the pharmaceutical industry and the industries involved in the production of devices, medical supplies and equipment. Here are some of the major differences.

Perhaps the most significant difference is the way in which the consumer pays for the products involved. Consumers paid directly 85 percent of the more than $6 billion spent at retail for 1.5 billion drug prescriptions filled in 1971. In contrast some mode of indirect payment was involved for 84 percent of the consumable supplies and equipment used during illnesses in the same year. Prosthetic devices, including eyeglasses, which are paid for directly, accounted for the remaining 16 percent. Supplies are said to be paid for indirectly when they are part of a consolidated bill presented by a hospital or clinic or when they are part of a bill paid by an insurance carrier or other third party. In either case the patient is usually unaware of the details.

A corollary of the mode of payment leads to the second major difference between the drug houses and the makers of medical supplies: the degree of product visibility. The general public is aware of and concerned about such issues as the safety of oral contraceptives, price-fixing in antibiotics and the debate over brand-name v. generic-name prescription writing. The public has little or no interest, however, in such matters as proof of safety and effectiveness of equipment used for patient care or the unnecessary duplication of costly equipment by hospitals located in the same area. One thinks, for example, of the fad for installing hyperbaric chambers in hospital operating rooms in the mid-1960's. Costing upward of $100,000 per installation, their value to the patient undergoing surgery now appears marginal.

Product visibility, or lack of it, helps to explain the third major difference between the part of the industry that produces drugs and the part that produces supplies and equipment. Whereas the Government subjects drug makers to heavy regulation, it has only recently begun to regulate the makers of medical supplies and equipment.

The fourth major difference between the two parts of the industry is in profitability. The pharmaceutical houses outperform all other major American industries in net profit after taxes as a percent of stockholders' equity. The drug companies regularly show a return of about 18 percent, a figure two-thirds higher than the average rate of return for all manufacturing concerns in the decade 1960–1970. Although the consolidated data are not available for direct comparison, it is evident from the annual reports of the major companies in the medical supplies and equipment business that their rates of return are closer to the industrial average of 11 percent than to the drug companies' 18 percent. These, then, are the two major segments of the medical business: one highly visible, highly profitable and highly controversial, the other almost hidden from view, returning only average profits and making few "waves." Let us now take a closer look at the two segments.

The pharmaceutical industry manufactures two major classes of products: proprietary drugs sold freely over the counter and ethical drugs, which require a prescription. Ethical pharmaceuticals are further subdivided into brand-name and generic products. The former are patented products manufactured by the larger companies; the latter are substances on which the patent has usually expired and that bear a uniform chemical name regardless of the source.

In 1971, according to surveys conducted by the magazine *Drug Topics,* the dollar volume of all packaged medicines sold at retail without a prescription was $2.9 billion. Of this total cough and cold "remedies" accounted for $619 million, headache nostrums for $600 million and mouthwashes and gargles for $240 million. Many observers question the desirability of this traffic in drugs that are mostly marginal in their effectiveness. Although they are heavily advertised as being capable of relieving and even curing various target ailments, the claims are rarely supported by objective studies. The Federal Trade Commission has begun to look closely at the curative claims made for these over-the-counter drugs in television and newspaper advertisements.

Meanwhile the prescription drug industry is enjoying an unbroken rise in sales. The value of ethical-drug shipments in 1971 was $4.11 billion, an increase of more than 100 percent in 10 years, with no leveling off in sight. If Congress were to enact some kind of comprehensive national health-insurance plan that would include payment for prescription drugs, total sales could jump 20 to 25 percent almost overnight.

I shall leave it to other authors . . . to question whether Americans really need 1.5 billion drug prescriptions per year or an average of 20 per family. I shall limit my remarks to the way the industry uses its sales dollars.

It is estimated that the ethical-drug houses currently spend $1.2 billion per year on advertising and promotion. This represents about $1 in every $4 they receive for their products at wholesale and is nearly four times what they spend annually on research and development. Virtually none of the marketing expenditures are directed at the consumer who buys the product. They are directed at the physician who writes the prescription and at the pharmacist who, with increasing frequency, is in a position to select the brand when the prescription is written generically or when it allows him to substitute one brand for another.

Since the marketing costs come to about $4,000 per physician per year they are deemed excessive by many critics of the industry. The $1.2-billion figure includes the salaries of more than 21,000 "detail men," each of whom costs the industry an estimated $35,000 per year; their sole job is to make periodic calls on physicians, pharmacists and hospital purchasing agents to push their firm's products. Also included in the $1.2 billion are such costs as advertising in medical journals, exhibits at medical conventions, direct-mail pieces (including physicians' samples), seminars, educational films, brochures and the practice of allowing wholesalers, retailers and hospitals to return unsold merchandise for credit. How essential these expenditures are is a matter of judgment. That they add significantly to the nation's drug bill is undisputable.

During the past five years research costs in the pharmaceutical industry have averaged close to 6 percent of net sales, a figure comparable to that in other high-technology industries. In the same period the return on research investments, as measured by new products, has shown a steady decline. The decline followed the passage of the Kefauver-Harris amendments to the Federal Food, Drug, and Cosmetic Act of 1962, which substantially increased the Food and Drug Administration's regulating authority with respect to the testing and marketing of new drugs. The peak for

Figure 1.

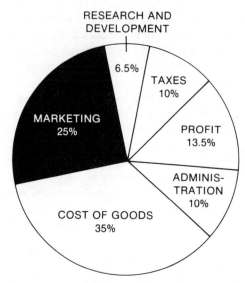

Breakdown of Sales Dollar is estimated for 1968 for 17 leading pharmaceutical houses. Although the industry takes pride in its large investment in research and development (some $400 million in 1968), the amount spent on marketing and promotion is nearly four times larger. The industry is second only to mining in profitability.

new chemical entities (63) was reached in 1959; the peaks for new combinations (253) and new dosage forms (109) had been reached a year earlier. By requiring that new drugs be efficacious as well as safe, the Kefauver-Harris amendments accelerated the decline in all three categories of new products. With 5,558 new products entering the marketplace between 1950 and 1962 the country needed not more combinations, new dosage forms and duplicate products but more effective drugs.

In spite of some predictions the amendments have not stifled drug research. The quest for new drugs continues apace. The total industry outlay for research and development exceeds $500 million per year, and the Federal Government spends $1.75 billion on drug testing alone.

Production costs in the pharmaceutical industry average a third of the manufacturer's sales dollar. The most significant portion of this expenditure, however, is related not to the cost of raw materials or to the manufacturing process itself but rather to the highly complex quality-control procedures required by Federal law. More than 8,000 workers, 16 percent of the industry's work force, are engaged in quality control.

Profitability has long been the hallmark of the pharmaceutical industry. Year after year the industry ranks first or second in after-tax income as a percentage of net worth. This profitability has been maintained by the drug industry even though drug prices have not climbed as rapidly as consumer prices in general. The drug industry has been able to limit price increases thanks in large part to the high degree of automatic control achieved in its manufacturing processes. At the same time the absence of price competition for most products has ensured continued high profits.

When the pharmaceutical industry is called on to defend its large profit margins, it responds that it is in a high-risk business in which vast sums are spent on research with little or no guarantee of return. Spokesmen for the drug industry often compare the search for new drugs with the drilling of wildcat wells in the oil industry. The fact is that during the past 25 years no major pharmaceutical house has been forced out of business. As one economist said in testimony before the Senate Select Committee on Small Business: "The high profitability reflects the absence of competition; the stability of profits demonstrates the absence of risk to investors. If risks were to exist, one would expect to see the high gains of some firms accompanied by occasional losses—to themselves or to others—but such evidence of risk is virtually nonexistent."

The industry's profitability has been maintained also in the face of rising Government interest in and control of its activities. Federal interest was aroused in the era of Theodore Roosevelt, when the blatant claims of many makers of patent medicines led to calls for Government regulation. Apart from the fact that the claims were often misleading and even dangerous, many of the nostrums contained opium derivatives, with the result that many people unwittingly became addicted to the drug. Harvey W. Wiley, a chemist in the Department of Agriculture, was one of the leaders in the effort to bring patent medicines under control. It was not until the publication of Upton Sinclair's novel *The Jungle,* however, that Congress responded by passing the Food and Drug Act of 1906. From this modest beginning the Federal role in drug regulation has grown to its present level. In each instance drug legislation granting new authority was precipitated by some crisis affecting the consumer.

In 1938, for example, it was the elixir of sulfanilamide disaster, in which the use of ethylene glycol as a solvent by a chemist with the S. E. Massengill Company led to the death of more than 100 persons, most of them small children. Congress swiftly enacted a law requiring that drugs by proved safe prior to marketing. Such legislation had been sought by the Executive Branch of the Government each year since 1933, only to be beaten back each time in Congress through the efforts of the drug-industry lobby.

In 1961, when the thalidomide tragedy struck in Europe, Richardson-Merrell, a major U.S. pharmaceutical manufacturer, had a new-drug application for thalidomide pending before the Food and Drug Administration. Thanks to the vigilance of Frances Oldham Kelsey, a physician and pharmacologist on the FDA staff, the application was held up and ultimately never issued. Congress again acted swiftly by passing the Kefauver-Harris amendments, which provided the FDA with an entire range of new authorities, including the requirement that all new drugs must be proved not only safe but also effective before being allowed to enter the marketplace. The FDA was also empowered to require periodic reports from manufacturers; to require that ethical-drug advertising be honest, with sufficient balance to give the physician information about a drug's side effects and contraindications as well as its potential benefits; to require immediate reporting of any unusual side effects during development work, and to review all drugs marketed between 1938 and 1962 to determine their efficacy as well as their safety.

Some observers believe that the pharmaceutical industry is now over-regulated and that bureaucratic interference with the industry has reached such a level that the American public is being denied certain drugs available overseas. The University of Chicago economist Milton Friedman has recently made this point forcefully, and with much publicity, by charging that FDA regulations are keeping important new drugs off the American market and that the U.S. is falling behind the rest of the world in the development of new drugs. Calling for repeal of the Kefauver-Harris amendments, Friedman pointed to the availability in Europe of two new drugs for heart patients, Practolol and Oxprenolol, as prime examples of why the present system should be changed.

Friedman's allegations were effectively refuted during recent Senate hearings by spokesmen from three organizations that rarely find themselves in total agreement about anything: the Food and Drug Administration, the American Medical Association and the Pharmaceutical Manufacturers Association. Spokesmen for these groups, along with a number of prominent heart and cancer specialists, made it quite clear that even though the U.S. has the most demanding requirements of any nation in the world, all safe and effective drugs, or their equivalents, are available here. (Practolol and Oxprenolol are not deemed safe.)

The companies that manufacture medical supplies, devices and equipment might be termed the hidden, or at least the unknown, segment of the medical business. When the patient is billed for blood tests or X rays, it probably does not occur to him that part of the fee is used to offset the purchase price of expensive analytical instruments or an X-ray camera. And who even cares that the doctor's bill must cover the cost of tongue depressors, Band-Aids, thermometers, disposable hypodermic syringes and the almost countless other impedimenta of medical practice?

In spite of their low profile, the companies that make these medical goods are enjoying the sharply rising expenditures on health care. For example, manufacturers of surgical dressings and instruments have annual sales of more than $500 million. This amount includes $163 million for adhesive tape, $127 million for compresses, gauze and other dressings, $88 million for elastic bandages and rolls containing plaster of Paris for making casts and $30 million for cotton balls. Sales of surgical instruments come to about $120 million per year.

Manufacturers of other kinds of medical supplies have annual sales of more than $2 billion. Sales are expected to reach $2.9 billion by 1975 and $4.2 billion by 1980. Products under this heading include anesthetics, parenteral solutions, syringes and needles, sutures, laboratory ware and reagents, thermometers, stethoscopes, sphygmomanometers, medical linen and X-ray supplies. (More square feet of photographic film are consumed in making X rays than are used by the motion-picture industry, which has recently led the Eastman Kodak Company to introduce a system for copying the standard 14-by-17-inch X-ray image on a "chip" about two inches square so that the silver in the original large negative can be recycled.)

The introduction of new technology, much of it made possible by solid-state electronics, has led to a sharp rise in the sales of medical and hospital equipment. The magazine *Electronics* predicts, for example, that sales will increase more than 50 percent between 1970 and 1975: from $530 million to $832 million. Sales of patient-monitoring systems will nearly triple in the same period: from $29 million to $80 million.

Sizable increases are also predicted for sales of such laboratory equipment as automatic clinical chemistry systems, blood-bank equipment, blood analyzers, chromatography systems, electrolyte-measuring instruments, automatic bloodcell counters, electron and light microscopes and spectrophotometers. Sales of these items, which were less than $200 million in 1968, may reach $380 million in 1975 and exceed $570 million in 1980, according to *Electronics*.

The use of new plastics and alloys has led to great advances in such surgical implants as artificial joints, bone plates, pins and arterial grafts. It is estimated that 100,000 arterial grafts will be inserted this year, along with 45,000 heart valves and 200,000 cerebrospinal-fluid shunts (mechanical devices for relieving excess aqueous pressure within the brain). It is estimated that 100,000 Americans are now equipped with electronic heart pacemakers and that 50,000 new installations will be made this year. More than three million women have now been fitted with intrauterine contraceptive devices (IUD's) in the form of rings, coils, loops, bows, springs and spirals.

During the remainder of the decade one can expect major progress in the development of assistive prosthetic and corrective devices, such as "radar" aids for the blind and artificial larynxes. Sales of devices in this category are expected to reach $640 million by 1975 and $890 million by 1980.

Many observers believe the medical supply industry is in the same position as the drug industry was in before the enactment of the 1938 legislation. There has been an enormous proliferation of medical devices (a recent FDA survey counted 12,000 devices made by 1,100 companies), but no Federal agency has yet been given the responsibility for determining either their safety or their efficacy. The International Organization for

Standardization has been pressing its member countries to exercise greater control over devices with the greatest potential for doing harm, particularly surgical implants. At the same time the FDA has been asking Congress to increase its control over the manufacture and sale of medical devices of all kinds.

In recent testimony before a Congressional subcommittee the then Acting FDA Commissioner Sherwin Gardner noted that under the limited powers granted the agency in 1938 most of its effort, until recently at least, had been devoted to removing obviously dangerous products from the market and controlling the promotion of "quack type" devices. "Because existing law imposes no statutory requirements for FDA to review the safety and effectiveness of medical devices prior to marketing," Gardner testified, "FDA has the burden of proof and must accumulate evidence sufficient to assure that it can sustain a court action."

An indication of the seriousness of the problem is that, even with such limited powers, the FDA in the first three months of this year seized more than 300 devices, ordered the recall of 35 different kinds of device (including several hundred heart pacemakers) and issued more than 1,800 advisory opinions (letters of warning or caution to manufacturers). A bill that is currently before Congress would enable the agency to require all manufacturers of medical devices to be registered with the FDA, to disclose all complaints received, to maintain records and submit reports (including clinical studies of safety and efficacy) and to recall, replace or repair defective devices. One would hope that adequate control legislation will for once in this country be enacted on its merits and not in response to a tragedy.

17

Centralizing Health Care

Dorothy Nelkin and David J. Edelman

A new 416-bed, one hundred million dollar municipal hospital is about to open in New York's north central Bronx after a delay of more than two years. This hospital (NCB) was built by New York City, adjacent to and connected with Montefiore Hospital and Medical Center, a privately owned voluntary (not-for-profit) hospital. It is located in a middle-class community in a part of the Bronx which already has more hospital beds than any other area in the borough. This community has been strongly antagonistic to the addition of new hospital facilities which would further contribute to congestion and the decline of the local neighborhood.

Ironically, NCB was built as a replacement for Morrisania Hospital in the central Bronx where, as the only viable social institution in the neighborhood, the hospital was an extremely important resource. Just as community organizations in the north central Bronx have opposed the construction of the new hospital, so groups in the west, central, and south Bronx have fought to maintain their medical services. And while the city administration seeks to close municipal hospitals that are a drain on its depleted budget, a new, modern facility has been the focus of a bitter dispute over its future management and its effect on other areas of the Bronx less well endowed with medical services.

Analyses

Some analysts attribute the fiasco leading to the construction of NCB Hospital to the imperialist ambitions of Montefiore's administration, which donated the land on which the new facility was built; others blame it on the inept character of New York City's health administration and the influence of private interests concerned with developing the health delivery system to their own advantage. This analysis will suggest rather that the problem of NCB reflects the relentless economic and administrative imperatives of technology-based medicine, imperatives that have driven the health care system to increased centralization in large-scale medical centers.

Montefiore, along with most modern medical planning groups, has long been committed to developing regionalized programs that would decentralize ambulatory primary care services while centralizing specialized care. But the development of ambulatory programs has failed to match the pace of centralization. We shall use this case to analyze the factors that encourage the trend toward centralization and the implications for efforts to organize more rational schemes for health care delivery.

Contradictions

Many contradictions have plagued the health delivery system since the rapid development of medical science has enhanced the importance and prestige of the modern hospital. At a time when the large urban hospital is the central unit in the delivery of health care, it is also a focus of angry public opposition, resented as a symbol of the inequities in the medical care system. At a time when the complexity of hospital administration requires expert technical management, there is increasing demand for public involvement by groups with no expertise but intense personal or political interest in the direction of hospital planning. And at a time when the urban teaching hospital is a center for remarkable medical and scientific achievements, it has become a battlefield for conflicts having little to do specifically with medicine as defined by the medical profession.

Concern with neighborhood quality, resentment of bureaucratic and expert authority, desire for community control, and—above all—fear that technological development is overriding human priorities are expressed in attacks on hospital policies. On the one hand, the university hospital, the "jewel" of the medical system, has been fervently described by Selig Greenberg in his *The Quality of Mercy* (1971) as

> the place where the latest benefits of science can best be obtained . . . [where] new weapons of healing are forged . . . where the exploration of the grim terrain of disease presents the great intellectual challenge and where apprentice physicians are trained to shift the balance in favor of the prolongation of life and vigor.

On the other hand, these strengths are bitterly criticized by the Health Policy Advisory Center as irrelevant to health care:

> The asserted ability of the major teaching hospitals to provide quality care has been apparent only for certain specialized and "interesting" treatment and diagnostic procedures. The empires' control has usually been antagonistic to the achievement of medical quality in social terms, i.e., comprehensive, low cost, patient-centered services (Barbara and John Ehrenreich, *The American Health Empire*, 1970).

These contradictions, apparent in the NCB dispute and numerous other controversies over hospital expansion, reflect the collision between the administrative imperatives that direct the policies of a large technology-based medical center and the social priorities of various groups that are affected by hospitals as they become increasingly important social institutions.

The Imperatives of Scientific Medicine

The remarkable development of medical technology, especially since World War II, contributed to the specialization of medicine. Between 1949 and 1973 the percentage of doctors who were specialists increased from 36 to 82 percent. In addition, the costs of technology generated administrative and organizational changes necessary to make economical use of expensive, specialized technical resources. Major institutional changes followed, in particular the decline of the entrepreneurial tradition in medicine and the concentration of health care services in an essentially industrial base—the modern voluntary teaching hospital.

The hospital is increasingly the center for the delivery of health care. Each year a higher proportion of physicians are salaried hospital employees, and a higher proportion of the total expenditures for personal health services are for hospital care (e.g., 33.1 percent in 1950 to 41.3 percent in 1973). Hospital admissions increased from 110.5 per 1,000 people in 1950 to 168 per 1,000 in 1974.

The technical complexity of scientific medicine creates financial and administrative imperatives that bear directly on the allocation of hospital services. First, a hospital must have a large and stable financial base; philanthropy, private insurance, or direct payment for service are no longer adequate sources of funds. Thus all hospitals, private as well as public, rely on public support through various health insurance schemes and contracts.

The spiraling costs of scientific medicine have brought hospitals into new relationships with state and local government bureaucracies, with serious implications for the allocation of medical resources. Ironically, while private hospitals receive increased public support, the public or municipal hospitals responsible largely for poor and long-term patients are approaching insolvency; and their medical services, subject to the vagaries of municipal budgets and obsolete civil service requirements, are deteriorating. Indeed, those poor with any choice flock to the voluntary hospitals, still further impoverishing the municipals which cannot maintain an adequate census. Thus, despite heavy government subsidization, the private sector increasingly dominates medical resources.

Second, all hospitals must secure a steady flow of patients to maintain maximum utilization of their technical facilities. Medical teams can work together effectively only with regular, practical experience. Thus each hospital must be able to draw on a large population of potential clients. If a hospital cannot fill its beds and fully utilize its equipment, it cannot afford to remain open. The tendency therefore is invariably to consolidate resources; centralization of hospital services appears necessary to avoid duplication and to meet the demands for modernization with reasonable economy.

In the trend toward consolidation the larger, better equipped teaching hospitals tend to grow, while smaller, marginal institutions close. And as municipal hospitals lose out in the "battle for beds," they may leave large areas with reduced access to medical services, raising difficult questions about the distribution of hospital care. Which communities stand to benefit from the medical center, and which will lose services from the concentration of medical resources? And what services must give way to support the cost of high-technology procedures?

Third, the high costs of scientific medicine have fostered a management style in which economic efficiency must be the primary goal. The economics of efficient management often dominate social goals, and priorities for health service programs may follow less from social need than from income produced. Thus costly programs for ambulatory care, promising neither remuneration nor prestige, tend to be of low priority for the modern hospital despite community needs.

Montefiore Hospital

The force of these imperatives is clear in the case of Montefiore Hospital and Medical Center in the Bronx. This center, including its affiliates, is the largest hospital complex in the Bronx. It is world renowned for its social service projects; indeed, the hospital has been a leader in the development of family health care centers and community medicine. Yet it is bitterly resented, accused by many people in its own community of neglecting local needs in favor of prestigious research, and criticized as an example of the negligence of high-technology institutions. Moreover, it is resented by other Bronx communities as contributing to the deterioration in the distribution of hospital services.

Administrative decisions at Montefiore are bound by the need for institutional survival. In a competitive, high-cost operation such as Montefiore financial security is necessarily the criteria underlying each decision; priorities begin with those programs that can "fill the beds" and attract a competent staff.

Furthermore, it is axiomatic among hospital administrators that a hospital must have a well-balanced mix of patients from different socioeconomic backgrounds, both to maintain this economic viability and to sustain continued technical excellence. Serving lower-class patients fulfills a sense of social purpose; but the medical school also has a pedagogical interest in the character of diverse pathologies, and it is often easier to study welfare patients who are less inclined than middle-class patients to object to the dual role of patient and "teaching material."

Serving private middle-class patients, however, is necessary for a healthy hospital economy. Medicaid and Blue Cross only reimburse the hospital for the cost of each service at a negotiated rate. More prosperous patients, who pay for medical services through Blue Shield or other private insurance arrangements, are reimbursed on an idemnity basis which allows the hospital to acquire risk capital to develop new programs. These private insurance plans bring in about one million dollars a year to Montefiore, half of which can be used for new programs.

Thus voluntary hospitals must make a special effort to maintain a socioeconomic balance. Montefiore, for instance, must attract competent doctors from the suburbs (e.g., Westchester) who will choose to hospitalize their private patients at Montefiore in preference to many other voluntary hospitals in the New York area.

A doctor's decision where to send a patient depends on several factors: the existence of appropriate technical facilities for the particular patient, the need to rationalize his own schedule, and convenience such as accessibility and parking. Thus Montefiore is under special pressure to continually modernize its technology in order to provide incentives that will outweigh its relative lack of convenience for many affiliated physicians. The hospital administration is firmly convinced that private doctors who commute from suburban areas will only maintain affiliation if Montefiore remains a prestige hospital providing high-quality, specialized care unavailable elsewhere and parking as well.

But keeping up with the rate of technological change in biomedicine creates its own problems. It requires regular acquisition of new and expensive equipment, involving not only high capital but teams of technicians and specialized practitioners. Staffing imposes demanding organizational requirements. Complex techniques such as open heart surgery, for example, require a highly coordinated team of about seventeen doctors and technicians; effective teamwork can be achieved only through the experience acquired by working together on a regular basis. A high rate of utilization is also necessary for the economic viability of costly technical facilities, and this viability requires a large population base from which patients will come to Montefiore and use its special services in preference to those of other hospitals.

Ambulatory care programs help broaden this population base. But Montefiore remains ambivalent about expanding those programs which impose a financial strain on hospital resources. Many ambulatory care patients are uninsured—the so-called "self-pay, no-pay" clients—and only 11 percent of hospital income is derived from this source, in contrast to the 70 percent from inpatient services. Economically pressured to fill its beds, Montefiore's outpatient services thus tend to have low priority.

Despite a liberal commitment to social medicine, surgery remains the high-prestige department. Martin Cherkasky, Montefiore's director, has observed that outpatient facilities often tend to be "by-passed by the talented physician." Ambulatory care is important as evidence that Montefiore is a forward-looking institution, but it is often called "the bastard child" or "hardly real medicine" by hospital doctors.

Faced with ambivalence from staff physicians as well as uncertain funding for social service programs, Montefiore has created its social programs in an ad hoc manner, implementing projects as funds for them become available. Although committed to ambulatory care and involved in several neighborhood family care centers, its outpatient activities are severely limited; basic ambulatory services remain located largely in the emergency rooms of the municipal hospitals throughout the Bronx.

As Montefiore seeks to expand its own population base in order to maintain full utilization of its facilities, it comes into direct conflict with these municipal hospitals which must also fill their beds to remain solvent. Thus Montefiore is engaged in continuing negotiations with public agencies, the city government, and other health care interests in what can only be labeled "the battle for the beds in the Bronx."

Battle for Beds in the Bronx

In May 1961 the Hospital Council of Greater New York, reporting on the health care situation in the Bronx, recommended replacing Lincoln and Morrisania hospitals, two aging city municipal institutions, and urged greater integration of the municipal and voluntary systems through affiliation agreements that would resolve the staffing and administrative problems of the municipals. The city would continue to administer the municipals and their nontechnical staff, but the voluntaries would provide professional services. During the 1960s seventeen of the city's nineteen municipal hospitals were thus affiliated with six medical schools and seven voluntary hospitals. As part of this citywide program, Montefiore agreed in 1962 to a professional affiliation contract with Morrisania Hospital, a 331-bed facility located in the central Bronx.

At this time Montefiore's administration voiced a serious reservation. How could a medical staff effectively serve Morrisania, over forty congested city blocks from the central hospital? It was argued that the distance to an affiliate must be minimized if doctors were to serve there, and that Morrisania was simply too far away. As part of the negotiated affiliation agreement, therefore, the New York City Department of Hospitals promised that instead of renovating the aging Morrisania, it would build a new replacement on land adjacent to Montefiore. Montefiore in turn promised to give land to the city for the new hospital, and plans were soon underway for a modern 416-bed municipal hospital actually attached to Montefiore.

Justification for this unusual agreement was provided by the Hospital Review and Planning Council of Southern New York in November 1966. Noting the deterioration of community hospitals, the council proposed that future planning of health care facilities should concentrate community health functions around a "medical service center," that is, a modern, well-equipped general hospital. The council proposed that funds earmarked to replace municipal hospitals be used instead to expand facilities near voluntary teaching hospitals. Thus the council endorsed New York City's decision to replace Morrisania Hospital on the land donated by Montefiore, since combining the two hospitals would provide a medical center of over one thousand beds.

By the time this report was issued, however, city health planners began to realize the ironies of forcing patients to commute from Morrisania to the new hospital instead of bringing doctors to the central Bronx. Health care studies were strongly suggesting the importance of decentralizing hospitals, emphasizing that they be located in areas of maximum service needs. These ideas became increasingly salient to city health planners as community concerns about losing Morrisania began to surface in the central Bronx.

In 1966 this area had lost three hundred beds with the closing of St. Francis, a Catholic hospital that had served mostly ward patients supported by city funds. This closing left a considerable burden on nearby Lincoln and Morrisania hospitals, both of which were already outmoded and overcrowded. As in most low-income urban areas, demands on the emergency rooms at both hospitals had increased dramatically, and thus the prospect of a further decrease of medical services was resisted. Yet the plan to replace Morrisania by North Central Bronx Hospital would further concentrate medical facilities in the more affluent part of the Bronx and reduce service in low-income areas with the greatest medical needs.

By January 1968 the Hospital Review and Planning Council that had earlier recommended replacing Morrisania had second thoughts; but by this time the city, supported by a technical study recommending that the new hospital be built, had spent $750,000 on plans. Thus in the summer of 1969 Montefiore transferred (for one dollar) 73,000 square feet of land appraised at $400,000, to the city for the purpose of building the new hospital. The contract included the agreement that NCB was to be physically connected to Montefiore Hospital and that its plans would be developed in consultation with the Montefiore staff. It was understood that Montefiore would provide all professional services to the new hospital, and that if that agreement should terminate the city would pay back the appraised value of the land. In addition, Montefiore held a purchase option to buy back the building if the city chose to use the property for other purposes.

A Lemon Built in the Wrong Place

Once construction actually began on the new hospital Montefiore found itself in the middle of a major controversy. Its own neighbors in the middle-class community of Norwood vigorously opposed any new construction. The new addition meant construction noise, traffic problems, and increased congestion. Neighborhood residents also feared that if the Montefiore-NCB Hospital complex became a specialized medical center for the entire Bronx, it would attract blacks and Puerto Ricans from the south. This situation, they feared, would lead to the further decline of a neighborhood already battling the early stages of transition as younger families moved to the suburbs, leaving vacant apartments.

The main issue, however, was the effect of the new hospital on the existing hospitals in the Bronx. The Morrisania community was especially upset that a decision about NCB, so vital to its interest in keeping Morrisania Hospital open, was reached without any involvement of its representatives. The community near Fordham Hospital, further west, saw its own plans to build a new hospital threatened by the construction of NCB and by the potential control of Montefiore as the dominant unit in an increasingly centralized system, a prediction confirmed two years later.

The concerns of various groups affected by the NCB decision were reinforced in April 1973 when a copy of a regional plan prepared by Montefiore was leaked to the *New York Post*. It turned out that in August 1972 the Health and Hospital Corporation (HHC) had commissioned Montefiore to study ways to rationalize the distribution of health care in the Bronx. With construction of NCB well under way the HHC president, Dr. Joseph T. English, had been worried about how best to use this facility to resolve the difficult problem of distributing hospital beds in the Bronx. A municipal hospital was not truly needed to serve patients in Montefiore's area, yet there it stood.

English's concerns were reinforced by growing criticism of HHC's role in improving regional health planning in New York. Montefiore Director Martin Cherkasky had long been the city's leading advocate of regional health care and had specifically proposed that the new NCB Hospital, adjacent to Montefiore, provide a unique opportunity to implement a regional plan. Thus English commissioned Montefiore to prepare a study that could serve as the basis for a regional system for the west Bronx, and in particular a study that would include the terms of managing NCB.

Despite the magnitude of any decision involving a publicly financed hospital, and the huge network of public and private medical facilities and community groups concerned with health care, all discussions and negotiations during the preparation of the regionalization plan were confidential. Even the HHC Board of Directors was not informed about the proposed regionalization study.

In this vulnerable situation the *Post* suddenly disclosed the existence of Montefiore's West Bronx Health Planning Study, a regionalization plan that called for dividing the west Bronx into ten areas, each with its group practice ambulatory care center serving forty thousand people. These centers would be backed by community hospitals, and all would be supported by a large regional medical center prepared to deliver complex services. The combined Montefiore-NCB complex would serve this purpose. The two hospitals would operate under a unified administration and with a single work force directed by Montefiore and audited by the HHC.

Nearly every health interest in the Bronx attacked. It was not that the study lacked professional competence; on the contrary, it was a thorough and rational document, based on careful analysis of the health needs of the west Bronx and the adequacy of existing health care institutions. Here was a document, supported by the president of the HHC and developed by Montefiore Hospital, that laid out a plan for the west Bronx that would affect health care throughout the entire borough. Moreover, the plan was so detailed that it was widely assumed that negotiations for its implementation were well under way.

Yet the plan was prepared in complete secrecy. Medical, political, community, and union leaders had not been consulted. That the regional plan proposed Montefiore-NCB as the dominant hospital unit in the region strengthened hostility. And the timetable indicating that negotiations were to be completed by May 1973 (only a month after the document's release), supported suspicions that the HHC had made a deal agreeing to grant Montefiore administrative authority over health care in the entire area.

By May 1973 NCB Hospital had become so controversial that HHC publicly labeled it "a lemon built in the wrong place," and Martin Cherkasky declared that he would not take NCB as a "gift." "I didn't ask for it," he said, "I don't need it; I don't want it."

The Municipals and Montefiore

Decisions about NCB and the future of Morrisania Hospital are part of the much larger problem of curtailing what has seemed to be an endless increase in the city health care budget. New York City's municipal hospital system has long been a source of financial strain for the city; and while the affiliation system had temporarily eased some administrative problems, the 1970s brought increasing economic strain. City government economists provoked efforts to rationalize the health delivery system by closing underused municipal hospitals and regionalizing specialized services. These decisions, affecting the allocation of health services, have been extremely controversial, and critics saw the voluntary hospitals gaining directly from the decline of the municipal system.

In this sensitive context the NCB decision became the focal point of the battle for beds in the Bronx. The disclosure of the West Bronx Health Planning Study and the realization that Montefiore might run NCB brought a deluge of position papers and studies from hospitals, communities, politicians, special commissions, and labor unions—all aware that NCB would vitally affect their interests. In July 1973 the HHC recommended that when NCB opened, three hundred beds in existing municipal hospitals should be eliminated and that Morrisania would have to close.

In the same month Bronx Borough President Robert Abram's Committee on Health Care in the Bronx distributed a 250-page collection of documents on the history of NCB, intended to portray a sordid picture of surreptitious negotiation. The committee proposed that a voluntary hospital *other* than Montefiore manage NCB under the governance of a special board of trustees with a majority of community representatives. In the light of evidence concerning the surplus of general care beds and the need for extended care facilities, Abrams further proposed using NCB as an independent extended care nursing and mental health facility. Such a hospital would not need expensive equipment; the money saved could then be used to pay back Montefiore for the appraised value of the land it had originally donated for NCB.

Increasingly concerned about disaffection among his constituents, Abrams also announced an alternate regionalization plan called the Bronx County Community Health Care Cooperative. Like Montefiore's West Bronx Health Planning Study, this plan was intended to end the dual standard of health care through better coordination of the health care system and to restructure the system by increasing the number of primary care units (i.e., neighborhood centers associated with community hospitals).

The plans, however, diverged in important ways. The Montefiore plan, reflecting the hospital's technical perspective, envisioned an organization directed entirely by a professional board and run with the regional NCB-Montefiore medical center as the core decision-making and coordinating unit. The emphasis was on efficiency of service. In contrast, Abram's plan sought a structure based on participation of community groups. It stressed the autonomy of each community hospital unit and the desirability of governance by community representation to insure accountability. The Bronx Community Health Care Cooperative would be an umbrella, not-for-profit public benefit corporation, responsible for planning and organizing the health system in response to local needs.

By October 1974 HHC, under continuing financial pressure to see that the total number of beds in the Bronx did not exceed demand, published another staff report that again proposed closing Morrisania Hospital once both the new Lincoln Hospital and NCB opened. The report calculated that the two new hospitals would increase the Bronx bed supply by 64 percent. Reduced occupancy rates in existing hospitals, declining population in the Bronx, plus reduction in the average length of hospital stays called for fewer services. Patients from the area near Morrisania Hospital, where the occupancy rate had declined from 86 percent in 1969 to 78.8 percent in 1974, could be transferred by special taxi or ambulance to NCB.

On April 30, 1975 one thousand people from community groups throughout the Bronx gathered to defend interests they felt were jeopardized by the HHC regionalization scheme. A neighborhood organizer from a Bronx community board expressed the community perspective in a statement to the Health and Hospital Corporation:

The fact is that the health needs of the population in the Bronx are so severe and so under-served that if all of the people requiring hospitalization for mental or physical ailments were hospitalized, there would be a shortage of beds for years to come.

. . . .

If Fordham Hospital and Morrisania Hospital are taken out of their communities, the Health and Hospital Corporation will have gone on record in favor of an expensive regionalization scheme which concentrates medical resources in locations which are inaccessible to the majority of the people who would need and use them.

The battle for the beds continues in the context of several factors. High-technology medicine has driven the cost of health care beyond the limits of the city budget and has contributed to the continued decline of municipal hospitals. With greater flexibility to respond to increased costs, the voluntaries are glad to absorb the extra patients resulting from a reduction in the total number of hospital beds—and they seek to improve and expand their own facilities. They do so, however, in a changing climate of public opinion: the battle for the beds has increased public mistrust of voluntary hospitals and further politicized the health planning process.

Problems of Regionalization

The dispute over NCB and the West Bronx Health Planning Study reflects the difference between technocratic and political perspectives of health care. Hospital administration is a professional activity devoted to applying scientific principles to the solution of the problems of illness. Centralized, autonomous planning with minimum interference is deemed necessary to provide a rational and efficient allocation of services. Professional expectations converge with the spiraling costs of specialized, technology-based medicine and the need for less wasteful organization to suggest the economic rationality of centralization.

From a social or political perspective, however, the value of centralization is less obvious. For communities affected by hospital decisions health is defined in broad terms, including social conditions, jobs, housing, and the quality of neighborhood life. The role of a hospital transcends the simple provision of scientific medicine as measured by procedures performed or patients processed. In contrast to Montefiore's technical perspective, the community views hospital planning as a social and political activity bearing on community well-being.

Such conflicting definitions underlie the long history of failure in efforts to rationalize the delivery of health care through regionalization schemes. Concepts of regionalization, similar to those proposed in the West Bronx Health Planning Study, have been advocated as the rational means to organize a health delivery system since the Dawson regional plan for Great Britain's health services in 1920. Such schemes are intended to combine the benefits of scientific planning and coordination with economies of scale by creating comprehensive, integrated hospital systems.

The core of a regionalized health care system is a high-technology medical center bringing together medical specialists, technical equipment, and other costly resources to deal with health problems requiring sophisticated and specialized care. Such a center would support a system of smaller, dispersed community hospitals that provide care for more routine cases. Neighborhood or ambulatory care centers would serve as the primary units—liaisons between individuals in the community and the regional health care system.

Regionalization would rationalize both the distribution of physician services and the allocation of hospital beds. It can potentially decrease the costs of operation by coordinating occupancy rates among hospitals with the allocation of personnel and technical resources. Joint administrative, accounting, and supply arrangements would bring economies of scale. Referring all highly specialized, episodic problems to a single high-technology regional medical center would avoid the wasteful duplication of costly equipment. Such plans are advocated as a natural outgrowth of technical progress: a means of scientific planning for the prudent allocation of resources.

Yet with all the sensible premises embodied in the concept of regional health care, no comprehensive system exists in the United States which even approximates the ideal. The reasons behind this apparent paradox are to be found in the political dimensions of regionalization plans and their anticipated effect on existing organizations and on the distribution of health care. The NCB-Montefiore case suggests that competing medical interests perceive highly rational regionalization plans simply as rationalizations for the expansion and development of medical empires.

Existing hospitals are reluctant to surrender their own development plans, and are unlikely to accept paternalistic governance by a central research and teaching hospital like Montefiore. They worry that regionalization would eliminate hospitals that are judged economically inefficient, regardless of local community needs. Moreover, the location of large medical centers is a sensitive question for community groups concerned with housing, employment, and neighborhood quality. These concerns are rooted in an astonishing degree of mistrust, exacerbated by the competitive pressures within the health industry with its prestige hierarchies based on specialized medicine. They preclude anything but incremental movement in the direction of regionalization.

The reaction to Montefiore's West Bronx Health Planning Study suggests the force of political opposition to regionalization plans. The study proposed that Montefiore-NCB, operating under a unified administration, would back up a regional system as the specialized, high-technology hospital. This proposition was logical since Montefiore, as the dominant medical center in the Bronx, was already well equipped with technical resources; but the response was immediate and hostile. It came from representatives of nearly every health-related agency in the Bronx, including community boards; the Bronx Medical Society; municipal, voluntary, and proprietary hospitals; and city health planning councils. These groups signed a press release calling the plan "a deceptive attempt to justify the questionable existence of the NCB Hospital located on the Montefiore premises" and demanding investigation of "Montefiore's use of taxpayers' money to enhance its own development."

Montefiore's neighboring community claimed that there had been no discussion with communities affected by the plan. The Bronx County Medical Society argued that the regionalization study failed to consider private sources of medical care. Regionalization, the society claimed, would foster discontinuous and impersonal hospital care. A Fordham Hospital organization deplored the "ill-conceived plan," accusing Montefiore of "secrecy and arrogance," of "having no concern for community health needs." Bronx Borough President Abrams rejected the plan as "a unilateral mechanism to justify the location of NCB on the Montefiore campus."

This overwhelmingly negative response, despite the general agreement on the need to develop community hospitals and ambulatory programs, suggests that regionalization fails to work in part because the motives of those people who are most interested are highly suspect. They are at the center of the system; they will benefit the most. The visionary concepts of regionalization plans are blocked not because the concepts themselves are perceived as undesirable, but because they fail to take into account the conflicts inherent in the present structure of competing public and private medical institutions.

Regionalization schemes neglect the difficulties of coordinating this dual system, and the best laid plans to disperse medical care in community hospitals merely seem to augment the power of central institutions. There is no doubt that medical centers will thrive, but there is also no confidence in their commitment to develop adequate community outreach programs that are the essence of a working regional scheme.

Hospital Imperatives

As the imperatives of costly technological development reinforce tendencies toward consolidation, the large medical centers stand only to gain, for they are insulated from effective political challenge. They will doubtless provide their clients with quality medical services, but at enormous public cost.

If changes in the organization of medical care are not to perpetuate the inequities in the health care delivery system, hospitals must cope with some of the most basic problems in a technological society: how to distribute the benefits of technology in a system dominated by private interests; how to consider the second-order impacts of technological development as an integral part of planning and still maintain solvency; and how to reconcile the needs of professionalism with the expectations of participation and accountability fundamental to a democratic society.

Financing Medical Care

MEDICAL CARE IS BIG BUSINESS in the United States. Billions of dollars are spent each year on medical services, with nearly half of each dollar coming from public funds. Medical costs are a significant factor in the economy's inflationary spiral and, until quite recently, were practically unregulated. Most of the money spent on medical care in the United States is spent via *third-party payments* on a fee-for-service basis.[1] As differentiated from *direct* (or *out-of-pocket*) payments, third-party payments are those made through some form of insurance or charitable organization for someone's medical care. Third-party payments have increased steadily over the past thirty years; in 1950, 32 percent of personal health care expenditures were made via third-party payments; in 1965 that figure was up to 48 percent; and by 1974 the ratio of third-party payments had increased to 65 percent (*Medical Care Chart Book*, 1976: 117). Almost all third-party payments are made by public or private insurance. The insurance industry, thus, is central to the financing of medical care services in this country. This section examines the role of insurance in financing medical care and the influence of the insurance industry on the present-day organization of medical services.

The original method of paying for medical services directly or individually, in money or in kind, has today been replaced by payment via insurance. Essentially, insurance is a form of "mass financing" that ensures that medical care providers will be paid and people will be able to obtain or pay for the medical care they need. Insurance involves the regular collection of small amounts of money (premiums) from a large number of people. That money is put into a pool, and when any of the insured people get sick, that pool (the insurance company) pays for their medical services either directly or indirectly by sending the money to provider or patient.

Although most people in the United States are covered by some form of third-party insurance, many millions of Americans are not. In addition, even having an insurance plan does not mean that all of one's medical costs are paid for by that plan.

The United States has both private and public insurance programs. Public insurance programs, including Medicare and Medicaid, are funded primarily by monies collected by federal, state, or local governments in the form of taxes. The nation has two types of private insurance organizations: *nonprofit* tax-exempt Blue Cross and Blue Shield plans and for-profit *commercial* insurance companies.

Blue Cross and Blue Shield emerged out of the Great Depression of the 1930s as mechanisms to assure the payment of medical bills to hospitals (Blue Cross) and physicians (Blue Shield). The Blues (Blue Cross and Blue Shield) were developed as community plans through which people made small "pre-payments" on a regular (generally monthly) basis. If they became sick their hospital bills were paid directly by the insurance plan.

Although there were commercial insurance companies as early as the nineteenth century, it wasn't until after World War II that the commercials really expanded in this country. Blue Cross and Blue Shield originally set the price of insurance premiums by what was called "community rating," giving everybody within a community the chance to purchase insurance at the same price. Commercials, on the other hand, based their price on "experience rating." Experience rating bases the price of insurance premiums on the statistical likelihood of the insured needing medical care. People less likely to need medical care are charged less for premiums than people more likely to need it. Experience rating allowed the commercials to undercut the Blues and capture a large segment of the labor union insurance market in the 1950s and 1960s by offering younger, healthier workers lower rates than could the Blues. In order to compete with the commercials, Blue Cross and Blue Shield eventually abandoned community rating and began using experience rating as well. One unfortunate result of the spread of experience rating has been that those who most need insurance coverage—the old, the sick—are least able to afford or obtain it (Bodenheimer et al., 1974: 583–584).

Medicare and Medicaid were passed by Congress in 1965 as ammendments to the Social Security Act. Medicare pays for the medical care of people over sixty-five years of age (and of other qualified recipients of Social Security) and Medicaid pays for the care of those who qualify as too poor to pay their own medical costs. However, commercial and nonprofit insurance companies act as intermediaries in these government programs. Instead of the providers of medical care being paid directly by public funds, these funds are channeled through the (private) insurance industry. For example, 93 percent of Medicare payments to hospitals and 53 percent of Medicare payments to nursing homes are administered by Blue Cross. The Blues also act as intermediaries in most Medicaid programs (which are state controlled). Public funding via private insurance companies has resulted in enormous increases in the costs of both of these public insurance programs, high profits for the insurance intermediaries and their beneficiaries (e.g., physicians, hospitals), and near exhaustion of available public funds for the continuation of Medicare and Medicaid. In fact, cutbacks in these programs in the form of increased costs and decreased coverage have resulted in the inability of both of these programs to pay for many of the medical needs of those they were intended to help (Bodenheimer et al., 1974; Davis, 1975).

The first article in this section, "Capitalizing on Illness: The Health Insurance Industry," by Thomas Bodenheimer, Steven Cummings, and Elizabeth Harding, presents significant information about the consequences of the various types of insurance plans in the United States. In particular, the authors argue that the profit-making basis of the private insurance sector not only severely limits insurance benefits, but has also contributed to the high cost and maldistribution of medical care services in this country.

In "Blue Cross—What Went Wrong?," Sylvia A. Law traces the historical development of Blue Cross and its close connection with the hospital industry. That history, she concludes, is one of unchecked growth and unnecessary expenditures in which, despite its public status as a tax-exempt corporation, Blue Cross has been able to make millions of dollars without public accountability or control. In large measure this has resulted from the administrative domination of Blue Cross by representatives of the American Hospital Association and other medical care providers. She outlines suggestions for reform within the current Blue Cross structure and raises as well the more fundamental question of to whom Blue Cross should be accountable.

The article by Elliott A. Krause, "The Failure of Medicaid," is a short but succinct analysis of how the "voucher" system of Medicaid failed to correct the "two-class medical system," in which the poor receive different quality care than the non-poor. He argues that the decision to run Medicaid through the fragmented welfare system "doomed it from the start as a strategy for change." Like Medicare (see Davis, 1975), Medicaid only reinforced the inequalities in the medical care system, rather than providing, as was theoretically intended, a system of equal medical care for all, regardless of social class, race, or age.

Notes

1. Fee-for-service is a central feature of the economic organization of medicine in our society. Since medical providers are paid a fee for every service they provide, many critics argue that a fee-for-service system creates a financial incentive to deliver unnecessary services, making medical care more profitable and costly.

References

Bodenheimer, Thomas, Steven Cummings, and Elizabeth Harding. 1974. "Capitalizing on illness: The health insurance industry." International Journal of Health Services 4, 4: 583–598.

Davis, Karen. 1975. "Equal treatment and unequal benefits: The Medicare program." Milbank Memorial Fund Quarterly 53, 4: 449–88.

Medical Care Chart Book. Sixth Edition. 1976. School of Public Health, Department of Medical Care Organization, University of Michigan. Data on third-party payments computed from Chart D-15: 117.

18

Capitalizing on Illness: The Health Insurance Industry

Thomas Bodenheimer, Steven Cummings, and Elizabeth Harding

For an insurance company, illness is not a frightening and uncomfortable experience, it is a golden opportunity. And today, when people are willing to spend a great deal of money to avoid possible financial ruin through illness, payment for health care at the time of illness is gradually being replaced by the mass financing of private health insurance: regular collection of small amounts of money from everyone to pay for the care of people who are sick. The questions then remain: How much money is collected and from whom? What types of institutions receive and pay out the money? How much is paid out and to whom?

It is our contention in this article that private health insurance institutions have taken the progressive concept of mass financing and have used it for their own benefit and that of the health care providers. They are indeed capitalizing on people's illness.

. . . .

What People Get from Health Insurance

About 160 million Americans presently hold private health insurance policies. Many buy the insurance as part of a group such as a company, union, or professional organization, with their premiums often being deducted automatically from their paychecks. About 40 million have the far more expensive individual health insurance, and these people tend to be employees without access to a group, the unemployed, the self-employed and sporadically employed, and the elderly or sick.

Many insurance policies will not insure or will only partially insure the ill. Blue Cross states in one policy, "If at the time your application is reviewed a condition is found which excludes you from enrollment, you may be given an opportunity to join with a waiver for that condition." In other words, if you are sick, you can buy our policy and your medical expenses will be covered, but only if you get a different illness.

The elderly, under experience rating, pay more for health insurance. A Prudential policy offering hospital coverage costs $318.36 per year for a 26-year-old female and $482.36 for a 58-year-old female. Women are generally charged more than men for the same coverage because they use medical care more frequently. And people with chronic illness such as high blood pressure or diabetes must pay more for insurance, if they can obtain insurance at all.

All types of health insurance have deductibles and uncovered or partially covered care. Deductibles refer to the amount the consumer must pay for services before the insurance company will pay. Medicare patients are required to pay the first $84 of their hospital bill and the first $60 a year of their doctors' bills. A major medical plan offered by Connecticut General begins paying for covered services after the consumer has paid a $750 deductible. A similar plan by Prudential has a $400 deductible, and Equitable offers major medical plans with from $500 to $2000 deductibles.

Insurance companies generally make patients pay part of the costs of services. Partially covered care is expressed in two ways: the first is called co-insurance—we pay 80 percent and you pay 20 percent; the second is limited coverage—we pay for 60 days of care, you pay the rest. Insurance salesmen call this "sharing the risk with us." Medicare requires patients to pay $21 per day of their hospital bill for the 61st to 90th hospital day, $10.50 per day for the 21st to 100th nursing home day, and 20 percent of the bill for visits to the doctor. A group Blue Cross plan requires the policyholder to pay 20 percent for almost all services received outside the hospital, and 20 percent of the hospital bill after 70 days; the plan pays only $100 for outpatient psychiatric care. Innumerable additional examples could be listed.

Every insurance policy leaves many medical services uncovered. The best examples of such services are dental care, outpatient psychiatric care, preventive care, and outpatient drugs. Medicare fails to pay for eye and hearing examinations, glasses or hearing aids, routine checkups, and outpatient drugs. A Connecticut General major medical insurance policy pays for no outpatient care at all. A group basic benefit plan offered by Equitable pays for no visits to doctors' offices, no psychiatric care, no dental care, and no outpatient drugs.

About 20 percent of the population has no private surgical and hospital insurance, 28 percent has no in-the-hospital physician insurance, 55 percent has no insurance for physician visits, 48 percent has no insurance for prescribed drugs, and 93 percent has no dental insurance (1).

An average family of four has the following medical needs: yearly physical examinations by a doctor for all members, four visits to the doctor for illness, a yearly dental checkup and needed dental work, prescription drugs for three members, and an eye examination and glasses for one member. The standard insurance policy will pay for none of these services and costs the family about $350 per year.

Private insurance advocates claim that deductibles, uncovered, and partially covered care prevent the consumer from "overusing" health facilities. In reality, however, two studies show that out-of-pocket payments mainly prevent lower-income people from using needed services (2). With the average person covered for only 42 percent of health costs (1), and with these costs rising each year, out-of-pocket expenses even for insured middle-class people can be financially disastrous as the following examples show (3):

- In 1969 the daughter of two federal government employees had a sudden attack of intestinal disease with complications in the liver and lungs. She was hospitalized for 44 days, with a bill of $7571. Even with her parents' comparatively good insurance, the family had to pay $1550 out-of-pocket.
- In 1965 an engineer was stricken with kidney disease. In three months he ran up medical bills of $24,000. His Blue Cross and Blue Shield policies left $9000 unpaid. The patient lost his $3000 in savings, sold his car and some furniture, moved to a small apartment, and went on welfare.

· ·

Commercial Insurance Companies

Unlike the Blues [Blue Cross, Blue Shield], which were put together to assure the payment of bills to the hospitals and doctors, commercial insurance companies sell health insurance purely for the purpose of making a profit. About 1000 companies offer health insurance, with about 115 million people holding some type of commercial policy. In 1972, the commercials took in $14.3 billion in premium income (4). Thus the total volume of commercial insurance is somewhat greater than that of the Blues, though no one commercial company comes close to Blue Cross in size.

The ten largest commercial health insurers are Aetna, Travelers, Metropolitan Life, Prudential, CNA, Equitable, Mutual of Omaha, Connecticut General, John Hancock, and Provident. In 1970, Aetna took in over a billion dollars in health premiums (5).

Most of the top health insurance companies are also the biggest life insurers. These giants represent an enormous concentration of wealth and political power in America. Prudential and Metropolitan Life, the two largest, each have $30 billion in assets, making them far bigger than General Motors, Standard Oil of New Jersey, and ITT, and the equals of Bank of America and Chase Manhattan Bank. In 1970, supposedly a bad year for health insurance, the life insurance business boomed. In that year Prudential and Metropolitan Life received premium income (life, accident, health, and other policies) of almost $4 billion each and net income from investments of $1.4 billion each (5).

The major insurance companies are closely tied to the largest U.S. banks and manufacturing corporations through enormous financial empires. The Rockefeller family interests control or heavily influence the Metropolitan Life and Equitable insurance companies, Chase Manhattan Bank, Standard Oil, Mobil Oil, IBM, and numerous other corporations. The Morgan empire (the legacy of J. P. Morgan) includes the Prudential Insurance Company, the Bankers Trust and Morgan Guarantee Trust banks, General Electric, and U.S. Steel. Of 28 directors of Metropolitan Life, 23 sit on the boards of banking institutions, particularly Chase Manhattan. Eighteen of Prudential's 29 directors sit on bank boards. Half of Equitable's directors are on bank boards with an especially close relation with Chase Manhattan (6).

These facts are given in order to make the point that commercial health insurance policy is ultimately set by very rich and influential people in U.S. society. The money that comes into the hands of these companies, constituting one-half of the net savings of individuals in America (7), is used in several ways: (a) to make huge loans ($185 million daily) to corporations, thus supplying much of the money needed for corporate expansion; (b) to buy large blocks of stock in corporations so that the insurance company can effectively control the corporations; (c) to finance real estate developments and urban high-rise buildings; and (d) to influence politicians through campaign contributions and other favors (for example, W. Clement Stone, chairman of Combined Insurance, the thirteenth largest health insurer, gave $1 million to Richard Nixon's 1968 campaign, another million to the 1972 campaign, and received a preferential ruling from the Price Commission in 1971 to raise insurance rates) (8).

Commerical insurance companies have a different relationship with doctors and hospitals than do the Blues. Whereas the Blues make contracts with hospitals and doctors regarding how much they will pay, a commercial company contracts with the patient and does not deal with the providers directly. Thus patients often have to fight to collect the money from their insurance company.

Commercial companies formerly paid the patient only a stipulated sum of money for each service, for example, $50 per hospital day despite the fact that the daily charge might be $80. Many individual policies are still written this way. One plan advertized in a San Francisco newspaper pays $100 per week ($14.28 per day) for hospital care while hospital rates are around $100 per day. The advertisement contained the sentence: "When hospital emergency strikes, you can say 'Thank Heaven, we didn't have to borrow a cent.' "

However, commercial group plans have generally changed due to competition among themselves and with the Blues. Many of these plans now pay the full daily hospital rate, though with the usual deductibles, coinsurance, and limitations. Commercials thus have become concerned with the rapid rise in hospital charges since they too must pay out more when the rates go up.

In 1972, commercial companies collected $14.3 billion in insurance premiums and paid out $10.6 billion in benefit payments (4). On the average, group policies pay out in benefits 96 percent of the premiums collected, whereas individual policies pay out only 51 percent. Clearly, individual plans pay far fewer benefits and thus are of less value to the buyer than are group plans (9). Different companies pay out higher or lower percentages of their premium income depending on whether they have more or less group coverage. In 1970, Aetna and Travelers paid out 90 percent of their premium income; these companies overwhelmingly sell group insurance. Metropolitan Life and Prudential paid out around 85 percent of premiums, whereas Mutual of Omaha paid only 73 percent and Combined Insurance (run by former President Nixon's friend W. Clement Stone) paid out only 43 percent of its largely individual premiums (5).

In light of the profit orientation of insurance companies, it may come as a surprise that in 1970, the commercial insurance industry spent $600 million more in benefits and administrative costs than it collected in premiums. Aetna, the largest commercial insurer, collected $1 billion in 1970 premiums, paid out $984 million in benefits, spent millions more in administration, and consequently lost $13 million on its health insurance. In 1969 Aetna lost $28 million on health insurance; in 1968, $16 million; and in 1967 it gained $6 million. In 1970 Travelers lost $41 million in health insurance; Metropolitan Life lost $18 million; Connecticut General lost $37 million; and Combined Insurance gained $16 million (5). By 1972, however, the companies as a whole were doing better, as we will describe later.

Are health insurance companies really losing money? The answer is no. First, commercial health insurance is closely linked to life and other forms of insurance. A large amount of group commercial insurance (perhaps $2–3 billion a year) is bought by companies who pay for workmen's compensation, disability, life, accident, and health insurance for their employees. These companies generally study the policies of several insurers and buy all the insurance in a package from one insurance company. Thus, an insurance company that makes a good offer on health insurance will sell more of the highly profitable life insurance, and the apparent health insurance losses are actually bringing in greater profits in other types of insurance.

Secondly, the health insurance losses do not take investment income into account. When Aetna collects $1 billion in health insurance premiums, it does not pay this money out in benefits right away. The money is available for investment, which produces a profitable return. Aetna's total investment income in 1970 was $344 million (5). Since 55 percent of Aetna's premiums are from health insurance, one can assume that Aetna earned $190 million in investments from its health business. Thus the $13 million in "losses" is erased, and Aetna actually profited immensely from its health insurance.

What's Wrong with Private Health Insurance?

Private health insurance does great harm to the U.S. health care system for a number of reasons:

- The insurance companies siphon off billions of dollars of people's money for health care. In 1972, the insurance industry collected $25.7 billion in health premiums and paid out $21 billion in benefits (12, pp. 35, 45). Fully $4.7 billion in one year was wasted in administrative costs, high executive salaries, competitive advertizing, sales promotion, and profits. A publicly financed health system based on salaries and budgeting rather than fee-for-service and individual claims could save a large portion of this sum.
- Twenty-five million people (12 percent of the population) are entirely without private insurance, Medicare, or Medicaid, and unable to afford needed health care (10). Many more have grossly inadequate insurance, with the result that inability to meet medical expenses is the number one cause of personal bankruptcy in the country (11).
- Insurance companies, especially the Blues, have helped to keep the cost of medical care high and rising. The Blues, in both private and public programs, have tended to pay anything hospitals and doctors asked for. Blue Cross provides over 50 percent of hospital income, so that it does have the power to say "no" to rising hospital rates. However, although a tendency toward more cost-consciousness is beginning, by and large no major changes have occurred, and those changes that have taken place tend to make care less accessible to consumers.
- Insurance companies have helped to grossly distort medical practice, with expensive and dangerous effects. The best known distortion is the push of health insurance toward hospitalization. Many more people have hospital insurance than insurance for ambulatory care. Therefore, patients are hospitalized for minor diagnostic tests and treatment which could be done outside the hospital. It is estimated that 30 percent of days spent in the hospital are unnecessary (12). A more significant distortion has been the push toward surgery. Many more people have surgical insurance than insurance for nonsurgical physician services. Thus the tendency of surgeons to over-operate is reinforced by the insurance structure. Two million unnecessary operations are performed in the U.S. each year, resulting in at least 10,000 needless deaths (13, 14).

References

1. Mueller, M. S. Private health insurance in 1971: Health care services, enrollment, and finances. *Social Security Bulletin* 36(2): 3–22, 1973.
2. Of paying and queuing. *Notes on Health Politics* 1: 1–2, September 1, 1973.
3. Hoyt, E. *Your Health Insurance: A Story of Failure.* The John Day Company, New York, 1970.
4. *Source Book of Health Insurance Data,* pp. 36, 43. Health Insurance Institute, New York, 1973–1974.
5. *Best's Insurance Reports, Life-Health, 1971.* A. M. Best Company, Morristown, N.J., 1971.
6. Menshikov, S. *Millionaires and Managers.* Progress Publishers, Moscow, 1969.
7. Perlo, V. *The Empire of High Finance.* International Publishers, New York, 1957.
8. Rich Nixon contributor: Price favoritism denied. *San Francisco Chronicle,* p. 6, October 6, 1972.
9. *Basic Facts on the Health Industry.* House Committee on Ways and Means, June 1971.
10. Health care message from the President of the United States. *Congressional Record* 120: H540, February 6, 1974.
11. Americans who lack insurance coverage. *San Francisco Sunday Examiner and Chronicle,* p. A22, May 6, 1973.
12. Testimony of Dr. Amos Johnson, past president of the American Association of General Practice, before the Senate Antitrust and Monopoly Subcommittee, February 24, 1970.
13. A protest on surgery deaths. *San Francisco Chronicle,* p. 10. December 17, 1971.
14. Unneeded surgeries put at 2 million a year. *Washington Post,* p. 1, July 18, 1972.

19

Blue Cross—What Went Wrong?

Sylvia A. Law

It is widely acknowledged that the American health care crisis is primarily one of organization, administration, and accountability. Blue Cross is at the heart of the administration of the present medical care delivery system.[1] Over $22 billion a year, about one-third of the national health care dollar, are spent in hospitals.[2] Blue Cross provides about half of hospital revenues, administering over $11 billion in 1970. Public funds comprised over half of Blue Cross payments to hospitals—$4.9 billion under Medicare, $1.2 billion under Medicaid, and $545 million under other federally financed programs.[3]

Blue Cross is a complex animal, impossible to characterize in a few words. For example, it may be seen as the financing arm of American hospitals, with a primary obligation to provide them, on an equitable basis, with a stable source of income to be utilized as they judge necessary. If this is regarded as its primary role, then Blue Cross's responsibilities to subscribers and to the public are to offer hospital insurance benefits at competitive rates, to maintain a financially sound rate structure, and to pay hospitals promptly for services provided to subscribers. Alternatively, Blue Cross may be seen as a quasi-public agency with primary responsibility to the public and to its subscribers. If this is its primary role, then its obligations are to offer benefits that will enable subscribers to obtain quality health care services economically, to monitor the quality of care provided subscribers in participating hospitals, to utilize the collective power of its payments to encourage hospitals to establish programs that will best meet subscribers' health needs, and to refuse to reimburse hospitals for charges that are excessive or do not meet subscribers' needs. Finally, with respect to the public funds it administers, Blue Cross may legitimately be viewed as an agent of the government, with an obligation to carry out the policies of Congress and of the administrative agencies responsible for publicly financed medical programs. Confusion as to the proper role of Blue Cross is common and pervades the organization itself, the state regulatory agencies, Congress, and the Department of Health, Education and Welfare.

In a nutshell . . . Blue Cross is most accurately characterized today as the financing arm of American hospitals. . . .

A Unique American Institution

Blue Cross is the child of the Depression and the American Hospital Association. The period from 1875 to 1915 was one of major development of medical institutions in this country, and by 1920 the now familiar pattern of community voluntary hospitals and local autonomy in health matters was established.[4] During the 1920s there was growing recognition of the need for some mechanism by which middle income people could finance extraordinary costs of hospitalization. Hospital insurance was virtually nonexistent.[5] In October 1927, the president of the American Hospital Association described the organization's "ultimate objective" as

> providing hospitalization for the great bulk of people of moderate means . . . [who are] confronted with the necessity of amassing a debt or the alternative of casting aside all pride and accepting the provisions that are intended for the poor . . . Let us keep in mind the *raison d'être* of our existence, vis.: the provision of hospitalization for the patient of moderate means, consisting of 80 percent of the entire population. The wise solution of this great problem will inscribe the name of the American Hospital Association in the hearts of the people for all time.[6]

The solution most often proposed then was public education; people should be taught to save for large medical expenses.[7] The Depression, however, provided the impetus for a movement away from public education toward the development of the comprehensive Blue Cross network. Hospitals were hard hit by the Depression. In one year, from 1929 to 1930, the average hospital receipts per patient fell from $236.12 to $59.26. Average percent of occupancy fell from 71.28 percent to 64.12 percent. Average deficits as a percentage of disbursements rose from 15.2 percent to 20.6 percent.[8] The hospitals had an immediate interest in developing a stable source of payment for services and also had the technical and financial resources to create such a program. Of 39 Blue Cross plans established in the early 1930s, 22 obtained all of their initial funds from hospitals, and five were partially financed by hospitals.[9]

There was by that time a variety of small, voluntary plans for the prepayment of medical expenses, including the predictable expenses incident to childbirth.[10] The largest of these plans, and the one generally credited as the progenitor of Blue Cross, was initiated in 1929 by Dr. Justin Ford Kimball in Dallas, Texas. As executive vice president of Baylor University, Dr. Kimball found the unpaid bills of many local school-teachers among the accounts receivable of the university's medical facilities. In order to assure payment to the university, he enrolled 1,250 teachers in a program to prepay fifty cents a month for 21 days of semi-private hospitalization at the Baylor University Hospital.[11]

Under the Baylor plan and other early programs, subscribers could receive services only at the hospital that had organized the prepayment program. Most state insurance commissioners regarded these single hospital programs as group contracts for the sale of services by the hospitals to subscribing members and hence not subject to legal requirements applicable to insurance companies.[12] However, in some states insurance officials ruled that single hospital prepayment plans presented serious limitations to individuals and physicians by forcing them to select a hospital at the time of enrollment rather than at the time of illness. Consequently, during 1932 and 1933 "free choice" plans that covered care at a number of hospitals were organized in several cities. While the applicability of insurance laws to single hospital prepayment plans was an open question, the free choice plans were more clearly a form of insurance. The legal issue came sharply into focus when the United Hospital Fund of New York and the Cleveland Hospital Council were told that they would have to establish either a mutual or stock insurance company before making prepaid care available to the public.[13]

In response to this problem, the American Hospital Association and local hospital organizations sought state legislation to create a special class of nonprofit corporation and of hospital insurance. In 1932, Dr. C. Rufus Rorem, associate director of the Julius Rosenwald Fund, studied the existing group hospital prepayment programs. He was also retained by the AHA to promote hospital prepayment and to seek the necessary enabling legislation. The following year the AHA promulgated seven "standards which should characterize group hospitalization plans." The standards were: (1) emphasis on public welfare, (2) limitation to hospital services, (3) freedom of choice of hospital and physician by subscriber, (4) nonprofit sponsorship, (5) compliance with legal requirements, (6) economic soundness, and (7) dignified and ethical administration.[14] In 1936, the AHA obtained a grant from the Rosenwald Fund to finance a special Committee on Hospital Service, and Dr. Rorem became its first executive director. In 1938 the committee established fourteen standards for nonprofit hospital care plans, including, for the first time, the requirement that the plan be approved by the AHA.[15]

The special enabling legislation sought by the AHA conferred the following advantages and privileges on the proposed hospital service corporations: exemption from the general insurance laws of the state; status as a charitable and benevolent organization; exemption from the obligation of maintaining the reserves required of commercial insurers; and tax exemption. The major justification offered in support of the special enabling legislation was the promise of service to the community, and particularly to low income families.[16] The AHA House of Delegates, in a 1939 resolution supporting the development of hospital service plans, cited the need for a program that would provide hospitalization "among the low income groups" and noted that such plans "would reduce the need for taxation and philanthropy."[17] Dr. Rorem explained:

> Hospital service plans are unique, historically and geographically. . . . They deal with a service which has long been recognized as a community responsibility. *Hospital care must be provided for all persons regardless of their ability to pay.* Such a responsibility cannot and should not be assumed by a private insurance company, the first concern of which should be the financial interests of the policyholders and stockholders . . . Government controlled hospitalization or health insurance is a second alternative to the nonprofit hospital service plan. . . . *But low-cost hospital service plans may reach many persons employed at low incomes who would otherwise require the aid of philanthropy or taxation.*[18] (Emphasis added.)

In 1934 the first hospital service plan enabling act was adopted by the New York state legislature.[19] With the support of the AHA, the bill had been promoted by the New York United Hospital Fund—a coalition of civic leaders, hospital administrators, hospital trustees, and physicians.[20] The New York act served as a model for other states, and by 1945 similar laws had been adopted in 35 states.[21] Currently 48 states have special enabling legislation for hospital service organizations,[22] and in 20 states such corporations are exempt from taxation.[23] Individual Blue Cross plans and the Blue Cross Association (BCA), the national trade association, are also exempt from the payment of federal taxes.[24]

. . . .

From the 1930s on, the American Hospital Association sought to promote and control the development of monopolistic Blue Cross organizations. Preferred corporate status and tax treatment were important in the growth of Blue Cross and these publicly conferred advantages were intensified by the private policy and control of the AHA. The enabling acts do not refer to Blue Cross by name but rather allow the establishment of "hospital service corporations." Although theoretically there could be several competing hospital service corporations in any one area, the enabling acts typically require that the corporation establish cooperative agreements with the majority of hospitals in the area served. Furthermore, AHA policy has required that, in order to use the Blue Cross emblem, a hospital service corporation must establish agreements with 75 percent of the area hospital,[25] and the AHA generally authorized use of the emblem by only one hospital service corporation in any given area.[26] Thus, historically, the combination of public enabling legislation and the private power of the AHA has assured that there is only one Blue Cross organization in any given area and that it is, to some degree, controlled by the hospitals.

By 1938, 1.4 million people in the United States had enrolled in 38 Blue Cross plans. Private insurance companies provided hospital insurance to only 1 million people. During the forties Blue Cross expanded at a rapid pace; the private health insurance industry also grew, but more slowly. Several factors contributed to the rapid growth of Blue Cross: it began writing contracts with employers and contracts having nationwide coverage; health insurance increasingly became a matter for collective bargaining, with labor supporting Blue Cross; and employment and wages mushroomed during World War II.[27] In 1945 Blue Cross claimed 61 percent of the hospital insurance market, compared with the insurance companies' 33 percent. But in 1951, for the first time, the number of people with private commerical hospital insurance (40.0 million) surpassed the number enrolled in Blue Cross plans (37.4 million),[28] and throughout the fifties and sixties Blue Cross was unsuccessful in competing with the commercial companies. At the end of 1969 Blue Cross had an enrollment of 67.2 million, or 37 percent of the civilian population under 65, while the commercial insurance companies provided hospital coverage to 100 million people, or 57 percent of the civilian population under 65.[29] The passage of Medicare and Medicaid legislation in 1965, however, gave Blue Cross a boost that reestablished its dominance in terms of hospital payments as a whole.

Two major characteristics have distinguished Blue Cross from most commercial insurance companies: payment of service benefits to hospitals rather than cash benefits to the individual insured; and community rating, that is, the provision of benefits to all members of the community at the same rate, rather than higher rates to high risk groups.

The Blue Cross commitment to the payment of service benefits to hospitals means, simply, that while commercial insurers generally pay the individual a fixed dollar amount per day or period of hospitalization, and the individual bears primary responsibility for the payment of the hospital bill, Blue Cross gives the subscriber the assurance it will settle his bill with the hospital, with the subscriber bearing responsibility only for the coinsurance, or deductible, specified in the policy. The original American Hospital Association standards for the approval of hospital service plans required that, "Benefits in member hospitals should be expressed in 'service contracts,' which describe specifically the types and amounts of hospital services to which the subscribers are entitled."[30] Over the years, however, as a result of competitive pressures, an increasing number of Blue Cross plans have offered subscribers indemnity rather than service contracts.[31]

The second major distinction between Blue Cross and commercial insurers was the Blue Cross promise of service to the community. Initially all Blue Cross plans offered hospital insurance to all members of the community at uniform rates,[32] one rate for individuals and one rate for families, while commercial companies offered more favorable rates to those groups and individuals who were actuarially less likely to make claims.[33] Since low income families and the aged tend to utilize hospital services more than the general population, these groups are helped by community rating.[34] During World War II, as organized labor began to press for more adequate health benefits and other insurance companies began to compete for this growing business, Blue Cross, after a decade of internal struggle, abandoned its commitment to community rating.[35] Today most Blue Cross plans offer group experience-rated contracts, particularly for larger group policies, as well as community-rated policies for those individuals who are not able to obtain a group policy through their work or otherwise.[36]

The adoption of experience rating was probably inevitable if Blue Cross was to compete successfully with the commercial insurers for the business of the low risk customer.[37] The alternatives were to persuade low risk groups that Blue Cross was so useful as an organization serving the entire community that low risk customers should subsidize the costs of the higher risk groups or to offer a service so excellent that high risk groups could be subsidized without fatal competitive disadvantage.[38] Either of these alternatives would have been very difficult. Since a return to strict community rating is unlikely, the current major issue is whether Blue Cross deserves its favored status under state and federal law.

. . . .

Local Plans, the Blue Cross Association and the American Hospital Association

Membership in the national Blue Cross organization is critical to a local Blue Cross plan. The advantages of membership include: use of the official Blue Cross emblem and seal; the right to exclusive provision of Blue Cross benefits within a territorial area; the national advertising, public relations, and lobbying; the use of information gathering, processing, and dissemination apparatus; and mechanisms for coordination of national accounts and for the transfer and acceptance of subscribers who move from one plan's territory to another's. With the advent of Medicare, membership in the national organization became even more valuable. The national Blue Cross Association (BCA) contracted with the Social Security Administration for the administration of the Medicare program, and the BCA now serves as protector and interpreter for local plans vis-à-vis the federal government.

The name "Blue Cross" and the Blue Cross insignia were owned by the

American Hospital Association until 1972.[39] The relationship between the AHA and Blue Cross plans has been close throughout Blue Cross history, as we have seen. In 1936, as part of its effort to promote the establishment of prepaid hospitalization plans, the AHA created a Committee on Hospital Services, which in 1946 became the Blue Cross Commission of the AHA.[40] Until 1957, the commission performed the national coordinating function among Blue Cross plans. In 1960, most of the commission's functions were transferred to the Blue Cross Association, a nonprofit Illinois corporation. The BCA and AHA maintained close coordination through interlocking directorates, with the AHA designating three members on the BCA board and BCA designating two members on the AHA board. Other functions, including the administration of the approval program for use of the Blue Cross insignia, were retained by the AHA. In 1971, the AHA and Blue Cross agreed in principle that the ownership of the Blue Cross name and insignia should be transferred to the BCA, and this transfer became effective on June 30, 1972.[41] The two groups also agreed to eliminate their interlocking directorates and substitute a joint committee to facilitate communication between them.[42] AHA officials stated that the change was made as a "response to changing public attitudes" and emphasized that it did not represent a "cooling off" in the close relationships between Blue Cross and the AHA.[43]

. . . .

In 1971, the Subcommittee on Antitrust and Monopoly of the Senate Committee on the Judiciary heard extensive testimony on the operation of BCA review of local plan performance, with particular reference to the Richmond, Virginia, plan. The hearings revealed that BCA's claim of national review of local plans is predominantly public relations puffing. Testimony showed that throughout the late sixties the administrative costs of the Virginia plan were among the highest of any Blue Cross plan in the nation.[44] Subsequent investigations prompted by public and congressional concern revealed gross mismanagement. For example, the plan had 119 rented automobiles and could not account for their use.[45] It paid for staff memberships in various country clubs and owned stock in a country club.[46] Two years after Medicare began, the plan moved into an $8 million office building. One million dollars was spent to decorate and furnish the building, and most of the purchases were made, without competitive bidding, from a firm whose sales manager was chairman of the Building Committee of the Blue Cross board.[47] The plan paid $198,000 to a profit-making data processing organization but received no identifiable service. The assistant general manager of the plan was also a member of the board of the data processing organization, but he never revealed this relationship, because he believed that there was no conflict of interest.[48]

In October 1968, while these policies were in effect, the Richmond plan was given a "Total Plan Review" by the BCA. This review was described as

> a review and analysis of the overall corporate structure of the plan, its organization, objectives, future plans and management controls, especially as they related to the effectiveness of the administrative system. Particular emphasis was given to the support function of data processing and financial activities.[49]

The final report, while noting low productivity and high cost per claim, was laudatory.

> The team was particularly impressed with the overall corporate structure and organization of the plan . . . The executive management group of the Richmond plan displays a progressive and confident attitude. . . . There is an atmosphere which is conducive to innovation and change aimed at improvement. . . .
> It was favorably noted that a good start has been made toward greater refinement of the budget, cost accounting, etc. in the financial area. The Richmond plan has made great strides towards attracting and retaining qualified personnel. This is true with respect to physical surroundings, progressive atmosphere, etc.[50]

Despite this clean bill of health, by early 1970 public attention prompted the BCA to reexamine the plan. Internal BCA memos subpoenaed by the Senate committee revealed that the 1970 investigation was primarily concerned with public appearances. One national official recommended that a BCA team be sent in "in the interest of preserving the National reputation as opposed to assisting the Plan." Another BCA offical visiting Richmond concluded that BCA should

> refrain from moving in since we know the bad news that might erupt. . . . Richmond could blow up. It is a real "can of worms." But we know enough bad things without necessarily sending in a team to get more information. However, I also recognize that the National Associations must preserve their dignity and be prepared to answer questions. . . . Nevertheless, this is another case of "locking the barn door after the horse has departed.[51]

It seems that local malfeasance is a subject for national concern only when it approaches the level of scandal or illegality. Even then BCA efforts are directed first toward preventing adverse publicity, then toward correcting the problems.

. . . .

While corporate waste through high administrative costs is significant, it is not the central issue in evaluating Blue Cross performance. In Richmond, administrative costs represented only 5.4 percent of the earned subscriber income, the balance being payments to hospitals.[52] The key issue of public concern should be what Blue Cross does to ensure that hospital costs are reasonable. Not surprisingly, the evidence was that the Richmond plan did not pursue any form of hospital cost control. The executive director of the plan was asked, "What if your audit [of hospital books] indicated clearly wasteful practices? What do you do?" He responded, "Well, Mr. Chairman, I am not aware of our audits ever uncovering wasteful charges, and I really wouldn't know what we would do if we ran into them."[53]

Because of the difficulty in obtaining information about the internal operations of Blue Cross, it is not possible to know whether the Richmond operation is typical. Probably it is not.[54] However, such mismanagement is not unique. For example, the General Accounting Office and a subcommittee of the House Committee on Government Operations found that during 1966–67, Washington, D.C., Blue Cross kept an average of more than $10 million in federal funds in noninterest-bearing accounts in Washington banks. Larger amounts, estimated in excess of $15 million, were kept in noninterest-bearing accounts from 1961–1965.[55] Several members of the Blue Cross board, including the treasurer, were officers and board members of the banks in which the monies were deposited.[56] From 1963 until 1971 Illinois Blue Cross had between $7 and $15 million deposited in noninterest-bearing accounts in a bank at which the chairman of the board served as senior vice president and an additional $2 million in noninterest-bearing accounts in a second bank, one of the officers of which was also on the Blue Cross board.[57]

Periodic investigations by congressional committees are obviously an ineffective means to discover whether plans operate efficiently or to encourage such operation. As the facts concerning the mismanagement of the Richmond plan unfolded, the Subcommittee on Antitrust and Monopoly grappled to find some mechanism of public accountability—some means by which the interests of the public and of subscribers could be protected. Senator Hart asked, "There isn't any outside discipline, either the Virginia Corporation Commission or legislative body or the National Blue Cross, that could do other than sort of wonder. Nobody could correct, is that right, the absent internal discipline?" The chief executive officer responded, "Mr. Chairman, I would say you are absolutely right, but that responsibility rests purely on the shoulders of the boards of directors. . . . The moment they found the level of spending which they couldn't quite stand, they acted immediately."[58]

It is extraordinarily difficult to obtain concrete information about Blue Cross operations. The BCA and published materials do not provide even basic information on the practices of various plans with respect to reimbursement of hospitals, claims review, determination of subscriber rates, governance, or state and federal regulation. Because of the lack of public information and the importance of concrete data on which to base an analysis and evaluation of Blue Cross, the author, on January 20, 1972, distributed a twelve-page questionnaire, covering the subjects listed above, to each Blue Cross plan. On February 1, 1972, D. Eugene Sibery, executive vice president of the BCA, wrote that the national association would be responding to the questionnaire on behalf of the local plans. Its response to most questions was that information was unavailable.[59] The questionnaire had originally been directed to the local plans precisely because the author was unable to obtain the information sought from the BCA and understood that the BCA did not have the data. Local plans may have been reluctant to provide information even if the BCA had not intervened.[60] BCA intervention assured the unavailability of the information.

Blue Cross Boards of Directors

The local Blue Cross board has the primary—and often the sole—responsibility for determining policy and assuring accountability within the plan. For example, the local board determines whether the plan shall offer community rates to all subscribers or experience rates based on the particular utilization patterns of groups of subscribers. It decides whether the plan shall offer benefits only for inpatient hospital services or provide more comprehensive benefits, including coverage for less expensive forms of care. It determines whether the plan shall pay hospitals whatever they ask or use the economic power of payments to force cost control and otherwise shape local hospital planning. It is responsible for establishing procedures for subscriber complaints and for determining the governing structure of the organization.

In the 1960s, the assertion that Blue Cross boards were publicly responsive was a major selling point in persuading Congress to give Blue Cross a key role in the Medicare program.[61] Although citizen control of local Blue Cross policy has always been emphasized in Blue Cross rhetoric, it is only within the past few years that there has been serious scrutiny of the actual composition of Blue Cross boards. Two major issues have been raised. First, what role, if any, should providers of service have on the board? Second, do the standards and procedures for the selection of public members of the board adequately ensure that they will represent public and subscriber interests?

Hospital representatives currently dominate Blue Cross boards. The AHA Standards for Approval, now taken over by the BCA, require that at least one-third of the board members represent the contracting hospitals, and some enabling acts require hospital representatives on the board.[62] In 1970, according to BCA figures, 56 percent of the members of local boards were health care providers, 42 percent representing hospitals and 14 percent representing the medical profession.[63]

A case can be made that hospital representatives have no proper role on

Blue Cross boards. Because the federal and state governments have delegated to Blue Cross the public functions of: (1) paying for publicly financed hospital care; (2) determining the reasonableness of hospital costs; and (3) using payment processes to encourage rational planning and utilization patterns, the place of provider representatives on Blue Cross boards can certainly be questioned. For example, the chairman of the Massachusetts Rate Setting Commission and special counsel for health affairs commented:

> If we regard Blue Cross as having a responsibility to "regulate" hospital costs—
> and I most certainly do—then we can look upon this arrangement as those who
> are regulated actually being the regulators of themselves. The counterbalancing
> and resolution of discrete interests which should be the heart of any regulatory
> process is lacking.[64]

. . . .

The criticism of provider members on Blue Cross boards is not primarily that they are self-dealing or necessarily incapable of avoiding conflicts of interest.[65] Rather, the problem is that provider representatives are primarily responsible to hospitals rather than to subscribers or the public. It is unrealistic to expect that, as Blue Cross board members, hospital representatives will challenge hospital policies on cost control, area planning, or reorientation of services, when these are policies they have developed. Hospital representatives will seek to maintain the autonomy of the hospital.[66]

. . . .

As presently constituted, even the public board members often do not protect or reflect subscriber interests. Although in 1970, 44 percent of the members of local plan boards were "public" representatives, examination reveals that under present structures public representatives are an elite group with little resemblance to subscribers. In most Blue Cross plans public representatives are selected by the incumbent board.[67] In twenty-one plans they are selected by the hospital representatives.[68] In Washington, D.C., the public representatives are appointed by the commissioner of the district. Subscribers elect public representatives in only eight plans, including the Philadelphia plan.[69]

Compared to other plans the Philadelphia board has democratic selection procedures. Subscribers have always been able to vote for a small minority of board members. However, in 1970 and 1971 the plan bylaws were amended to allow subscribers to vote for all but four of the 34 board members, with nominations being made by the incumbent board or by petition with 300 subscriber signatures. In 1971 and 1972 subscribers nominated candidates to run against the nominees of the board. Through advertisements in local newspapers and through contacts with large organizations holding group contracts, the plan management solicited proxy votes for the board's candidates. In both years the plan refused subscriber requests to publish a ballot that would allow subscribers to cast votes for the insurgent candidates and to publish information about the position of various candidates on questions of plan policy. In 1971, the subscriber candidates received over 1,000 votes, but the management slate won with about 3,000 votes. In 1972, the subscriber candidates received over 4,000 votes, but management had increased its effort and obtained 16,000 proxy votes.[70] During the intervening year there had been substantial adverse publicity about Blue Cross, as Insurance Commissioner Herbert Denenberg criticized the plan for failure to hold down hospital costs. It is difficult to believe that the fivefold jump in votes for the incumbent board reflected a vote of confidence or popularity. The number of votes obtained by the management appears to reflect the amount of management resources devoted to the collection of proxies rather than subscriber endorsement of management policy and competence. The subscriber candidates had no financial support but depended on volunteer efforts of those concerned about Blue Cross policy. There are no limitations on the resources which the plan can devote to insuring the election of a board that will support current policies and management.[71]

The Philadelphia plan directors are not representative of the plan's subscribers. Twelve of the 34 directors are directors of banking and financial institutions. Two sit on the boards of major real estate companies, one is the president of a company with major interests in hospital supply, and others are business executives.[72] Two directors represent organized labor. The typical board member is white, male, over 40, and wealthy; departures from this norm are few. The Philadelphia board does not even reflect the broad range of the city's hospitals; in 1970 five of the city's most influential hospitals had more than one representative on the board.[73]

The pattern in Philadelphia is typical of the rest of the country. Blue Cross Association data show that the 824 members of local plan boards designated as public and consumer representatives include: 311 business executives, 116 physicians and surgeons, 90 retired people, 73 bankers, 54 lawyers, 39 labor leaders, 34 university and school officials, 23 investment advisers, 17 religious leaders, 8 real estate men, and 59 people in a variety of other positions.[74] Of these public representatives, only 18 are women.

Labor representatives on Blue Cross boards are often cited as the representatives of ordinary subscribers. There is no evidence that they have played such a role.[75] Further examination of labor members of Blue Cross boards is needed. One hypothesis is that labor representatives have been content to obtain relatively favorable rate treatment for their own members.[76] Blue Cross critics charge that community-rated subscribers, who pay substantially higher rates, subsidize the organized experience-rated subscribers.[77] No one would be the wiser if a plan were to offer favorable group rates based not on experience but on political influence, representation on the plan board, or other extraneous factors. Only Blue Cross has the information needed to determine whether such discriminatory rate setting exists. Insurance commissioners do not obtain sufficient information to know whether experience rates are justified on the basis of actual experience and administrative savings resulting from the group contract; certainly community-rated subscribers do not have access to such information.[78] Aggressive scrutiny of Blue Cross policies and pursuit of institutional reform would require enormous effort and tenacity and could quickly put labor representatives into direct conflict with plan administration and board members from the hospitals. Given that labor representatives constitute such a small minority on a Blue Cross board and given that they are accountable to a constituency that is probably not demanding reforms in the Blue Cross structure, it would not be surprising to find labor members playing a quiet role in Blue Cross governance.[79]

Within the present Blue Cross board structures, there are some reforms that can and should be instituted. It would be a fairly simple matter for the BCA, state insurance departments, or the federal government as administrator of Medicare to gather and publicize information on the affiliations of Blue Cross directors and on the major organizations with which the plan contracts and banks. Simply gathering such information and making it public would do much to curb the more flagrant abuses of Blue Cross power.

The more fundamental question of who governs Blue Cross, and to whom it should be accountable, requires a more comprehensive solution. It is an illusion to believe that effective public control of an institution as complex and influential as Blue Cross could be achieved easily or with minor reforms. . . .

References

1. See Herman M. and Anne R. Somers, "Private Health Insurance: Problems, Pressures, and Prospects," 46 *Calif. L. Rev.* 508, 555–57 (1958). See also L. Barrett, "Retreat From Idealism: Blue Cross," *The Nation*, Jan. 9, 1960, pp. 26–32; E. T. Chase, "Can Blue Cross Survive Its Own Success?" 21 *The Reporter* 18–19 (Oct. 29, 1959).
2. *Basic Facts on the Health Industry,* Report by the Staff of the House Committee on Ways and Means, 92nd. Cong., 1st. Sess., 1971, pp. 8 and 42.
3. Figures for Medicare and other federal programs are from SSA, BHI, *Quarterly Report to Providers* (1970). Medicaid figures are from internal data, Research and Development Dept., Blue Cross Association.
4. Dr. Odin W. Anderson, quoted in F. R. Hedinger, *The Social Role of Blue*

Cross as a Device for Financing the Costs of Hospital Care, Health Care Research Series, No. 2, Iowa, p. 3 (1966). Hereinafter cited as Hedinger.

5. For a description of pre-Blue Cross hospital insurance, see T. J. Richardson, "The Origin and Development of Group Hospitalization in the United States, 1890–1940," 20 *University of Missouri Studies,* No. 3, pp. 15–18 (1945). See also Hedinger, supra n. 4, at pp. 6–9; Robert Eilers, *Regulation of Blue Cross and Blue Shield Plans,* Huebner Foundation Studies (Homewood, Ill.: Irwin, 1963): 8–9.

6. R. G. Brodrick, M.D., Presidential Address, *Bulletin of the American Hospital Association,* October, 1927, pp. 25–27.

7. "Economic preparedness of the individual in connection with the use of the modern hospital is largely a matter of public education and training . . . Practicable and easy plans might well be formulated to encourage use of the item 'sickness' in the family budget as actively as the items 'Insurance' and even 'Clothes' are budgeted." Asa S. Bacon, "Hospital Budget-Savings Plan for Prospective Mothers," *Bulletin of the American Hospital Association,* January 1928, p. 68.

8. "A Statistical Analysis of 2,717 Hospitals," *Bulletin of the American Hospital Association,* July 1931, p. 68.

9. Louis S. Reed, *Health Insurance: the Next Step in Social Security* (N.Y.: Harper, 1937), p. 189.

10. See Hedinger, supra n. 4, at pp. 4–13.

11. Justin Ford Kimball, "Prepayment and Hospital," *Bulletin of the American Hospital Association,* July 1934, pp. 44. On the early history of Blue Cross, see also Duncan M. MacIntyre, *Voluntary Health Insurance and Rate Making* (Ithaca, N.Y.: Cornell University Press, 1962), pp. 166 et seq.; HEW, SSA, *Private Health Insurance and Medical Care* (1968); O. W. Anderson, *State Enabling Legislation for Non-Profit Hospital and Medical Plans,* Public Health Economics, Research Series, No. 1 (Ann Arbor, Mich.: University of Michigan, 1944).

12. Harry Becker, ed., *Financing Hospital Care in the United States* (N.Y.: McGraw-Hill, 1955), p. 7.

13. R. Rorem, *Non-Profit Hospital Service Plans* (Chicago: Commission on Hospital Service, 1940), p. 29.

14. Reported in Hedinger, supra n. 4, at p. 11.

15. *Hospitals, Journal of The American Hospital Association,* February 1938, p. 77. Item 14 stated: "A hospital care insurance plan should meet with the general approval of the Committee on Hospital Service of the American Hospital Association."

16. Hedinger, supra n. 4, at p. 52, says: "This social characteristic anticipated the enrollment of low income members of the community and their being provided with protection equal to that received by the more affluent community members at a lower cost. The implication, if not the stated goal, of this element as recognized by various state lawmakers was that Blue Cross would serve as an income redistribution device, a role, customarily reserved for governmental action, and more particularly, governmentally owned or controlled social insurance and public assistance schemes."

17. Rorem, supra n. 13, at pp. 92–93.
18. Dr. Odin W. Anderson, an early historian of the health insurance industry, states that the Blue Cross plans adopted the following characteristics "to differentiate themselves from the private insurance companies," and to justify the competitive advantage granted to them under the special enabling legislation:

    1. They were incorporated as nonprofit organizations, and, therefore, had no stockholders or profits for individuals.
    2. Their boards of directors represented hospitals, physicians, and the general public.
    3. They were supervised by state insurance departments.
    4. As nonprofit corporations they held low cash reserves since hospitals were assumed to provide a reserve of service instead of cash.
    5. They placed emphasis on hospital benefits in the form of service rather than a cash indemnity.
    6. They placed all employees on salaries and offered no commissions to salesmen.

    Odin W. Anderson, "The Development of Health Services and Public Policy in the United States, 1875–1965" (unpublished manuscript), chap. XV, quoted in Hedinger, supra n. 4, at p. 17.
19. N.Y. Laws 1934, c. 595, adding Art 14, §§452–461, to the New York Insurance Law. Amended, June 15, 1939, and recodified, Art. IX-C, §§250–259.
20. Hedinger, supra n. 4, at p. 51.
21. Nathan Sinai, Odin W. Anderson, and Melvin L. Dollar, *Health Insurance in the United States* (N.Y.: Commonwealth Fund, 1946), p. 46. In 1939 the Blue Cross Commission of the American Hospital Association developed a Model Law to Enable the Formation of Non-Profit Hospital and/or Medical Service Plan. Eilers, supra n. 5, at p. 101.
22. *Ala. Code* tit. 28, §§304–316 (Supp. 1969); *Alaska Stat.* §§21.20.140–.20.200; *Ariz. Rev. Stat. Ann.* §20-821 to -840 (Supp. 1973); *Ark. Stat. Ann.* §§66–4901 to -4920 (Supp. 1971); *Cal. Ins. Code* §§11491-11517 (West 1972); *Colo. Rev. Stat. Ann.* §72-24-1 to -24-25 (Supp. 1967); *Conn. Gen. Stat. Rev.* §§33-157 to -167 (Supp. 1973); *Del. Code Ann.* tit. 18, §§6301–6309 (Insurance Pamphlet 1971); *Fla Stat.* §§641.01–641.38; *Ga. Code* §56-1701 to -1721 (Supp. 1972); *Hawaii Rev. Stat.* §433-1 to -19 (Supp. 1972); *Idaho Code* §41-3401 to -3436 (Supp. 1972); *Ill. Rev. Stat.* ch. 32, §551–562 and 595–624 (Supp. 1973); *Iowa Code* §§514.1-.18 (Supp. 1973); *Kan. Stat. Ann.* §§40-1800 to -1816 (Supp. 1972); *Ky. Rev. Stat. Ann.* §§304.32-010 to .32-270 (Supp. 1972); *La. Rev. Stat.* §§22.1661-.1663 (Supp. 1973); *Me. Rev. Stat. Ann.* tit. 24, §§2301–2315 (Supp. 1973); *Md. Ann. Code* art. 48A, §§354–361A (Supp. 1973); *Mass. Gen Laws* ch. 176A, §§1–30 (Supp. 1973); *Mich. Comp. Laws Ann.* §§550.501–.517 (Supp. 1973); *Minn. Stat. Ann.* §§62C.01–.23 (Supp. 1973); *Miss. Code Ann.* §§83-41-1 to -41-9 (Supp. 1973); *Mo. Stat. Ann.* §§354.010 to .175 (Supp. 1974); *Mont. Rev. Codes Ann.* §§15-2301 to -2397 (Supp. 1973); *Neb. Rev. Stat.* §§21-1509 to -1521 (1970); *Nev. Rev. Stat.* §§696.010–.300; *N.H. Rev. Stat. Ann.* §§419:1–:12 (Supp. 1972); *N.J. Stat. Ann.* §§17:48-1 to 48-18

(Supp. 1973); *N.M. Stat. Ann.* §§58-25-1 to -25-49 (Supp. 1973); *N.Y. Ins. Law* §§250–260 (McKinney Supp. 1973); *N.C. Gen. Stat.* §57-1 to -20 (Supp. 1971); *N.D. Cent. Code* §§26-26-01 to -26-14 (Supp. 1973); *Ohio Rev. Code Ann.* §§1739.01-.15 (Supp. 1972); *Okla. Stat. Ann.* tit. 36, §§2601–2621; *Ore. Rev. Stat.* §§750.005–.065 (Supp. 1972); *Pa. Stat. Ann.* tit. 40, §§6101–6127 (Supp. 1973); *R.I. Gen. Laws Ann.* §§27-19-1 to -19-16 (Supp. 1972); *S.C. Code Ann.* §§37-441 to -445 (Supp. 1971); *S.D. Compiled Laws Ann.* §§58-40-1 to -40-19 (Supp. 1973); *Tenn. Code Ann.* §§56-3001 to -3018 (Supp. 1972); *Tex Rev. Civ. Stat.* art. 20.01–.21 (Supp. 1972–1973); *Utah Code Ann.* §§31-37-1 to -37-26 (Supp. 1973); *Vt. Stat. Ann.* tit. 8, §§4511–4522 (Supp. 1973); *Va. Code Ann.* §§32-195.1 to -195.20:1 (1973); *Wash. Rev. Code Ann.* §§48.44.010–.44.220 (Supp. 1972); *W. Va. Code Ann.* §§33-24-1 to -24-11 (Supp. 1973); *Wisc. Stat. Ann.* §182.032 (Supp. 1973).

23. *Ariz. Rev. Stat. Ann.* §20–837 (Supp. 1973); *Ark. Stat. Ann.* §§66–4917, -4918 (special 1% tax); *Cal. Ins. Code* §11493.5 (West 1972); *Conn. Gen. Stat. Rev.* §33–165 (Supp. 1973); *Ga. Code* §56–1718 (Supp. 1972); *Idaho Code* §41–3427; *Ill. Rev. Stat.* ch. 32, §562; *Ky. Rev. Stat. Ann.* §136.395 (Supp. 1972); *La. Rev. Stat.* §22:1661 (Supp. 1973); *Me. Rev. Stat. Ann.* tit. 24, §2311 (Supp. 1973); *Mass. Gen. Laws* ch. 176A, §19; *Mich. Comp. Laws Ann.* §550.515; *N.J. Stat. Ann.* §17:48–18; *N.Y. Ins. Law* §251 (McKinney Supp. 1973); *N.C. Gen. Stat.* §57-14 (Supp. 1971); *Ohio Rev. Code Ann.* §1739.07; *Okla. Stat. Ann.,* tit. 36, §2617; *Vt. Stat. Ann.* tit. 8, §4518; *W. Va. Stat. Ann.* §33-24-4; *Wisc. Stat. Ann.* §182.032(8).

24. The federal tax exemption is provided under §501(c)(4), Int. Rev. Code of 1954, for "civic leagues or organizations not organized for profit but operated exclusively for the promotion of social welfare."

25. Approval Program for Blue Cross Plans, AHA, 2M-12/70-1575, 1964, Standard No. 5.

26. There has been some overlap in the territorial jurisdiction of two Illinois Blue Cross plans. The Illinois Supreme Court struck down a provision of the state enabling act requiring hospital service corporations to obtain contracts with at least 30% of the hospitals in the area served.

   The court described the situation saying: "[In 1957 the Illinois Hospital Association] formulated a policy to solve a problem which had concerned it for 'several years.' The problem was whether the two Illinois Blue Cross Plans, one known as the 'Chicago' plan and the other, the plaintiff in this case, known as the 'Rockford' plan, should be allowed to operate concurrently in the same areas in the State. 'On this question,' the Association stated, 'it is the opinion of the Board of Trustees that the public is better served and confusion avoided if only one Blue Cross Plan operates in a given area.' Since the plans were unable to 'agree upon territories,' the Association directed the attention of its members to [the state enabling law requirement], and recommended that no member hospital have a contract with more than one Blue Cross Plan. 'If this is done, the Plan not selected would be restricted from operating in that County under the provisions of the State Statues.' " *Illinois Hospital Service, Inc. v. Gerber,* 18 Ill. 2d 531, 165 N.E.2d 279 (1960).

   On June 30, 1972, the function of authorizing use of the Blue Cross insignia was transferred from the AHA to the BCA. As of this writing, the BCA is using the same authorization standards as the AHA, although the standards are being reviewed and some revisions will be made. Telephone interview with Robert L. Mickelsen, Senior Director, Approval and Licensure Program, Blue Cross Association, June 28, 1973.

27. Hedinger, supra n. 4, at p. 24; MacIntyre, supra n. 11, at p. 155.

28. Harry Becker, ed., *Financing Hospital Care in the United States* (N.Y.: McGraw-Hill, 1955), pp. 8–11.

29. *Research and Statistic Note,* No. 17 (Washington, D.C.: HEW, SSA, Oct. 13, 1965), p. 6; M. S. Mueller, "Enrollment, Coverage and Financial Experience of Blue Cross and Blue Shield Plans, 1969," *Research and Statistic Note,* No. 4 (Washington, D.C.: HEW, SSA, April 21, 1971), p. 4; *National Health Insurance Proposals,* Hearings before the House Committee on Ways and Means, 92nd Cong., 1st Sess., p. 342 (1971).

30. R. Rorem, *Non-Profit Hospital Service Plans,* supra n. 13, at p. 24.

31. Herman M. and Anne R. Somers, *Doctors, Patients, and Health Insurance* (Washington, D.C.: The Brookings Institution, 1961), p. 304.

32. Eilers, supra n. 5, at p. 89; MacIntyre, supra n. 11, at p. 154. The commitment to provide equal rates to the entire community was expressed in general terms, and the term *community rating* was not coined until the late forties. For example, "Hospital service plans have based their rate structures upon the anticipated utilization of hospital service for the community as a whole . . . The plans have felt that if their project is one community-wide in nature, no special consideration could be given to units making up the community." Norby, "Hospital Service Plans: Their Contract Provisions and Administrative Procedures," 6 *Law and Cont. Prob.* 545, 557 (1939). See also J. Stuart, "Blue Cross and Insurance: The Difference," 33 *Hospitals* 51 (Feb. 16, 1959).

33. See O. D. Dickerson, *Health Insurance,* 3d ed. (Homewood, Ill.: Irwin, 1968), ch. 18, pp. 568–601; Frank Joseph Angell, *Health Insurance* (N.Y.: Ronald Press, 1963), pp. 363–66 and 478–90; and Edwin J. Faulkner, *Health Insurance* (N.Y.: McGraw-Hill, 1960), ch. 11, pp. 364–405, for an explanation of rate setting by commercial insurers. Moral, racist, and sexist factors not based on actuarial experience have played a role in selection of risks and determination of rates. See generally Edwin J. Faulkner, *Accident-and-Health Insurance* (N.Y.: McGraw-Hill, 1940), pp. 115–19 and 126–27.

The Baylor plan did not purport to serve the whole community. One early report commented, "Employees who are underpaid and overworked are not considered good risks and applications are not solicited from such groups." Further, "although every member insured at this hospital pays a rate of 50¢ per month, all do not receive the same accommodations. Employees of the so-called lower classes, such as laborers, porters, etc. are given hospital treatment in ward beds at the rate of $3 per day. This discrimination has led to some criticism in the community." "Group Hospital Insurance Plan," a paper read Oct. 13, 1932, before the Hospital Conference of the City of New York by Frank Van Dyk, Executive Secretary, Hospital Council of Essex County, Newark, New Jersey, p. 10.

34. The number of persons hospitalized per 1,000 population per year are the following, broken down by family income:

Family Income	Total Persons Hospitalized per 1,000 population
All incomes	96
Under $3,000	123
$3,000–$4,999	107
$5,000–$6,999	97
$7,000–$9,999	94
$10,000 and over	82

The number of persons hospitalized per 1,000 population per year are the following, broken down by age:

Age	Total Persons Hospitalized per 1,000 population
All ages	96
Under 15 years	51
15–44	113
45–64	102
65 years and over	155

HEW, Public Health Service, Health Services and Mental Health Administration, National Center for Health Statistics, *Persons Hospitalized by Number of Hospital Episodes and Days in a Year, United States—1968,* National Health Survey, Series 10, Number 64, DHEW Publication No. (HSM) 72–1029, p. 4 (1971).

35. On pressure by organized labor for experience rating see MacIntyre, supra n. 11 at pp. 155 et seq.; Hedinger, supra n. 4, at pp. 65 et seq. As late as 1953 a special Blue Cross committee was appointed to consider whether Blue Cross was "a community social agency or an insurance company," whether plans should ban or outlaw experience rating outright, and if no agreement could be reached on an outright ban whether Blue Cross should ban future use of experience rating. The annual national Blue Cross meeting adopted a resolution stating that the "overwhelming majority of Blue Cross Plans have not deviated from presently known Blue Cross practices to the point of offering experience rating" and urging "those Plans not yet engaged in experience rating programs to make an honest effort to withstand the pressures which arise for experience rating." MacIntyre, supra n. 11, at p. 161.

36. Unpublished data provided by the Public Relations Department of the Blue Cross Association, 840 N. Lake Shore Drive, Chicago, Ill. 60611. The Vermont-New Hampshire plan has remained committed to community rating.

37. Dickerson, supra n. 33, at p. 329. See George E. McLean, "An Actuarial Analysis of a Prospective Experience Rating Approach for Group Hospital-Surgical-Medical Coverage," 48 *Proceedings of the Casualty Actuarial Society* 155.

38. A 1964 report by the Subcommittee on Health of the Elderly of the Senate

Special Committee on the Aging studied the problem of Blue Cross moves toward experience rating and concluded, "Blue Cross and its older subscribers are in very serious trouble. . . . The route of experience rating and abandonment of service benefits is nothing less than a complete denial of the basic reasons for the existence of Blue Cross. There is, however, an alternative— enactment of a program of hospital insurance benefits for the elderly financed through the social security mechanism." *Blue Cross and Private Health Insurance Coverage of Older Americans,* 88th Cong., 2d Sess. p. 35 (1964).

39. U.S. Service Mark Registration Number 554,448, registered Feb. 5, 1952; No. 554,817, registered Feb. 12, 1952; and 554,818, registered Feb. 12, 1952.

40. "The name 'Commission on Hospital Service' was subsequently changed to 'Hospital Service Plan Commission' and, finally, to 'Blue Cross Commission' in 1946. Legally, the Blue Cross Commission was a subordinate trust of the American Hospital Association. The Board of Trustees of the AHA could disapprove any course of action of the commission. Thus, the Blue Cross Commission was in a literal sense an arm or 'commission' of the American Hospital Association." Eilers, supra n. 5, at p. 58.

41. "AHA and Blue Cross Split but Still a Twosome," *Medical World News,* Sept. 10, 1971, p. 20; Telephone interview with Robert L. Mickelsen, Director, Division of Blue Cross Approvals, June 28, 1973. (Prior to the transfer Mr. Mickelsen was an employee of the AHA, with the title Blue Cross Specialist.)

42. Bylaws, AHA and BCA. The 1971 organizational changes are reported in *AHA Convention Daily,* Aug. 25, 1971; *Modern Hospital,* September 1971, p. 37.

43. *Modern Hospital,* ibid. In June 1972 the AHA committee searching for a new president of that organization recommended Walter J. McNerney, President of BCA. *Washington Report on Medicine and Health,* No. 1305, July 3, 1972. The committee's recommendation was not accepted.

44. BCA maintains information on some factors that provide some indication of plan functioning, at least relative to other plans, for example administrative expense per claim, staff ratios, productivity. An internal BCA memo dated May 1971 stated that the figures for the Virginia plan have "been unsatisfactory for some time and each periodic reading shows greater deterioration." Testimony of Walter J. McNerney, *High Cost of Hospitalization,* Hearings before the Subcommittee on Antitrust and Monopoly of the Senate Committee of the Judiciary, 91st Cong., 2nd Sess., Pt. 2, p. 51 (January 1971). Hereinafter cited as Hart Committee Hearings.

45. Id. at pp. 31, 54.

46. Ibid.

47. Id. at pp. 32–33, 61.

48. Id. at pp. 36–37, 48.

49. Id. at p. 188.

50. Id. at pp. 188–89.

51. Id. at p. 55. Another BCA memo, dated May 11, 1970, stated, "The uncontrolled increase in administrative cost has created an explosive situation regarding Medicare and could generate bad publicity coupled with SSA and Congressional reactions even worse than those encountered by the Washington D.C. plan." Id. at p. 51.

52. *Blue Cross-Blue Shield Fact Book 1972* (Chicago, BCA), p. 12.
53. Hart Committee Hearings, supra n. 44, at p. 26.
54. For example, the Evaluation of Part A Intermediary Performance, SSA, March 19, 1971, based on the 18 months ending December 1970, indicated that the Richmond plan was one of the three Blue Cross plans in the nation that had an "unsatisfactory" composite of unit cost per bill processed. The other plans with an unsatisfactory rating were New York City and Puerto Rico. In addition, seven plans were evaluated as having "substandard" costs per bill processed: Buffalo, N.Y.; District of Columbia; Maryland; Minnesota; New Mexico; Los Angeles, California; Jamestown, N.Y.
55. The Washington Blue Cross is called Group Health Association Inc. See *Administration of Federal Health Benefit Programs,* Hearings before a Subcommittee of the House Committee on Government Operations, 91st Cong., 2nd Sess., pp. 274–75 (1970).
56. Id. at 274–75. The chairman of the board and president of the National Savings and Trust Co. was also a member of the Blue Cross board, its treasurer for over ten years, and a member of both its Executive and Finance and Investment committees. That bank was the primary one used by Blue Cross and also served as investment custodian for all of the funds of the organization. Id. at pp. 228, 261. Other members of the Blue Cross board were officers of other banks, some of which were beneficiaries of Blue Cross noninterest-bearing accounts. Id. at p. 252.
57. The chairman of the Illinois Blue Cross board was senior vice president of the Continental Illinois National Bank of Chicago until recently. When he joined the board in 1947, Blue Cross had less than $1 million on deposit. By 1963, when he became chairman of the board, the plan's balances at Continental had passed $7 million. On December 31, 1971, the plan had $15.3 million on deposit. In addition, the plan has more than $2 million in noninterest-bearing accounts in the Northern Trust Company, one of whose officers is also on the Blue Cross board. In 1971, perhaps in response to the 1970 congressional investigation of Washington Blue Cross, Continental paid Blue Cross interest amounting to $375,339. A. Bajonski, "The Blue Cross Double Cross," 5 *Chi. Journalism Rev.,* No. 2, p. 4 (February 1972), and A. Bajonski, "Further Notes on the Blue Cross Double Cross," 5 *Chi Journalism Rev.* no. 6, p. 19 (June 1972).
58. Hart Committee Hearings, supra n. 44, at pp. 40–41.
59. The BCA responded that information was not available on the following subjects: amount of Blue Cross payments to hospitals under Medicaid; number of days of work on hand; percentage of Medicaid claims reviewed for medical necessity; breakdown of the types of personnel involved in claims review work; percentages of claims for payment for hospital and nursing home care that were questioned and/or rejected; whether member hospitals had functioning utilization review committees and whether those committees utilized length of stay data; rate of hospital usage by experience-rated groups; comparative information on rates to community-and experience-rated subscribers; increases in rates to community-rated subscribers. The questionnaire, BCA response, and related correspondence are available from the Health Law Project, 133 So. 36th Street, Philadelphia, Penn. 19174.

60. For example, Philadelphia Blue Cross takes the position that information concerning per diem costs and charges should be made available only to the professional public, because the general public is not in a position to evaluate such information and public disclosure would be unfair to the physicians and hospitals involved. See Sen. Abraham Ribicoff, *The American Medical Machine* (N.Y.: Saturday Review Press, 1972), p. 98.

61. In 1965, Walter McNerney described the members of Blue Cross boards: "the majority are public representatives, and these reflect labor, management, the church, and various facets in the community, and they all serve without pay." Executive Hearings before the House Committee on Ways and Means, 89th Cong., 1st Sess., Pt. 1., p. 181. Before the Senate Finance Committee, he stated, "Blue Cross plans, like many hospitals, were started by thousands of public servants, many of whom were not professionally involved in health. They were labor leaders, businessmen, educators and legislators who saw a vital need to help their fellow citizens have access to health care. They organized hospitals. They wrote, sponsored, and passed enabling legislation authorizing Blue Cross plans. These laws declared public policy to include the functioning of these plans as a public policy, using some of the principles of insurance, but dedicated to obtaining total community membership." Hearings on H.R. 6675 before the Senate Finance Committee, 89th Cong., 1st Sess., Pt. 1 (1965).

    Asked, "who is it that sets the salaries and provides the costs that are necessary," McNerney responded, "It is a community board. For example, we might have on the board a group of the top industrialists and labor people in the town, representatives of the churches. We might, for example, have people who are providers of care. These people will establish the basic policy of this operation." Hearings on H.R. 3920 before the House Committee on Ways and Means, 88th Cong., 1st and 2nd Sess., Pt. 3, p. 2072.

62. For example, *N.J. Stat. Ann* §17:48-5 (Supp. 1973); *Calif. Stat. Ann. Insurance* §11498 (1972); *Wisc. Stat. Ann* §182.032(3)(a) (1957); *N.Y. Ins. Law* §250.1-a (Supp. 1973).

63. Hart Committee Hearings, supra n. 44, Pt. 2, p. 184. These figures do not include hospital trustees as public representatives. Over the past 25 years there has been a slight decrease in the proportion of provider representatives.

	Hospital	*Medical*
1945	55%	17%
1959	51%	17%
1965	45%	14%
1967	44%	14%
1968	43%	17%
1969	43%	16%

64. Id. at p. 131.

65. The Massachusetts rate chairman noted, "without in any sense suggesting wrong doing on the part of these 11 [provider representatives on the Blue Cross board]—many of whom are known to me personally as fine, honorable men who act only according to deeply held convictions—I believe their mere

duality of roles weakens the resolve of Blue Cross in its dealings with the hospitals." Hart Committee Hearings, supra n. 44, at p. 131.

66. See Sen. Edward Kennedy, *In Critical Condition* (N.Y.: Simon and Schuster, 1972), pp. 209–10.

67. According to BCA data, the board of directors or corporate membership selects the public board members in 44 plans. Hart Committee Hearings, supra n. 44, at pp. 177–82. Often the only "members" of the Blue Cross corporation are the board of directors. Boards are sometimes casually self-perpetuating. For example, J. N. Stanberry, an Illinois Blue Cross director emeritus and retired vice president of Illinois Bell, says, "when I left the Blue Cross board, I suggested my successor at Bell to take my place, and the other directors said it was all right with them." Andrew Bajonski, "The Blue Cross Double Cross," 5 *Chi. Journalism Rev.,* No. 2, p. 4 (February 1972).

68. Hart Committee Hearings, supra n. 44, at pp. 178 et seq. Plans in which the hospital representatives select the public board members include: Los Angeles; Atlanta; Des Moines; Sioux City; Kentucky; New Orleans; Michigan; Minnesota; Kansas City, Mo.; St. Louis; Montana; North Dakota; Canton, Ohio; Lima, Ohio; Youngstown, Ohio; Allentown, Pa.; Chattanooga; Memphis; Parkersburg, West Va.; and Wheeling, West Va.

69. Ibid. In Maine, Nebraska, and Puerto Rico the public representatives are nominated and elected by the subscribers. In Kansas and Wilkes-Barre, Pa., the public representatives are elected by the corporate members chosen from the Subscriber Advisory Board, which represents subscribers in each county served. In Mississippi and Oklahoma the subscribers select public members from a list nominated by the board.

70. See *Philadelphia Inquirer,* Jan. 30, 1972, p. 26; Feb. 14, 1971, p. F17, col. 1; Feb. 23, 1972, p. 17; *Philadelphia Bulletin,* Jan 26, 1972, p. 9; Feb. 23, 1972, p. 38, col. 4. After the 1972 election it was revealed that the plan management learned of two additional vacancies just prior to the election. The board appointed a former plan executive and a businessman to fill the positions. Subscribers unsuccessfully urged the seating of those receiving the next highest vote in the election. Minutes, Associated Hospital Service of Philadelphia, Consumer Advisory Committee Meeting, May 1, 1972.

71. On Sept. 28, 1972, the Consumer Advisory Board of Philadelphia Blue Cross recommended that the bylaws be amended to provide that no employee of Blue Cross should be allowed to solicit proxy votes. The proposal was rejected. Minutes, Associated Hospital Service, Nov. 22, 1972. The bylaws were amended to provide for the listing of candidates nominated by petition in newspaper advertisements, but the board refused to accept the consumers' recommendation that proxy forms be provided for insurgent as well as management candidates. The board also rejected a consumer rcommendation limiting office to six years.

72. Major affiliations of the public board members include food companies (e.g. Horn & Hardart, Tasty Baking Co., Campbell Soups), insurance companies (e.g. Penn Mutual Life Insurance, Fidelity Mutual Life, Lumberman's Mutual Life Insurance), and other businesses such as Sears, Roebuck, and Co., Quaker Chemical, etc. Detailed data on each member of the Philadelphia plan board is

compiled in an unpublished paper, "Conflicts of Interest on the 1970 Blue Cross of Greater Philadelphia Board," on file at the Health Law Project, 133 So. 36th Street, Philadelphia, Penn. 19174.

73. The 32-person board had 6 physicians, 1 hospital administrator, 15 hospital trustees, and 3 former hospital trustees. Thomas Jefferson University Hospital had 4 representatives; Albert Einstein Medical Center had 3; Temple University Hospital, Pennsylvania Medical College, and Germantown Hospital and Dispensary each had 2. The Hospital of the University of Pennsylvania had only 1 trustee on the board; however, 3 Blue Cross directors were trustees of the university. Ibid.

74. The information upon which this tabulation is based was presented in *Physician Training Facilities and Health Maintenance Organization,* Hearings before the Subcommittee on Health of the Senate Committee on Labor and Public Welfare, 92nd Cong., 1st Sess., Pt. 3, pp. 1043 ff. (Nov. 2, 1971). The other positions listed included: 1 agricultural agent, 1 farm commissioner, 2 farmers, 1 rancher, 5 executive secretaries, 4 secretaries, 1 research nurse, 1 chemist, 2 manufacturers, 1 trustee, 1 congressman, 2 accountants, 1 civic worker, 1 health officer, 5 superintendents, 2 radio and TV staff, 1 office manager, 1 machinery worker, 1 biologist, 3 editors, 5 publishers, 3 hospital officials, 1 comptroller, 3 CPAs, 1 salvage worker, 1 coal operator, 2 supervisors, an executive and an employee of PRWRA (an unidentified Puerto Rican organization), 1 Blue Cross official, 2 government employees, and 1 police officer.

75. For example, although there were labor representatives on the board of the Washington, D.C., and Illinois plans, and an official of George Washington University on the Finance Committee of the Washington board, there was no evidence that these people raised questions about the plan's deposits in noninterest-bearing accounts. *Administration of Federal Health Benefit Programs,* supra n. 55, at p. 228.

76. Walter J. McNerney states, "If you examine what has animated Blue Cross over the years, you would find, for example . . . that in Michigan the greatest impact on Michigan Blue Cross is derived from the United Auto Workers . . . and other labor unions in that State who were very explicit about what they wanted and the conditions under which they wanted them. In Western Pennsylvania it was steel, and in Cleveland, similarly, and so on around the country. . . . Eighty percent of our business is through groups. We have seven out of the ten largest industries enrolled in this country and if there is any dominancy, it certainly comes from that source." Hart Committee Hearings, supra n. 44, at p. 220. Harry Becker, a health economist long associated with Blue Cross and organized labor, estimates that the single most important objective of Blue Cross plan subscriber relations is to keep the blue chip accounts happy. Interview, May 6, 1971, New York, N.Y.

77. C. Silberstein, "Non-Group and Small Group Coverage: What's Available and How Much Does it Cost?" (Unpublished ms, Nov. 11, 1971). See also *The American Health Empire,* A Report from the Health Policy Advisory Center (N.Y.: Random House, 1970), pp. 151–54.

78. The New York Insurance Department recently proposed regulations that

would require insurance companies to maintain experience data for determining rates. Proposed Amendments to 11 N.Y.C.R.R. 52, issued Dec. 20, 1972.
79. Harry Becker explains that labor representatives impressed by the opportunity to meet, work, and socialize with financial and professional leaders take an accommodating and unquestioning role in exchange for amiable relationships on the board. Supra n. 76.

20

The Failure of Medicaid

Elliott A. Krause

. . . .

A ... major strategy for changing the delivery of services to the poor was a "voucher" strategy: specifically the Medicaid program. The *problem,* as diagnosed by those who advocated the voucher strategy, was that the poor are *poor,* that is, without the money or the insurance coverage to buy services in the top level of the two-class medical system. Given the money to buy care anywhere (the ticket or the voucher) the poor would go away from the undersystem and it would wither away, as they cashed the vouchers in at nonprofit voluntary hospitals and doctor's offices.

When the Medicare/Medicaid legislation was passed during the Johnson era, in 1965, it was a three-part law, the first two parts of which created a medical insurance system for the middle-class elderly, administered through the Social Security Administration; and the third part of which—Medicaid—was to be administered in Washington by the *welfare* divisions of HEW. In theory, the "vouchers" would be payments both for those on welfare and those *not* on welfare but too poor to pay for their own care in the top-level system. They were to be called the "medically indigent." With the new Medicaid money, they could theoretically go anywhere, and say, as if they had Mastercharge or BankAmericard, "Take me, too, Medicaid will pay for it." The private physician, or voluntary hospital, would then get paid by the local welfare department or the state government for the services they gave. This was the strategy—and it didn't work. The reasons are our present subject.

To begin with, when the original Medicaid law was passed, no strong central administration was set up at HEW to run the program, so each state could and did decide for themselves who would be eligible to use the new vouchers. Wealthier and more progressive states such as New York and California were more generous here to their poor, and also were able to demand and get more federal "matching funds" (money to match what they put up as states) than states which had not moved so fast. Soon the demands for money just from these states alone in the first year and a half of the program, outran the lawmakers' estimated cost of the program for the whole nation.[1] Then there was the critical issue of whether this was really a "voucher" system, or whether it was simply to be another element in the existing welfare system. Did the poor have a *right* to this money, or would it be up to each welfare department, in each state, to decide who the "deserving poor" would be? *The decision to run the program through the Federal Welfare Bureau, and then in each state through the welfare departments, which was a decision made at the beginning of the Medicaid program, doomed it from the start as a strategy for change.* For the program was to be run by the low prestige welfare system, which had already been under fire for years, and which itself was a major element in harassing the poor in many poverty areas. One year after the program began, Stevens and Stevens concluded that

> HEW itself inevitably gave priority, insofar as there were clear priorities, to run Medicare, which as a prestige operation run by the powerful Social Security Administration as part of the Social Security program was the darling of the politicians and the electorate. Without real power within the Department and without a clearly defined political constituency, MSA and Medicaid found themselves the whipping boys for rising medical costs and rising "welfare" expenditures for which they were, at most, only partially responsible.[2]

As the costs of the program shot up, the screams of antiwelfare politicians bounced off the walls in Congress and quickly led to cutbacks in the overall program. Campaigns to sign the poor up in the program were followed a year or so later by the disqualifications of many of the "medically indigent" who no longer qualified as the maximum income level for qualification in the program began to *drop*. Power struggles began: the new Welfare Rights organizations were campaigning for higher rates for welfare clients in general, and for more people being allowed on Medicaid, while at the same time the politicians and the American middle class, motivated in part by racist considerations, fought against what they called "welfare cheating." Soon it became evident that hospitals and private physicians were in some cases getting rich on Medicaid payments, that profit-making nursing homes were springing up everywhere to take advantage of the federal money (in 1969, 14,470 out of the nation's 18,910 nursing homes were private profit-making ones),[3] and that fraud levels by physicians were approaching five to seven percent of the cases in New York City. An investigation found the practice of "mass visits"—a physician walking past a line of forty patients and charging for a visit to each one. Unnecessary medication and tests were often prescribed—sometimes to a drugstore or lab that gave a kick-back to the physician.[4]

The beginning year of the Medicaid program was a time of expansion. The second period, from 1967 to 1969, was a time of cutback in payments and restriction of the program down to those on welfare, in many places. By 1970, there was also a stronger focus on the fraud of providers. Neither the escalation of costs nor the fraud made the program popular with the voter, and unpopularity in political terms does not mean a bright future for any program. But regardless of the politics which were determining the programs's fate from year to year, the most essential aspect of the experiment in the first place was to have been that the poor would be treated the same as anyone else in the society; that they could get the same care that others could. But to be poor in America is to be a hostage of the welfare system, and to have to beg for health-care vouchers just as one has to beg for a bed or an extra few dollars for children's clothes. There was no due process of law for several years, and a welfare worker could and did sometimes decide to deny Medicaid support to a particular client as a way of punishing him or her. Even today, it is hard to get the "hearing" that is the right of the client without a storefront lawyer at one's side in the welfare office. Stevens and Stevens present this from the welfare client's point of view:

> As welfare or near-welfare recipients, Medicaid patients were often treated as social dependents rather than "consumers," even in the thick of the consumer movement. Not only did recipients frequently find it humiliating trying to get on Medicaid, they often faced humiliation when they had a complaint about the program, or there was some doubt about their continued eligibility.... Regulation of recipients has thus largely been repressive rather than protective.[5]

But what of the ability to buy out of the bottom system? Several limitations on this have been important, and they relate directly to the overall patterns of service and the strength of the elements of the existing two-class system. First, since costs far outran predictions, many states got far behind on their bill paying. Since the private physician and the voluntary hospital have control over who they want to take, and since after a while the Medicaid voucher system began to look very much like a $3 bill, the signs began to go up over all the metropolitan areas: "Medicaid cards not honored here." Others, who *specialized* in Medicaid patients, did so for money and not for service, cutting corners to the point were their "private" care was, if anything, worse than that which the poor were getting in the public hospitals. The poor could not afford the trip to the suburbs and its hospitals, and doctors' offices; many soon became suspicious of the new "Medicaid factories." So they took their vouchers to the only place left—the city hospital. Because of bureaucratic politics in Washington, for many years they couldn't even cash them in at neighborhood health centers of the OEO [Office of Economic Opportunity] type. And welfare workers, holding power over the poor, could and did tell them where to get medical care. Few people could argue with them, because they did not know their rights. In the Harvard comprehensive care project . . . some poor patients would not join even when urged by the project staff because, they said, "Their welfare worker wouldn't allow them to." Robertson and his group, with all the resources of a major medical center and a special project, could not win the battle against the local welfare department:

> It is also known that long after the Medicare-Medicaid legislation, which allowed welfare families to use whatever facilities they wished, some welfare workers had not conveyed this information to their clients and were continuing to urge them to use City Hospital. Since the families in our sample used many facilities, these admonitions were not always effective but some may have been confused by being told different things regarding their rights.[6]

The final chapter in the Medicaid story is the fiscal crisis of the state in the mid-seventies. Here the working class is set against the poor by the refusal of the capitalist class to pay more in taxes to support social service, in a situation where they are under pressure from world competition from socialist and Third-World activity. Since the white- and blue-collar workers will not pay the bill either—for they cannot and still have money left for consumption—massive cutbacks become necessary to the service for the poor. In 1975 Massachusetts, a generally liberal state, removed all general relief recipients from the Medicaid program. They were officially made charity cases and from the time of the action on, have had to beg their medical care wherever they can find it, with no reimbursement for those giving it to them.

To sum up, the voucher strategy shared with the comprehensive service demonstration strategy and the OEO Neighborhood Health Center strategy certain assumptions and certain fates. As ideas, by well-meaning liberal theorists, they were attempts to rearrange the pattern of services delivered to the poor and increase the quality of these services; that is, to deal with the two-class system. But the existing interest groups, and the overall structural pressures bearing on the capitalist class, went to work on Medicaid even more quickly and thoroughly than in the other two main areas . . . (OEO and demonstrations of comprehensive care). The money in the other two areas was trivial in comparison to that involved in the Medicaid program. Political opposition to the creation of genuine equal opportunity in health care for the poor, and an alignment of the main system elements causing the trouble in the first place, plus the profit motivation of the private system, led to the quick deflection of the program from its original goal. Thousands of poor people have had greater support through Medicaid, even more than were helped with the OEO Neighborhood Health Centers and the "comprehensive care" demonstrations. But the program simply channeled money into one existing element in the lower class of the medical system. If anything, the hand of the agencies dealing with the poor was strengthened by the program, as was the two-class system itself. And evenually, by the mid-seventies, the fiscal crisis of the capitalist state—especially in the cities—sounded the death knell of the program, even as a *support* system for the lower class.

References

1. Robert and Rosemary Stevens, *Welfare Medicine in America. A Case Study of Medicaid* (New York: Free Press, 1974), pp. 73–128.
2. Ibid.
3. U.S. Government Statistics, HEW, National Center for Health Services Research, Rockville, Md., 1971.
4. See Lowell E. Bellin, "*Realpolitik* in the Health Care Arena: Standard-setting of Professional Services." *American Journal of Public Health*, 59 (1969): 820–824.
5. Stevens and Stevens, *op. cit.*, p. 199.
6. Leon S. Robertson et al., *Changing the Medical Care System* (New York: Praeger, 1974): p. 55.

Racism and Sexism in Medical Care

The suppression of the social, economic, and political desires of American women
and racial minorities and the exploitation of their labor are two primary characteristics of American society; despite legislation and judicial decisions, women
and minorities continue to be discriminated against. Nowhere is discrimination
more prevalent than in the treatment which women and minorities receive at the
hands of the health industry. Whether as providers or consumers, they are ex-
ploited, abused, and discriminated against. (Weaver and Garett, 1978: 677)

AMERICAN SOCIETY IS STRATIFIED, layered with groups who have
differing amounts of power, privilege, access to job and educational opportunities, different incomes, and different conditions of
living. This stratification is not a "natural" product of society, nor
is it a result of mere chance. Indeed, certain forms of institutionalized inequality are both cause and effect of unequal health care
among the populations of American society. This section examines
the consequences of racism and sexism on the American medical
system and on the health of women and nonwhites.

The medical labor force is a microcosm of social stratification
in America, with women and nonwhites kept to the "lower rungs"
of the medical hierarchy. Almost all physicians are white (approximately 90 percent). Almost all nurses are women, and most of the
higher ranking nurses (RN's) are white. But the lower status and
lower paying jobs of nursing aides and orderlies are increasingly
being filled by minority women. Almost all men who work in
these lower status jobs are nonwhite as well. In 1970 only 2.2
percent of all physicians were black, 3.7 percent were of Spanish
heritage (Hispanic) and 9.4 percent were female (DHEW, 1975).
On the other hand, 84.8 percent of nursing aides, orderlies, and
attendants that same year were female, 24.2 percent of those
workers were black, and 3.8 percent were of Spanish heritage
(Chicanos or Puerto Ricans) (DHEW, 1975).

While the past decade has seen a great deal of publicity about
the impact of "affirmative action" on opening up educational opportunities, the absolute and proportionate numbers of women

and nonwhites in the medical profession remain low compared to their numbers in the population as a whole (Weaver and Garrett, 1978: 678). In fact, the percentage of black applicants accepted into medical school actually decreased from 51.4 percent in 1970–1971 to 38.6 percent in 1977–1978, although the potential pool of qualified nonwhite applicants entering colleges and universities increased (Strelnick, 1980). Despite evidence to the contrary, medical school personnel continue to promote myths about why medicine has failed to improve the representation of nonwhites and, by and large, blame this state of affairs on those discriminated against. And, according to a report by the United States General Accounting Office, the Department of Health, Education and Welfare has failed to enforce affirmative action and nondiscrimination rules (Strelnick, 1980, citing General Accounting Office, 1975).

One indicator of a medical school's willingness to accept nonwhites and women as students is the composition of its faculty and, in turn, the representation of nonwhites and women on faculty admissions committees. The percentage of black, Hispanic and Native-American medical school faculty has remained the same 2.6 percent since 1971–1972. Women currently constitute about the same 15.2 percent of medical school faculties as they did in 1965–1966 (although the percentage dropped and rose during this period). However, since 70 percent of medical school librarians are women, their representation throughout medical school faculties, and in particular as administrators of medical schools, is quite low. In addition, when women are on medical school faculties, they are disproportionately represented in the lower faculty ranks (Strelnick, 1980).

While women have made greater relative improvements in their representation in medical school classes than nonwhites (they currently constitute about 25 percent of students entering medical school classes), they continue to be underrepresented in proportion to their numbers in the population. Women who manage to complete medical school are concentrated in certain, generally stereotypically "female" specialties, including pediatrics and psychiatry, and are underrepresented in the more prestigious and powerful surgical specialties. Indeed, it has been found that gender stereotypes among young male physicians has been increasing rather than decreasing (Quadagno, 1976). Sadly, while there is good evidence that women and nonwhites are more likely to serve those patient populations who most need medical care, their underrepresentation in certain medical areas and specialties undercuts their potential for mitigating the unequal distribution of medical care.

In addition to racism and sexism, there is a continued under-representation of people (of all races, both women and men) from working-class and low economic background in medical schools. In fact, several studies have found that lower class students have had to have higher grades than upper class students to gain entrance to medical schools, and that children of families who earn more than $50,000 per year are admitted to medical schools at higher rates than any other group (Strelnick, 1980 citing Gee, 1959, and Dagenais and Rosinski, 1977). Class background is also a strong predictor of a medical student's choice of specialization, with children of wealthier families more likely to opt to become specialists and children of poorer backgrounds more likely to become primary care physicians (Strelnick, 1980: 10).

Racism and sexism (and class oppression) combine to deliver a "double whammy" to minority women who work in medical care services. Comparing the salaries of males and females who are relatively low-paid health technicians, for example, we find that nonwhite men have the economic advantage over their nonwhite female counterparts. Such a pay differential between men and women holds for all occupational levels within the medical care labor force. It also holds for all occupations throughout the country as a whole. A recent Department of Labor study indicated that women earn about 57¢ for every $1.00 earned by men, whether they are professors, janitors, or physicians, a differential that has been growing in recent years (Sexton, 1977).

Until recently there has been little information about the nature and consequences of racism and sexism in the medical care industry. We do know that discrimination works in a number of ways, some more obvious or overt than others. For example, for many years medical schools set "quotas" on the numbers of women and blacks they would accept (if any) each year. Further, informal mechanisms of prejudice and discrimination operate within medical schools. We know, for example, that women are often ignored, harassed and otherwise mistreated and informally denied needed faculty support (Campbell, 1973; Quadagno, 1976). In addition, early patterns of discrimination are evident in the "tracking" of nonwhites and females out of preparatory science sequences as early as junior high school, making it impossible for them to have obtained the academic backgrounds to qualify for admission to medical school should they later decide they want to become physicians. In addition, lack of available scholarships makes it impossible for many people from working class and low economic backgrounds to attend medical schools even if they do have the necessary intellectual capacities and academic qualifications.[1]

Both racism and sexism directly affect the health of women and nonwhites. The most obvious effects of racism can be seen in mortality statistics. In his article, "Suffer the Children: Some Effects of Racism on the Health of Black Infants," Wornie L. Reed points out that there is a relationship between institutionalized racism and the inordinately high death rates for black infants in the United States. Such high death rates serve as a gross but reliable indicator of the generally poor health suffered by many if not most blacks in this country. As Reed notes, even when controlling for the effects of social class, black people are less healthy than whites as a population. One conclusion we might draw from this is that the effects of racism compound the known pathological consequences of poverty.

In addition to the direct effects of racism on health, there are added burdens for nonwhite persons who go into a medical care system in which the primary care-givers are white. The problems stemming from ethnic and racial differences may be compounded by prejudice, as when, for example, large numbers of poor black and Hispanic women are sterilized without their knowledge or permission by white, male physicians (Dreifus, 1977).

Sexism, like racism, has had direct consequences on the health and medical experiences of women. Sexist practices eliminated the early dominance of American women in providing health care for one another and thus contributed to the ignorance of many women (even today) about their own bodies and health needs (Ehrenreich and English, 1973). During the nineteenth century, organized medicine gained a strong dominance over the treatment of women, and proceeded to promulgate erroneous and damaging conceptualizations of women as sickly, irrational creatures who are always at the mercy of their reproductive organs (Barker-Benfield, 1976; Wertz and Wertz, 1977). In the selection in this section, "The Sexual Politics of Sickness," Barbara Ehrenreich and Deirdre English explore the history of the rise of these "scientific" explanations of women's health and illness experiences and of the creation of elitist assumptions about the "fragile" nature of upper class women, a nature first believed to be dominated by reproductive organs and, later, by psychological processes innate to women. The creation of the "cult of invalidism" among upper class women in the nineteenth century—at the same time working class women were considered capable of working long, hard hours in sweatshops and factories—can be seen as an example of physicians' functioning as agents of social control: in this case, by keeping women (of both classes) "in their place," both overtly and subtly, through a socialization process in which many women came to accept being sickly as their proper role and in which many more unquestioningly accepted the physician's claim to "expertise" in treating women's health and sexual problems.

While the grossest biases about the role of women's sexuality and reproductive capacities diminished in the twentieth century, the dominance of male physicians with their own sexist assumptions continues to affect the treatment procedures, conceptualizations, and "cures" given to women (Weiss, 1975). For example, childbirth under modern medicine has moved from being considered a normal, healthy event to a "pathological" process to be made "safe" only by the interventions and controls of the expert physician (Arms, 1975; Wertz and Wertz, 1977). Lest we think that medical sexism is an historical artifact, Diana Scully and Pauline Bart provide us with a contemporary example in "A Funny Thing Happened on the Way to the Orifice: Women in Gynecology Textbooks." They analyze how medical textbooks depict women and directly and indirectly influence what it is that physicians learn about women and their sexuality. Biases developed in the nineteenth century are still taught today as scientific fact, despite empirical evidence to the contrary now readily available to physicians.

Together, these selections give ample evidence that the medical profession's knowledge and treatment of women, like its treatment of nonwhites and the poor, are deeply biased by its own stereotypic assumptions, thus reinforcing the very sexism and racism which gave rise to those assumptions in the first place.

Note

1. For years the American Medical Association fought efforts to establish scholarships for poorer medical students, notwithstanding the fact that most medical

schools require their students not hold an outside job while attending school. While some scholarship monies have become available in recent years, scholarships are still extremely limited.

References

Arms, Suzanne. 1975. Immaculate Deception. Boston: Houghton Mifflin, Co.

Barker-Benfield, G. J. 1976. The Horrors of the Half-Known Life. New York: Harper and Row.

Campbell, Margaret. 1973. "Why Would a Girl Go Into Medicine?" Old Westbury, New York: The Feminist Press.

Dagenais, Fred, and Edwin F. Rosinski. 1977. "Social class level, performance, and values in medical school." Proceedings of the 16th Annual Conference on Research in Medical Education. Washington, D.C. (November).

Department of Health, Education and Welfare. 1975. Decennial Census Data for Selected Health Occupations: United States, 1970. Washington, D.C.: Government Printing Office (HRA 76-1231).

Dreifus, Claudia. 1977. "Sterilizing the poor." Reprinted from The Progressive, 1975 in Claudia Dreifus (Ed.), Seizing Our Bodies. New York: Random House.

Ehrenreich, Barbara, and Deirdre English. 1973. Witches, Midwives and Nurses. Old Westbury, New York: The Feminist Press.

Gee, Helen H. 1959. "Differential characteristics of student bodies: Implications for the study of medical education." Berkeley, Calif., Field Service Center and Center for the Study of Higher Education.

General Accounting Office. 1975. Comptroller General's Report to the Honorable Ronald V. Dellums, "More assurances needed that colleges and universities with government contracts provide equal employment opportunity." Washington, D.C.: Government Printing Office (August 25).

Quadagno, Jill. 1976. "Occupational sex-typing and internal labor market distributions: An assessment of medical specialties." Social Problems 23 (April): 442–445.

Sexton, Patricia Cayo. 1977. Women and Work. U.S. Department of Labor, R&D Monograph 46, Employment and Training Administration.

Strelnick, Hal. 1980. "Bakke-ing up the wrong tree." Health/PAC Bulletin 11, 3 (January-February).

Weaver, Jerry, and Sharon Garret. 1978. "Sexism and racism in the American health care industry: A comparative analysis." International Journal of Health Services 8, 4: 677–703.

Weiss, Kay. 1975. "What medical students learn about women." Off Our Backs, April/May. (Reprinted pp. 212–22 in Dreifus [Ed.], 1977.)

Wertz, Richard, and Dorothy Wertz. 1977. Lying-In, A History of Childbirth in America. New York: Schocken Books.

21

Suffer the Children: Some Effects of Racism on the Health of Black Infants

Wornie L. Reed

The life expectancy of Americans is greater now than ever before, mostly as a result of the increasing survival rate of infants. From this we may conclude that the overall health status of the population has improved, most probably as the result of improvements in the social environment (e.g., sanitation and nutrition) and developments in medical technology and the delivery of medical services. We may also assume that these improvements in general health and in medical services have occurred similarly for all Americans. However, we cannot assume that these improvements have occurred evenly across all population subgroups. In truth, these improvements in health have not been consistent across the board, especially in regards to black Americans. Although black Americans have benefited from these developments through improved health status, as would be expected, the true test of how these developments have affected this subgroup is to examine how blacks have fared relative to other subgroups, especially white Americans. This kind of examination reveals differential effects, with blacks consistently receiving the short end. The causes of this differentiation can be traced to institutional racism.

Institutional racism is to be distinguished from race prejudice and individual racism which, respectively, refer to individual attitudes and individual behaviors (Jones 1972). Institutional racism is racism inherent in and manifested in the outcomes of institutional operations.

> Institutional racism can be defined as those established laws, customs, and practices which systematically reflect and produce racial inequities in American society. If racist consequences accrue to institutional laws, customs, or practices, the institution is racist *whether or not the individuals maintaining those practices have racist intentions*. Institutional racism can be either overt or covert (corresponding to *de jure* and *de facto*, respectively) and either intentional or unintentional. (Jones 1972: 131; emphasis in original.)

Detailed treatments of institutional racism can be found in Carmichael and Hamilton (1967), Knowles and Prewitt (1969), and United States Commission on Civil Disorders (1968).

Several health problems can be used to illustrate the disadvantaged position of blacks, including hypertension, which is 235 percent higher in blacks than in whites, and sickle-cell anemia, a genetic disease found mostly in blacks. The debilitating effects of hypertension in the black community—including major incapacity through increased incidence of strokes—suggest a need for more research and more community screening programs than currently exist. Although the belated attention to sickle-cell anemia over the past decade has resulted in the creation of more basic research programs in this disease, it has also resulted in the creation of a potential mechanism for further racism. Many blacks have expressed considerable concern about the programs' thrust toward mandatory genetic screening programs (Wilkinson 1974).

The health problems of black Americans may best be illustrated, however, by examining infant mortality (i.e., children dying before one year of age).

> One of the most critical indices used nationally and internationally to interpret the status of a population group is the infant mortality rate. The infant mortality rate is the number of children dying before one year of age per 1,000 live births. The sensitivity of this index is that it provides clues to the nutritional status of the mother and the family, the housing condition, the health care situation, the income level and the overall socio-economic condition. In other words, a high infant mortality rate is indicative of an overall deprivation which impinges on the health of a population group. (Darity and Pitt, 1979: 128.)

In fact, the largest factor in increasing life expectancy has been the reduction in infant mortality in the general population. Thus, the high black infant mortality rate is to some degree reflected in the differential between life expectancies of blacks and whites.

Infant Mortality

As we look at infant mortality, it may be helpful to remember that it is but the tip of the iceberg and indicative of a more general problem of unhealthy infants. The two primary causes of infant mortality are low birth weight and congenital disorders, with low birth weight leading to other problems, including mental retardation, birth defects, growth and developmental problems, blindness, autism, cerebral palsy, and epilepsy (U. S. Department of Health, Education and Welfare, 1979).

Among selected industrialized countries, the United States ranked 10th in infant mortality in 1971, and 10th in 1976 (see Table 1), even though the rate of infant mortality was declining in all these countries. Why does

Table 1.
Infant Mortality Rates: Selected Countries, 1976 (Rates per 1,000 live births)

Country	Infant Mortality Rate
Sweden	8.7
Japan	9.3
Switzerland	10.5
Netherlands	10.5
France	12.5
England and Wales	14.0
German Democratic Republic	14.1
Australia	14.3
Canada	14.3
United States	15.2
German Federal Republic	17.4
Italy	19.1
Israel	22.9

SOURCE: U. S. DHEW. Health-United States 1978. Washington, D. C.: Department of Health, Education and Welfare (DHEW Publication No. 78-1232).

the United States lag behind nine other industrialized countries in infant mortality rates? Clearly, one major reason is the high death rate among nonwhite infants (Metropolitan Life, 1970).

Table 2 shows that although both white and black infant mortality rates have decreased substantially over the period between 1950 and 1976, the gap between black and white rates has increased. In 1950, the black infant mortality rate exceeded the white rate by less than two-thirds; yet, in 1976, the black rate exceeded the white rate by almost one hundred percent. Further, the black rate has not decreased as rapidly as that of other nonwhites. In 1950, the black rate was some 20 percent less than the rate for other nonwhites, yet it was nearly twice as high twenty years later in 1970. The decrease among other nonwhites has been mostly the result of a crash health program among Native Americans, which program's success demonstrates the capability of the Federal Government to further equity when it wishes to do so (Darity and Pitt, 1979).

Race and Infant Mortality

To understand the relationship between racism and infant mortality it is necessary to examine some of the factors related to poor infant health. One factor long associated with poor infant health and infant mortality is social class. Consequently, a common explanation for high black infant

Table 2.
Infant Mortality Rates by Race: United States 1950–1974 (Rates per 1,000 live births)

Year	All Races	White	Black	All Races Excluding Black and White	Ratio Black/White
1950	29.2	26.8	43.9	55.2	1.64
1955	26.4	23.6	43.1	38.4	1.83
1960	26.0	22.9	44.3	31.2	1.93
1965	24.7	21.5	41.7	26.0	1.94
1970	20.0	17.8	32.6	16.3	1.83
1975	16.1	14.2	26.8	NA*	1.89
1976	15.2	13.3	26.2	NA*	1.97

*Not Ascertained.

SOURCE: *Health of the Disadvantaged—Chart Book,* DHEW Pub. No. (HRA) 77-628, 1977.

mortality is the greater proportion of blacks who are poor. In point of fact, infant mortality rates are known to be sensitive to economic instability (Brenner, 1973). However, there is an excess of black infant mortality *beyond* that explained by socioeconomic status.

Data in Table 3, which show the inverse relationships between infant mortality and socioeconomic status (SES), also show a race effect over and above the class effect. First, the black infant mortality rate greatly exceeds the white rate in each category of the socioeconomic indices. Further examination of the table shows that the highest SES blacks have higher rates of infant mortality than the lowest SES whites. In fact, blacks with some college education have more infant mortality than whites with no more than an eighth grade education. In addition, the rate for blacks earning greater than $7,000, in 1964–1966, was greater than that of whites earning under $3,000.

To understand the many tentacles of racism and how they affect infant mortality, it is helpful to look at: (1) processes that develop conditions conducive to poor infant health, (2) processes that affect acquisition of requisite health care services, and (3) processes constituting the response of the medical care system to the problem of poor infant health. As we shall see, institutional racism places black infants in "triple jeopardy."

Class Inequity

One of the factors contributing to the high black infant mortality rate is economic discrimination. One result of economic discrimination/racism is the "placement" of a disproportionately high number of blacks and other nonwhites into the lower socioeconomic status groups. For example, 40

Table 3.
Infant Mortality Rates by Race and Socioeconomic Status: United States 1964–1966 (Rates per 1,000 Live Births)

Socioeconomic Index	All Races	White	Black
Father's Education			
Grade 8 or Less	33.0	30.3	42.4
Grades 9–11	27.4	23.9	44.8
Grade 12	19.0	17.6	32.2
1–3 Years of College	20.6	19.0	37.6
4 Years College or More	17.4	17.0	*
Mother's Education			
Grade 8 or Less	35.2	32.0	45.9
Grades 9–11	27.7	24.6	41.7
Grade 12	19.5	18.0	34.5
1–3 Years of College	15.9	15.0	32.1
4 Years College or More	20.0	19.6	*
Family Income			
Under $3,000	32.1	27.3	42.5
$3,000–4,999	25.1	22.1	46.8
5,000–6,999	18.1	17.8	22.0
7,000–9,999	19.9	19.2	37.6
10,000 or More	19.9	19.4	*

*Numbers too small for estimation.
SOURCE: National Center for Health Statistics, Series 22, No. 14.

percent of blacks are below the poverty level compared to only 10 percent of whites. As shown above, infant mortality is directly connected with socioeconomic status; and more blacks are poor because of institutional racism, which limits opportunity structures (United States Commission on Civil Disorders, 1968).

Residential Segregation

The development of the so-called black ghettoes is another of the racist processes that contributes to the black population being so greatly "at risk" to infant mortality.

> What white Americans have never fully understood—but what the Negro can never forget—is that white society is deeply implicated in the ghetto. White institutions created it, white institutions maintain it, and white society condones it. (U.S. Commission on Civil Disorders, 1968: 2.)

In 1910, some 73 percent of the black population in the United States were living in rural areas. Fifty years later the proportions reversed; some

73 percent of the black population lived in urban areas (Taeuber and Taeuber 1965). Like the European immigrants of earlier decades, blacks took the lowest status positions in the urban social structure. And, also like the European immigrants, blacks were restricted in their opportunities for housing. This residential segregation ("ghettoization") created a new urban underclass, in this case an underclass defined by race.

However, in sharp contrast to the immigrants, blacks remained at the bottom of the social structure. Black ghettoes expanded instead of disappearing. As black populations grew, residential boundaries were redrawn in ever widening circles, consistently circumscribing the area.

The restriction of blacks to circumscribed areas is more than a matter of economics. Regardless of income, blacks have been limited to well-defined housing areas. Taeuber and Taeuber (1965:2–3) studied the patterns of racial residential segregation and reached this conclusion:

> The poverty of urban Negroes is often regarded as contributory to their residential segregation. Because low-cost housing tends to be segregated from high-cost housing, any low-income group within the city will be residentially segregated to some extent from those with higher incomes. Economic factors, however, cannot account for more than a small portion of observed levels of racial residential segregation. Regardless of their economic status, Negroes rarely live in "white" residential areas, while whites, no matter how poor, rarely live in "Negro" residential areas. In recent decades Negroes have been much more successful in securing improvements in economic status than in obtaining housing on a less segregated basis. Continued economic gains by Negroes are not likely to alter substantially the prevalent patterns of racial residential segregation.

Taeuber (1968) found that whites and blacks were very highly segregated from each other regardless of social class. Updating these findings and using data from the 1970 United States Census as well as the 1950 and 1960 censuses, Shimkus (1978) found that racial residential segregation was still quite high regardless of occupation. In fact, racial residential segregation is much higher than gross occupational segregation.

This ghettoization is the result of social processes that clearly represent institutional racism. Blackwell (1975) discusses several techniques that worked to bring about the ghettoization of blacks in the United States. Among these are government policy, the operation of the real estate system, zoning laws, restrictive covenants, and violence against blacks.

The federal government itself has greatly contributed to housing discrimination. The Federal Housing Administration, created during the new deal in the 1930s, had an official policy of redlining and segregating residential areas. Its handbook explicitly discouraged the granting of mortgages for houses located in racially mixed residential areas. Further, although the Housing Act of 1937 brought the beginning of public housing for the poor, few blacks were permitted to occupy this housing. Ironically, a current method of racial exclusion is the establishment of zoning ordinances to keep public housing out of predominately "white" areas, since many blacks now occupy public housing.

Another problem area has been the real estate system. White agents generally refused to sell blacks housing that was located in racially mixed areas. Indeed, for a considerable period of time there were no black real estate agents, and when an association of black real estate agents was eventually formed, they were forbidden to label themselves as "realtors," thus limiting their credibility and acceptability. (They became "realtists"!)

State and local zoning laws were—and are—used as instruments of ghettoization. In the early part of this century, zoning laws dealt explicitly with race, specifically excluding blacks from occupying housing in certain areas. Nowadays, racist zoning ordinances are much more subtle, using such stand-in devices as lot size, unit size, land use, and family size to block entry of blacks into residential areas.

Restrictive covenants, agreements in housing purchase contracts that the property will not be sold to persons in specified racial, religious and ethnic groups, were permitted by the courts until the 1950s, thus giving legal sanction to a very powerful mechanism for racial exclusion.

When all else failed, physical violence was often used to restrict the residential movement of blacks. Although this method of restriction is somewhat less common today, it is by no means a thing of the past, a fact amply testified to by current newspaper reports.

All of these actions have combined to create and to maintain black ghettoized areas and to affect the lives of the residents through socio-environmental and other factors associated with ghettoes. The high mortality rate of black infants is but one consequence, albeit a particularly severe one, of institutional racism.

Ghettoization may indirectly affect infant mortality in several ways. One way is through environmental factors such as overcrowding, poor housing, and lack of sanitary environment. These conditions, typical of black ghettoes, are associated with high rates of infant mortality. Yankauer (1950) found that both white and nonwhite infant mortality rates whithin ghettoized areas rise as levels of segregation increase. While early infant deaths (neonatal mortality) and fetal deaths are related to the health of pregnant women, infant deaths between the end of the first month of life and the first year (post-neonatal mortality) are related to the environmental health as well as the medical care of infants (Stockwell, 1962; Chabot et al., 1975). Another way that ghettoization affects infant mortality is through subordinating, segregating, and precluding blacks from health facilities. Few medical facilities exist in these areas, and many existing ones are characterized by well-known barriers to access, such as travel time to the facility, waiting time to make appointments, and waiting time in the facility, before seeing a health care provider. These barriers contribute to a tendency to underutilize medical facilities.

The Medical Care System

Since high infant mortality implies inadequate medical care and since some studies find barriers to utilization within the health care delivery system itself (Reissman 1974; Dutton 1978; Bullough 1972), it is instructive to examine the health care delivery system vis-à-vis its response to the high black infant mortality rate.

First, we will look at relative access to prenatal care, and then discuss two developments that illustrate inappropriateness of response by the medical system to black infant mortality: (1) the rapid growth of federally supported family planning clinics, and (2) the suggested cutback in training of new physicians.

Prenatal Care

The infant mortality rate of a community has long been regarded as one of the most sensitive indicators of the general health of the population and of the effectiveness of prevailing medical care. It can also be viewed as an indirect measure of the adequacy of prenatal care programs. (National Center for Health Statistics, 1970: 14.)

Prenatal care is a significant factor in infant birth weight: most evidence shows birth weight and prematurity to be highly associated with high infant morbidity and mortality (National Center for Health Statistics, 1972; Kessner et al., 1973). A national study by the National Center for Health Statistics (1972) showed that infants weighing 2,500 grams or less at birth had an infant mortality rate 17 times higher than that of infants weighing over 2,500 grams. A much smaller percentage of white infants than nonwhite infants are born weighing less than 2,500 grams. For example, in 1970, 13.3 percent of all nonwhite babies had low birth weight compared to only 6.8 percent of white babies. Table 4 provides an estimate of what the infant mortality rate would have been for a given poverty-race group if the proportion of low birth weight babies was the same as in a standard population. The observed low birth weight rate for the total United States in 1960 was 7.8 percent. If the percent of low birth weight babies for nonwhites in poverty areas had been 7.8 instead of the observed 15.1, then the infant mortality rate would have been 22.0 instead of the actual 33.5 per 1,000 live births. Thus, the infant mortality rate of nonwhites in poverty areas would be over 50 percent less (National Center for Health Statistics, 1976).

Birth weight, well established as a factor in infant mortality, is affected by both the timing and the amount of prenatal medical visits. As shown in Table 5, over 22 percent of infants of all races for which no prenatal care is obtained will have low birth weight as against less than 3.3 percent if the pregnant woman has between thirteen and sixteen medical visits. Also,

Table 4.
Observed and Birth-Weight-Adjusted
Infant Mortality Rates, by Poverty Status
of Area of Residence and Race: United
States, 1969–1971 Average (Rates per
1,000 live births)

| | Infant Mortality Rates | |
Area and Race	*Observed*	*Adjusted*
Poverty Areas		
White	24.2	21.8
Nonwhite	33.5	22.0
Nonpoverty		
White	17.4	18.4
Nonwhite	27.0	20.3

SOURCE: National Center for Health Statistics,
1970:15.

if prenatal care is obtained during the first three months, the percentage of low birth weight babies will be smaller than if prenatal care begins later than the third month.

According to standards offered by the American College of Obstetricians and Gynecologists (cited in National Center for Health Statistics, 1978), pregnant women should ideally have approximately thirteen prenatal visits for a full-term pregnancy, with more visits if health problems occur. A minimum standard is nine visits. Yet, on the average, only slightly more than half of black mothers meet this standard compared to three-fourths of white mothers (National Center for Health Statistics, 1978a). Approximately twice the proportion of black mothers in comparison to white mothers received late care (in the third trimester) or no care at all. Obviously, lack of prenatal care among pregnant black women must be viewed as a serious problem.

Family Planning Clinics

From 1970 through 1975 the number of federally supported family planning clinics increased from 890 to 4,940, with an eightfold increase in patients (National Center for Health Statistics, 1978b), a growth rate that has caused some concern. This concern is not an argument against the use of, or the need for, family planning, family planning clinics, or abortion. However, one might question the growth and location of these family planning clinics compared to the growth and location of programs for prenatal care. The question is whether family planning clinics were a greater need than prenatal programs.

Table 5.
Percent of Infants of Low Birth Weight, by Number of
Prenatal Visits and Race: 37 States and the District of
Columbia, 1975

Number of Prenatal Visits	All Races*	White	Black
Total	7.4	6.2	13.2
No Visits	22.2	18.9	27.9
1 to 4 Visits	19.6	18.5	22.4
5 to 8 Visits	11.5	10.8	14.0
9 to 12 Visits	4.9	4.3	9.0
13 to 16 Visits	3.3	2.9	7.1

*Includes races other than white and black.
SOURCE: National Center for Health Statistics, 1978a, p. 23.

The intended user group for these clinics is suggested by the following data from the National Center for Health Statistics (1979a). Of black women 15–55 years of age in the population, approximately 144 per 1,000 had enrolled by 1976 in family planning clinics compared to only 44 per 1,000 white women in this group. Fewer black women than whites used any kind of family planning services (46.2 percent compared to 59.2 percent), yet proportionately more black women enrolled in these public clinics. The racial breakdown between the users of private physicians and family planning clinics illustrates this further. Seventeen percent of the currently married fecund (physiologically able to reproduce) black women, 15 to 44 years of age, used these clinics compared to only 8.3 percent of white women in the same age group. On the other hand, only 29.1 percent of married fecund black women in the 15–44 age group used private physicians against 50.8 percent of white women in this category (National Center for Health Statistics, 1979b). So, during the period of time in which the gap between black and white infant mortality rates was increasing, and while more prenatal services and a better allocation of resources were being requested, there was a rapid increase in public family planning clinics accessible to black women.

Of course, family planning programs and legalized abortion did result in a reduction in black as well as white infant mortality (Roghmann, 1975; Pakter and Nelson, 1974; Lee et al., 1980). They did so by decreasing the incidence of low birth weight babies, the high risk group. On the other hand, there was no improvement in the weight distribution of live births in the United States between 1950 and 1975. Although proportionately as many low birth weight babies were born in 1975 as in 1950, birth weight specific neonatal mortality declined during this period, and it did so at an accelerated pace after the launching of maternal and infant care projects in

1964. The bulk of the evidence suggests that credit for much of the improvement in birth weight specific mortality should be given to maternal and infant care projects and not to abortion or family planning (Lee et al., 1980). The conclusion one must draw is that more, and better, perinatal care might produce more reductions in infant mortality. This would, of course, be beneficial to the black community, which has twice the rate of low birth weight babies as whites.

Limitations on Training Physicians

In the face of the growing concern for the relative lack of medical services in the ghettoized areas, two recent health-policy pronouncements by federal officials forecast the intention to reverse the policy of encouraging medical schools to increase their enrollments. Secretary of Health, Education and Welfare Califano (cited in Darity and Pitt, 1979), referring to a "glut of doctors," proposed that medical schools reduce the size of their classes. In addition, an official from the Office of Management and Budget discussed proposed drastic cuts in health program financing, including those programs that helped black and other minority students to attend medical schools. Yet, data suggest that the black community is underserved rather than "glutted." To the black community, these proposed cutbacks and the current maldistribution of physicians are unfavorable systematic responses to black infant mortality—and further indications of institutional racism.

Discussion

The approximately 15 percent infant mortality rate of the early 1900s was reduced to about 3 percent in the 1950s (through measures such as improved sanitation, personal hygiene, and nutrition) and to approximately 1½ percent in the mid-1970s. Some health policy investigators (McNamara et al., 1978) suggest that a national goal of 1 percent or less (as in Sweden, Japan, Switzerland and the Netherlands) through intensive public intervention will be difficult and quite costly to achieve. This may very well be true. However, it would surely seem that enlightened public policy should attempt to alleviate the great racial inequities in infant mortality, where the current rate in the black community is approximately equivalent to the white rate in the 1950s. Some 6,000 black infants die each year who would be living if the infant mortality rate observed for black infants in a geographic region was as low as that for white infants in the same area (Kovar, 1979).

Generally, reformers suggest attacks on poverty-related factors. These include nutritional programs for poor pregnant mothers and infants, programs to train paramedical personnel to educate expectant mothers on the benefits of prenatal and preventive care, and, most importantly, the provision of free medical care for all poor expectant mothers and for children up to one year of age (Seham 1970).

Maternity and Infant Care (MIC) projects have been quite successful at reaching vulnerable populations and in bringing about subsequent declines in low birth weight incidence and infant mortality (DHEW, 1979). Some urban MIC programs are attacking the problem by better coordination of programs and by outreach programs, including casefinding and surveillance (Gentry, 1979). One study showed that a community health center with an outreach program in prenatal care was used nearly twice as readily as a hospital-based health center program (Birch and Wolfe, 1976).

While some MIC clinics, properly located and staffed, are having success in reducing local infant mortality, many local prenatal programs are understaffed, fragmented, and unsuccessful at reaching pregnant women early enough. Although maternal and infant care providers tend to be confident that good prenatal care helps, some are pessimistic about major progress without direct efforts to eliminate economic and social problems. For example, one local program director feels that "the most effective thing we could do is raise the employment level among young adults. That might do more than all the new hospitals and prenatal units and doctors combined" (Freivogel, 1979).

This assessment returns to center stage the background issue—racial discrimination in economic and social institutions, or institutional racism. With teenage unemployment reaching epidemic proportions in the black community—currently greater than among any other population group in recent American history—and with no program or social policy to reverse this trend, the prognosis for improvement in the black infant mortality rate looks bleak, even if some of the other problems raised above are solved.

References

Birch, J. S., and S. Wolfe, 1976, "New and Traditional Sources of Care Evaluated by Recently Pregnant Women." Public Health Reports 91: 413.

Blackwell, J. 1975. The Black Community. New York: Harper and Row Publishers.

Brenner, M. H. 1973. "Fetal, Infant and Maternal Mortality During Periods of Economic Instability." International Journal of Health Services 3: 145–159.

Bullough, B. 1972. "Poverty, Ethnic Identity and Preventive Health Care." Journal of Health and Social Behavior 13: 347–59.

Carmichael, S., and C. Hamilton. 1967. Black Power: The Politics of Liberation in America. New York: Random House.

Chabot, M., J. Garfinkel, and M. W. Pratt. 1975. "Urbanization and Differentials in White and Nonwhite Infant Mortality." Pediatrics 56: 777–81.

Darity, W. A., and E. W. Pitt. 1979. "Health Status of Black Americans." In

National Urban League, The State of Black America—1979. Washington, D.C.: National Urban League.

Dutton, D. B. 1978. "Explaining the Low Use of Health Services by the Poor: Costs, Attitudes, or Delivery Systems?" American Sociological Review 43 (June): 348–68.

Freivogel, M. W. 1979. "Infant Death Rate Stays Grim Statistic Here." St. Louis Post-Dispatch, November 18, Section A, 1R.

Gentry, J. T. 1979. "Approaches to Reducing Infant Mortality." Urban Health 8: 27–30.

Jones, J. M. 1972. Prejudice and Racism. Reading, Mass.: Addison-Wesley Publishing Company.

Kessner, D. M., J. Singer, C. E. Kalk, and E. R. Schlesinger. 1973. Contrasts in Health Status. Vol. I. Infant Death: An Analysis by Maternal Risk and Health Care. Washington: Institute of Medicine, National Academy of Sciences.

Knowles, L. and K. Prewitt. 1969. Institutional Racism in America. Englewood Cliffs, N.J.: Prentice Hall.

Kovar, M. G. 1979. "Mortality of Black Infants in the United States." Phylon XXXVIII: 370–97.

Lee, K., N. Paneth, L. M. Gartner, M. A. Pearlman, and L. Gruss. 1980. "Neonatal Mortality: An Analysis of the Recent Improvement in the United States." American Journal of Public Health 70 (1): 15–21.

McNamara, J. J., S. Blumenthal, and C. Landers. 1978. "Trends in Infant Mortality in New York City Health Areas Served by Children and Youth Projects." Bulletin of the New York Academy of Medicine 54: 484–98.

Metropolitan Life. 1970. Statistical Bulletin. 51: 2.

National Center for Health Statistics. 1970. Selected Vital and Health Statistics in Poverty and Nonpoverty Areas of 19 Large Cities, United States 1969–71. Vital and Health Statistics. Series 21, Number 26. Washington, D.C.: U. S. Department of Health, Education and Welfare.

1972. A Study of Infant Mortality from Linked Records by Birth Weight. Series 20, No. 12 (May).

1976. Selected Vital and Health Statistics in Poverty and Nonpoverty Areas of 19 Large Cities, United States, 1969–71.

1978a. Prenatal Care. United States, 1969–75. Vital and Health Statistics. Series 21, Number 33. Washington, D.C.: U. S. Department of Health, Education and Welfare.

1978b. Background and Development of the National Reporting System for Family Planning Services. Vital and Health Statistics. Series 1, Number 13. Washington, D. C.: U.S. Department of Health, Education and Welfare.

1979a. Office Visits for Family Planning, National Ambulatory Medical Care Survey: United States, 1977. Advance Data from Vital and Health Statistics of the National Center for Health Statistics. Number 49. Washington, D.C.: U.S. Department of Health, Education and Welfare.

1979b. Use of Family Planning Services by Currently Married Women 15–44 Years of Age: United States, 1973 and 1976. Advance Data from Vital and Health Statistics of the National Center for Health Statistics. Number 45. Washington, D.C.: U.S. Department of Health, Education and Welfare.

Pakter, J. and F. Nelson. 1974. "Factors in the Unpredicted Decline in Infant Mortality in New York City." Bulletin of the New York Academy of Medicine 50: 839–68.

Riessman, C. K. 1974. "The Use of Health Services by the Poor." Social Policy 5: 41–9.

Roghmann, K. 1975. "Impact of New York State Abortion Law." Chapter 8 in Child Health and the Community. New York: Wiley.

Seham, M. 1973. Blacks and American Medical Care. Minneapolis: University of Minnesota Press.

Shimkus, A. A. 1978. "Residential Segregation by Occupation and Race in Ten Urbanized Areas, 1950–1970." American Sociological Review 43 (1): 81–93.

Stockwell, E. G. 1962. "Infant Mortality and Socio-economic Status: A Changing Relation." Milbank Memorial Fund Quarterly 40: 101–11.

Taeuber, K. E., and A. F. Taeuber. 1965. Negroes in Cities. Chicago: Aldine.

Taeuber, K. E. 1968. "The Effect of Income Redistribution on Racial Residential Segregation." Urban Affairs Quarterly 4: 5–14.

U. S. Commission on Civil Disorders. 1968. Report of the National Advisory Commission on Civil Disorders. New York: Bantam Books.

U. S. Department of Health, Education and Welfare. 1979. Healthy People: The Surgeon General's Report on Health Promotion and Disease Prevention. Washington, D.C.: U.S. Government Printing Office (DHEW Publication No. 79–55071).

Wilkinson, D. Y. 1974. "For Whose Benefit? Politics and Sickle Cell." The Black Scholar 8 (5): 26–31.

Yankauer, A. 1950. "The Relationship of Fetal and Infant Mortality to Residential Segregation." American Sociological Review 15: 644–48.

22

The Sexual Politics of Sickness

Barbara Ehrenreich and Deirdre English

When Charlotte Perkins Gilman collapsed with a "nervous disorder," the physician she sought out for help was Dr. S. Weir Mitchell, "the greatest nerve specialist in the country." It was Dr. Mitchell—female specialist, part-time novelist, and member of Philadelphia's high society—who had once screened Osler for a faculty position, and, finding him appropriately discreet in the disposal of cherry-pie pits, admitted the young doctor to medicine's inner circles. When Gilman met him, in the eighteen eighties, he was at the height of his career, earning over $60,000 per year (the equivalent of over $300,000 in today's dollars). His renown for the treatment of female nervous disorders had by this time led to a marked alteration of character. According to an otherwise fond biographer, his vanity "had become colossal. It was fed by torrents of adulation, incessant and exaggerated, every day, almost every hour...."[1]

Gilman approached the great man with "utmost confidence." A friend of her mother's lent her one hundred dollars for the trip to Philadelphia and Mitchell's treatment. In preparation, Gilman methodically wrote out a complete history of her case. She had observed, for example, that her sickness vanished when she was away from her home, her husband, and her child, and returned as soon as she came back to them. But Dr. Mitchell dismissed her prepared history as evidence of "self-conceit." He did not want information from his patients; he wanted "complete obedience." Gilman quotes his prescription for her:

> "Live as domestic a life as possible. Have your child with you all the time." (Be it remarked that if I did but dress the baby it left me shaking and crying—certainly far from a healthy companionship for her, to say nothing of the effect on me.) "Lie down an hour after each meal. Have but two hours intellectual life a day. And never touch pen, brush or pencil as long as you live."[2]

Gilman dutifully returned home and for some months attempted to follow Dr. Mitchell's orders to the letter. The result, in her words was—

> ... [I] came perilously close to losing my mind. The mental agony grew so unbearable that I would sit blankly moving my head from side to side... I would crawl into remote closets and under beds—to hide from the grinding pressure of that distress....[3]

Finally, in a "moment of clear vision" Gilman understood the source of her illness: she did not want to be a *wife;* she wanted to be a writer and an activist. So, discarding S. Weir Mitchell's prescription and divorcing her husband, she took off for California with her baby, her pen, her brush and pencil. But she never forgot Mitchell and his near-lethal "cure." Three years after her recovery she wrote *The Yellow Wallpaper*[4] a fictionalized account of her own illness and descent into madness. If that story had any influence on S. Weir Mitchell's method of treatment, she wrote after a long life of accomplishments, "I have not lived in vain."[5]

Charlotte Perkins Gilman was fortunate enough to have had a "moment of clear vision" in which she understood what was happening to her. Thousands of other women, like Gilman, were finding themselves in a new position of dependency on the male medical profession—and with no alternative sources of information or counsel. The medical profession was consolidating its monopoly over healing, and now the woman who felt sick, or tired or simply depressed would no longer seek help from a friend or female healer, but from a male physician. The general theory which guided the doctors' practice as well as their public pronouncements was that women were, by nature, weak, dependent, and diseased. Thus would the doctors attempt to secure their victory over the female healer: with the "scientific" evidence that woman's essential nature was not to be a strong, competent help-giver, but to be a *patient*.

A Mysterious Epidemic

In fact at the time there were reasons to think that the doctors' theory was not so farfetched. Women were decidedly sickly, though not for the reasons the doctors advanced. In the mid- and late nineteenth century a curious epidemic seemed to be sweeping through the middle- and upper-class female population both in the United States and England. Diaries and journals from the time give us hundreds of examples of women slipping into hopeless invalidism. For example, when Catherine Beecher, the educator, finished a tour in 1871 which included visits to dozens of relatives, friends and former students, she reported "a terrible decay of female health all over the land," which was "increasing in a most alarming ratio." The notes from her travels go like this:

> Milwaukee, Wis. Mrs. A. frequent sick headaches. Mrs. B. very feeble. Mrs. S. well, except chills. Mrs. L. poor health constantly. Mrs. D. subject to frequent headaches. Mrs. B. very poor health . . .
>
> Mrs. H. pelvic disorders and a cough. Mrs. B. always sick. Do not know one perfectly healthy woman in the place. . . .[6]

Doctors found a variety of diagnostic labels for the wave of invalidism gripping the female population: "Neurasthenia," "nervous prostration," "hyperesthesia," "cardiac inadequacy," "dyspepsia," "rheumatism," and "hysteria." The symptoms included headache, muscular aches, weakness, depression, menstrual difficulties, indigestion, etc., and usually a general debility requiring constant rest. S. Weir Mitchell described it as follows:

> The woman grows pale and thin, eats little, or if she eats does not profit by it. Everything wearies her,—to sew, to write, to read, to walk,—and by and by the sofa or the bed is her only comfort. Every effort is paid for dearly, and she describes herself as aching and sore, as sleeping ill, and as needing constant stimulus and endless tonics. . . . If such a person is emotional she does not fail to become more so, and even the firmest women lose self-control at last under incessant feebleness.[7]

The syndrome was never fatal, but neither was it curable in most cases, the victims sometimes patiently outliving both husbands and physicians.

Women who recovered to lead full and active lives—like Charlotte Perkins Gilman and Jane Addams—were the exceptions. Ann Greene Phillips—a feminist and abolitionist in the eighteen thirties—first took ill during her courtship. Five years after her marriage, she retired to bed, more or less permanently. S. Weir Mitchell's unmarried sister fell prey to an unspecified "great pain" shortly after taking over housekeeping for her brother (whose first wife had just died), and embarked on a life of invalidism. Alice James began her career of invalidism at the age of nineteen, always amazing her older brothers, Henry (the novelist) and William (the psychologist), with the stubborn intractability of her condition: "Oh, woe, woe is me!" she wrote in her diary:

> . . . all hopes of peace and rest are vanishing—nothing but the dreary snail-like climb up a little way, so as to be able to run down again! And then these doctors tell you that you will die or *recover!* But you *don't* recover. I have been at these alterations since I was nineteen and I am neither dead nor recovered. As I am now forty-two, there has surely been time for either process.[8]

The sufferings of these women were real enough. Ann Phillips wrote, ". . . life is a burden to me, I do not know what to do. I am tired of suffering. I have no faith in anything."[9] Some thought that if the illness wouldn't kill them, they would do the job themselves. Alice James discussed suicide with her father, and rejoiced, at the age of forty-three, when informed she had developed breast cancer and would die within months: "I count it the greatest good fortune to have these few months so full of interest and instruction in the knowledge of my approaching death."[10] Mary Galloway shot herself in the head while being attended in her apartment by a physician and a nurse. She was thirty-one years old, the daughter of a bank and utility company president. According to the New York *Times* account (April 10, 1905), "She had been a chronic dyspeptic since 1895, and that is the only reason known for her suicide."[11]

Marriage: The Sexual Economic Relation

In the second half of the nineteenth century the vague syndrome gripping middle- and upper-class women had become so widespread as to represent not so much a disease in the medical sense as a way of life. More precisely, the way this type of woman was expected to live predisposed her to sickness, and sickness in turn predisposed her to continue to live as she was expected to. The delicate, affluent lady, who was completely dependent on her husband, set the sexual romanticist ideal of femininity for women of all classes.

Clear-headed feminists like Charlotte Perkins Gilman and Olive Schreiner saw a link between female invalidism and the economic situation of women in the upper classes. As they observed, poor women did not suffer from the syndrome. The problem in the middle to upper classes was that marriage had become a "sexuo-economic relation" in which women performed sexual and reproductive duties for financial support. It was a relationship which Olive Schreiner bluntly called "female parasitism."

To Gilman's pragmatic mind, the affluent wife appeared to be a sort of tragic evolutionary anomaly, something like the dodo. She did not work: that is, there was no serious, productive work to do in the home, and the tasks which were left—keeping house, cooking and minding the children—she left as much as possible to the domestic help. She was, biologically speaking, specialized for one function and one alone—sex. Hence the elaborate costume—bustles, false fronts, wasp waists—which caricatured the natural female form. Her job was to bear the heirs of the businessman, lawyer, or professor she had married, which is what gave her a claim to any share of his income. When Gilman, in her depression, turned away from her own baby, it was because she already understood, in a half-conscious way, that the baby was living proof of her economic dependence—and as it seemed to her, sexual degradation.

A "lady" had one other important function, as Veblen pointed out with acerbity in the *Theory of the Leisure Class*. And that was to do precisely nothing, that is nothing of any economic or social consequence.[12] A successful man could have no better social ornament than an idle wife. Her delicacy, her culture, her childlike ignorance of the male world gave a man the "class" which money alone could not buy. A virtuous wife spent a hushed and peaceful life indoors, sewing, sketching, planning menus, and supervising the servants and children. The more adventurous might fill their leisure with shopping excursions, luncheons, balls, and novels. A "lady" could be charming, but never brilliant; interested, but not intense. Dr. Mitchell's second wife, Mary Cadwalader, was perhaps a model of her type: she "made no pretense at brilliancy; her first thought was to be a foil to her husband. . . ."[13] By no means was such a lady to concern herself with politics, business, international affairs, or the aching injustices of the industrial work world.

But not even the most sheltered woman lived on an island detached from the "real" world of men. Schreiner described the larger context:

> Behind the phenomenon of female parasitism has always lain another and yet larger social phenomenon . . . the subjugation of large bodies of other human creatures, either as slaves, subject races, or classes; and as a result of the excessive labors of those classes there has always been an accumulation of unearned wealth in the hands of the dominant class or race. *It has invariably been by feeding on this wealth, the result of forced or ill-paid labor,* that the female of the dominant race or class has in the past lost her activity and has come to exist purely through the passive performance of her sexual functions.[14]
> (Emphasis in original)

The leisured lady, whether she knew it or not and whether she cared or not, inhabited the same social universe as dirt-poor black sharecroppers, six-year-old children working fourteen-hour days for subsubsistence wages, young men mutilated by unsafe machinery or mine explosions, girls forced into prostitution by the threat of starvation. At no time in American history was the contradiction between ostentatious wealth and unrelenting poverty, between idleness and exhaustion, starker than it was then in the second half of the nineteenth century. There were riots in the cities, insurrections in the mines, rumors of subversion and assassination. Even the secure business or professional man could not be sure that he too would not be struck down by an economic downturn, a wily competitor, or (as seemed likely at times) a social revolution.

The genteel lady of leisure was as much a part of the industrial social order as her husband or his employees. As Schreiner pointed out, it was ultimately the wealth extracted in the world of work that enabled a man to afford a more or less ornamental wife. And it was the very harshness of that outside world that led men to see the home as a refuge—"a sacred place, a vestal temple," a "tent pitch'd in a world not right," presided over by a a gentle, ethereal wife. A popular home health guide advised that

> . . . [man's] feelings are frequently lacerated to the utmost point of endurance, by collisions, irritations, and disappointments. To recover his equanimity and composure, home must be a place of repose, of peace, of cheerfulness, of comfort; then his soul renews its strength, and will go forth, with fresh vigor, to encounter the labor and troubles of the world.[15]

No doubt the suffocating atmosphere of sexual romanticism bred a kind of nervous hypochondria. We will never know, for example, if Alice James's lifelong illness had a "real" organic basis. But we know that, unlike her brothers, she was never encouraged to go to college or to develop her gift for writing. She was high-strung and imaginative, but *she* could not be brilliant or productive. Illness was perhaps the only honorable retreat from a world of achievement which (it seemed at the time) nature had not equipped her to enter.

For many other women, to various degrees, sickness became a part of life, even a way of filling time. The sexuo-economic relation confined women to the life of the body, so it was to the body that they directed their energies and intellect. Rich women frequented resortlike health spas and the offices of elegant specialists like S. Weir Mitchell. A magazine cartoon from the eighteen seventies shows two "ladies of fashion" meeting in an ornately appointed waiting room. "What, *you* here, Lizzie? Why, ain't you well?" asks the first patient. "Perfectly thanks!" answers the second. "But what's the matter with *you,* dear?" "Oh, nothing whatever! I'm as right as possible dear."[16] For less well-off women there were patent medicines, family doctors, and, starting in the eighteen fifties, a steady stream of popular advice books, written by doctors, on the subject of female health. It was acceptable, even stylish, to retire to bed with "sick headaches," "nerves" and various unmentionable "female troubles," and that indefinable nervous disorder "neurasthenia" was considered, in some circles, to be a mark of intellect and sensitivity. Dr. Mary Putnam Jacobi, a female regular physician, observed impatiently in 1895:

> ... it is considered natural and almost laudable to break down under all conceivable varieties of strain—a winter dissipation, a houseful of servants, a quarrel with a female friend, not to speak of more legitimate reasons. . . . Women who expect to go to bed every menstrual period expect to collapse if by chance they find themselves on their feet for a few hours during such a crisis. Constantly considering their nerves, urged to consider them by well-intentioned but short-sighted advisors, they pretty soon become nothing but a bundle of nerves.[17]

But if sickness was a reaction, on women's part, to a difficult situation, it was not a way out. If you have to be idle, you might as well be sick, and sickness, in turn, legitimates idleness. From the romantic perspective, the sick woman was not that far off from the ideal woman anyway. A morbid aesthetic developed, in which sickness was seen as a source of female beauty, and beauty—in the high-fashion sense—was in fact a source of sickness. Over and over, nineteenth-century romantic paintings feature the beautiful invalid, sensuously drooping on her cushions, eyes fixed tremulously at her husband or physician, or already gazing into the Beyond. Literature aimed at female readers lingered on the romantic pathos of illness and death; popular women's magazines featured such stories as "The Grave of My Friend" and "Song of Dying." Society ladies cultivated a sickly countenance by drinking vinegar in quantity or, more effectively, arsenic.[18] The loveliest heroines were those who died young, like Beth in *Little Women,* too good and too pure for life in this world.

Meanwhile, the requirements of fashion insured that the well-dressed woman would actually be as frail and ornamental as she looked. The style of wearing tight-laced corsets, which was *de rigeur* throughout the last half of the century, has to be ranked somewhere close to the old Chinese practice of foot-binding for its crippling effects on the female body. A fashionable woman's corsets exerted, on the average, twenty-one pounds of pressure on her internal organs, and extremes of up to eighty-eight pounds had been measured.[19] (Add to this the fact that a well-dressed woman wore an average of thirty-seven pounds of street clothing in the winter months, of which nineteen pounds were suspended from her tortured waist.[20]) Some of the short-term results of tight-lacing were shortness of breath, constipation, weakness, and a tendency to violent indigestion. Among the long-term effects were bent or fractured ribs, displacement of the liver, and uterine prolapse (in some cases, the uterus would be gradually forced, by the pressure of the corset, out through the vagina).

The morbidity of nineteenth-century tastes in female beauty reveals the hostility which never lies too far below the surface of sexual romanticism. To be sure, the romantic spirit puts woman on a pedestal and ascribes to her every tender viture absent from the Market. But carried to an extreme the demand that woman be a *negation* of man's world left almost nothing for women to actually *be:* if men are busy, she is idle; if men are rough, she is gentle; if men are strong, she is frail; if men are rational, she is irrational; and so on. The logic which insists that femininity is negative masculinity necessarily romanticizes the moribund woman and encourages a kind of paternalistic necrophilia. In the nineteenth century this tendency becomes overt, and the romantic spirit holds up as its ideal—the *sick* woman, the invalid who lives at the edge of death.

Femininity as a Disease

The medical profession threw itself with gusto on the languid figure of the female invalid. In the home of an invalid lady, "the house physician like a house fly is in chronic attention"[21] and the doctors fairly swarmed after wealthy patients. Few were so successful as S. Weir Mitchell in establishing himself as *the* doctor for hundreds of loyal clients. Yet the doctors' constant ministrations and interventions—surgical, electrical, hydropathic, mesmeric, chemical—seemed to be of little use. In fact, it would have been difficult, in many cases, to distinguish the *cure* from the *disease*. Charlotte Perkins Gilman of course saw the connection. The ailing heroine of *The Yellow Wallpaper,* who is being treated by her physician-husband, hints at the fearful truth:

> John is a physician, and *perhaps*—(I would not say it to a living soul, of course, but this is dead paper and a great relief to my mind)—*perhaps* that is one reason I do not get well faster.[22]

In fact, the theories which guided the doctor's practice from the late nineteenth century to the early twentieth century held that woman's *normal* state was to be sick. This was not advanced as an empirical observation, but as physiological fact. Medicine had "discovered" that female functions were inherently pathological. Menstruation, that perennial source of alarm to the male imagination, provided both the evidence and the explanation. Menstruation was a serious threat throughout life—so was the lack of it. According to Dr. Engelmann, president of the American Gynecology Society in 1900:

> Many a young life is battered and forever crippled on the breakers of puberty; if it crosses these unharmed and is not dashed to pieces on the rock of childbirth, it may still ground on the ever-recurring shallows of menstruation, and lastly upon the final bar of the menopause ere protection is found in the unruffled waters of the harbor beyond reach of sexual storms.[23]

Popular advice books written by physicians took on a somber tone as they entered into "the female functions" or "the diseases of women."

> It is impossible to form a correct opinion of the mental and physical suffering frequently endured from her sexual condition, caused by her monthly periods, which it has pleased her Heavenly Father to attach to woman. . . .[24]

Ignoring the existence of thousands of working women, the doctors assumed that every woman was prepared to set aside a week or five days every month as a period of invalidism. Dr. W. C. Taylor, in his book *A Physician's Counsels to Woman in Health and Disease,* gave a warning typical of those found in popular health books of the time:

> We cannot too emphatically urge the importance of regarding these monthly returns as periods of ill health, as days when the ordinary occupations are to be suspended or modified. . . . Long walks, dancing, shopping, riding and parties should be avoided at this time of month invariably and under all circumstances. . . .[25]

As late as 1916, Dr. Winfield Scott Hall was advising:

> All heavy exercise should be omitted during the menstrual week . . . a girl should not only retire earlier at this time, but ought to stay out of school from one to three days as the case may be, resting the mind and taking extra hours of rest and sleep.[26]

Similarly, a pregnant woman was "indisposed," throughout the full nine months. The medical theory of "prenatal impressions" required her to avoid all "shocking, painful or unbeautiful sights," intellectual stimulation, angry or lustful thoughts, and even her husband's alcohol and tobacco-laden breath—lest the baby be deformed or stunted in the womb. Doctors stressed the pathological nature of childbirth itself—an argument which also was essential to their campaign against midwives. After delivery, they insisted on a protracted period of convalescence mirroring the "confinement" which preceded birth. (Childbirth, in the hands of the medical men, no doubt was "pathological," and doctors had far less concern about prenatal nutrition than they did about prenatal "impressions.") Finally after all this, a woman could only look forward to menopause, portrayed in the medical literature as a terminal illness—the "death of the woman in the woman."

Now it must be said in the doctor's defense that women of a hundred years ago *were,* in some ways, sicker than the women of today. Quite apart from tight-lacing, arsenic-nipping, and fashionable cases of neurasthenia, women faced certain bodily risks which men did not share. In 1915 (the first year for which national figures are available) 61 women died for every 10,000 live babies born, compared to 2 per 10,000 today, and the maternal mortality rates were doubtless higher in the nineteenth century.[27] Without adequate, and usually without any, means of contraception, a married woman could expect to face the risk of childbirth repeatedly through her fertile years. After each childbirth a woman might suffer any number of gynecological complications, such as prolapsed (slipped) uterus or irreparable pelvic tear, which would be with her for the rest of her life.

Another special risk to women came from tuberculosis, the "white plague." In the mid-nineteenth century, TB raged at epidemic proportions, and it continued to be a major threat until well into the twentieth century. Everyone was affected, but women, especially young women, were particularly vulnerable, often dying at rates twice as high as those of men of their age group. For every hundred women aged twenty in 1865, more than five would be dead from TB by the age of thirty, and more than eight would be dead by the age of fifty.[28]

So, from a statistical point of view, there was some justification for the doctors' theory of innate female frailty. But there was also, from the doctors' point of view, a strong commercial justification for regarding women as sick. This was the period of the profession's most severe "population crisis." The theory of female frailty obviously disqualified women as healers. "One shudders to think of the conclusions arrived at by female bacteriologists or histologists," wrote one doctor, "at the period when their entire system, both physical and mental, is, so to speak, 'unstrung,' to say nothing of the terrible mistakes which a lady surgeon might make under similar conditions."[29] At the same time the theory made women highly qualified as patients. The sickly, nervous women of the upper or middle class with their unending, but fortunately non-fatal, ills, became a natural "client caste" to the developing medical profession.

Meanwhile, the health of women who were *not* potential patients—poor women—received next to no attention from the medical profession. Poor women must have been at least as susceptible as wealthy women to the "sexual storms" doctors saw in menstruation, pregnancy, etc.; and they were definitely much more susceptible to the hazards of childbearing, tuberculosis, and, of course, industrial diseases. From all that we know, sickness, exhaustion, and injury were routine in the life of the working-class woman. Contagious diseases always hit the homes of the poor first and hardest. Pregnancy, in the fifth- or sixth-floor walk-up flat, really was debilitating, and childbirth, in a crowded tenement room, was often a frantic ordeal. Emma Goldman, who was a trained midwife as well as an anarchist leader, described "the fierce, blind struggle of the women of the poor against frequent pregnancies" and told of the agony of seeing children grow up "sickly and undernourished"—if they survived infancy at all.[30] For the woman who labored outside her home, working conditions took an enormous toll. An 1884 report of an investigation of "The Working Girls of Boston," by the Massachusetts Bureau of Statistics of Labor, stated:

... the health of many girls is so poor as to necessitate long rests, one girl being out a year on this account. Another girl in poor health was obliged to leave her work, while one reports that it is not possible for her to work the year round, as she could not stand the strain, not being at all strong.[31]

Still, however sick or tired working-class women might have been, they certainly did not have the time or money to support a cult of invalidism. Employers gave no time off for pregnancy or recovery from childbirth, much less for menstrual periods, though the wives of these same employers often retired to bed on all these occasions. A day's absence from work could cost a woman her job, and at home there was no comfortable chaise longue to collapse on while servants managed the household and doctors managed the illness. An 1889 study from Massachusetts described one working woman's life:

Constant application to work, often until 12 at night and sometimes on Sundays (equivalent to nine ordinary working days a week), affected her health and injured her eyesight. She ... was ordered by the doctor to suspend work ... but she must earn money, and so she has kept on working. Her eyes weep constantly, she cannot see across the room and "the air seems always in a whirl" before her ... [she] owed when seen three months' board for self and children ... She hopes something may be done for working girls and women, for, however strong they may be in the beginning, "they cannot stand white slavery for ever."[32]

But the medical profession as a whole—and no doubt there were many honorable exceptions—sturdily maintained that it was affluent women who were most delicate and most in need of medical attention. "Civilization" had made the middle-class woman sickly; her physical frailty went hand-in-white-gloved-hand with her superior modesty, refinement, and sensitivity. Working-class women were robust, just as they were supposedly "coarse" and immodest. Dr. Lucien Warner, a popular medical authority, wrote in 1874, "It is not then hard work and privation which make the women of our country invalids, but circumstances and habits intimately connected with the so-called blessings of wealth and refinement."

Someone had to be well enough to do the work, though, and working-class women, Dr. Warner noted with relief, were *not* invalids: "The African negress, who toils beside her husband in the fields of the south, and Bridget, who washes, and scrubs and toils in our homes at the north, enjoy for the most part good health, with comparative immunity from uterine disease."[33] And a Dr. Sylvanus Stall observed:

At war, at work, or at play, the white man is superior to the savage, and his culture has continually improved his condition. But with woman the rule is reversed. Her squaw sister will endure effort, exposure and hardship which would kill the white woman. Education which has resulted in developing and strengthening the physical nature of man has been perverted through folly and fashion to render woman weaker and weaker.[34]

In practice, the same doctors who zealously indulged the ills of wealthy patients had no time to spare for the poor. When Emma Goldman asked the doctors she knew whether they had any contraceptive information she could offer the poor, their answers included, "The poor have only themselves to blame; they indulge their appetites too much," and "When she [the poor woman] uses her brains more, her procreative organs will function less."[35] A Dr. Palmer Dudley ruled out poor women as subjects for gynecological surgery on the simple ground that they lacked the leisure required for successful treatment:

> ... the hardworking, daily-toiling woman is not as fit a subject for [gynecological surgery] as the woman so situated in life as to be able to conserve her strength and if necessary, to take a long rest, in order to secure the best results.[36]

So the logic was complete: better-off women were sickly because of their refined and civilized lifestyle. Fortunately, however, this same lifestyle made them amenable to lengthy medical treatment. Poor and working-class women were inherently stronger, and this was also fortunate, since their lifestyle disqualified them from lengthy medical treatment anyway. The theory of innate female sickness, skewed so as to account for class differences in ability to pay for medical care, meshed conveniently with the doctors' commercial self-interest.

The feminists of the late nineteenth century, themselves deeply concerned about female invalidism, were quick to place at least part of the blame on the doctors' interests. Elizabeth Garrett Anderson, an American woman doctor, argued that the extent of female invalidism was much exaggerated by male doctors and that women's natural functions were not really all that debilitating. In the working classes, she observed, work went on during menstruation "without intermission, and, as a rule, without ill effects."[37] Mary Livermore, a women's suffrage worker, spoke against "the monstrous assumption that woman is a natural invalid," and denounced "the unclean army of 'gynecologists' who seem desirous to convince women that they possess but one set of organs—and that these are always diseased."[38] And Dr. Mary Putnam Jacobi put the matter most forcefully when she wrote in 1895, "I think, finally, it is in the increased attention paid to women, and especially in their new function as lucrative patients, scarcely imagined a hundred years ago, that we find explanation for much of the ill-health among women, freshly discovered today...."[39]

The Dictatorship of the Ovaries

It was medicine's task to translate the [nineteenth-century] evolutionary theory of women into the language of flesh and blood, tissues and organs. The result was a theory which put woman's mind, body and soul in the thrall of her all-powerful reproductive organs. "The Uterus, it must be remembered," Dr. F. Hollick wrote, "is the *controlling* organ in the female body, being the most excitable of all, and so intimately connected, by the ramifications of its numerous nerves, with every other part."[40] Professor M. L. Holbrook, addressing a medical society in 1870, observed that it seemed "as if the Almighty, in creating the female sex, *had taken the uterus and built up a woman around it.*"[41] (Emphasis in original.)

To other medical theorists, it was the ovaries which occupied center stage. Dr. G. L. Austin's 1883 book of advice for "maiden, wife and mother" asserts that the ovaries "give woman all her characteristics of body and mind."[42] This passage written in 1870 by Dr. W. W. Bliss is, if somewhat overwrought, nonetheless typical:

> Accepting, then, these views of the gigantic power and influence of the ovaries over the whole animal economy of woman,—that they are the most powerful agents in all the commotions of her system; that on them rest her intellectual standing in society, her physical perfection, and all that lends beauty to those fine and delicate contours which are constant objects of admiration, all that is great, noble and beautiful, all that is voluptuous, tender, and endearing; that her fidelity, her devotedness, her perpetual vigilance, forecast, and all those qualities of mind and disposition which inspire respect and love and fit her as the safest counsellor and friend of man, spring from the ovaries,—*what must be their influence and power over the great vocation of woman and the august purposes of her existence when these organs have become compromised through disease!*[43] (Emphasis in original.)

According to this "psychology of the ovary" woman's entire personality was directed by the ovaries, and any abnormalities, from irritability to insanity, could be traced to some ovarian disease. Dr. Bliss added, with unbecoming spitefulness, that "the influence of the ovaries over the mind is displayed in woman's artfulness and dissimulation."

It should be emphasized, before we follow the workings of the uterus and ovaries any further, that woman's total submission to the "sex function" did not make her a *sexual* being. The medical model of female nature, embodied in the "psychology of the ovary," drew a rigid distinction between reproductivity and sexuality. Women were urged by the health books and the doctors to indulge in deep preoccupation with themselves as "The Sex"; they were to devote themselves to developing their reproductive powers and their maternal instincts. Yet doctors said they had no predilection for the sex act itself. Even a woman physician, Dr. Mary Wood-Allen wrote (perhaps from experience), that women embrace their husbands "without a particle of sex desire."[44] Hygiene manuals stated that the more cultured the woman, "the more is the sensual refined away from her nature," and warned against "any spasmodic convulsion" on a woman's part during intercourse lest it interfere with conception. Female sexuality was seen as unwomanly and possibly even detrimental to the supreme function of reproduction.

The doctors themselves never seemed entirely convinced, though, that the uterus and ovaries had successfully stamped out female sexuality. Underneath the complacent denials of female sexual feelings, there lurked the age-old male fascination with woman's "insatiable lust," which, once awakened, might turn out to be uncontrollable. Doctors dwelt on cases in which women were destroyed by their cravings; one doctor claimed to have discovered a case of "virgin nymphomania." The twenty-five-year-old British physician Robert Brudenell Carter leaves us with this tantalizing observation on his female patients:

> . . . no one who has realized the amount of moral evil wrought in girls . . . whose prurient desires have been increased by Indian hemp and partially gratified by medical manipulations, can deny that remedy is worse than disease. I have . . . seen young unmarried women, of the middle class of society, reduced by the constant use of the speculum to the mental and moral condition of prostitutes; seeking to give themselves the same indulgence by the practice of solitary vice; and asking every medical practitioner . . . to institute an examination of the sexual organs.[45]

But if the uterus and ovaries could not be counted on to suppress all sexual strivings, they were still sufficiently in control to be blamed for all possible female disorders, from headaches to sore throats and indigestion. Dr. M. E. Dirix wrote in 1869:

> Thus, women are treated for diseases of the stomach, liver, kidneys, heart, lungs, etc.; yet, in most instances, these diseases will be found on due investigation, to be, in reality, no diseases at all, but merely the sympathetic reactions or the symptoms of one disease, namely, a disease of the womb.[46]

Even tuberculosis could be traced to the capricious ovaries. When men were consumptive, doctors sought some environmental factor, such as overexposure, to explain the disease. But for women it was a result of reproductive malfunction. Dr. Azell Ames wrote in 1875:

> It being beyond doubt that consumption . . . is itself produced by the failure of the [menstrual] function in the forming girls . . . one has been the parent of the other with interchangeable priority. [Actually, as we know today, it is true that consumption may *result* in suspension of the menses.][47]

Since the reproductive organs were the source of disease, they were the obvious target in the treatment of disease. Any symptom—backaches, irritability, indigestion, etc.—could provoke a medical assault on the sexual organs. Historian Ann Douglas Wood describes the "local treatments" used in the mid-nineteenth century for almost any female complaint:

> This [local] treatment had four stages, although not every case went through all four: a manual investigation, "leeching," "injections," and "cauterization." Dewees [an American medical professor] and Bennet, a famous English gynecologist widely read in America, both advocated placing the leeches right on the vulva or the neck of the uterus, although Bennet cautioned the doctor to count them as they dropped off when satiated, lest he "lose" some. Bennet had known adventurous leeches to advance into the cervical cavity of the uterus itself, and he noted, "I think I have scarcely ever seen more acute pain than that experienced by several of my patients under these circumstances." Less distressing to a 20th century mind, but perhaps even more senseless, were the "injections" into the uterus advocated by these doctors. The uterus became a kind of catch-all, or what one exasperated doctor referred to as a "Chinese toy shop": Water, milk and water, linseed tea, and "decoction of marshmellow . . . tepid or cold" found their way inside nervous women patients. The final step, performed at this time, one must remember, with no anesthetic but a little opium or alcohol, was cauterization, either through the application of nitrate of silver, or, in cases of more severe infection, through the use of much stronger hydrate of potassa, or even the "actual cautery," a "white-hot iron" instrument.[48]

In the second half of the century, these fumbling experiments with the female interior gave way to the more decisive technique of surgery—aimed increasingly at the control of female personality disorders. There had been a brief fad of clitoridectomy (removal of the clitoris) in the sixties, following the introduction of the operation by the English physician Isaac Baker Brown. Although most doctors frowned on the practice of removing the clitoris, they tended to agree that it might be necessary in cases of nymphomania, intractable masturbation, or "unnatural growth" of that organ. (The last clitoridectomy we know of in the United States was performed in 1948 on a child of five, as a cure for masturbation.)

The most common form of surgical intervention in the female personality was ovariotomy, removal of the ovaries—or "female castration." In 1906 a leading gynecological surgeon estimated that there were 150,000 women in the United States who had lost their ovaries under the knife. Some doctors boasted that they had removed from fifteen hundred to two thousand ovaries apiece.[49] According to historian G. J. Barker-Benfield:

> Among the indications were troublesomeness, eating like a ploughman, masturbation, attempted suicide, erotic tendencies, persecution mania, simple "cussedness," and dysmenorrhea [painful menstruation]. Most apparent in the enormous variety of symptoms doctors took to indicate castration was a strong current of sexual appetitiveness on the part of women.[50]

The rationale for the operation flowed directly from the theory of the "psychology of the ovary": since the ovaries controlled the personality, they must be responsible for any psychological disorders; conversely, psychological disorders were a sure sign of ovarian disease. Ergo, the organs must be removed.

One might think, given the all-powerful role of the ovaries, that an ovaryless women would be like a rudderless ship—desexed and directionless. But on the contrary, the proponents of ovariotomy argued, a woman who was relieved of a diseased ovary would be a *better* woman. One 1893 advocate of the operation claimed that "patients are improved, some of them cured; . . . the moral sense of the patient is elevated . . . she becomes tractable, orderly, industrious, and cleanly."[51] Patients were often brought in by their husbands, who complained of their unruly behavior. Doctors also claimed that women—troublesome but still sane enough to recognize their problem—often "came to us pleading to have their ovaries removed."[52] The operation was judged successful if the woman was restored to a placid contentment with her domestic functions.

The overwhelming majority of women who had leeches or hot steel applied to their cervices, or who had their clitorises or ovaries removed, were women of the middle to upper classes, for after all, these procedures cost money. But it should not be imagined that poor women were spared the gynecologist's exotic catalog of tortures simply because they couldn't pay. The pioneering work in gynecological surgery had been performed by Marion Sims on black female slaves he kept for the sole purpose of surgical experimentation. He operated on one of them thirty times in four years, being foiled over and over by postoperative infections.[53] After moving to New York, Sims continued his experimentation on indigent Irish women in the wards of New York Women's Hospital. So, though middle-class women suffered most from the doctors' actual practice, it was poor and black women who had suffered through the brutal period of experimentation.

. . . .

Subverting the Sick Role: Hysteria

The romance of the doctor and the female invalid comes to full bloom (and almost to consummation) in the practice of S. Weir Mitchell. But . . . there is a nastier side to this affair. An angry, punitive tone has come into his voice; the possibility of physical force has been raised. As time goes on and the invalids pile up in the boudoirs of American cities and recirculate through the health spas and consulting rooms, the punitive tone grows louder. Medicine is caught in a contradiction of its own making, and begins to turn against the patient.

Doctors had established that women are sick, that this sickness is innate, and stems from the very possession of a uterus and ovaries. They had thus eliminated the duality of "sickness" and "health" for the female sex;

there was only a drawn-out half-life, tossed steadily by the "storms" of reproductivity toward a more total kind of rest. But at the same time, doctors *were* expected to cure. The development of commercial medicine, with its aggressive, instrumental approach to healing, required some public faith that doctors could *do something,* that they could fix things. Certainly Charlotte Perkins Gilman had expected to be cured. The husbands, fathers, sisters, etc. of thousands of female invalids expected doctors to provide cures. A medical strategy of disease by decree, followed by "cures" which either mimicked the symptoms or caused new ones, might be successful for a few decades. But it had no long-term commercial viability.

The problem went deeper, though, than the issue of the doctors' commercial credibility. There was a contradiction in the romantic ideal of femininity which medicine had worked so hard to construct. Medicine had insisted that woman was sick *and* that her life centered on the reproductive function. But these are contradictory propositions. If you are sick enough, you cannot reproduce. The female role in reproduction requires stamina, and if you count in all the activities of child raising and running a house, it requires full-blown, energetic *health*. Sickness and reproductivity, the twin pillars of nineteenth-century femininity, could not stand together.

In fact, toward the end of the century, it seemed that sickness had been winning out over reproductivity. The birth rate for whites shrank by a half between 1800 and 1900, and the drop was most precipitous among white Anglo-Saxon Protestants—the "better" class of people. Meanwhile blacks and European immigrants appeared to be breeding prolifically, and despite their much higher death rates, the fear arose that they might actually replace the "native stock." Professor Edwin Conklin of Princeton wrote:

> The cause for alarm is the declining birth rate among the best elements of a population, while it continues to increase among the poorer elements. The descendants of the Puritans and the Cavaliers . . . are already disappearing, and in a few centuries at most, will have given place to more fertile races. . . .[54]

And in 1903 President Theodore Roosevelt thundered to the nation the danger of "race suicide":

> Among human beings, as among all other living creatures, if the best specimens do not, and the poorer specimens do, propagate, the type [race] will go down. If Americans of the old stock lead lives of celibate selfishness . . . or if the married are afflicted by that base fear of living which, whether for the sake of themselves or of their children, forbids them to have more than one or two children, disaster awaits the nation.[55]

G. Stanley Hall and other expert observers easily connected the falling WASP birth rate to the epidemic of female invalidism:

> In the United States as a whole from 1860–'90 the birth-rate declined from 25.61 to 19.22. Many women are so exhausted before marriage that after

> bearing one or two children they become wrecks, and while there is perhaps a
> growing dread of parturition or of the bother of children, many of the best
> women feel they have not stamina enough. . . .[56]

He went on to suggest that "if women do not improve," men would have
to "have recourse to emigrant wives" or perhaps there would have to be a
"new rape of the Sabines."

The genetic challenge posed by the "poorer elements" cast an unflatter-
ing light on the female invalid. No matter whether she was "really" suffering, she was clearly not doing her duty. Sympathy begins to give way to
the suspicion that she might be deliberately *malingering*. S. Weir Mitchell
revealed his private judgment of his patients in his novels, which dwelt on
the grasping, selfish invalid, who uses her illness to gain power over
others. In *Roland Blake* (1886) the evil invalid "Octapia" tries to squeeze
the life out of her gentle cousin Olivia. In *Constance Trescot* (1905) the
heroine is a domineering, driven woman, who ruins her husband's life and
then relapses into invalidism in an attempt to hold on to her patient sister
Susan:

> By degrees Susan also learned that Constance relied on her misfortune and her
> long illness to insure to her an excess of sympathetic affection and unremitting
> service. The discoveries thus made troubled the less selfish sister. . . .[57]

The story ends in a stinging rejection for Constance, as Susan leaves her to
get married and assume the more womanly role of serving a man. Little
did Dr. Mitchell's patients suspect that his ideal woman was not the delicate lady on the bed, but the motherly figure of the nurse in the background! (In fact, Mitchell's rest cure was implicitly based on the idea that
his patients were malingerers.) As he explained it, the idea was to provide
the patient with a drawn-out experience of invalidism, but without any of
the pleasures and perquisites which usually went with that condition.

> To lie abed half the day, and sew a little and read a little, and be interesting
> and excite sympathy, is all very well, but when they are bidden to stay in bed a
> a month and neither to read, write, nor sew, and to have one nurse,—who is
> not a relative,—then rest becomes for some women a rather bitter medicine,
> and they are glad enough to accept the order to rise and go about when the
> doctor issues a mandate . . .[58]

Many women probably *were* using the sick role as a way to escape
their reproductive and domestic duties. For the woman to whom sex really
was repugnant, and yet a "duty," or for any woman who wanted to avoid
pregnancy, sickness was a way out—and there were few others. The available methods of contraception were unreliable, and not always that available either.[59] Abortion was illegal and risky. So female invalidism may be
a direct ancestor of the nocturnal "headache" which so plagued husbands
in the mid-twentieth century.

The suspicion of malingering—whether to avoid pregnancy or gain attention—cast a pall over the doctor-patient relationship. If a woman was really sick (as the doctors said she ought to be), then the doctor's efforts, however ineffective, must be construed as appropriate, justifiable, and of course reimbursable. But if she was *not* sick, then the doctor was being made a fool of. His manly, professional attempts at treatment were simply part of a charade directed by and starring the female patient. But how could you tell the real invalids from the frauds? And what did you do when no amount of drugging, cutting, resting, or sheer bullying seemed to make the woman well?

Doctors had wanted women to be sick, but now they found themselves locked in a power struggle with the not-so-feeble patient: Was the illness a construction of the medical imagination, a figment of the patient's imagination, or something "real" which nevertheless eluded the mightiest efforts of medical science? What, after all, was behind "neurasthenia," "hyperesthesia," or the dozens of other labels attached to female invalidism?

But it took a specific syndrome to make the ambiguities in the doctor-patient relationship unbearable, and to finally break the gynecologists' monopoly of the female psyche. This syndrome was hysteria. In many ways, hysteria epitomized the cult of female invalidism. It affected middle- and upper-class women almost exclusively; it had no discernible organic basis; and it was totally resistant to medical treatment. But unlike the more common pattern of invalidism, hysteria was episodic. It came and went in unpredictable, and frequently violent, fits.

According to contemporary descriptions, the victim of hysteria might either faint or throw her limbs about uncontrollably. Her back might arch, with her entire body becoming rigid, or she might beat her chest, tear her hair or attempt to bite herself and others. Aside from fits and fainting, the disease took a variety of forms: hysterical loss of voice, loss of appetite, hysterical coughing or sneezing, and, of course, hysterical screaming, laughing, and crying. The disease spread wildly, not only in the United States, but in England and throughout Europe.

Doctors became obsessed with this "most confusing, mysterious and rebellious of diseases." In some ways, it was the ideal disease for the doctors: it was never fatal, and it required an almost endless amount of medical attention. But it was not an ideal disease from the point of view of the husband and family of the afflicted woman. Gentle invalidism had been one thing; violent fits were quite another. So hysteria put the doctors on the spot. It was essential to their professional self-esteem either to find an organic basis for the disease, and cure it, or to expose it as a clever charade.

There was plenty of evidence for the latter point of view. With mounting suspicion, the medical literature began to observe that hysterics never had fits when alone, and only when there was something soft to fall on. One doctor accused them of pinning their hair in such a way that it would fall luxuriantly when they fainted. The hysterical "type" began to be characterized as a "petty tyrant" with a "taste for power" over her husband, servants, and children, and, if possible, her doctor.

In historian Carroll Smith-Rosenberg's interpretation, the doctor's accusations had some truth to them: the hysterical fit, for many women, must have been the only acceptable outburst—of rage, of despair, or simply of *energy*—possible.[60] Alice James, whose lifelong illness began with a bout of hysteria in adolescence, described her condition as a struggle against uncontrollable physical energy:

> Conceive of never being without the sense that if you let yourself go for a moment . . . you must abandon it all, let the dykes break and the flood sweep in, acknowledging yourself abjectly impotent before the immutable laws. When all one's moral and natural stock-in-trade is a temperament forbidding the abandonment of an inch or the relaxation of a muscle, 'tis a never-ending fight. When the fancy took me of a morning at school to *study* my lessons by way of variety instead of shrieking or wiggling through the most impossible sensations of upheaval, violent revolt in my head overtook me, so that I had to "abandon" my brain as it were.[61]

On the whole, however, doctors did continue to insist that hysteria was a real disease—a disease of the uterus, in fact. (Hysteria comes from the Greek word for uterus.) They remained unshaken in their conviction that their own house calls and high physician's fees were absolutely necessary; yet at the same time, in their treatment and in their writing, doctors assumed an increasingly angry and threatening attitude. One doctor wrote, "It will sometimes be advisable to speak in a decided tone, in the presence of the patient, of the necessity of shaving the head, or of giving her a cold shower bath, should she not be soon relieved." He then gave a "scientific" rationalization for this treatment by saying, "The sedative influence of fear may allay, as I have known it to do, the excitement of the nervous centers. . . ."[62]

Carroll Smith-Rosenberg writes that doctors recommended suffocating hysterical women until their fits stopped, beating them across the face and body with wet towels, and embarrassing them in front of family and friends. She quotes Dr. F. C. Skey: "Ridicule to a woman of sensitive mind, is a powerful weapon . . . but there is not an emotion equal to fear and the threat of personal chastisement. . . . They will listen to the voice of authority." The more women became hysterical, the more doctors became punitive toward the disease; and at the same time, they began to see the disease everywhere themselves until they were diagnosing every independent act by a woman, especially a women's rights action, as "hysterical."

With hysteria, the cult of female invalidism was carried to its logical conclusion. Society had assigned affluent women to a life of confinement and inactivity, and medicine had justified this assignment by describing women as innately sick. In the epidemic of hysteria, women were both accepting their inherent "sickness" *and* finding a way to rebel against an intolerable social role. Sickness, having become a way of life, became a way of rebellion, and medical treatment, which had always had strong overtones of coercion, revealed itself as frankly and brutally repressive.

But the deadlock over hysteria was to usher in a new era in the experts' relationship to women. While the conflict between hysterical women and their doctors was escalating in America, Sigmund Freud, in Vienna, was beginning to work on a treatment that would remove the disease altogether from the arena of gynecology.

Freud's cure eliminated the confounding question of whether or not the woman was faking: in either case it was a mental disorder. Psychoanalysis, as Thomas Szasz has pointed out, insists that "malingering *is* an illness—in fact, an illness 'more serious' than hysteria."[63] Freud banished the traumatic "cures" and legitimized a doctor-patient relationship based solely on talking. His therapy urged the patient to confess her resentments and rebelliousness, and then at last to accept her role as a woman. Freud's insight into hysteria at once marked off a new medical speciality: "Psychoanalysis," in the words of feminist historian Carroll Smith-Rosenberg, "is the child of the hysterical woman." In the course of the twentieth century psychologists and psychiatrists would replace doctors as the dominant experts in the lives of women.

For decades into the twentieth century doctors would continue to view menstruation, pregnancy, and menopause as physical diseases and intellectual liabilities. Adolescent girls would still be advised to study less, and mature women would be treated indiscriminately to hysterectomies, the modern substitute for ovariotomies. The female reproductive organs would continue to be viewed as a kind of frontier for chemical and surgical expansionism, untested drugs, and reckless experimentation. But the debate over the Woman Question would never again be phrased in such crudely materialistic terms as those set forth by nineteenth-century medical theory—with brains "battling" uteruses for control of woman's nature. The psychological interpretation of hysteria, and eventually of "neurasthenia" and the other vague syndromes of female invalidism, established once and for all that the brain was in command. The experts of the twentieth century would accept woman's intelligence and energy: the question would no longer be what a woman *could* do, but, rather, what a woman *ought* to do.

References

1. Anna Robeson Burr, *Weir Mitchell: His Life and Letters* (New York: Duffield and Co., 1929), p. 289.
2. Charlotte Perkins Gilman, *The Living of Charlotte Perkins Gilman: An Autobiography* (New York: Harper Colophon Books, 1975), p. 96.

3. Gilman, loc. cit.
4. Charlotte Perkins Gilman, *The Yellow Wallpaper* (Old Westbury, New York: The Feminist Press, 1973).
5. Gilman, *Autobiography,* p. 121.
6. Catherine Beecher, "Statistics of Female Health," in Gail Parker (ed.), *The Oven Birds: American Women on Womanhood 1820–1920* (Garden City, New York: Doubleday/Anchor, 1972), p. 165.
7. Ilza Veith, *Hysteria: The History of a Disease* (Chicago and London: The University of Chicago Press, 1965), p. 216.
8. Quoted in F. O. Matthiessen, *The James Family* (New York: Alfred A. Knopf, 1961), p. 272.
9. Quoted in Irving H. Bartlett, *Wendell Phillips: Brahmin Radical* (Boston: Beacon Press, 1961), p. 78.
10. Quoted in Leon Edel (ed.), *The Diary of Alice James* (New York: Dodd, Mead, 1964), p. 14.
11. We thank medical historian Rick Brown for sharing this story with us.
12. Thorstein Veblen, *Theory of the Leisure Class* (New York: Modern Library, 1934).
13. Burr, op. cit., p. 176.
14. Olive Schreiner, *Woman and Labor* (New York: Frederick A. Stokes, 1911), p. 98.
15. John C. Gunn, M.D., *Gunn's New Family Physician* (New York: Saalfield Publishing, 1924), p. 120.
16. New York Public Library Picture Collection, no source given.
17. Dr. Mary Putnam Jacobi, "On Female Invalidism," in Nancy F. Cott (ed.), *Root of Bitterness: Documents of the Social History of American Women* (New York: E. P. Dutton, 1972), p. 307.
18. John S. Haller, Jr., and Robin M. Haller, *The Physician and Sexuality in Victorian America* (Urbana, Illinois: University of Illinois Press, 1974), pp. 143–44.
19. Ibid., p. 168.
20. Ibid., p. 31.
21. Ibid., p. 28.
22. Gilman, *The Yellow Wallpaper,* pp. 9–10.
23. Quoted in G. Stanley Hall, *Adolescence, Vol. II* (New York: D. Appleton, 1905), p. 588.
24. Gunn, op. cit., p. 421.
25. W. C. Taylor, M.D., *A Physician's Counsels to Woman in Health and Disease* (Springfield: W. J. Holland and Co., 1871), pp. 284–85.
26. Winfield Scott Hall, Ph.D., M.D., *Sexual Knowledge* (Philadelphia: John C. Winston, 1916), pp. 202–3.
27. U. S. Bureau of the Census, *Historical Statistics of the United States, Colonial Times to 1957,* Washington, D.C., 1960, p. 25.
28. Rachel Gillett Fruchter, "Women's Weakness: Consumption and Women in the 19th Century," Columbia University School of Public Health, unpublished paper, 1973.
29. Haller and Haller, op. cit., p. 59.

30. Emma Goldman, *Living My Life,* Vol. I (New York: Dover Publications, Inc., 1970, first published 1931), pp. 185–86.
31. Carroll D. Wright, *The Working Girls of Boston* (Boston: Wright and Potter Printing, State Printers, 1889), p. 71.
32. Ibid., pp. 117–18.
33. Lucien C. Warner, M.D., *A Popular Treatise on the Functions and Diseases of Woman* (New York: Manhattan Publishing, 1874), p. 109.
34. Quoted in Dr. Alice Moqué, "The Mistakes of Mothers," *Proceedings of the National Congress of Mothers Second Annual Convention,* Washington, D. C., May 1898, p. 43.
35. Goldman, op. cit., p. 187.
36. Quoted in G. J. Barker-Benfield, *The Horrors of the Half-Known Life: Male Attitudes Toward Women and Sexuality in Nineteenth-Century America* (New York: Harper & Row, 1976), p. 128.
37. Quoted in Elaine and English Showalter, "Victorian Women and Menstruation," in Martha Vicinus (ed.), *Suffer and Be Still: Women in the Victorian Age* (Bloomington: Indiana University Press, 1972), p. 43.
38. "Mary Livermore's Recommendatory Letter," in Cott, op. cit., p. 292.
39. Mary Putnam Jacobi, M.D., in Cott, op. cit., p. 307.
40. Frederick Hollick, M.D., *The Diseases of Women, Their Cause and Cure Familiarly Explained* (New York: T. W. Strong, 1849).
41. Quoted in Ann Douglas Wood, "The 'Fashionable Diseases': Women's Complaints and their Treatment in Nineteenth-Century America," *Journal of Interdisciplinary History* 4, Summer 1973, p. 29.
42. Quoted in Rita Arditti, "Women as Objects: Science and Sexual Politics," *Science for the People,* September 1974, p. 8.
43. W. W. Bliss, *Woman and Her Thirty-Years' Pilgrimage* (Boston: B. B. Russell, 1870), p. 96.
44. Quoted in Haller and Haller, op. cit., p. 101.
45. Quoted in Veith, op. cit., p. 205.
46. M. E. Dirix, M.D., *Woman's Complete Guide to Health* (New York: W. A. Townsend and Adams, 1869), pp. 23–24.
47. Quoted in Fruchter, op. cit.
48. Wood, op. cit., p. 30.
49. Barker-Benfield, op. cit., pp. 121–24.
50. Ben Barker-Benfield, "The Spermatic Economy: A Nineteenth Century View of Sexuality," *Feminist Studies* 1, Summer 1972, pp. 45–74.
51. It is unlikely that the operation had this effect on a woman's personality. It would have produced the symptoms of menopause, which do not include any established personality changes. Barker-Benfield, *Horrors of the Half-Known Life,* p. 122.
52. Ibid., p. 30.
53. Ibid., pp. 96–102.
54. Quoted in Theodore Roosevelt, "Birth Reform, From the Positive, Not the Negative Side," in *Complete Works of Theodore Roosevelt,* Vol. XIX (New York: Scribner, 1926), p. 163.
55. Roosevelt, op. cit., p. 161.

56. Hall, op. cit., p. 579.
57. S. Weir Mitchell, *Constance Trescot* (New York: The Century Co., 1905), p. 382.
58. Quoted in Veith, op. cit., p. 217.
59. See Linda Gordon, *Woman's Body, Woman's Right: A Social History of Birth Control in America* (New York: Grossman, 1977).
60. Carroll Smith-Rosenberg, "The Hysterical Woman: Sex Roles in Nineteenth Century America," *Social Research,* 39, Winter 1972, pp. 652–78.
61. Quoted in Matthiessen, op. cit., p. 276.
62. Dirix, op. cit., p. 60.
63. Thomas S. Szasz, *The Myth of Mental Illness* (New York: Dell, 1961), p. 48.

23

A Funny Thing Happened on the Way to the Orifice: Women in Gynecology Textbooks

Diana Scully and Pauline Bart

The gynecologist is our society's official specialist on women, legitimately commenting on their psyches as well as on the illnesses of their reproductive tracts (Novak, Jones, and Jones 1970; Green 1971).[1] Nevertheless, gynecologists are overwhelmingly male (93.4% [*Time* 1972, p. 89]); and the tools of the sociology of knowledge suggest that one's perspectives are constrained by one's place in the social structure and thus gynecologists may not adequately represent the worldview and the interests of the group they are supposed to attend and advocate. Indeed, examination of gynecology textbooks, one of the primary professional socialization agents for practitioners in the field, revealed a persistent bias toward greater concern with the patient's husband than with the patient herself. Women are consistently described as anatomically destined to reproduce, nurture, and keep their husbands happy. So gynecology appears to be another of the forces committed to maintaining traditional sex-role stereotypes, in the interest of men and from a male perspective.[2]

The contents of 27 general gynecology texts published in the United

States since 1943 were analyzed. Complete lists of texts and authors were obtained from the Index Catalog of the Library of the Surgeon General's Office, National Library of Medicine. We attempted to read all the texts available, rather than to sample (27 books out of 32). To allow for emergent trends based on new information about female sexuality, the books were divided into three periods; pre-Kinsey, 1943–52 (six of nine were used); post-Kinsey, pre-Masters and Johnson, 1953–62 (nine of 10 were used); post-Masters and Johnson, 1963–72 (12 of 14 were used). Only the latest edition of each text was read. The numbers represent authors active in the field rather than total volumes published.

1943–53[3]

In this period, prior to the work of Kinsey and Masters and Johnson, there was little empirical data about female sexuality. Of the four books in this group, two did not index female sexuality. One of the four (Janney 1950) presented a strikingly egalitarian approach to sexuality. Two others are characterized by a double standard. Thus Cooke stated: "The fundamental biologic factor in women is the urge of motherhood balanced by the fact that sexual pleasure is entirely secondary or even absent" (Cooke 1943, pp. 59–60). Since women were assumed to be "almost universally generally frigid," while the male "is created to fertilize as many females as possible and has an infinite appetite and capacity for intercourse" (Cooke 1943, p. 60), two texts instruct gynecologists to teach their patients to fake orgasm. "It is good advice to recommend to the women the advantage of *innocent simulation* [italics added] of sex responsiveness, and as a matter of fact many women in their desire to please their husbands learned the advantage of such innocent deception" (Novak and Novak 1952, p. 572; Lowrie 1952, p. 671).

The Kinsey Era, 1953–62

Once Kinsey et al. published *Sexual Behavior in the Human Female* (1953), the medical field had an authoritative and definitive (albeit from a nonrandom sample) source of information on the female. For the most part, these texts used Kinsey's report selectively; findings which reinforced old stereotypes were repeated, but the revolutionary findings significant for women were ignored. For example, one often finds in the textbooks that the male sets the sexual pace in marital coitus, but nowhere is it mentioned that women are multiorgasmic, a Kinsey finding which raises questions concerning the gynecologist's belief in the stronger male sex drive.

Though Kinsey is not usually credited with the discovery, he debunked

Table 1.
Female Sexuality and Orgasm in Three Decades of Gynecology Texts

	1943–52		1953–62		1963–72	
	N	% of Indexed Item (N)	N	% of Indexed Item (N)	N	% of Indexed Item (N)
Texts which indexed female sexuality	(4)	...	(8)	...	(9)	...
Sex primarily for reproduction*	...	25 (1)	...	62 (5)	...	67 (6)
Male sex drive stronger	...	50 (2)	...	62 (5)	...	89 (8)
Women characterized as frigid	...	25 (1)	...	37 (3)	...	33 (3)
Female sexuality not indexed	(4)	...	(1)	...	(3)	...
Total texts	(6)	...	(9)	...	(12)	...
Text which indexed orgasm (clitoral-vaginal)	(4)	...	(4)	...	(4)	...
Vaginal mature response	...	0	...	75 (3)	...	50 (2)†
Not discussed in these terms	...	75 (3)†	...	25 (1)	...	0
Orgasm not indexed	(2)	...	(5)	...	(8)	...
Total texts	(6)	...	(9)	...	(12)	...

*Of those books in which female sexuality was indexed, some had more than one reference area. Therefore the total number of references is greater than the number of books.
†One text in the 1963–72 period indicated the clitoris to be the seat of sensation, and two texts, one in the 1963–72 and one in the 1943–52 period, indicated no difference in clitoral and vaginal orgasm.

the myth of the vaginal orgasm. "The literature usually implies that the vagina itself should be the center of sensory stimulation but this as we have seen is a physical and physiologic impossibility for nearly all females" (Kinsey 1952, p. 582).

Gynecologists, however, have tenaciously clung to the idea of the vaginal orgasm as the appropriate response and labeled "frigid" and immature those patients who could not experience it. The content analysis (see table 1) showed that no text read in any of the three decades said that portions of the vagina had no nerve endings and lacked sensation (a Kinsey finding); only one, in the 1963–72 decade, said that the clitoris was the seat of sensation; three in the second decade and two in the most current decade said that the vaginal response was the "mature response"; and two, one in the current decade and one in the 1952–63 period, stated the vagina and clitoris were equally sensitive. For example: "Investigators of sexual behavior distinguished between clitoral and vaginal orgasm, the first playing a dominant role in childhood sexuality and in masturbation and the latter in the normal mature and sexually active women. ... The limitation of sexual satisfaction to one part of the external genitalia is apparently due to habit and aversion to normal cohabitation" (Ruben 1965, p. 77). Indeed as late as 1965, gynecology texts were reporting the vagina as the main erogenous zone (Greenhill 1965, p. 496). In 1962: "The transference of sensations from the clitoris to the vagina is completed only in part and frequently not at all. . . . If there has been much manual stimulation of the clitoris *it* (italics added) may be reluctant to abandon control, or the vagina may be unwilling to accept the combined role of arbiter of sensation and vehicle for reproduction" (Parsons and Sommers 1962, pp. 501–2). But, even if she is "truly frigid . . . the marital relations may proceed without *disturbing* (italics added) either partner" (Parsons and Sommers 1962, p. 494).

1963–72

In the early 1960s reports began to flow from the laboratories of Masters and Johnson, and, though their findings are not generally quoted, there has been some indirect influence. Two-thirds (eight) of the books of that decade failed to discuss the issue of the clitoral versus vaginal orgasm. Eight continued to state, contrary to Masters and Johnson's findings, that the male sex drive was stronger; and half (six) still maintained that procreation was the major function of sex for the female. Two said that most women were "frigid," and another stated that one-third were sexually unresponsive. Two repeated that the vaginal orgasm was the only mature response (Greenhill 1965; Jeffcoate 1967).

Although sex roles are never indexed, we learn from reading the texts that when they deal with the subject, the traditional female sex role is preferred (nine out of 12 in the recent decade). Thus Jeffcoate states: "An important feature of sex desire in the man is the urge to dominate the women and subjugate her to his will; in the women acquiescence to the masterful takes a high place" (Jeffcoate 1967, p. 726). In 1971 we read: "The traits that compose the core of the female personality are feminine narcissism, masochism and passivity" (Willson 1971, p. 43).

So it appears that in gynecology texts the basic underlying image of woman and her "normal adult female role in the marital relationship" (Green 1971, p. 436) has changed little even though new data contradicting such views have been available. A 1970 text states: "The frequency of intercourse depends entirely upon the male sex drive. . . . The bride should be advised to allow her husband's sex drive to set their pace and she should attempt to gear hers satisfactorily to his. If she finds after several months or years that this is not possible, she is advised to consult her physician as soon as she realizes there is a real problem" (Novak, Jones, and Jones 1970, pp. 662–63).

The gynecologist's self-image as helpful to women combined with unbelievable condescension is epitomized in this remark: "If like all human beings, he [the gynecologist] is made in the image of the Almighty, and if he is kind, then his kindness and concern for his patient may provide her with a glimpse of God's image" (Scott 1968, p. 25).

Summary

A review of 27 gynecology texts written from 1943 to 1972 shows that they are written, as a sociology-of-knowledge framework would lead us to expect, from a male viewpoint. Traditional views of female sexuality and personality are presented generally unsullied by the findings of Kinsey and Masters and Johnson, though the latter resulted in some changes in rhetoric.

In the last two decades at least one-half of the texts that indexed the topics stated that the male sex drive was stronger than the female's; she was interested in sex for procreation more than for recreation. In addition, they said most women were "frigid" and that the vaginal orgasm was the "mature" response. Gynecologists, our society's official experts on women, think of themselves as the woman's friend. With friends like that, who needs enemies?

Notes

1. We thank Marlyn Grossman for a careful reading of this paper and valuable criticism. Another version of this paper was presented at the American Sociological Association meetings in 1972. A longer version is available from the authors. This paper is on file at the Women's History Research Center in Berkeley, Calif.
2. There is a growing literature detailing the emphasis on traditional sex roles in works ranging from children's story and school books through college history and sociology texts and academic disciplines (e.g., Ehrlich 1971; Weitzman et al. 1972).
3. Our analysis is based not only on indexed items but on a general reading of the texts.

References

* Behrman, Samuel J., and John R. C. Gosling. 1959. *Fundamentals of Gynecology.* New York: Oxford University Press.
* Benson, Ralph C. 1971. *Handbook of Obstetrics and Gynecology.* Los Altos, Calif.: Lange Medical Publishers.

  * One of the 27 gynecology textbooks used in this study.

* Brewer, John I., and Edwin J. DeCosts. 1967. *Textbook of Gynecology*. Baltimore: Williams & Wilkens.
* Cooke, Willard R. 1943. *Essentials of Gynecology*. Philadelphia: Lippincott.
* Crossen, Robert James. 1953. *Diseases of Women*. Saint Louis: Mosby.
* Curtis, A. H. 1946. *A Textbook of Gynecology*. Philadelphia: Saunders.
* Danforth, David. 1971. *Textbook of Obstetrics and Gynecology*. New York: Hoeber.
* Davis, Henry Carl, ed. 1964. *Gynecology and Obstetrics*. 3 vols. Hagarstown, Md.: Prior.
Ehrlich, Carol. 1971. "The Male Sociologist's Burden: The Place of Women in Marriage and Family Texts." *Journal of Marriage and the Family* 33:421–30.
* Gray, Laman. 1960. *A Textbook of Gynecology*. Springfield, Ill.: Thomas.
* Green, Thomas H. 1971. *Gynecology: Essentials of Clinical Practice*. Boston: Little, Brown.
* Greenhill, J. P. 1965. *Office Gynecology*. Chicago: Yearbook Medical Publishers.
* Huffman, John Williams. 1962. *Gynecology and Obstetrics*. Philadelphia: Saunders.
* Janney, James C. 1950. *Medical Gynecology*. Philadelphia: Saunders.
* Jeffcoate, Thomas. 1967. *Principles of Gynecology*. London: Butterworth.
* Kimbrough, Robert A., ed. 1965. *Gynecology*. Philadelphia: Lippincott.
Kinsey, Alfred C., et al. 1953. *Sexual Behavior in the Human Female*. New York: Simon & Schuster.
* Kistner, R. W. 1964. *Gynecology*. Chicago: Yearbook Medical Publishers.
* Lowrie, Robert J. 1952. *Gynecology, Diseases and Minor Surgery*. Springfield, Ill.: Thomas.
* Meigs, J. V., and S. H. Sturgis. 1963. *Progress in Gynecology*. New York: Grune & Stratton.
* Novak, Edmund R., Georgeanna Seegar Jones, and Howard W. Jones. 1970. *Novak's Textbook of Gynecology*. Baltimore: Williams & Wilkens.
Novak, Emil, and Edmund R. Novak. 1952. *Textbook of Gynecology*. Baltimore: Williams & Wilkens.
* Parsons, Langdon, and Sheldon C. Sommers. 1962. *Gynecology*. Philadelphia: Saunders.
* Pettit, Mary DeWitt. 1962. *Gynecologic Diagnosis and Treatment*. New York: McGraw-Hill.
* Reich, Walter, and M. Nechtow. 1957. *Practical Gynecology*. Philadelphia: Lippincott.
* Rubin, I. C., and Josef Novak. 1956. *Integrated Gynecology: Principles and Practice*. New York: McGraw-Hill.
Scott C. Russell. 1968. *The World of a Gynecologist*. London: Oliver & Boyd.
Scott, William A., and H. Brookfield Van Wyck. 1946. *The Essentials of Obstetrics and Gynecology*. Philadelphia: Lea and Febiger.
* Taylor, Edward Stewart. 1962. *Essentials of Gynecology*. Philadelphia: Lea and Febiger.
Weitzman, Lenore J., Deborah Eifler, Elizabeth Hokada, and Catherine Ross. 1972. "Sex Role Socialization in Picture Books for Preschool Children," *American Journal of Sociology* 77 (May):1125–50.
* Wharton, L. R. 1943. *Gynecology*. Philadelphia: Saunders.
* Willson, James Robert. 1971. *Obstetrics and Gynecology*. St. Louis: Mosby.

Medicine in Practice

THE SOCIAL ORGANIZATION OF MEDICINE is manifested on the interactional as well as the structural levels of society. There is an established and rich tradition of studying medical work "first hand" in medical settings, through participant-observation, interviewing, or both. Researchers go "where the action is"—in this case amongst doctors and patients to see just how social life (i.e., medical care) happens. Such studies are time-consuming and difficult (see Danziger, 1979) but are the only way to penetrate the structure of medical care and reveal the sociological texture of medical practice. For it is here that the structure of medicine shapes the type of care that is delivered.

There are at least three general foci for these qualitative studies. Some studies focus on the organization of the institution itself, such as a mental hospital (Goffman, 1961) or a nursing home (Gubrium, 1975). Others examine the delivery of services or practitioner-patient interaction ranging from childbirth (Shaw, 1974) to dying (Sudnow, 1967). A third general focus is on collegial relations among professionals (e.g., Freidson, 1975; Bosk, 1979). All of these studies give us a window on the backstage world of medical organization. No matter what the focus, they bring to life the processes through which organizations operate and how participants manage in their situations. It is worth noting also that most of these close-up studies end up with the researchers taking a critical stance toward the organization and practice of medicine.

The four articles in this section reveal different yet overlapping aspects of medicine in practice. The papers represent a range of medical settings and situations: outpatient obstetric encounters, an emergency room, a hospital surgical service, and a physician review committee. As well as illuminating the texture of medical practice, they individually and together raise a number of significant sociological issues.

In her study of the prenatal care of women, "The Uses of Expertise in Doctor-Patient Encounters During Pregnancy," Sandra Klein Danziger shows how the doctor's monopoly of medical knowledge, which manifests itself in an asymmetrical relationship between doctor and patient, is used by the physician to control the medical encounter. The women's health movement, among other health reform movements, has recognized the implications of the use of medical expertise as an instrument of power and has begun to challenge it.

In the second article, "Some Contingencies of the Moral Evaluation and Control of Clientele: The Case of the Hospital Emergency Service," Julius A. Roth demonstrates how everyday "prejudices" and evaluations by the staff of a patient's social worth affect the type of treatment people receive. (For another example of this process, see Sudnow, 1967.) Emergency room staff make moral judgments of patients' worthiness based on their evaluations of the patients' social attributes and the "appropriateness" of their demands on the staff. This not only reinforces and amplifies existing inequalities in medical care and services, but creates new ones.

Judith Lorber's study, "Good Patients and Problem Patients: Conformity and Deviance in a General Hospital" also shows physicians and medical staff making social evaluations that affect treatment. In her study of patients receiving elective surgery in a large urban hospital, Lorber describes how the medical staff defines "good" patients and "problem" patients in terms of the amount of "trouble" they cause for the staff. Problem patients are those who are uncooperative, complaining and demanding, while good patients are those who are compliant and take little staff time. Patients who interrupt well-established medical work routines are likely to reap the consequences of being labeled a problem patient.

The final article in this section is "Medical Mortality Review: A Cordial Affair" by Marcia Millman. Millman takes us into the "backrooms" of medicine and describes how physicians deal with medical mistakes among their colleagues. It appears that the mortality review is essentially designed to neutralize physicians' mistakes (although, of course, not their effect on the patient) and to maintain the medical social structure.[1] It is the "professional dominance" of physicians that insulates them from outside review of their mistakes and confines medical errors to the purview of the physician's peers. It is not surprising, especially given the potential for malpractice suits, that physicians try to neutralize the meaning of their mistakes and downplay their importance, but the problem of accountability for medical error remains a central issue in the reform of medical care.

All four articles highlight the structure of medical practice. Each illustrates how the social organization of medicine constrains and shapes the physician's work. Aside from delivering services, it appears that a very important element of the physician's task is sustaining the medical order in which services are delivered.

Note

1. In a recent study, Bosk (1979) conceptualizes different types of medical errors and implies that neutralization of mistakes may be less widespread than indicated by Millman's findings.

References

Bosk, Charles L. 1979. Forgive and Remember: Managing Medical Failure. Chicago: University of Chicago Press.

Danziger, Sandra Klein. 1979. "On doctor watching: Fieldwork in medical settings." Urban Life 7 (January): 513–31.

Freidson, Eliot. 1975. Doctoring Together: A Study of Professional Social Control. New York: Elsevier.

Goffman, Erving. 1961. Asylums. New York: Doubleday.

Gubrium, Jabar. 1975. Living and Dying at Murray Manor. New York: St. Martin's Press.

Shaw, Nancy Stoller. 1974. Forced Labor: Maternity Care in the United States. New York: Pergamon.

Sudnow, David. 1967. Passing On: The Social Organization of Dying. Englewood Cliffs, N.J.: Prentice-Hall.

24
The Uses of Expertise in Doctor-Patient Encounters During Pregnancy

Sandra Klein Danziger

Doctor-patient relationships typically bring together two people with very different interests. One is preoccupied with his/her work concerns, while the other is absorbed in his/her own personal well-being. In our society the state of the individual's well-being is largely in the hands of experts, who assess its status and designate ways to improve it. That people turn to others as experts implies that these others are in some sense "special". They have privileged access to knowledge, resources and skills that presumably can benefit the lay person. How such expertise is employed conversationally in the course of delivering medical care to pregnant women is the focus of this paper.

In theory, every interactional encounter between a physician and patient, whether surgery or a blood test is administered, whether contraception or chemotherapy is prescribed, is a situation in which medical information may be exchanged. How much information is given and how closely it approximates the physician's "real" assessment of the situation may depend in part upon two interactional factors: (a) the doctor's expressed interest in imparting expertise to the patient; and (b) the compatibility between this interest of the doctor and that of the patient in receiving the medical information or expertise.

An asymmetry between lay person and expert arises, then, from the former having to satisfy two conditions of the interaction. The lay person wants both to appear compatible with the expert and meet the need for which the expert's help is sought. In other words, suppose person A wants advice from expert B. In order for A to get B to give the desired quality and quantity of advice, A must fit into B's notions of the type of patient with the type of problem that warrants this particular type of advice giving. In contrast to the Parsonian notion of the medical professional's affective/value neutrality, I am suggesting that people in our society may expect doctors to hold rather typified views of their patients. Because of this, they assume a particular patient role when interacting with medical experts. They attempt to defer in a passive or submissive manner. One implication of their taking this role position is that doctors are permitted a more active role in controlling or structuring the course of an interaction sequence with a patient.

Two major variables, setting of the interaction and behavioral role repertoire of the individuals, obviously contribute to this asymmetry. First, the import of the factor of locale (and social organization thereof) cannot be underestimated. Compare the situation in which all medical encounters take place on the physician's turf, i.e. where the one person practices on a daily, routine basis and the other "visits" only infrequently and/or irregularly, with what may be the case when the doctor makes house calls, visits to settings where patients live and/or work. See Mehl (1) for a discussion of these differences with regard to home vs hospital childbirth. The other important point to be made here is that the amount of deference vs control exhibited during the encounter may or may not be related to what either party does in other situations. The most persistently aggressive patient may turn out to be most compliant in terms of carrying out a prescribed treatment regimen. Likewise, the most submissive patient in an encounter may be the most noncompliant when out of the doctor's office. See Lorber (2) for an analysis of behavioral compliance to the patient role and medical outcomes.

Many other factors influence the degree of asymmetry between the status positions of doctor and patient. Some of these have been addressed elsewhere, such as socioeconomic background in Duff and Hollingshead (3), ethnicity in Shuval (4) and Zola (5), age, marital status and family size in Shaw (6) and gender in Nathanson (7). My interest here is to elucidate some patterns of *effects* of this status discrepancy in terms of one particular product of medical interactions, the information transmitted. In examining what occurs within this frame of interaction, I am characterizing the doctor and patient as engaged in a parry and thrust situation, giving each other cues about the amount of information sharing that is appropriate. The result is based on what the doctor indicates is appropriate and how this coincides with the patient's expressed interest in obtaining the expertise. The model rests on a theoretical assertion of structural asymmetry, the assumption that the doctor wields more power in controlling the course of conversation, that the patient is for two reasons the more deferential interaction partner.

Within this framework, then, we may conceptualize a continuum of interactional postures doctors can assume with respect to providing information and those that patients can assume with reference to seeking or receiving information. First of all, the doctor is in the autonomous position of having a monopoly on the applied uses of medical scientific knowledge, as argued in Freidson (8). In the encounter with the patient, a physician has the prerogative to define what is therapeutic and what is outside the bounds of consideration, what aspects of the case shall be deemed relevant and irrelevant, and what topics are open and what topics are not open for discussion between doctor and patient. Topical autonomy is also demonstrated in Roth (9), Davis (10) and Daniels (11). In this scheme, there are three styles in which doctors can express their orientation toward the imparting of knowledge. They can perform their services as medical experts, as medical counselors, or as medical coparticipants. Ort (12) and Sorenson (13) posit similar continuums. The expert acts as a technician and exhibits little willingness to discuss his/her plan of action and to impart knowledge to the client. The counselor displays more general, rather than merely technical wisdom. He/she is more informative in the doctor-patient encounter, authoritatively guiding the client through the therapeutic process. The coparticipant acts with recognition of the client's need for valid information about his/her condition and encourages patient involvement in medical decision making.

The client or patient, on the other hand, is in an inferior position *vis-á-vis* the doctor with respect to information. Lacking the professional's knowledge, skills and resources is what presumably brings him/her to professional services in the first place. For other plausible reasons see Zola (14). Patients can interpret their role as recipient of services (see also Haug [15]) in one of three ways: as mere passive recipients; as active-dependent recipients; or as potentially knowledgeable participants. For a variety of reasons, the passive recipient does not seek information from the physician and is unresponsive to any attempt by the physician to impart knowledge. The active-dependent recipient seeks assurance that the doctor is reliable and competent. A minimum amount of information is sought, enough to convince the patient satisfactorily of the physician's ability to handle the therapeutic process. This patient is unlike the third type, the potentially knowledgeable participant, whose interest in the doctor's expertise exceeds this minimum, and who exhibits a willingness to share in the responsibility of decision making, provides information and asks for feedback from the doctor. Physicians and patients thus act out the encounter in ways which convey their respective notions of how expert knowledge is to be shared. See Table 1.

Field Data on Pregnancy

To illustrate the various uses of expertise that occur when each party adopts one of these positions, field data on prenatal medical care in a U.S. midwestern city will be presented. Ethnographic observation was conducted over an eight-month period in 1975–1976 in two clinic and three

Table 1.
Positions on Information Sharing

	Doctor	Patient
Not interested	Expert	Passive recipient
In limited favor	Counselor	Active-dependent recipient
Strongly in favor	Teaching coparticipant	Potentially knowledgeable participant

hospital settings where specialist obstetrician-gynecologists and family medical practitioners work. One clinic was a medical-school-based teaching institution, while the other was organized as a private group practice. In studying the activities and interactions of doctors and nurses with "low-risk"[1] patients and spouses of patients, I utilized two observation strategies. First, I followed staff members through the course of a workday or clinic session in which they would see up to 15–20 patients who were at all stages of the childbearing process. Then, I followed longitudinally a subsample of a dozen women, attending all of their medical encounters from mid-pregnancy through their labor and delivery. The data include descriptions and conversations from 100 to 150 episodes of early and initial-to-late prenatal care provided by a total of seven physicians to more than 30 patients.

Behavior toward expertise may have some special characteristics in the case of medical care during pregnancy. First of all, in obstetrics the doctor-patient relationship is frequently a male-female one. Knowledge is less likely to flow freely between the two participants when the physician's authority is reinforced by his maleness and the woman is in the role of recipient. The feminist literature abounds with descriptions of the way sex role typifications are exacerbated in health care services to women (16–19). Secondly, as McKinlay (20) and others have described it, pregnancy is a unique and ambiguous state for women. Being pregnant is not a usual condition; nor is it a medically pathological state. In pregnancy, compared to other situations in which people utilize doctors' services, relatively little medical intervention takes place. In its place, it is likely that a great deal of emphasis is placed on preventive health education during doctor-patient interactions. Thirdly, child-bearing women seem to feel an increased sense of vulnerability and need for supportive relationships from their families and their physicians (21, 22). Among the sample of women observed as patients in this study, I noticed a consistent avoidance of potential conflict with obstetrical care providers, physicians and nurses. Such avoidance may diminish the patient's efforts to obtain knowledge during encounters.[2]

Finally, certain dramaturgical aspects of prenatal care may further heighten the status asymmetry between doctor and patient. See Emerson

(23) for an analysis of these contingencies in gynecological care. In all of these visits, the doctor has some routine technical tasks of monitoring the woman's and baby's vital signs and progressing development. For the most part, the woman was perched on an exam table while the doctor was standing over her performing these physical manipulations. S/he may have examined further for medical risks, such as to check for edema, and/or inquired about symptoms indicative of risk factors or onset of labor. The woman was usually dressed but with her abdomen exposed for physical access. The physician was almost always in medical garb. Toward the end of pregnancy, s/he may perform from one to several internal pelvic examinations, for which the woman is half-naked and draped, braced on stirrups. In these, the doctor assessed a woman's "progress" in terms of whether or not labor was imminent.

The pronouncement on these occasions was invariably ambiguous in this data set, e.g. "well you're probably not going into labor soon", or "you still might go any day now". More precise information about factors that facilitate ease or promote difficulty during labor was obtained and sometimes conveyed to patients, but doctors were generally quite guarded in their predictions. Symbolic aspects of doctor-patient interaction such as clothing and the manner in which tasks are performed are likely to affect the frequency with which participants adopt the various positions on information sharing, as are other background factors of personality and situation.

In examining what actually transpires during a patient's visit to the doctor, it is useful to note first how little time is spent on information transmittal. For example, Waitzkin (24) found in a pretest study that less than a minute of a 20-minute session was devoted on the average to communicating information about illness. Within this portion of each visit, the variability in information outcomes may fall into one of nine categories, given the position of each participant.

Depending on which participant takes the initiative, the informing occasion takes two forms. One instance is that of the patient asking a question or bringing up a topic for discussion. The physician, on the other hand, is likely to initiate information sharing at a juncture in the session between completing one set of tasks and starting another, such as between the routine physical check and the charting of notes on the patient's medical record. S/he may typically comment upon the patient's progress or situation, describe a procedure or physiological development, or ask the patient if s/he has any questions or troubles to present to the doctor.

Each example from the data is thus characterized by either a patient's inquiry for medical information or a doctor's offering of information. Each participant's contribution to the exchange is classified as exemplifying one of the three relative positions of interest in sharing expertise. This is derived from what is said between the participants directly in the en-

Table 2.
Conversational Uses of Expertise

Type of patient behavior	Type of physician behavior		
	Expert	*Counselor*	*Coparticipant*
Passive recipient	Perfunctory 1,1	1,2	Hostile: antagonistic 1,3
Active-dependent recipient	2,1	Protective 2,2	2,3
Potentially knowledgeable participant	Hostile: arrogant 3,1	3,2	Educative 3,3

counters and from descriptive accounts of the observer's interactions with either patient or doctor. The range of possible outcomes is presented in Table 2.

Each of the nine cells represents a different conversational use of expertise, five of which will be illustrated with pregnancy data. These five have been chosen because they represent the three cases of compatible expressions and the two cases of incompatibility in the extreme.

Perfunctory Use

When the doctor[3] acts as a technical expert and the patient as a passive recipient (cell 1,1), the doctor's preexisting monopoly of knowledge does not change, and little information is transmitted during the encounter. This situation is characteristic of the perfunctory relationship, in which services are provided in a way similar to the way plumbers fix plumbing and mechanics repair cars. To such experts providing information to the owner of the car is extraneous to the job of getting the engine running. The perfunctory interchange between doctor and patient emphasizes that the service is a technical matter; communication never advances beyond the expert obtaining medical history and physical information and the patient describing symptoms or asking how to take prescribed medication. The person in the recipient status is treated as a work object, that which is to be operated on; the model of the surgical relationship (see Szasz and Hollander's models in Wilson and Bloom [25]) fits most closely into this category of exchange. The following example from the data on prenatal care illustrates perfunctory information sharing. Relatively little knowledge is imparted in this situation, a routine late pregnancy visit by a woman who suspected she was in labor. The doctor determined that it was "just" a case of stomach flu.

Well, other than that [the flu and the fact that she isn't in labor], everything looks good. Your blood pressure's good, you're growing, the baby's fine. You've lost a pound; that's probably from the flu. . . . Well, I think you'll probably go in a day or so, but you ought to go ahead and make another appointment for next week. Dr. —— will want to do a pelvic exam if you don't, so just in case . . .

No interpretation of the situation was sought or volunteered. He read off the checklist of things he was recording on the chart without responding to the fact that she had been up all night with cramps, nausea and diarrhea. When she came in, the patient told the nurse that she was uncertain whether she was both sick and in labor; she left with the knowledge that she was only sick and still waiting for labor. The doctor pronounced her condition without elaborating and without expressing any personal sympathy. This perfunctory provision of service thus resulted in no transmission of expertise and no patient involvement in the decision or assessment process.

Protective Use

When the doctor acts as a counselor and the patient as an active-dependent recipient (cell 2,2), the result is the sharing of some knowledge in conjunction with a reaffirmation of the doctor's controlling authority. This provision of information-with-reassurance falls in the category of protective outcomes. Services are rendered in a style characteristic of the benefactor-beneficiary relationship. The source of the benefactor's knowledge remains inaccessible to the patient. Many variations in counseling styles from the manner of a high priest or generalized wise man to that of a more mundane problem solver like a tax accountant, are characterized by this information sharing with assurance. The expertise is applied in a way that emphasizes the special importance of the professional and the deficiencies of the lay person. In medicine, reassuring patients is considered to have great therapeutic value; the profession's ethics give higher priority to courtesy and kindliness than to the patient's right to know. The result is that the information given sometimes does not match the doctor's actual perception of the situation. This is especially common during labor and delivery, when patients are often told only how "well" they are doing, despite the fact that the doctor may be worried and may even be planning contingency strategies for intervening in the birth process.

For example, doctors often assume that the question "How am I doing?" carries an implicit answer, i.e. that patients *want* to be told, "You're doing fine". Doctors presume that patients who ask this do not necessarily want to know what the doctor *really* thinks. One physician commented to me about a patient's question, "some people just beg you to lie to them". Such a patient differs from a passive and nonquestioning patient in seeking some kind of information from the doctor. Whichever party initiates the imparting of information and/or the provision of reassurance, they both respond compatibly in the protective use of expertise. This may be contrasted with the situations represented by any of the other four cells in the table: 1,2; 2,1; 3,2; and 2,3. In each of these, only one party initiates assurance-provision, and the other acts with more or less interest in sharing information. The result that is negotiated is marred by less acceptance of the doctor's authority to define the situation than in the more compatible protective case. The following exchange between a doctor and a patient's husband during the woman's regular prenatal visit illustrates protective information sharing. At this point in the session, the doctor has just explained her situation by telling them that with suspected preeclampsia,[4] he advises women to get a lot of rest.

> HUSBAND: Why wouldn't they just go ahead and induce her then?
> DOCTOR: Okay . . . her symptoms aren't really clear enough to suggest something like that is warranted . . . (talk of symptoms) . . . You know, if it were really something we were concerned about, we would start to think of her pregnancy as causing excess strain. But my thinking at this point is that everything is really coming along well but that we just want to make sure it stays that way.
> HUSBAND: Well, you know more about this than I do, but I just couldn't understand why wait when this thing seemed, you know, like it was pretty serious.
> DOCTOR: Oh, gee, I hope I didn't alarm you. Were you very worried,————?
> PATIENT: Well, uh . . .
> HUSBAND: She sure was . . .
> DOCTOR: Well we can't have you worried; that defeats the whole purpose. . . . I hope it's clear now that we aren't terribly concerned and there's nothing to be afraid of, but we just want you to stay well. . . .

The doctor expends most of his verbal energy on assuring them that they need not worry. Deferring to the doctor's superior knowledge, the husband is readily convinced not to press for more information. This doctor told me that he purposely did not go into much detail about induction, that he did not want to be too specific in the event that he changed his mind about its necessity. He was protecting his own autonomy to act without having to justify his decision to the patient. Likewise, the patient displays satisfaction in hearing that the doctor has his reasons, but does not persist in being told what they are.

Educative Use

Another category of compatible behaviors occurs when both parties participate in the sharing of expertise: the doctor acts as coparticipant and the patient as potentially knowledgeable participant (cell 3,3). The product of educative relationships is cooperative decision making and a relatively open feedback situation. Like teachers with students, doctors in this type of interaction spend time explaining procedures to patients, emphasizing the importance of the patient's understanding and involvement in the therapeutic process. The patient expresses interest in acquiring his/her own perspective on the problem at hand, rather than merely deferring to the opinion of the professional. Both parties treat the learning process as intrinsic to the provision of service. The following excerpt from the data— a discussion of breastfeeding during a regular prenatal visit—illustrates the mutual sharing of both information and decision making.

> PATIENT: Oh, I have something else. I'm planning to try to breastfeed the thing and . . . when do they have you start, right away or after a day or so?
> DOCTOR: Whenever you want to.
> PATIENT: Well, which is best?
> DOCTOR: Oh, it depends. It's better for the milk coming in to start as soon as possible. But if you're not up to it, you don't have to. . . .
> PATIENT: But then do they give it formula?
> DOCTOR: No, not necessarily. Listen, the whole thing about breastfeeding is *not* to worry about it and to really want to do it. If you have *any* doubts about it, chances are you'll have trouble.
> PATIENT: Well, I'm not hung up over it or anything. I've got a friend who is really uptight and I can't understand that at all. No, that's not for me. But how do the gals over there in the nursery react to it?
> DOCTOR: Well, we have really come full swing. You know, way back when, it used to be that if you didn't breastfeed, it was somehow not right. Then, it got to if you did breastfeed, it just wasn't nice or something. Now, we're back to if you don't, you're almost bad. It doesn't matter really one way or the other. I've seen healthy babies on both. I've seen psychologically sound, good relationships both ways. So it's really up to you to do what suits you best. Sooo. . . .
> PATIENT: So! Okay, that's all my questions, then. . . .

In this instance, the patient is left to decide what to consider therapeutic. The doctor merely presents the choice and suggests that she follow her own emotional feelings about it. She is clearly free to question him further on the issue. The woman's expressed interest in knowing is compatible with doctor's view of her as the able and competent decision maker with whom the ultimate responsibility for this matter should rest.

Hostile Uses

The previous three categories represent the results of the most compatible behaviors of doctor and patient. The next two types of uses of expertise occur when the doctor and patient act most dissimilarly with respect to information sharing. The situation of the antagonistic type of hostility occurs when the doctor acts as a coparticipant and the patient as the passive recipient (cell 1,3). This occurs, for example, when the patient is unwilling to comply with medical orders and the physician tries to convince the patient of the seriousness of the situation. The information as to severity of condition is perceived by the doctor as intrinsic to the provision of service while it is irrelevant for the patient.

The arrogant type of hostility occurs when the doctor acts as mere technical expert and the patient acts as potentially knowledgeable participant (cell 3,1). Conflict can result from a patient's wanting to know more than the doctor wants to discuss with her/him. Both types of exchanges can result in the doctor's attempting to resolve the conflict and achieve control of the situation by distorting the information given. In both cases, the patient's expressed attitude toward information is defined by the doctor as inappropriate: in the case of antagonism, the doctor may try to convince the patient of the dangers of not following the prescribed medical regimen, perhaps by exaggerating these dangers beyond what the doctor "really" thinks they are; in the case of arrogance, the doctor may put down the patient's expressed wish for medical information by invoking his or her own superior authoritative wisdom, implying that the patient has overstepped his/her limits. Examples of both types are provided from the data. The following exchange illustrates hostile: antagonistic (cell 1,3).

> DOCTOR: You obviously didn't do any of the things I told you. Your pressure's up.
> PATIENT: (*Sheepish*) I guess I didn't.
> DOCTOR: I'll tell you, you keep this up and I'll put you in the hospital. And if you think that's a threat, it's because it is. I'm threatening you to make you realize that you just cannot continue like this. Now what kinds of excuses are you going to give me for not doing what you're supposed to? (*Pause*) No excuses?
> PATIENT: I've been busy? (*Sheepish giggle again*).
> DOCTOR: Busy? You should be busy *resting* and that's all you should be doing! Did you have high blood pressure with your last pregnancy?
> PATIENT: No, I don't think so. They didn't make a big deal out of it, so I would think not.
> DOCTOR: Well, it is a big deal. It's the way mothers and babies die. Does your husband know you're supposed to be taking it easy?
> PATIENT: Well, yes, but. . .
> DOCTOR: This has got to stop. You are to do absolutely nothing except rest two hours in the morning, two hours in the afternoon, and be in bed every night by 9 o'clock.
> PATIENT: My little girl isn't even in bed by then.
> DOCTOR: Well, her father will have to stay up with her but not you. And if you can't do this, I'll put you in the hospital and put nurses on you who won't let you out of bed. . .

The harangue continued at length, with the doctor giving reasons for reacting so strongly, emphasizing that there is little he can do, that only she can do something about it. His reactions were exaggerated from the beginning, when he accused her of not heeding his advice; in fact, he had not previously warned her of her pressure elevation. In this exchange, the patient acted dumbfounded, and the doctor showered her with information on the severity of her situation and on what needed to be done, resulting in hostility and overly negative information. The last example of a situation in prenatal care illustrates the hostile: arrogant exchange (cell 3,1).

PATIENT: The nurse was saying they're doing the Leboyer method at the hospital?

DOCTOR: Leboyer, huh?

PATIENT: Yes. I was wondering what your opinion of it was.

DOCTOR: My opinion? Of Leboyer? It's unscientific. I'm tired of being told I'm cruel to babies! We don't do that bath business; nor would I do deliveries in the dark without gloves. So, I'm not the least bit interested in it.

PATIENT: Well, what about the things like nursing on the table right away? I thought we had talked about that earlier and you seemed to say that might be okay.

DOCTOR: You can breastfeed whenever you want and as much as you want. I don't care, that's fine with me.

PATIENT: Hmm, okay.

First, the doctor puts the idea completely out of the question by invoking the canons of science. He simply cannot go along with such "nonsense" so she must not press the issue. The patient then tries another angle, which he permits as a reasonable request. The doctor leaves no room for discussion, but rather insists that his authority is unbendable. He later commented to me that "people who want it (Leboyer) are neurotic, and they want me to do some sort of magic that will change things." The patient's question was indicative of the fact that her attitude about participation was incongruous with her doctor's. The result was hostility and truncated communication with him biasing his comments with ridicule of the patient's ideas, thereby refusing to consider her input in the therapeutic process.

Other Uses

The four other outcomes represented in Table 2 occur when only one of the two participants takes a middle-range position on the continuum. When the patient acts as active-dependent recipient with either an expert-acting doctor (cell 2,1) or a coparticipating doctor (cell 2,3), or when the doctor acts as counselor with either a passive (cell 1,2) or a potentially knowledgeable patient (cell 3,2), the resulting conversational use of expertise is more variable than in the cases of clearly compatible or incompatible expressions. In these situations, more subtle nuances of interaction are likely to determine the outcomes. The positions taken by each member are only slightly different from each other, which makes it probable that a host of other factors influence the results. The cases illustrating these categories might thus be quite dissimilar from one another depending upon who initiates what type of information sharing.

For example, in cell 2,1, the patient could ask for reassurance and receive a negative response from the technician type of doctor such as, "Don't be silly, there is nothing to worry about". On the other hand, a doctor could be acting perfunctorily, to which the patient responds by requesting assurance. The result of this could be a polite, efficient "everything's going to be just fine". The products of such interactions are thus more subject to negotiation and less stable than the patterns described in the preceding five cells.

Summary

In summary, I have typologized doctor-patient encounters in terms of the participants' behavior with respect to expertise and the resulting quality and quantity of information exchanged. Of the nine possible classes of outcomes, five were illustrated with data on care during pregnancy. For any single doctor-patient relationship, the type of exchanges that are engaged in can vary over the course of the pregnancy, birth and postpartum period, and can even be mixed within a single encounter. The primary focus here has been to distinguish analytically the ranges of possible uses of expertise that result from the expressions of different interests in sharing knowledge.

In the first category, expertise is used perfunctorily. In the illustration, the doctor seems obliged to conduct some minimal amount of conversation, so he whips out an assessment of the patient's status. The discussion is apparently extrinsic to the rendering of his services. He merely verbalizes some pieces of his assessment while jotting down his notes on the medical record. The patient expresses no further interest in the information.

In the second category, expertise is used protectively. The doctor restricts his answer to a limited patient inquiry to a variation on the theme of "just leave these things to me and everything will be fine". This allows the doctor greater autonomy by asking the patient to entrust her/himself to the physician. The lack of further questioning from the patient, or in the example given the patient's spouse, appears to confirm the fact that this is all the information s/he is interested in obtaining.

In the third category, the transmittal of information is an intrinsic part of the delivery of the expert's services. The expertise is used to enhance the patient's decision-making responsibility for a therapeutic matter. The patient initiates the discussion of medical policy on breastfeeding, and the physician, despite his message about potential problems, conveys that it is primarily a matter of personal choice.

In the fourth and fifth categories of informing interactions, expertise is used to maximize the physician's power over the patient or, put differently, the lay person's dependency on the expert's control. Information is conveyed from the doctor with hostility of two types. In antagonistic situations, s/he provides an assessment of the patient's health status which exaggerates her problems by accusing her of noncompliance and threatening her with a description of the risks she runs by not abiding by doctor's orders. A more balanced assessment would describe the outcome potential both for doing what the doctor suggests and for not complying, thereby leaving the choice and risk taking up to the patient herself. In the illustration, however, the doctor told her only that if she did not heed his advice, she could die. In all likelihood, he was interpreting her passivity in the encounter as a confirmation of her negligence. He framed his expertise in an argument that suggested that she had no choice but to submit to his authority.

Finally, in the arrogant type of hostile exchange, the physician reacts negatively to a patient's request for information. She asks what he thinks of a procedure; he interprets her interest as troublesome, as a misguided or inappropriate interest in medical expertise. He responds by distorting the weight of scientific evidence and refusing to entertain her request. Actually, the absurdity or merit of the Leboyer procedure has not been conclusively demonstrated. The doctor masks his intolerance of the patient's input by claiming his privileged access to superior knowledge. He uses his expertise to deny the patient the prerogative to question him on his own territory as he defines it.

Implications

The work settings through which the delivery of health care is "produced" have been extensively examined in the literature. Despite this fact, McKinlay (26) notes the lack of "empirical attempts to explore the various ways in which aspects of professional behavior may influence client-professional encounters". One way in which medical work has been illuminated is in terms of the social relations of one of its special resources, knowledge. Throughout the work of Freidson runs this theme of medicine's privileged monopoly on an ever-encroaching arena of expertise.

His analysis of the profession (8) raises the issue of the fine line between technical expertise and privileged social power. Medicine is viewed as a particular case of an occupational group with autonomy over itself as well as control over an enormous range of occupations in the hierarchy of the health industry. This autonomy, granted to the profession by society, is exercised in the practical routines of medical work in a way that violates the very conditions upon which it is guaranteed—that members will be self-regulating. Not only do clinicians practice avoidance of control over each other, but they are also segregated from each other in a way that reinforces this nonregulation and legitimizes it. The consequences are especially dangerous in the case of this type of consulting profession, since the expanding sphere of medical authority is growing at an unprecedented rate with very little pressure for physicians to become accountable to each other, much less to other groups in society.

Some of his suggestions of the dangers of medical control are based upon the work done by Scheff and others on illness as social deviance, particularly those illnesses classified as mental disorders. In *Being Mentally Ill,* Scheff (27) claims that "the medical metaphor of 'mental illness' suggests a determinate process which occurs within the individual: the unfolding and development of disease". This is sometimes a prejudgment of the issue that socially problematic behavior is symptomatic of existing underlying disorder.

The role of physicians in the process of deviance amplification or secondary career is developed as a uniquely biased type of official authority. The prevailing norm for medical decision rules in cases of diagnostic uncertainty is that it is better to judge a well person sick than a sick person well. To the extent that the public and physicians are biased toward diagnosis and treatment, the creation of illness or secondary deviation will occur.

A most recent extension of this argument has been conceptualized by Conrad as the process of "medicalization of deviance" (28). When an issue is discovered to fall within the rubric of the medical model of intervention, it is desocialized and consequently depoliticized. The crux of the issue of the "coming of the therapeutic state" thesis is for me the question of the peculiarity of this form of social control. How the medical model succeeds in controlling behavior is not so much an issue of use of pharmacological agents or surgical implementation. It is a matter of their occasioned legitimation in terms of the definition of the situation.

An understanding of this legitimation process requires an interactional perspective on what transpires in medical settings. Most of the studies of doctor-patient relationships, however, are not characterized by this dynamic orientation. Instead, these seek largely to explain the finding that communication between doctors and patients is problematic and filled with gaps (see for example Duff and Hollingshead [3]). Such "failures" in communication appear to produce patient dissatisfaction and varying degrees of lack of concern among physicians. In general, doctors are said to minimize the importance of the problem or to make excuses for it by referring to the harried nature of their daily clinical work.

Researchers have replied by suggesting the profound potential detriments to patient welfare that can stem from cognitive difficulties with health problems (see Skipper and Leonard [29] and Leventhal [30]).

Others have framed the issue in terms of compliance (2) perhaps on the grounds that if doctors are not aroused by the specter of psychosomatic effects, they may "buy" the issue as significant for patients' motivation to carry out courses of therapy. Of most interest are the studies that have located the source of the problem in the attitudes and orientations of physicians toward their work (see for example Shuval [4], Waitzkin and Stoeckle [31], Waitzkin [24] and Comaroff [32]). However, what doctors and patients may want or expect of their interactions with one another is a different issue than: (1) what occurs during ongoing, situated transactions; and (2) how expected-actual discrepancies are resolved. Whether and, more importantly, how patients struggle to obtain more information and doctors actively engage in withholding information are unsubstantiated by a lack of empirical data.

Many theoretical models have been developed that depict this interaction process (Parsons [33], Freidson [34], Wilson and Bloom [25], Waitzkin and Stoeckle [31] and Leventhal [30]). The contributions of Glaser and Strauss (35), Davis (10) and Roth (9, 36, 37) all provide documentation of one processual aspect of these encounters. Each substantiates that information about prognosis is selectively conveyed to patients, resulting in a variety of consequences for the patient's perception and management of his/her illness. None of these, however, provides a framework to examine the way selective conveyances are produced in the course of the interactional encounter. While some even go so far as to categorize the content of what is conveyed, they do not analyze how it is that these information transmissions "work".

The question addressed with this model is thus not why communication "fails", but precisely how it is done and with what contextual implications. I have described both structural and negotiated interactional features that contribute to the power of medical expertise. Several dimensions of this typology lend themselves to further analysis.

Further Applications of the Model

First of all, the model suggests several hypotheses about relative frequencies of various uses of expertise. One could compare interactions in different settings or with patients at different stages of illness or with different types of problems. One could vary the doctor or professional expert variables as well as the patient or context characteristics in order to test for differences in information transmission. Were this particular data set large enough, I could compare the frequency of informing positions taken by the specialists and the family doctors and hold constant the stage of pregnancy, or the social status of the patient, or the number of patient-initiated requests for information. Another application of the model has to do with the way historical and societal pressures affect the quality of these interactions. Changing frequencies of types of exchanges occurring between one type of experts and their clientele might reflect changes in society or in technology.

In terms of longitudinal changes, one might expect that if the feminist movement is having an impact on medicine, it should become evident in a changing frequency of the different types of doctor-patient exchanges in obstetrics and gynecology (see also Kaiser and Kaiser [38]). While the *protective* patterns are currently the most common ones, we would expect feminist women to intensify their assertions of participatory rights in encounters with doctors. This would increase the number of *hostile: arrogant* and/or *educative* relationships, depending on doctors' reactions to the heightened interest of patients in medical knowledge and decision making.

Among other potentially influential factors are the changing technology of obstetrical medical care and the growing advocacy of patient's rights, particularly in the "natural childbirth" movement. These two factors are probably creating opposing pressures on physicians. While the scientific and technological advances encourage them to be more like experts, more medically specialized and problem oriented, the consumer rights groups demand that they be more like counselors or perhaps coparticipants, more family oriented and attuned to social-psychological and emotional considerations. The changing cultural contexts of medicine and of pregnancy and birth provide different notions of the way expertise should be used and thus have implications for the types of doctor-patient relationships that will proliferate and decline.

Notes

The research for this paper was supported by a predoctoral Health Services Research Traineeship, National Institutes of Health, directed by George Psathas, Boston University, and by a postdoctoral traineeship from N.I.M.H., directed by David Mechanic. The author wishes to acknowledge the excellent comments of Diane Brown, Sol Levine, Camille Smith, Howard Waitzkin and two anonymous journal referees.

1. The term "low risk" designates the absence of well-known risk factors and forecasts these pregnancies as uneventful or uncomplicated.
2. A psychiatrist I spoke with supported this notion, which is also a popular belief: women hold their obstetricians in extraordinary regard and place them on a pedestal. Many reasons could be offered for this perception which are beyond the scope of this paper.
3. In the quoted excerpts from the data, all doctors are referred to by the pro-

noun "he." While a few of the physicians in the study were women, revealing them as such would risk violating their anonymity.
4. Preeclampsia is a pathological condition of late pregnancy, characterized by hypertension, swelling and protein in the urine.

References

1. Mehl, L. E. Options in maternity care. *Women and Health* 2. 29, 1977.
2. Lorber J. Good patients and problem patients: conformity and deviance in a general hospital. *J. Hlth soc. Behav.* **16**, 213, 1975.
3. Duff R. S. and Hollingshead A. B. *Sickness and Society.* Harper & Row, New York, 1968.
4. Shuval J. T. *Social Functions of Medical Practice.* Jossey-Bass, San Francisco, 1970.
5. Zola I. K. Problems of communication, diagnosis and patient care, *J. med. Educ.* **38**, 829, 1963.
6. Shaw N. S. *Forced Labor: Maternity Care in the United States.* Pergamon Press, New York, 1974.
7. Nathanson C. A. Illness and the feminine role: a theoretical review. *Soc. Sci. Med.* **9**, 57, 1975.
8. Freidson E. *Profession of Medicine,* Dodd-Mead, New York, 1972.
9. Roth J. A. Staff and client control strategies in urban hospital emergency services. *Urban Life Cult.* **1**, 39, 1972.
10. Davis F. Uncertainty in medical prognosis, clinical and functional. *Am. J. Sociol.* **66**, 41, 1960.
11. Daniels A. K. Advisory and coercive functions in psychiatry. *Sociol. Work Occupn* **2**, 55, 1975.
12. Ort R. S. *et al.* The doctor-patient relationship as described by physicians and medical students. *J. Hlth hum. Behav.* **5**, 25, 1964.
13. Sorenson J. R. Biomedical innovation, uncertainty, and doctor-patient interaction. *J. Hlth soc. Behav.* **15**, 366, 1974.
14. Zola I. K. Pathways to the doctor—from person to patient. *Soc. Sci. Med.* **7**, 677, 1973.
15. Haug M. R. The deprofessionalization of everyone? *Sociol. Focus* **8**, 201, 1975.
16. Ehrenreich B. and English D. *Complaints and Disorders: The Sexual Politics of Sickness* The Feminist Press, New York, 1973.
17. Frankfort E. *Vaginal Politics,* Quadrangle, New York, 1972.
18. Chesler P. *Women and Madness,* Doubleday, New York, 1972.
19. Boston Women's Health Collective. *Our Bodies, Ourselves.* Simon & Schuster, New York, 1971.
20. McKinlay J. B. The sick role—illness and pregnancy. *Soc. Sci. Med* **6**, 561, 1972.
21. Benedek T. The psychobiology of pregnancy. In *Parenthood—Its Psychology*

and Psychobiology (Edited by Anthony E. J. and Benedek T.) Little-Brown, Boston, 1970.

22. Newton N. Emotions of pregnancy. *Clin. Obstet. Gynec.* **6**, 639, 1963.
23. Emerson J. Behavior in private places: sustaining definitions of reality in gynecological examinations. In *Recent Sociology* No. 2 (Edited by Dreitzel H. P.) p. 74. Macmillan, London, 1970.
24. Waitzkin H. Information control and the micropolitics of health care: summary of an ongoing research project. *Soc. Sci. Med.* **10**, 263, 1976.
25. Wilson R. and Bloom S. Patient practitioner relationships. In *Handbook of Medical Sociology* 2nd edn. (Edited by Freeman H. E. *et al.*) p. 315. Prentice-Hall. Englewood Cliffs, 1972.
26. McKinlay J. B. Some approaches and problems in the study of the uses of services—an overview. *J. Hlth soc. Behav.* **13**, 137, 1972.
27. Scheff T. J. *Being Mentally Ill,* p. 31. Aldine, Chicago, 1966.
28. Conrad P. The discovery of hyperkinesis: notes on the medicalization of deviant behavior. *Social Probl.* **23**, 19, 1975.
29. Skipper J. K. and Leonard R. C. Children, stress, and hospitalization: a field experiment. *J. Hlth soc. Behav.* **9**, 275, 1968.
30. Leventhal H. The consequences of depersonalization during illness and treatment: an information-processing model. In *Humanizing Health Care* (Edited by Howard J. and Strauss A.) p. 119. Wiley-Interscience, New York, 1975.
31. Waitzkin H. and Stoeckle J. D. The communication of information about illness: clinical, sociological, and methodological considerations. *Adv. psychosom. Med.* **8**, 180, 1972.
32. Comaroff J. Communicating information about nonfatal illness: the strategies of a group of general practitioners. *Sociol. Rev.* **24**, 269, 1976.
33. Parsons T. *The Social System.* Free Press. New York, 1951.
34. Freidson E. *Professional Dominance: The Social Structure of Medical Care.* Atherton, New York, 1970.
35. Glaser B. and Strauss A. Awareness contexts and social interaction. In *Social Psychology Through Symbolic Interaction* (Edited by Stone G. and Farberman H.) p. 336. Blaisdell, New York. 1970.
36. Roth J. A. *Timetables Structuring the Passage of Time in Hospital Treatment and Other Careers.* Bobbs-Merrill, Indianapolis, 1963.
37. Roth J. A. Some contingencies of the moral evaluation and control of clientele: the case of the emergency hospital service. *Am. J. Sociol.* **77**, 839, 1972.
38. Kaiser B. L. and Kaiser I. H. The challenges of the women's movement to American gynecology. *Am. J. Obstet. Gynec.* **120**, 652, 1974.

25

Some Contingencies of the Moral Evaluation and Control of Clientele: The Case of the Hospital Emergency Service

Julius A. Roth

The moral evaluation of patients by staff members has been explored in detail in the case of "mental illness" (Scheff 1966, chap. 5; Strauss et al. 1964, chaps. 8 and 12; Belknap 1956; Scheff 1964; Goffman 1961, pp. 125–70, 321–86; Hollingshead and Redlich 1958; Szasz 1960). The assumption is made by some (especially Thomas Szasz) that mental illness is a special case which readily allows moral judgments to be made because there are no technical criteria to be applied and because psychiatric concepts in their historical development have been a pseudoscientific replacement of moral judgments. Charles Perrow (1965) stresses lack of technology as a factor which forces psychiatric practitioners to fall back on commonsense concepts of humanitarianism which open the way to moral evaluations of the clientele.

I contend that the diagnosis and treatment of mental illness and the "care" of mental patients are not unique in incorporating moral judgments of the clientele, but are only obvious examples of a more general phenomenon which exists no matter what the historical development or the present state of the technology. Glaser and Strauss (1964) put forward such a notion when they demonstrated how the "social worth" of a dying patient affects the nursing care he will receive. I would add that moral evaluation also has a direct effect on a physician's diagnosis and treatment recommendations. This is obvious in extreme cases, such as when a monarch or the president of the United States is attended by teams of highly qualified diagnosticians to insure a detailed and accurate diagnosis and has outstanding specialists flown to his bedside to carry out the treatment. I will discuss some aspects of this same process as it applies on a day-to-day basis in a routine hospital operation involving more "ordinary" patients.

The data are taken from observations of six hospital emergency services in two parts of the country—one northeastern location and one West Coast location. My co-workers and I spent several periods of time (spread over two or three months in each case) in the emergency department of each of the hospitals. In one hospital we worked as intake clerks over a period of three months. At other times we observed areas in the emergency unit without initiating any interaction with patients, visitors, or personnel. At other points we followed patients through the emergency service from their first appearance to discharge or inpatient admission, interviewing patient and staff during the process. During these periods of observation, notes were also kept on relevant conversations with staff members.

The hospital emergency service is a setting where a minimum of information is available about the character of each patient and a long-term relationship with the patient is usually not contemplated. Even under these conditions, judgments about a patient's moral fitness and the appropriateness of his visit to an emergency service are constantly made, and staff action concerning the patient—including diagnosis, treatment, and disposition of the case—are, in part, affected by these judgments.

The Deserving and the Undeserving

The evaluation of patients and visitors by emergency-ward staff may be conveniently thought of in two categories: (1) The application by the staff of concepts of social worth common in the larger society. (2) Staff members' concepts of their appropriate work role. In this section I will take up the first of these.

There is a popular myth (generated in part by some sociological writing) that persons engaged in providing professional services, especially medical care, do not permit the commonly accepted concepts of social worth in our culture to affect their relationship to the clientele. An on-the-spot description of *any* service profession—medicine, education, law, social welfare, etc.—should disabuse us of this notion. There is no evidence that professional training succeeds in creating a universalistic moral neutrality (Becker et al. 1961, pp. 323–27). On the contrary, we are on much safer ground to assume that those engaged in dispensing professional services (or any other services) will apply the evaluations of social worth common to their culture and will modify their services with respect to those evaluations *unless discouraged from doing so by the organizational arrangements under which they work.* Some such organizational arrangements do exist on emergency wards. The rapid turnover and impersonality of the operation is in itself a protection for many patients who might be devalued if more were known about them. In public hospitals, at least, there is a rule that *all* patients presenting themselves at the registration desk must be seen by a doctor, and clerks and nurses know that violation of this rule, if discovered, can get them into serious trouble. (Despite this, patients are occasionally refused registration, usually because they are morally repugnant to the clerk.) Such arrangements restrict the behavior of the staff only to a limited extent, however. There remains a great deal of room for expressing one's valuation of the patient in the details of processing and treatment.

One common concept of social worth held by emergency-ward personnel is that the young are more valuable than the old. This is exemplified most dramatically in the marked differences in efforts to resuscitate young and old patients (Glaser and Strauss 1964; Sudnow 1967, pp. 100–109). "Welfare cases" who are sponging off the taxpayer—especially if they represent the product of an immoral life (such as a woman with illegitimate children to support)—do not deserve the best care. Perons of higher status in the larger society are likely to be accorded more respectful treatment in the emergency ward just as they often are in other service or customer relationships, and conversely those of lower status are treated with less consideration. (The fact that higher-status persons are more likely to make an effective complaint or even file lawsuits may be an additional reason for such differential treatment.)

Of course, staff members vary in the manner and degree to which they apply these cultural concepts of social worth in determining the quality of their service to the clientele. The point is that they are in a position to alter the nature of their service in terms of such differentiation, and all of them—porters, clerks, nursing personnel, physicians—do so to some extent. Despite some variations, we did in fact find widespread agreement on the negative evaluation of some categories of patients—evaluations which directly affected the treatment provided. Those who are the first to process a patient play a crucial role in moral categorization because staff members at later stages of the processing are inclined to accept earlier categories without question unless they detect clear-cut evidence to the contrary. Thus, registration clerks can often determine how long a person will have to wait and what kind of treatment area he is sent to, and, occasionally, can even prevent a person from seeing a doctor at all. Some patients have been morally categorized by policemen or ambulance crewmen before they even arrive at the hospital—categorization which affects the priority and kind of service given.

In the public urban hospital emergency service, the clientele is heavily skewed toward the lower end of the socioeconomic scale, and nonwhite and non-Anglo ethnic groups are greatly overrepresented. Also, many patients are in the position of supplicating the staff for help, sometimes for a condition for which the patient can be held responsible. With such a population, the staff can readily maintain a stance of moral superiority. They see the bulk of the patients as people undeserving of the services available to them. Staff members maintain that they need not tolerate any abuse or disobedience from patients or visitors. Patients and visitors may be issued orders which they are expected to obey. The staff can, and sometimes does, shout down patients and visitors and threaten them with ejection from the premises. The staff demands protection against possible attack and also against the possibility of lawsuits, which are invariably classified as unjustified. There is no need to be polite to the clientele and, in fact, some clerks frequently engage patients and visitors in arguments. The staff also feels justified in refusing service to those who complain or resist treatment or refuse to follow procedures or make trouble in any other way. From time to time the clients are referred to as "garbage," "scum," "liars," "deadbeats," people who "come out from under the rocks," by doctors, nurses, aides, clerks, and even housekeepers who sweep the floor. When we spent the first several days of a new medical year with a new group of interns on one emergency service, we found that an important part of the orientation was directed toward telling the interns that the patients were not to be trusted and did not have to be treated politely. At another public hospital, new registration clerks were told during their first few days of work that they would have to learn not to accept the word of patients but to treat everything they say with suspicion.

Despite the general negative conception of the clientele, differentiations are made between patients on the basis of clues which they present. Since this is typically a fleeting relationship where the staff member has little or no background information about the patient, evaluations must usually be made quickly on the basis of readily perceivable clues. Race, age, mode of dress, language and accents and word usage, and the manner in which the client addresses and responds to staff members are all immediate clues on which staff base their initial evaluations. A little questioning brings out other information which may be used for or against a patient: financial status, type of employment, insurance protection, use of private-practice doctors, nature of medical complaint, legitimacy of children, marital status, previous use of hospital services. In the case of unconscious or seriously ill or injured patients, a search of the wallet or handbag often provides informative clues about social worth.

Some characteristics consistently turn staff against patients and affect the quality of care given. Dirty, smelly patients cause considerable comment among the staff, and efforts are made to isolate them or get rid of them. Those dressed as hippies or women with scanty clothing (unless there is a "good excuse," e.g., a woman drowned while swimming) are frowned upon and are more likely to be kept waiting and to be rushed through when they *are* attended to. We observed hints that certain ethnic groups are discriminated against, but this is difficult to detect nowadays because everyone is extremely sensitive to the possibility of accusations of racial discrimination. If a woman with a child is tabbed a "welfare case" (from her dress, speech, and manner, or in the explicit form of a welfare card which she presents), the clerk is likely to ask, "Is there a father in the house?" while better-dressed, better-spoken women with children are questioned more discreetly.

Attributes and Categories: A Reciprocal Relationship

On one level, it is true to say that the staff's moral evaluation of a patient influences the kind of treatment he gets in the emergency room. But this kind of causal explanation obscures important aspects of the network of interrelationships involved. On another, the definition of devalued or favored categories and the attributes of the patient reinforce each other in a reciprocal manner.

Take, for example, patients who are labeled as drunks. They are more consistently treated as undeserving than any other category of patient. They are frequently handled as if they were baggage when they are brought in by police; those with lacerations are often roughly treated by physicians; they are usually treated only for drunkenness and obvious surgical repair without being examined for other pathology; no one believes their stories; their statements are ridiculed; they are treated in an abusive or jocular manner; they are ignored for long periods of time; in one hospital they are placed in a room separate from most other patients. Emergency-ward personnel frequently comment on how they hate to take care of drunks.

Thus, it might seem that the staff is applying a simple moral syllogism: drunks do not deserve to be cared for, this patient is drunk, therefore, he does not deserve good treatment. *But* how do we know that he is a drunk? By the way he is treated. Police take him directly to the drunk room. If we ask why the police define him as drunk, they may answer that they smell alcohol on his breath. But not all people with alcohol on their breath are picked up by the police and taken to a hospital emergency room. The explanation must come in terms of some part of the patient's background—he was in a lower-class neighborhood, his style of dress was dirty and sloppy, he was unattended by any friend or family member, and so on. When he comes to the emergency room *he has already been defined as a drunk*. There is no reason for the emergency-room personnel to challenge this definition—it is routine procedure and it usually proves correct insofar as they know. There is nothing to do for drunks except to give them routine medications and let them sleep it off. To avoid upsetting the rest of the emergency room, there is a room set aside for them. The police have a standard procedure of taking drunks to that room, and the clerks place them there if they come in on their own and are defined as drunk on the basis, not only of their breath odor (and occasionally there is no breath odor in someone defined as drunk), but in terms of their dress, manner, and absence of protectors. The physicians, having more pressing matters, tend to leave the drunks until last. Of course, they may miss some pathology which could cause unconsciousness or confusion because they believe the standard proves correct in the great majority of cases. They really do not know *how* often it does not prove correct since they do not check up closely enough to uncover other forms of pathology in most cases, and the low social status of the patients and the fact that they are seldom accompanied by anyone who will protect them means that complaints about inadequate examination will be rare. There *are* occasional challenges by doctors—"How do you know he's drunk?"—but in most cases the busy schedule of the house officer leaves little time for such luxuries as a careful examination of patients who have already been defined as drunks by others. Once the drunk label has been accepted by the emergency-room staff, a more careful examination is not likely to be made unless some particularly arresting new information appears (for example, the patient has convulsions, a relative appears to tell them that he has diabetes, an examination of his wallet shows him to be a solid citizen), and the more subtle pathologies are not likely to be discovered.

Thus, it is just as true to say that the *label* of "drunk" is accepted by hospital personnel because of the way the patient is treated as it is to say that he is treated in a certain way because he is drunk. Occasional cases show how persons with alcohol on their breath will not be treated as drunks. When an obviously middle-class man (obvious in terms of his dress, speech, and demands for service) was brought in after an automobile accident, he was not put in the drunk room, although he had a definite alcohol odor, but was given relatively quick treatment in one of the other examining rooms and addressed throughout in a polite manner.

Most drunks are men. A common negative evaluation for women is PID (pelvic inflammatory disease). This is not just a medical diagnostic category, but, by implication, a moral judgment. There are many women with difficult-to-diagnose abdominal pains and fever. If they are Negro, young, unmarried, lower class in appearance and speech, and have no one along to champion their cause, doctors frequently make the assumption that they have before them the end results of a dissolute sex life, unwanted pregnancy and perhaps venereal disease, illegal abortion, and consequent infection of the reproductive organs. The label PID is then attached and the patient relegated to a group less deserving of prompt and considerate treatment. This is *not* the same thing as saying a diagnosis of PID leads to rejection by medical personnel.

We observed one patient who had been defined as a troublemaker because of his abusive language and his insistence that he be released immediately. When he began to behave in a strange manner (random thrashing about), the police were promptly called to control him and they threatened him with arrest. A patient who was not defined as a trouble-maker and exhibited like behavior prompted an effort on the part of the staff to provide a medical explanation for his actions. Here again, we see that the category into which the patient has been placed may have more effect on determining the decisions of medical personnel than does his immediate behavior.

Thus, it is not simply a matter of finding which "objective" pathological states medical personnel like or dislike dealing with. The very definition of these pathological states depends in part on how the patient is categorized in moral terms by the screening and treatment personnel.

The Legitimate and the Illegitimate

The second type of evaluation is that related to the staff members' concept of their appropriate work roles (Strauss et al. 1964, chap. 13). Every worker has a notion of what demands are appropriate to his position. When demands fall outside that boundary, he feels that the claim is illegitimate. What he does about it depends on a number of factors, including his alternatives, his power to control the behavior of others, and his power to select his clientele (more on this later).

The interns and residents who usually man the larger urban emergency services like to think of this assignment as a part of their training which will give them a kind of experience different from the outpatient department or inpatient wards. Here they hope to get some practice in resuscitation, in treating traumatic injuries, in diagnosing and treating medical emergencies. When patients who are no different from those they have seen *ad nauseam* in the outpatient department present themselves at the emergency ward, the doctors in training believe that their services are being misused. Also, once on the emergency ward, the patient is expected to be "cooperative" so that the doctor is not blocked in his effort to carry out his tasks. Nurses, clerks, and others play "little doctor" and to this extent share the concepts of the boundaries of legitimacy of the doctors. But, in addition to the broadly shared perspective, each work specialty has its own notions of appropriate patient attributes and behavior based on their own work demands. Thus, clerks expect patients to cooperate in getting forms filled out. Patients with a "good reason," unconsciousness, for example, are excused from cooperating with clerical procedures, but other patients who are unable to give requested information or who protest against certain questions bring upon themselves condemnation by the clerks who believe that a person who subverts their efforts to complete their tasks has no business on the emergency ward.

A universal complaint among those who operate emergency services is that hospital emergency rooms are "abused" by the public—or rather by a portion of the public. This is particularly the case in the city and county hospitals and voluntary hospitals with training programs subsidized by public funds which handle the bulk of emergency cases in urban areas. The great majority of cases are thought of as too minor or lacking in urgency to warrant a visit to the emergency room. They are "outpatient cases" (OPD cases), that is, patients who could wait until the outpatient department is open, or if they can afford private care, they could wait until a physician is holding his regular office hours. Patients should not use the emergency room just because it gives quicker service than the outpatient department or because the hours are more convenient (since it is open all the time). Pediatricians complain about their day filled with "sore throats and snotty noses." Medical interns and residents complain about all the people presenting longstanding or chronic diseases which, though sometimes serious, do not belong in the emergency room. In every hospital—both public and private—where we made observations or conducted interviews, we repeatedly heard the same kinds of "atrocity stories": a patient with a sore throat of two-weeks' duration comes in at 3:00 A.M. on Sunday and expects immediate treatment from an intern whom he has got out of bed (or such variations as an itch of 75-days' duration, a congenital defect in a one-year-old child—always coming in at an extremely inconvenient hour).

Directors of emergency services recognize that some of their preoccupation with cases which are not "true emergencies" is not simply a matter of "abuse" by patients, but the result of tasks imposed upon them by other agencies—for example, giving routine antibiotic injections on weekends, caring for abandoned children, giving routine blood transfusions, receiving inpatient admissions, giving gamma globulin, providing venereal disease follow-up, examining jail prisoners, arranging nursing-home dispositions for the aged. But the blame for most of their difficulty is placed upon the self-referred patient who, according to the emergency-room staff, does not make appropriate use of their service.

The OPD case typically gets hurried, routine processing with little effort at a careful diagnostic work-up or sophisticated treatment unless he happens to strike the doctor as an interesting case (in which case he is no longer classified as an OPD case). Thus, pediatric residents move rapidly through their mass of sore throats and snotty noses with a quick look in ears and throat with the otolaryngoscope, a swab wiped in the throat to be sent to the laboratory, and if the child does not have a high fever (the nurse has already taken his temperature), the parent is told to check on the laboratory results the next day, the emergency-ward form is marked "URI" (upper respiratory infection), and the next child moves up on the treadmill. If a patient or a visitor had given anyone trouble, his care is likely to deteriorate below the routine level. Often, doctors define their task in OPD cases as simply a stopgap until the patient gets to OPD on a subsequent day, and therefore a careful work-up is not considered necessary.

Medical cases are more often considered illegitimate than surgical cases. In our public hospital tabulations, the diagnostic categories highest in the illegitimate category were gynecology, genito-urinary, dental, and "other medical." The lowest in proportion of illegitimate cases were pediatrics (another bit of evidence that children are more acceptable patients than adults), beatings and stabbings, industrial injuries, auto accidents, other accidents, and "other surgical." Much of the surgical work is suturing lacerations and making other repairs. Although these are not necessarily serious in terms of danger to life (very few were), such injuries were seen by the staff as needing prompt attention (certainly within 24 hours) to reduce the risk of infection and to avoid scarring or other deformity.

It is not surprising that in surgical cases the attributes and behavior of the patients are of lesser consequence than in medical cases. The ease with which the condition can be defined and the routine nature of the treatment (treating minor lacerations becomes so routine that anyone thinks he can do it—medical students, aides, volunteers) means that the characteristics and behavior of the patient can be largely ignored unless he becomes extremely disruptive. (Even violence can be restrained and the treatment continued without much trouble.) Certain other things are handled with routine efficiency—high fevers in children, asthma, overdose, maternity cases. It is significant that standard rules can be and have been laid down in such cases so that everyone—clerks, nurses, doctors (and patients once they have gone through the experience)—knows just how to proceed. In such cases, the issue of legitimacy seldom arises.

We find no similar routines with set rules in the case of complaints of abdominal pains, delusions, muscle spasms, depression, or digestive upset. Here the process of diagnosis is much more subtle and complex, the question of urgency much more debatable and uncertain. The way is left open for all emergency-ward staff members involved to make a judgment about whether the case is appropriate to and deserving of their service. Unless the patient is a "regular," no one on the emergency service is likely to have background information on the patient, and the staff will have to rely entirely on clues garnered from his mode of arrival, his appearance, his behavior, the kind of people who accompany him, and so on. The interpretation of these clues then becomes crucial to further treatment and, to the casual observer, may appear to be the *cause* of such treatment.

It is also not surprising that "psychiatric cases" are usually considered illegitimate. Interns and residents do not (unless they are planning to go into psychiatry) find such cases useful for practicing their diagnostic and treatment skills,[1] and therefore regard such patients as an unwelcome intrusion. But what constitutes a psychiatric case is not based on unvarying criteria. An effort is usually made to place a patient in a more explicit medical category. For example, a wrist slashing is a surgical case requiring suturing. An adult who takes an overdose of sleeping pills is a medical case requiring lavage and perhaps antidotes. Only when a patient is troublesome—violent, threatening suicide, disturbing other patients—is the doctor forced to define him as a psychiatric case about whom a further decision must be made. (In some clinics, psychiatrists are attempting to broaden the definition by making interns and residents aware of more subtle cues for justifying a psychiatric referral and providing them with a consulting service to deal with such cases. However, they must provide a prompt response when called upon, or their service will soon go unused.)

It is no accident either that in the private hospitals (especially those without medical school or public clinic affiliation) the legitimacy of a patient depends largely on his relationship to the private medical system. A standard opening question to the incoming patient in such hospitals is, "Who is your doctor?" A patient is automatically legitimate if referred by a physician on the hospital staff (or the physician's nurse, receptionist, or answering service). If he has not been referred, but gives the name of a staff doctor whom the nurse can reach and who agrees to handle the case, the patient is also legitimate. However, if he does not give a staff doctor's name, he falls under suspicion. The hospital services, including the emergency room, are designed primarily to serve the private physicians on the staff. A patient who does not fit into this scheme threatens to upset the works. It is the receptionist's or receiving nurse's job to try to establish the proper relationship by determining whether the case warrants the service of the contract physician or the doctor on emergency call, and if so, to see to it that the patient gets into the hands of an attending staff doctor for follow-up treatment if necessary. Any patient whose circumstances make this process difficult or impossible becomes illegitimate. This accounts for the bitter denunciation of the "welfare cases"[2] and the effort to deny admission to people without medical insurance or other readily tappable funds. (Most physicians on the hospital staff do not want such people as patients, and feel they have been tricked if a colleague talks them into accepting them as patients; neither does the hospital administration want them as inpatients.) Also, such hospitals have no routine mechanism for dealing with welfare cases, as have the public hospitals which can either give free treatment or refer the patient to a social worker on the premises. Such patients are commonly dealt with by transferring them to a public clinic or hospital if their condition permits.

The negative evaluation of patients is strongest when they combine an undeserving character with illegitimate demands. Thus, a patient presenting a minor medical complaint at an inconvenient hour is more vigorously condemned if he is a welfare case than if he is a "respectable citizen." On the other hand, a "real emergency" can overcome moral repugnance.

Thus, when a presumed criminal suffering a severe abdominal bullet wound inflicted by police was brought into one emergency ward, the staff quickly mobilized in a vigorous effort to prevent death because this is the kind of case the staff sees as justifying the existence of their unit. The same patient brought in with a minor injury would almost certainly have been treated as a moral outcast. Even in the case of "real emergencies," however, moral evaluation is not absent. Although the police prisoner with the bullet wound received prompt, expert attention, the effort was treated simply as a technical matter—an opportunity to display one's skill in keeping a severely traumatized person alive. When the same emergency ward received a prominent local citizen who had been stabbed by thugs while he was trying to protect his wife, the staff again provided a crash effort to save his life, but in this case they were obviously greatly upset by their failure, not simply a failure of technical skills but the loss of a worthy person who was the victim of a vicious act. One may speculate whether this difference in staff evaluations of the two victims may have resulted in an extra effort in the case of the respected citizen despite the appearance of a similar effort in the two cases.

Staff Estimates of "Legitimate" Demands

As is common in relationships between a work group and its clientele, the members of the work group tend to exaggerate their difficulties with the clients when they generalize about them. In conversations, we would typically hear estimates of 70 percent–90 percent as the proportion of patients who were using the emergency service inappropriately. Yet, when we actually followed cases through the clinic, we found the majority were being treated as if they were legitimate. In one voluntary hospital with an intern and residency training program, we classified all cases we followed during our time on the emergency room as legitimate or illegitimate whenever we had any evidence of subjective definition by staff members, either by what they said about the patient or the manner in which they treated the patient. Among those cases suitable for classification, 42 were treated as legitimate, 15 as illegitimate, and in 24 cases there was insufficient evidence to make a classification. Thus, the illegitimate proportion was about 20 percent–25 percent depending on whether one used as a base the total definite legitimate and illegitimate cases or also included the unknowns. In a very active public hospital emergency room we did not use direct observation of each case, but rather developed a conception of what kind of diagnostic categories were usually considered legitimate or illegitimate by the clinic staff and then classified the total consensus for two days according to diagnostic categories. By this method, 23 percent of 938 patients were classified as illegitimate. This constitutes a minimum figure because diagnostic category was not the only basis for an evaluation, and some other patients were almost certainly regarded as illegitimate by the staff. But it *does* suggest that only a minority were regarded as illegitimate.

The number of specific undesirable or inappropriate categories of patients were also consistently exaggerated. Thus, while in the public hospital the interns complained about all the drunks among the men and all the reproductive organ infections among the women ("The choice between the male and the female service is really a choice between alcoholics and PIDs," according to one intern), drunks made up only 6 percent of the total emergency-room population and the gynecology patients 2 percent. Venereal disease was also considered a common type of case by clerks, nurses, and doctors, but in fact made up only about 1 percent of the total E.R. census. Psychiatric cases were referred to as a constant trouble, but, in fact, made up only a little over 2 percent of the total. Some doctors believed infections and long-standing illnesses were common among the E.R. population and used this as evidence of neglect of health by the lower classes. Here again, however, the actual numbers were low—these two categories made up a little more than 3 percent of the total census. In two small private hospitals, the staffs were particularly bitter toward "welfare cases" whom they regarded as a constant nuisance. However, we often spent an entire shift (eight hours) in the emergency rooms of these hospitals without seeing a single patient so classified.

Workers justify the rewards received for their labors in part by the burdens which they must endure on the job. One of the burdens of service occupations is a clientele which makes life hard for the workers. Thus, the workers tend to select for public presentation those aspects of the clientele which cause them difficulty. Teachers' talk deals disproportionately with disruptive and incompetent students, policemen's talk with dangerous criminals and difficult civilians, janitors' talk with inconsiderate tenants. A case-by-case analysis of client contacts is likely to demonstrate in each instance that the examples discussed by the staff are not representative of their total clientele.

Control of Inappropriate Demands for Service

When members of a service occupation or service organization are faced with undesirable or illegitimate clients, what can they do? One possible procedure is to select clients they like and avoid those they do not like. The selecting may be done in categorical terms, as when universities admit undergraduate students who meet given grade and test standards. Or it may be done on the basis of detailed information about specific individuals, as when a graduate department selects particular students on the basis of academic record, recommendations from colleagues, and personal information about the student. Of course, such selection is not made on a unidimensional basis and the selecting agent must often decide what weight to give conflicting factors. (Thus, a medical specialist may be willing to take on a patient who is morally repugnant because the patient has a medical condition the specialist is anxious to observe, study, or experiment with.) But there is an assumption that the more highly individualized the selection and the more detailed the information on which it is based, the more likely one is to obtain a desirable clientele. Along with this process goes the notion of "selection errors." Thus, when a patient is classed as a good risk for a physical rehabilitation program, he may later be classed as a selection error if doctors uncover some pathology which contraindicates exercise, or if the patient proves so uncooperative that physical therapists are unable to conduct any training, or if he requires so much nursing care that ward personnel claim that he "doesn't belong" on a rehabilitation unit (Roth and Eddy 1967, pp. 57–61).

Selectivity is a relative matter. A well-known law firm specializing in a given field can accept only those clients whose demands fit readily into the firm's desired scheme of work organization and who are able to pay well for the service given. The solo criminal lawyer in a marginal practice may, for financial reasons, take on almost every case he can get, even though he may despise the majority of his clients and wish he did not have to deal with them (Smigel 1964; Wood 1967). A common occupational or organizational aspiration is to reach a position where one can be highly selective of one's clientele. In fact, such power of selection is a common basis for rating schools, law firms, hospitals, and practitioners of all sorts.[3]

If one cannot be selective in a positive sense, one may still be selective in a negative sense by avoiding some potentially undesirable clients. Hotels, restaurants, and places of entertainment may specifically exclude certain categories of persons as guests, or more generally reserve the right to refuse service to anyone they choose. Cab drivers will sometimes avoid a presumed "bad fare" by pretending another engagement or just not seeing him. Cab driving, incidentally, is a good example of a line of work where judgments about clients must often be made in a split second on the basis of immediate superficial clues—clues based not only on the behavior and appearance of the client himself, but also on such surrounding factors as the area, destination, and time of day (Davis 1959: Henslin 1968, pp. 138–58). Ambulance crewmen sometimes manage to avoid a "bad load," perhaps making a decision before going to the scene on the basis of the call source or neighborhood, or perhaps refusing to carry an undesirable patient if they can find a "good excuse" (Douglas 1969, pp. 234–78).

Medical personnel and organizations vary greatly in their capacity to select clients. Special units in teaching hospitals and specialized outpatient clinics often are able to restrict their patients to those they have individually screened and selected. The more run-of-the-mill hospital ward or clinic is less selective, but still has a screening process to keep out certain categories of patients. Of all medical care units, public hospital emergency wards probably exercise the least selectivity of all. Not only are they open to the public at all times with signs pointing the way, but the rule that everyone demanding care must be seen provides no legal "out" for the staff when faced with inappropriate or repugnant patients (although persons accompanying patients can be, and often are, prevented from entering the treatment areas and are isolated or ejected if troublesome). In addition, the emergency ward serves a residual function for the rest of the hospital and often for other parts of the medical-care system. Any case which does not fit into some other program is sent to the emergency ward. When other clinics and offices close for the day or the weekend, their patients who cannot wait for the next open hours are directed to the emergency service. It is precisely this unselective influx of anyone and everyone bringing a wide spectrum of medical and social defects that elicits the bitter complaints of emergency-service personnel. Of course, they are not completely without selective power. They occasionally violate the rules and refuse to accept a patient. And even after registration, some patients can be so discouraged in the early stages of processing that they leave. Proprietary hospitals transfer some patients to public hospitals. But compared with other parts of the medical-care system, the emergency-service personnel, especially in public hospitals, have very limited power of selection and must resign themselves to dealings with many people that they believe should not be there and that in many cases they have a strong aversion to.

What recourse does a service occupation or organization have when its members have little or no control over the selection of its clients? If you cannot pick the clients you like, perhaps you can transform those you *do* get somewhere closer to the image of desirable client. This is particularly likely to occur if it is a long-term or repeated relationship so that the worker can reap the benefit of the "training" he gives the client. We tentatively put forth this proposition: *The amount of trouble one is willing to go to to train his clientele depends on how much power of selection he has. The easier it is for one to avoid or get rid of poor clients (that is, those clients whose behavior or attributes conflict with one's conception of his proper work role), the less interested one is in putting time and energy into training clients to conform more closely to one's ideal. And, of course, the converse.*

Janitors have to endure a clientele (that is, tenants) they have no hand in selecting. Nor can a janitor get rid of bad tenants (unless he buys the building and evicts them, as happens on rare occasions). Ray Gold (1964, pp. 1–50) describes how janitors try to turn "bad tenants" into more tolerable ones by teaching them not to make inappropriate demands. Tenants must be taught not to call at certain hours, not to expect the janitor to make certain repairs, not to expect him to remove certain kinds of garbage, to expect cleaning services only on given days and in given areas, to expect heat only at certain times, and so on. Each occasion on which the janitor is able to make his point that a given demand is inappropriate contributes to making those demands from the same tenant less likely in the future and increases the janitor's control over his work load and work pacing. One finds much the same long-term effort on the part of mental hospital staffs who indoctrinate inmates on the behavior and demands associated with "good patients"—who will be rewarded with privileges and discharge—and behavior associated with "bad patients"—who will be denied these rewards (Stanton and Schwartz 1954, pp. 280–89; Belknap 1956, chaps. 9 and 10). Prisons and schools are other examples of such long-term teaching of clients.[4]

The form that "client-training" takes depends in part on the time perspective of the trainers. Emergency-ward personnel do not have the longtime perspective of the mental hospital staff, teachers, or janitors. Despite the fact that the majority of patients have been to the same emergency ward previously and will probably be back again at some future time, the staff, with rare exceptions, treats each case as an episode which will be completed when the patient is discharged. Therefore, they seldom make a direct effort to affect the patient's future use of their services. They are, however, interested in directing the immediate behavior of clients so that it will fit into their concept of proper priorities (in terms of their evaluation of the clients) and the proper conduct of an emergency service, including the work demands made upon them. Since they do not conceive of having time for gradual socialization of the clients, they rely heavily on demands for immediate compliance. Thus, patients demanding attention, if not deemed by staff to be urgent cases or particularly deserving, will be told to wait their turn and may even be threatened with refusal of treatment if they are persistent. Visitors are promptly ordered to a waiting room and are reminded of where they belong if they wander into a restricted area. Patients are expected to respond promptly when called, answer questions put to them by the staff, prepare for examination when asked, and cooperate with the examination as directed without wasting the staff's time. Failure to comply promptly may bring a warning that they will be left waiting or even refused further care if they do not cooperate, and the more negative the staff evaluation of the patient, the more likely he is to be threatened.[5]

Nursing staff in proprietary hospitals dealing with the private patients of attending physicians do not have as authoritative a position vis-à-vis their clients as public hospital staff have: therefore, the demands for prompt compliance with staff directions must be used sparingly. In such a case more surreptitious forms of control are used. The most common device is keeping the patient waiting at some step or steps in his processing or treatment. Since the patient usually has no way of checking the validity of the reason given for the wait, this is a relatively safe way that a nurse can control the demands made on her and also serves as a way of "getting even" with those who make inappropriate demands or whom she regards as undeserving for some other reason.

In general, we might expect that: *The longer the time perspective of the trainers, the more the training will take the form of efforts toward progressive socialization in the desired direction; the shorter the time perspective of the trainers, the more the training will take the form of overt coercion ("giving orders") if the trainers have sufficient power over the clients, and efforts at surreptitious but immediate control if they lack such power.*

Conclusion

When a person presents himself at an emergency department (or is brought there by others), he inevitably sets off a process by which his worthiness and legitimacy are weighed and become a factor in his treatment. It is doubtful that one can obtain any service of consequence anywhere without going through this process. The evidence from widely varying services indicates that the servers do not dispense their service in a uniform manner to everyone who presents himself, but make judgments about the worthiness of the person and the appropriateness of his demands and take these judgments into account when performing the service. In large and complex service organizations, the judgments made at one point in the system often shape the judgments at another.

The structure of a service organization will affect the manner and degree to which the servers can vary their service in terms of their moral evaluation of the client. This study has not explored this issue in detail. A useful future research direction would be the investigation of how a system of service may be structured to control the discretion of the servers as to whom they must serve and how they must serve them. This paper offered some suggestions concerning the means of controlling the inappropriate demands of a clientele. The examples I used to illustrate the relationships of power of selection and the nature of training of clients are few and limited in scope. An effort should be made to determine whether these formulations (or modifications thereof) apply in a wider variety of occupational settings.

Notes

The study on which this paper is based was supported by National Institutes of Health grants HM 00437 and HM 00517, Division of Hospital and Medical

Facilities. Dorothy J. Douglas, currently at the University of Connecticut Health Center, worked with me and made major contributions to this study.

1. The authors of *Boys in White* (Becker et al. 1961, pp. 327–38) make the same point. A "crock" is a patient from whom the students cannot learn anything because there is no definable physical pathology which can be tracked down and treated.
2. "Welfare cases" include not only those who present welfare cards, but all who are suspected of trying to work the system to get free or low-priced care.
3. I am glossing over some of the intraorganizational complexities of the process. Often different categories of organizational personnel vary greatly in their participation in the selection of the clientele. Thus, on a hospital rehabilitation unit, the doctors may select the patients, but the nurses must take care of patients they have no direct part in selecting. Nurses can influence future selection only by complaining to the doctors that they have "too many" of certain kinds of difficult patients or by trying to convince doctors to transfer inappropriate patients. These attempts at influencing choice often fail because doctors and nurses have somewhat different criteria about what an appropriate patient is (Roth and Eddy 1967, pp. 57–61).
4. Of course, my brief presentation greatly oversimplifies the process. For example, much of the teaching is done by the clients rather than directly by the staff. But, ultimately, the sanctions are derived from staff efforts to control work demands and to express their moral evaluation of the clients.
5. Readers who are mainly interested in what happens on an emergency ward should not be misled into thinking that it is a scene of continuous orders and threats being shouted at patients and visitors. Most directives are matter-of-fact, and most clients comply promptly with directions most of the time. But when the staff's directive power is challenged, even inadvertently, the common response is a demand for immediate compliance. This situation arises frequently enough so that on a busy unit an observer can see instances almost every hour.

References

Becker, Howard S., Blanche Geer, Everett C. Hughes, and Anselm Strauss. 1961. *Boys in White.* Chicago: University of Chicago Press.

Belknap, Ivan. 1956. *Human Problems of a State Mental Hospital.* New York: McGraw-Hill.

Davis, Fred. 1959. "The Cab Driver and His Fare." *American Journal of Sociology* 65 (September): 158–65.

Douglas, Dorothy J. 1969. "Occupational and Therapeutic Contingencies of Ambulance Services in Metropolitan Areas." Ph.D. dissertation, University of California.

Glaser, Barney, and Anselm Strauss. 1964. "The Social Loss of Dying Patients." *American Journal of Nursing* 64 (June): 119–21.

Goffman, Erving. 1961. *Asylums.* New York: Doubleday.

Gold, Raymond L. 1964. "In the Basement—the Apartment-Building Janitor." In *The Human Shape of Work,* edited by Peter L. Berger. New York: Macmillan.

Henslin, James. 1968. "Trust and the Cab Driver." In *Sociology and Everyday Life,* edited by Marcello Truzzi. Englewood Cliffs, N.J.: Prentice-Hall.

Hollingshead, August B., and Frederick C. Redlich. 1958. *Social Class and Mental Illness.* New York: Wiley.

Perrow, Charles. 1965. "Hospitals, Technology, Structure, and Goals." In *Handbook of Organizations,* edited by James G. March. Chicago: Rand McNally.

Roth, Julius A., and Elizabeth M. Eddy. 1967. *Rehabilitation for the Unwanted.* New York: Atherton.

Scheff, Thomas J. 1964. "The Societal Reaction to Deviance: Ascriptive Elements in the Psychiatric Screening of Mental Patients in a Midwestern State." *Social Problems* 11 (Spring): 401–13.

———. 1966. *Being Mentally Ill.* Chicago: Aldine.

Smigel, Erwin. 1964. *Wall Street Lawyer.* New York: Free Press.

Stanton, Alfred, and Morris Schwartz. 1954. *The Mental Hospital.* New York: Basic.

Strauss, Anselm, Leonard Schatzman, Rue Bucher, Danuta Ehrlich, and Melvin Sabshin. 1964. *Psychiatric Ideologies and Institutions.* New York: Free Press.

Sudnow, David. 1967. *Passing On.* Englewood Cliffs, N.J.: Prentice-Hall.

Szasz, Thomas. 1960. "The Myth of Mental Illness." *American Psychologist* 15 (February): 113–18.

Wood, Arthur Lewis. 1967. *Criminal Lawyer.* New Haven, Conn.: College and Universities Press.

26

Good Patients and Problem Patients: Conformity and Deviance in a General Hospital

Judith Lorber

. . . .

From nurses' description of patients, Duff and Hollingshead (1968: 221–222, their emphasis) concluded that patients were divided into two categories—"problem" and "no problem." As they put it, "The definition of a *problem* is related to the degree to which the patient needed physical care or was unable to comply with orders." In other words, "... *problem* patients obstructed work and *no problem* patients facilitated work." In this study, the doctors' and nurses' choice of "good patient," "average patient," or "problem patient" on the self-administered questionnaire they were asked to fill out at the end of the patients' stay, plus their invited remarks on the questionnaire and in private conversation with the researcher, all bore out the relationship between the label of good or problem patient and the extent to which the patient made trouble for them. Patients who were considered cooperative, uncomplaining, and stoical by the doctors and nurses were generally labeled good patients, no matter what their procedure or postoperative complications.

For instance, the private-duty nurse who spent 36 nights caring for a young woman with extensive postoperative complications following a gallbladder removal wrote: "... A very good patient to my way of thinking because no matter how much pain, she was always pleasant and not disagreeable. She *tried at all times* [sic] to be cooperative even though the tension in her was great at all times." After 29 consecutive days of nursing a 55-year-old man who had a shunt operation for cirrhosis of the liver followed by almost fatal complications, the private-duty nurse said, "I really enjoyed taking care of him. He was never grouchy, always cooperative—even though he was sick." In talking of a 63-year-old woman who was vice-president of her local chapter of Cancer Care, and who had an extensive operation for cancer, her surgeon said to the researcher, "You sent me a questionnaire on the most cooperative patient I've seen in 35 years. . . . She had massive surgery—she had complications—but she never complains. She knows she had a malignancy, but she doesn't have to be reassured—she says, 'The axe had to fall sometime.' "

In contrast, patients whom the doctors and nurses felt were uncooperative, constantly complaining, overemotional, and dependent were frequently considered problem patients, whether they had routine or very serious surgery. For example, the resident and intern labeled a problem patient a 62-year-old man who had a hernia repair with no complications, but who had been extremely apprehensive about the operation. In the patient's medical record, the resident noted that he was "overreacting to his condition," and had "multiple complaints related to his personality." The intern simply called him "a *kvetch.*" A 74-year-old man who had a gallbladder removal with many post-operative complications, some psychosomatic, was labeled a problem patient by the surgeon, resident, intern, and day staff nurse. In the questionnaire, the resident said the patient's uncooperativeness made it difficult to perform routine procedures on him. The surgeon wrote that the patient was "lachrymose, combative, and generally impossible." To the researcher, the surgeon added that the patient had called him names, lied, and generally carried on.

Another patient considered a problem patient by her surgeon, the day staff nurse, and a private-duty nurse (but a good patient by the intern) was a pretty, 30-year-old divorcee. She told everyone about her family problems and described herself as a "devout coward." She had an uncomplicated gallbladder removal, but cried a lot and was given tranquilizers. The day head nurse said of her, "This patient seemed to have been pampered very much. She barely cooperated and seemed to have been extremely dependent on her mother. She was much more of a baby than most people having the same surgery."

The doctors and nurses on a case frequently did not agree on the evaluation of the patient. The same patient could be labeled good, problem, and average, and no patient was labeled a problem by every doctor or nurse who returned a questionnaire on him or her. The doctor or nurse who bore the brunt of the difficulty was usually the one who considered the patient a problem patient, while the others labeled him or her good or average. This supports the original contention that problem patients were those who created trouble for the medical staff.

A case in point was a young, well-educated man with a wife and child who was discovered to have a fast-growing, inoperable, and extremely painful form of cancer. He was very agitated before and after surgery, and he was demanding after surgery. But only the resident, with whom he fought over the question of pain medication, labeled him a problem pa-

Table 1.
Medical Staff Evaluations, by Patients' Attitudes[a]

		Patients' Attitudes		
Staff Evaluations		% Very Conforming (N=33)	% Moderately Conforming (N=42)	% Deviant (N=28)
Attending Physician	Good	67	74	64
	Problem	3	5	14
Resident	Good	36	41	46
	Problem	6	7	11
Intern	Good	46	52	36
	Problem	3	7	11
Day Staff Nurse	Good	33	38	39
	Problem	3	7	14

[a]Omits those labeled "average" and "no answer." Non-return of a questionnaire is an indication that the patient did not register one way or another; in general, the doctors and nurses were more inclined to fill out questionnaires for patients they either admired or found troublesome.

tient. The resident said of him, "Very argumentative about getting his own way." The patient needed little physical care, so the rest of the staff was able, in the words of the head nurse, to "humor him." The private-duty nurse on the case, a young woman, refused to fill out a questionnaire but told me, "I couldn't stand the man." She felt he was tyrannical and he thought her incompetent. With him for twelve hours a day, she would, of course, have borne the brunt of his troublesome behavior.

. . . While most patients were obedient and uncomplaining, patients with deviant attitudes toward the hospital-patient role were more argumentative and complained more than patients with conforming attitudes. Did the doctors and nurses more often label patients with deviant attitudes problem patients? Although the percentage differences were not large, they were in the expected direction: patients with deviant attitudes were most often labeled problem patients by the time they left the hospital, patients with moderately conforming attitudes less frequently, and patients with very conforming attitudes least of all. (See Table 1.)

Note, however, that very conforming patients were not labeled *good* patients to any great degree. One consequence of their uncomplaining, passive behavior might have been that they did not ask for help when they really needed it, so the nurses had to take time to do frequent checks on their physical status. For instance, a nurse wrote in the questionnaire of a 62-year-old woman who had very extensive abdominal surgery and was herself a nurse, "This patient was far too considerate of the nurses . . . she 'didn't want to bother' us and often remained quiet when in pain and had to be frequently checked for comfort." The nurse's use of quotation marks around the phrase "didn't want to bother" highlights the point that by not asking for needed attention, the patient, who should have known better, disrupted the usual routine. In this way the too stoical or too passive patient can also cause trouble.

Routine Management and Extraordinary Trouble

The analysis of the doctors' and nurses' evaluations of patients suggested that ease of management was the basic criterion for a label of good patient, and that patients who took time and attention felt to be unwarranted by their illness tended to be labeled problem patients. Robert Emerson (1971) points out that those troublemakers who can be managed routinely by social control agents are treated relatively leniently; only those who do not let themselves be managed routinely—who need extraordinary solutions to their problems—are singled out for stronger sanctions.

In the hospital studied, the medical staff expected a certain amount of complaining from surgical patients, particularly about pain. The most frequently mentioned method of handling *any* complaint was the use of sedative or narcotic drugs. Sixty-nine percent of the 499 questionnaires returned by the doctors and nurses mentioned drugs as the method used to handle complaints. The next most popular method was mentioned in only 34 percent of the returned questionnaires; it was talking to patients— reassuring, encouraging, explaining, ordering, scolding, and so on. Physical methods, such as turning, positioning, walking around, examining, making comfortable, and so on, were mentioned in 22 percent of the returned questionnaires, and methods that used mechanical devices were listed in 14 percent. (Mentions were multiple.) All the less favored methods took more time than the administration of a shot or oral dose of pain reliever or sedative every four hours.

Negative evaluations of relatively high percentages of patients who took up more time and were talked to fit in with the medical staff's own designation of which were the usual and which the less common methods of managing complaints. When the reports of amount of time spent with patients were cross-tabulated with evaluations of the patients, it was found that the patients with whom more time was spent were much more likely to to be labeled problem patients than those with whom average or less than average time was spent. The doctors labeled as problem patients from 25 to 36 percent of those they said took up more than the usual amount of time for that type of surgery. Between 80 and 91 percent of the patients the doctors said took up less than the average amount of time for their type of surgery were labeled good patients. In short, the less of the doctor's time the patient took, the better he or she was viewed.

Similarly, doctors and nurses were more likely to label problem patients

Table 2.
Medical Staff Evaluations of Patients, by Reports of Talking
to Patients[a]

Staff Evaluations		Questionnaire Responses	
		% Reporting Talk	% Reporting No Talk
Attending		N=20	N=71
Physician	Good	60	83
	Problem	10	7
Resident		N=29	N=44
	Good	45	66
	Problem	24	2
Intern		N=32	N=45
	Good	41	76
	Problem	13	7
Day Staff		N=25	N=46
Nurse	Good	36	63
	Problem	24	4

[a]Omits those labeled "average" and "no answer."

those they remembered having talked to, and less likely to label them good patients. Residents and day staff nurses, who had the responsibility for the daily management of the surgical wards, labeled as problem patients one-quarter of those they singled out as having been talked to. (See Table 2.)

The assumption that problem patients would be those who gave doctors and nurses the most trouble was borne out by other data, namely, the evaluations of patients having different types of procedures. Hernia-repair patients, who were so easy to care for they were virtually anonymous to the interns, residents, and nurses, were rarely labeled problem patients. Patients who had gallbladders removed or other moderately serious surgery, were most often described as problem patients by attending surgeons, residents and interns. Though medically routine, the postoperative condition of these patients called for a lot of attention, most of which was the residents' responsibility. It is not surprising that residents labeled as good patients only 19 percent of the moderately serious surgery cases. (See Table 3.)

To summarize, there are two variables involved in whether a doctor or nurse in charge views the patient as manageable by routine methods or as needing extraordinary solutions taking more time and attention. Patients manageable by routine methods are average—they make ordinary, ex-pected trouble. These patients have routine illnesses, no post-operative complications, are moderately cooperative, and only occasionally com-plain of pain or discomfort. (Some staff members labeled them good pa-tients, especially if they couldn't remember them too well.) Patients who

Table 3.
Medical Staff Evaluations of Patients, by Surgical Procedure[a]

| | | Type of Procedure | | | |
| | | % Routine (N=33) | % Moderately Serious (N=31) | % Very Serious No Cancer (N=14) | % Very Serious Cancer (N=25) |
Staff Evaluations					
Attending	Good	76	65	71	64
Physician	Problem	3	10	7	8
Resident	Good	46	19	43	60
	Problem	6	13	0	8
Intern	Good	39	36	64	56
	Problem	3	16	7	0
Day Staff	Good	42	29	36	40
Nurse	Problem	0	13	14	8

[a]Omits those labeled "average" and "no answer."

might be expected to cause extraordinary trouble because of the problematic nature of their illness, but who only cause ordinary trouble because of their extraordinary cooperativeness and cheerful stoicism, are frequently rewarded with the accolade "good patient" by doctors and nurses who do not ordinarily use that label, and "great patient" by the rest.

As for those labeled problem patients, they are of two types. The first has an ordinary illness but takes up more time and attention than is warranted by the medical condition because he or she is uncooperative and/or complains and argues much of the time. Doctors and nurses consider such behavior unnecessary and therefore extraordinary trouble, and the patient is soundly condemned. The second type of problem patient has an extraordinary medical status, such as severe complications, poor prognosis, or difficult diagnosis. Troublesome behavior of the sort described above, while not approved of, is somewhat forgiven as understandable given the patient's medical condition. The first kind of problem patient seems to be considered deliberately deviant—willfully causing extraordinary trouble; the second kind of problem patient seems to be considered an accidental deviant—responding with troublesome behavior to an extraordinary difficult situation beyond his or her control (cf. Lorber, 1967).

Possible Consequences of Being Labeled a Problem Patient

What do doctors and nurses do about those patients whose deviant behavior hinders their efficient routines? In the study reported here, patients whose behavior was troublesome and who did not respond to tranquilizers or sedation were sent home or recommended to a convalescent center where the nurses were trained to do psychotherapy. In one case, a staff psychiatrist was asked to see a troublesome dying patient who had been in psychiatric treatment before his illness. In short, deviant behavior on the part of these mostly middle-class, paying, short-term surgical patients was treated moderately permissively by the medical professionals who cared for them.

Indeed, the hospital tried various ways to meet the socio-economic needs of its patients. A "patient-relations nurse coordinator" had been appointed for the general surgical wards for a short time before this research was done. This role was modeled after the "clinical nurse specialist" who worked closely with the open-heart surgeon. (See Bandman, Wolpin, and Rehm, 1964.) On the general surgery wards, where there were many more attending surgeons and their patients to contend with, this nurse-liaison did not work out. It was said in personal communication during preliminary fieldwork that the medical personnel felt she was spying on them, while the patients did not feel their complaints were taken care of adequately.

Another short-lived experiment that took place just after the fieldwork was done was to allow all patients on the surgical wards the same all-day visiting hours as the private-room patients. This attempt to give patients additional support lasted about two months. Given the fact that with regular visiting hours, more complaints by patients were reported on the staff questionnaires by the evening staff nurses than any other shift (evening visits were the most popular), it is probable that patient-staff conflict was exacerbated, not eased, by the constant presence of relatives.

Other studies have found that the troublesome patient tends to be somewhat neglected by the medical staff. Interns have admitted giving "superior care to the better liked, with minimum but adequate care to those not liked" (Daniels, 1960:263). Those not liked were patients who tended to be complaining and uncooperative and to ask a lot of questions. Responding to hypothetical situations, 40 nurses said they would do more for the non-compliant patient in the short run, but in the long run, predicted they would do more for the compliant patient (Keller, 1971). In their study of dying patients, Glaser and Strauss (1965) found that nurses scolded, reprimanded, and then avoided those patients who asked a lot of questions, created emotional scenes, or refused to cooperate with hospital routines. Roth and Eddy (1967:106–109), in their study of rehabilitation patients, noted that abusive and uncooperative patients were discharged from the ward, and thus denied retraining. However, young patients with a greater chance of successful rehabilitation than older ones were treated more leniently. Roth's (1963a:41) research on long-term tuberculosis patients showed that "noisy agitation" sometimes resulted in slightly earlier discharge, especially if the staff felt the patient might leave against medical advice. But he also found hospitals with locked wards for "recalcitrant" patients whose medical status was still poor (Roth, 1963:25). The rare cooperative and cured patient who didn't want to leave the hospital left the staff in a complete quandary, and a psychiatrist was used as a last resort (Roth, 1963a:48).

Of all these responses to extraordinarily troublesome patients, the use of psychiatrists has the most potentially momentous consequences. Meyer and Mendelson (1961) studied 60 requests for psychiatric consultation with patients on medical and surgical wards, and found that a disruptive patient was first considered uncooperative or bad, but then defined as irrational and irresponsible, or "crazy," and a psychiatrist was called in. If a patient refuses to submit quietly to hospital routines and is referred to a psychiatrist because of disruptive behavior, he or she is labeled as someone with psychiatric problems. If the fact that he or she had seen a psychiatrist is entered into the medical records, the information becomes a permanent part of his or her future identity as a patient for all other professionals who have access to this set of records. His or her future behavior will be interpreted in the light of the putative psychiatric problems, and any opposition to the way he or she is treated will never be taken seriously. Even if the information is not officially recorded, ward scuttlebutt will certainly spread the word around—problem patients are discussed *ad infinitum*. For the remainder of the particular hospitalization, the patient will be treated as psychotic or neurotic, and not as someone with possible legitimate complaints (cf. Phillips, 1963, and Rosenhan, 1973).

Summary

On the basis of an attitude questionnaire administered to 103 surgical patients before their operations, this study found that most general-hospital patients enter the hospital feeling they should be obedient, cooperative, objective about their illness, and expect attention only if they are very ill. As other researchers have found, the better educated and younger patients tended to have more autonomous or deviant attitudes toward being a hospital patient. This study found that patients with deviant attitudes tended to argue more with the residents, interns, and nurses, and to complain more about minor discomforts as a way of getting attention.

Although patients feel that doctors and nurses always approve of obedience, cooperation, and undemandingness, a questionnaire administered to the medical staff at the end of the patients' stay in the hospital revealed that the staff's evaluations of the patients under their care depended on the amount of trouble these patients gave them. In general, cooperative, uncomplaining, and stoical patients *were* considered good patients, but the staff expected patients to make them aware of their needs; that is, to ask for attention when it was needed medically. Patients whom the doctors and nurses felt were uncooperative, overemotional, and who complained when it was not medically warranted were considered problem patients only by the staff member who had to bear the brunt of the trouble. Patients who did not respond to sedation or tranquilizers—the chief methods of handling complaints of pain and discomfort—but instead had to be reassured, encouraged, given explanations or exhortations, and who therefore took up more of the staff's time than they felt warranted by the extent of surgery, were also considered problem patients to a greater degree than those who took up an "average" amount of time and attention.

Patients who had the most routine surgery were usually labeled good patients, as were the very cooperative seriously ill patients. The patients who had surgery that is major and painful by lay standards, but routine by medical standards, were labeled problem patients to the greatest degree, particularly by the residents, who were primarily responsible for their care. (In this study, most of these patients were, in the doctors' words, "well-nourished" middle-aged women, which may have added to the impatience the residents, both male and female, showed with them.)

In sum, doctors and nurses expect to carry out their work by well-established routines, with a minimum of interruption from patients. Those patients who make no trouble at all, who do not interrupt the smoothness of medical routines, are likely to be considered *good* patients by the medical staff. In this study, good patients usually had routine surgery and were out of the hospital within a week, or had uncomplicated major surgery and accepted whatever was done to them cheerfully and cooperatively. Doctors and nurses tend to consider *average* patients those whose complaints are medically warranted, who respond to established routines for handling such complaints, and who therefore take up the expected amount of time for their type of illness. In this study, most of the average patients had uncomplicated major surgery, complained a fair amount about pain and discomfort, but were satisfied when their requests for attention were answered with pain medication every four hours for two or three days.

Problem patients are of two kinds. Those who are seriously ill, and who complain a great deal, are very emotional, anxious, and need a lot of reassurance, encouragement, and attention from the staff are problematic, but "forgivable" because the situation is not of their own making. In this study, they were often given the time and attention they demanded, particularly if they were grateful for it. Nonetheless, the extraordinary amount of time and attention they took up made them "problem patients." (Conversely, seriously ill patients who were extraordinarily cheerful, cooperative, uncomplaining, and objective about their illness were considered *great* patients and talked about after discharge as "ideal.") Patients who are *not* seriously ill in the staff's eyes, but who nevertheless act as if they are by complaining, crying, and refusing to cooperate with medical routines, are the most soundly condemned by the staff. Such problem patients, in this study, were tranquilized, sometimes discharged early, and, in one case, referred to a psychiatrist—types of response to wilfully troublesome patients other researchers have also found.

Thus, the consequences of deliberate deviance in the general hospital can be medical neglect or a stigmatizing label, while conformity to good-patient norms is usually a return home with only a surgical scar.

Note

This study was supported by U.S. Public Health Service Grant HS00013. For helpful criticisms on earlier drafts, I would like to thank Rose Coser, Arlene Daniels, Lynne Davidson, Eliot Freidson, Judith Gordon, Pamela Roby, and Gaye Tuchman. An abridged version of this paper with the same title was read at the 1974 American Sociological Association Meetings, Montreal, Canada.

References

Bandman, E., S. Wolpin and D. Rehm. 1964. "The patient-relations nurse coordinator." American Journal of Nursing 64 (September): 133–135.

Daniels, M. J. 1960. "Affect and its control in the medical intern." American Journal of Sociology 61 (November): 259–267.

Duff, Raymond S. and August B. Hollingshead. 1968. Sickness and Society. New York: Harper and Row.

Emerson, Robert M. 1971. "Trouble and unmanageability: Working notes on social control and practical action." Unpublished manuscript.

Glaser, Barney G. and Anselm L. Strauss. 1965. Awareness of Dying. Chicago: Aldine.

Keller, N. S. 1971. "Compliance, previous access and provision of services by registered nurses." Journal of Health and Social Behavior 12 (December): 321–330.

Lorber, J. 1967. "Deviance as performance: The case of illness." Social Problems 14 (Winter): 302–310.

Meyer, E. and M. Mendelson. 1961. "Psychiatric consultations with patients on medical and surgical wards: Patterns and processes." Psychiatry 24 (August): 197–220.

Phillips, D. L. 1963. "Rejection: A possible consequence of seeking help for mental disorders." American Sociological Review 28 (December): 963–972.

Rosenhan, D. L. 1973. "On being sane in insane places." Science 179 (January 19): 250–258.

Roth, Julius A. 1963. Timetables: Structuring the Passage of Time in Hospital Treatment and Other Careers. Indianapolis: Bobbs-Merrill.

Roth, Julius A. and Elizabeth M. Eddy. 1967. Rehabilitation for the Unwanted. New York: Atherton.

27

Medical Mortality Review: A Cordial Affair

Marcia Millman

. . . .

A mortality and morbidity conference for doctors bears some resemblance to a wedding or a funeral for members of a family. In all these ceremonies there is some feeling among those who attend that tact and restraint must be exercised if everyone is to leave on friendly terms. But steering a mortality meeting along on a pleasant and even course is occasionally difficult, for as in weddings and funerals, the very nature of the event often prompts participants to come dangerously close to saying to one another those upsetting things that are usually left unsaid.

Mortality meetings are regularly scheduled conferences at Lakeside Hospital[1]; they are held in a large auditorium to accommodate the entire medical staff (private attending physicians, house officers, and teaching staff). Their avowed purpose is to review, in fine detail, those medical cases that ended in an in-hospital patient death, and in which there is some question of error, failure, or general mismanagement on the part of the physicians involved. One of the implicit if unspoken concerns that always underlies the review is the question of whether the patient's death might have been avoided had the medical judgment been more sound, for what is usually involved in these cases is a question of misdiagnosis or of appropriate medical action taken too late.

In consideration of the delicacy of the occasion, the meetings are restricted to the medical staff of the hospital. Even the surgical staff is generally not invited. The surgical service has its own mortality meetings, and a surgeon would be considered meddlesome for attending a medical mortality conference simply out of curiosity. Only those surgeons who were directly involved in a particular case under consideration will be asked to attend a medical mortality meeting. Families are *not* informed that their deceased relative's case has been chosen for review. Although the meetings may be considerably embarrassing for the doctors involved, the Medical Mortality Conference is, at least on the surface, treated as an *educational* rather than a punitive affair. At Lakeside, the conferences are not investigations or formal hearings held to consider the competence of particular doctors, although they are often presented this way on television medical dramas. There are no formal sanctions applied to doctors at the end of these conferences. Rather, Mortality Review Conferences are "educational" sessions organized around reviewing particular cases rather than individual doctors, even though the cases are selected because there is disagreement over the appropriate treatment and often a question of physician error involved.

The Mortality Review Conference has a special quality of high tension, and the meetings are better attended than are those of the other regular teaching conferences. At Lakeside Hospital, the Chief of Medicine stands on the stage and presides over the Mortality Review Conference as a master of ceremonies. As the case is reviewed in chronological order, starting with the time of the patient admission to the hospital, and proceeding to the autopsy report, the chief calls on the various doctors who were involved in the case, asks them to step to the front of the auditorium, and instructs them to recall and explain what they did and what they thought at each moment in time. He counsels them not to jump ahead of the chronological order, nor to divulge information gained at a later time, in order not to spoil the final diagnosis for the members of the audience. As one after another of the staff testifies about how they were led to the same mistaken diagnosis, a convincing case for the justifiability of the error is implicitly presented and the responsibility for the mistake is spread so that no one doctor is made to look guilty of a mistake that anyone else wouldn't have made, and in fact, didn't make. As in a good detective story, the case is reconstructed to show that there was evidence for suspecting an outcome different from the one that turns out to be the true circumstance. Responsibility for the error is also neutralized by making much of unusual or misleading features of the case, or showing how the patient was himself to blame, because of uncooperative or neurotic behavior. Furthermore, by reviewing the case in fine detail the doctors restore their images as careful, methodical practitioners and thereby neutralize the actual sloppiness and carelessness made obvious by the mistake. The doctors' discomfort is further minimized by treating the review as an educational occasion rather than an investigatory event.

In order to appreciate the special atmosphere and significance of the Mortality Review, it is important to understand that doctors who work together ordinarily live by a gentlemen's agreement to overlook each other's mistakes. The aim is not merely to hide errors and incompetence from the patients and the public, but also to avoid interfering in one another's work and to avoid acknowledgment of the injury that has been done to patients. Such a conspiracy to look the other way regarding the failures of one's colleagues is not always recognized by the doctors for what it is, for a blindness to injury done to patients and a convincing set of justifications and excuses for medical mistakes are carefully built into their training and professional etiquette. Most doctors are therefore capable of comfortably viewing themselves as altruistic and highly responsible practitioners all the while they engage in collective rationalizations for ignoring and condoning each other's errors and incompetence.

Still, there are special occasions in the hospital routine, such as the Mortality Meeting, when doctors are gathered together to examine the sorts of unpleasant facts they would otherwise ignore. At these times a great deal of effort is expended to make the embarrassing facts seem less damaging. For if such medical incompetence or error were fully and publicly (among themselves) acknowledged, physician-colleagues might feel forced to take measures against one another, and this is one of the things they least like to do.

As the Chief of Medicine at Lakeside explained, "Eighty percent of the mistakes made around here are ignored or swept under the rug. I can only pick *certain* cases for mortality review—it's got to be a cordial affair."

Perhaps that description of the selection procedures for mortality review accounts for the curious fact that at Lakeside, most of the medical situations presented at these conferences conveniently seem to involve an illness that would have ended in the patient's death in any case, even if the correct diagnosis had been made immediately. There is a strange absence of cases reviewed in these meetings in which the patient would clearly have lived had it not been for the medical mismanagement. By selecting only those cases in which the physician's error was not fateful in an ultimate sense the discussion of mistakes largely becomes an academic affair.

Practicality rather than sentiment is the key to the tact and reserve with which doctors respond to each other's errors. A doctor's reluctance to criticize a colleague's mistakes to his face at a large meeting is not motivated out of respect or affection. Indeed, many doctors are willing, in small groups, to say that another physician (not present) is a menace or a terrible doctor. And even at the mortality review conferences, those doctors who are not involved in a case may occasionally sit back and enjoy the gentle roasting of a disliked work associate. The reluctance to point out and criticize another doctor's mistakes at an official meeting comes rather out of a fear of reprisal and a recognition of common interests. For each doctor knows that he has made some more or less terrible mistake in his career, and that he is likely to make others—mistakes, moreover, which will be obvious to his colleagues. That is why, in matters of peer regulation, doctors observe the Golden Rule.

So it is that mortality meetings are built upon a simultaneous admission and cover-up of mistakes. For although the avowed purpose of these meetings is to review mistakes and prevent their recurrence, in actuality the meetings are organized and conducted in ways that absolve the doctors from responsibility and guilt and provide the self-assuring but somewhat false appearance that physicians are monitoring each other and their standards of work. In case after case physician errors are systematically excused and justified, and their consequences made to look unimportant.

Before turning to some actual cases, it should be noted that despite the tact and sensitivity with which doctors treat each other's errors, a mortality meeting is not an entirely comfortable situation. Like a family trying collectively to ignore that the father is having an affair, or that the daughter is a drug addict, the doctors at a mortality meeting are often pushed to extreme displays of courtesy to overlook the worst and find good excuses for regrettable behavior.

Case No. 1: Jonathan Thomas

Jonathan Thomas was a thirty-four-year-old insurance salesman who had complained of abdominal pain and black stool (indicating gastrointestinal bleeding). His problem was diagnosed as a gastric ulcer and he was placed on a regimen of tranquilizers and an ulcer diet. His subsequent complaints were explained as being consistent with an ulcer and a neurotic personality. Ten months later Jonathan Thomas died of cancer spread throughout his abdominal cavity.

This was to be a particularly uncomfortable case for the staff to consider in Mortality Review because of a number of factors. First of all, the patient was a young man with a large family, and this made his life more valuable in the eyes of the doctors. Second, mistakes in diagnosis had been made repeatedly, and important information overlooked more than once. Third, a large number of people had been involved in this case, and while this offered the consolation of spreading out the responsibility, it also pointed out the weaknesses of the hospital consulting system. For if not one of a dozen physicians had caught the obvious errors, it was probably because each of the consultants involved in the case had been too accepting of each other's erroneous assumptions instead of carefully doing the diagnostic jobs they were supposed to be doing.

Notices about the mortality meeting had been distributed days beforehand and signs posted around the hospital. The chief's secretary had made sure that all the doctors involved in the case would be there for the review. As always, the meeting was held in the large theaterlike auditorium and members of the staff seated themselves in the rows of seats facing the stage in a steep incline.

The meeting was called to order by the Chief of Medicine, who welcomed everyone and made brief announcements of unrelated matters. Next, an intern described the hospital's mortality profile for the preceding month: he described how many patients had died in the hospital in each major disease category. Finally, the Chief of Medicine, Dr. Tanner, returned to the stage and introduced the Thomas case. As usual, the patient's history was reviewed in chronological order, each doctor being called to the front of the room to recall his thoughts and describe his participation at that moment in time in the case.

The early history was reviewed by Dr. Backman, the specialist in gastrointestinal disorders who had managed the case. Backman was highly respected and well-liked by most of the staff, and so there were no undertones of questioning his competence but rather friendly empathy for the usually careful physician who had made an uncharacteristic mistake. From the beginning, Backman explained, he had assumed that the gastrointestinal bleeding indicated by the black stool was caused by a stress-induced gastric ulcer: "What led us down the garden path last October was the fact that he was taking on added responsibility for his family's business. The sudden pain seemed to coincide with that, so we put him on an ulcer regimen and gave him tranquilizers and released him in satisfactory condition. After discharge, a GI series was negative, but epigastric pain reappeared and in April he reported severe upper left quadrant pains which became persistent."

Dr. Jenkins, one of the supervisors of the teaching program, interrupted: "Was this severe upper left quadrant pain different from the epigastric pain? Was it something new?"

Dr. Backman: "He described it as different. He had it at night, and it wasn't relieved with antacids."

Dr. Jenkins: "Well, didn't that make you uncomfortable with the diagnosis of gastric ulcer?"

Dr. Backman: "No, because he had resumed smoking and drinking now, and we suspected alcoholic hepatitis, because of his abnormal liver function test. He reported clay-colored stools and we readmitted him to the hospital. From the start of his admission he was quite agitated and needed more sedation, so we called in Dr. Sheingold (the Chief of Psychiatry)."

Dr. Sheingold had considered saying something about Dr. Backman's description of the patient as "drinking again." In fact, he knew the patient drank very little, only a few beers when he went bowling once a week, and it seemed unfair to imply that the man was drinking enough to justify a diagnosis of alcoholic hepatitis. The trouble, Sheingold felt, was that once the doctors decided to bring a psychiatrist into the case most of them no longer believed anything the patient said. And so it had been easy for the doctors to regard this patient as an alcoholic. Still, Dr. Sheingold had observed that Backman was one of the few doctors in the hospital who thought that psychiatry had anything to offer them in their treatment of medical patients, so he had refrained from objecting to the imputation of alcoholism.

Sheingold was motioned to the stage to report on his participation in the case. He began: "Yes, I was invited to walk down the garden path with the others. I talked with the patient on his fourth day of admission. His father-in-law had just retired and appointed the patient as director of the family insurance business. Mr. Thomas had never liked the business and found it morbid. Indeed, he had complicated feelings about his business exacerbated by a long history of depression. Ten years ago he had been responsible for an automobile accident in which his oldest daughter, then three years old, had died. So I was quite sure along with Dr. Backman that this was gastric ulcer disease, and I wrote that in my notes. I also noted that there was an unlikely chance of pancreatic carcinoma (cancer) because I knew that would be considered at some time, but I was quite sure that it was an ulcer."

Dr. Stevens, one of the department chiefs in medicine, had been upset with the reasoning in this case. As he explained, one of his pet peeves was the stupid use of psychiatry, especially by the GI doctors, and he had noticed that Backman was one of the frequent offenders in this regard because as a GI specialist Backman also considered himself something of an expert in the field of psychiatry. As Stevens described the situation, every time one of the GI doctors heard a patient complaint that couldn't be explained he called in a psychiatrist. Stevens wished they would instead just admit to the patient that they didn't know what was wrong, and explain that they would have to wait or do more tests. Instead, complained Stevens, a psychiatrist came in and spoke to the patient and *always* found a psychiatric complication. "And," concluded Stevens, "what did that tell you? That everyone has problems?"

Dr. Rosen, another internist on the hospital staff, was questioning Backman. "Why weren't the clay-colored stools considered? Didn't you believe him?"

Backman replied: "Well, the clay-colored stools could have been caused by the antacids he was taking, but to be perfectly frank, I didn't know how much credence I could give to his reports. He was quite upset and had gone into a rage about having to pay for the use of the television in his room. I should also add that he was now complaining about leg pain as well. He was re-endoscoped and a liver scan was taken. It showed an enlarged liver without focal abnormalities and the liver function was not impaired. A liver biopsy was normal, which surprised us. We expected to find alcoholic hepatitis. After the biopsy there was hemoptysis [coughing up blood]. We were concerned because that had never happened and we thought that bleeding from the liver biopsy might have gone into the lung area. We did a cholangiogram and it was normal, but we noted that he had an elevated alkaphosphotase level. We released him from the hospital once again on a bland diet with tranquilizers, and his discharge diagnosis was peptic ulcer."

Dr. Davis, one of the younger internists, directed more questions to Backman: "Why wasn't a surgical exploration done at this time?"

Backman smiled, shaking his head. "I'm not sure. I guess we weren't smart enough." Davis continued: "Why was no attention paid to the calf pain?" Backman answered: "The reason we ignored his complaints of leg pain was that his roommate in the hospital had thrombophlebitis in the leg. So when Thomas complained of it, it just seemed too coincidental and we figured it was just a hysterical reaction."

Dr. Sheingold was afraid that this case was certainly not going to encourage the doctors in the hospital to turn to the psychiatry department for help. It made him angry that the only situation in which most of the doctors considered psychiatry to be useful was for the management of what they considered a "crazy" patient, and once a patient in the hospital was seen by a psychiatrist the doctors would attribute to the patient all sorts of psychological mechanisms that had nothing to do with the patient's personality (in this case they were imputing "hysterical" behavior to a non-hysterical patient) and they wouldn't even read the notes that Sheingold wrote in the patient's chart about which psychological mechanisms were relevant. Also, since they didn't regard psychiatric illness as real, they always disliked patients with psychiatric symptoms. As Sheingold later explained, all the doctors had disliked this patient when they thought that he suffered only from an ulcer, and they had only decided that he was likable after they realized that he was "really" sick with cancer.

Backman was still explaining why he had released the patient despite abnormal laboratory findings. "Oh, and to finish your question about surgery—his abdominal pains went away after three days, so we didn't consider it any more." He leafed through the pages of the chart and continued. "He was readmitted the following week with a swollen foot, an enlarged liver, extensive thrombophlebitis." Backman nodded to Cohen, the cardiologist who had been consulted at this point. Cohen stood up and briefly spoke from his place in the audience. "I was asked to say whether the problem was due to pulmonary emboli or from hemoptysis to the lung from the liver biopsy. I thought he had pulmonary emboli."

Attention was now directed to the Chief of Surgery, who described his part in the case: "I saw him at this point and I knew something terrible was going on. He was going downhill rapidly. It looked like an abdominal mass. The plan was now to deal with his phlebitis—so here we were in a bind. We had a GI bleeder who had to be anticoagulated for his emboli [a treatment that would increase bleeding], and now he had shortness of breath. The problem in dealing with this patient was that he was dead opposed to surgery. He had been in the life insurance business all his life, and every time we talked about surgery he would say, 'Now my family's gonna be collect-

ing on my policy.' " The surgeon turned to Davis, who had earlier criticized
Backman for not calling a surgeon sooner. "I'll tell you why we didn't do an
exploratory laparotomy [surgical investigation] earlier. He was so frantic
and had been sick so long. He had abdominal pain, and calf pain and GI
bleeding. He dreaded surgery, and frankly I dreaded going in there. His wife
kept yelling at me, asking what was wrong, and when I said I didn't know
she called me stupid. I guess maybe we *were* stupid. Anyway that's why we
didn't do an exploratory earlier." In the back of the auditorium, some of the
medical residents were smiling and mumbling that the reason the Chief had
delayed surgery was that he hated to operate. Douglas had a reputation
among the younger aggressive doctors in the hospital of being too cautious
and slow to act. It was not clear whether Douglas noticed their remarks, and
he continued. "So we did a venous clip and when we later did an exploratory we saw that there was cancer all over. The patient died three days later,
and I just want to add here that according to the chart he was in severe
anguish on the last day of his life, and was not given the painkillers we had
prescribed, so we can thank our nurses for making the last day of his life as
miserable as possible." The surgeon nodded to the pathologist and the lights
were switched off. Color slides of the patient's affected organs were flashed
on the screen. Each one showed gross abnormalities from the spread of the
cancer. Throughout the auditorium murmurs could be heard at the exten-
siveness of the cancer, as if to emphasize that with so dramatic and perva-
sive a disease they as doctors could hardly have been expected to stop such
an invasion.

When the lights were turned on the surgeon drew the meeting to a close,
explaining how at that very moment the patient's brother was waiting in his
office; the brother had come to show him an article about a so-called
wonder drug, which was illegal, for curing cancer. Douglas added that he
had given the brother an appointment so that the man could yell at him for
having refused to try this illegal drug. Several doctors in the audience
laughed and shook their heads sympathetically, breaking into small groups
as they moved into the adjoining room for coffee and doughnuts.

The Thomas case, described above, illustrates how doctors often justify
their errors by pointing to misleading or unusual features of the case. By
demonstrating that they had good reason (though later shown to be mistaken) for doing what they did, they may avoid censure and discomfort,
and save face before their colleagues. Physical symptoms inconsistent with
the final diagnosis are the misleading cues which provide the most comforting and persuasive type of excuse for making the wrong diagnosis.
However, when physical justifications are unavailable, doctors often resort
to psychological and social evidence as the factors which misguided them
and justified their behavior. In these cases, the nonphysical evidence is
represented as being so convincing as to justify overlooking even physical
evidence which should have alerted doctors to the correct diagnosis. In the

Thomas case, for example, the doctors overlooked clear symptoms of organic disorder (such as the elevated alkaphosphotase level) because they were so convinced that the patient was neurotic and that his complaints and symptoms could be explained psychologically.

In other cases where physical findings are overlooked, or erroneously discounted, the physician will often excuse his embarrassing error by blaming the patient. If the patient can be "discredited" as crazy, alcoholic, obnoxious, uncooperative, or otherwise difficult or undeserving, then the responsibility for the medical error can be shifted away from the doctor to the patient. The physician's errors are made to seem understandable and inconsequential in a life fated for disaster by the patient's own doing. The following case illustrates this process.

Case No. 2: Alice McDonald

Mrs. McDonald was a fifty-year-old woman who died in the Emergency Room of a perforated duodenal ulcer which the staff failed to diagnose, despite her complaints of severe abdominal pain.

The case was introduced in the meeting by the intern who had seen her in the Emergency Room. He opened the discussion by describing her as "An obese, alcoholic woman of Irish extraction who was very uncooperative and used very abusive language," thereby fixing her in the minds of the physicians in the audience as the type of patient who is difficult to treat.

In explaining why they had not paid much attention to her complaints of abdominal pain, the doctors involved in the case made much of her appearance of being "mentally disconnected." Asked to be more specific about her mental state, both the intern and the medical doctor covering the Emergency Room that night stated that they remembered noting the smell of alcohol on her breath, and therefore felt they could dismiss her complaints as the ravings of a drunken woman.

Toward the end of the meeting someone in the audience offhandedly asked what the alcohol level in the blood had been at the time of the incident. Now the Chief of Medicine sheepishly admitted a fact that had been previously left unmentioned: although much had been made of this woman's drunkenness, the fact was that the alcohol level in the blood had been zero at the time of her examination.

This embarrassing fact was passed over quickly. No longer able to use her drunkenness as an excuse for their failure to take her complaints seriously, the doctors now turned more exclusively to emphasizing her angry, "disconnected" and uncooperative behavior toward them as the factor responsible for the poor treatment she received.

The power of the doctor's self-justification is highlighted in this case. For even after implicitly acknowledging that drunkenness was falsely attributed to the patient, the doctors continued to blame this woman's death on her own anger and abusive language, and ignored the possibility that such behavior was appropriate for a woman dying in great pain while the doctors around her treated her complaints as the fabrications of a hysterical alcoholic.

The case also illustrates how doctors may overlook important physical findings (which should indicate a serious illness) if they have already discounted the complaints by viewing the patient as a certain kind of neurotic individual. For a "neurotic" individual is viewed by doctors as an unreliable reporter, and once characterized this way, a patient's remarks are likely to be ignored. Indeed, these patients are commonly known among many doctors as "crocks" or "turkeys" and are considered undeserving of serious attention.

It is a complicated problem, for certainly doctors will occasionally meet with an anxious patient who will refuse to believe that he is in good health. But serious errors are often made as a result of characterizing patients as "crocks," for doctors are usually not in a position to correctly guess who is really sick and who isn't, from behavior alone. Furthermore, doctors appear to assign the label "crock" quite often on grounds of personal or prejudiced responses. They are more likely, for example, to dismiss a patient as neurotic and not really sick if the patient seems angry, mistrustful, or disrespectful to the doctor. The label "crock" also seems to be applied erroneously more often to women.

A third case reviewed in the Medical Mortality Conference illustrates another common pattern in neutralizing mistakes. Sometimes the patient may be viewed as so lacking in social value or otherwise so physically deteriorated that the question of a consequential medical mistake hardly occurs to anyone involved in the case. That is, the recognition of, and attention to, a medical mistake depends upon the doctor's seeing the patient as an individual having some value. The very definition of a mistake, by doctors, therefore, rests not on some universal and fixed standard of good or poor practice applied to every case, but the definition of a mistake rather shifts and slides according to the value of the patient as assessed by the doctors.

As this final Mortality Review case illustrates, the patient was viewed as so physically and socially worthless that the audience paid little attention to the one doctor among them who expressed distress at how the case had been handled.

Case No. 3: Freddy Grazzo

Freddy Grazzo had become a well-known patient in Lakeside Hospital, and his case the source of many jokes among the staff. He was a clear example of what many physicians think of as the "garbage" or deadwood of their work and clientele. Elderly, unmarried and unemployed, Freddy Grazzo lived in a rooming house and spent his days drinking beer with his friends. He had an undiagnosed illness that repeatedly brought him to the Emergency Room, close to death and in pulmonary edema (his lungs filled with fluid, and breathing with great difficulty). Each time, the resident or intern on duty would resuscitate him and have to do a "work-up" examination as part of the hospital admission. Within a day or two, "Freddy" (as he was called by doctors thirty years his junior) would be doing well enough to leave the hospital, but his furlough was always short: within a few days he would be back in the Emergency Room in the same condition.

Because of his surprising ability to survive one after another of these emergencies Freddy had acquired a wide reputation in the hospital. Any one of these attacks might have ended his life, so it had become something of a standing hospital joke when his emergency admissions began to number in the twenties. Word would spread in the hospital that Freddy was back, and the interns and residents would laugh bitterly about how they had to waste their fine talents on old broken men who would never get better.

Still, over the course of twenty-five admissions a bit of abstract affection for Freddy Grazzo had developed among the staff. As he would be rushed into the Emergency Room, gasping for air, the nurses would tease him that he should be fixed up with Mary O'Leary, who was the female record-breaking survivor of Emergency Room resuscitations. At daily reports to the Chief of Medicine the residents would describe his condition as the "paddle syndrome": like a ball attached to a paddle, he was released from the hospital, went down the street to the nearest bar and soon bounced back into the hospital again.

If the annoyance that the staff felt for this patient were weighed against the amusement, it would have to be said that annoyance prevailed. When Freddy Grazzo arrived in the Emergency Room for the twenty-third time, the charge nurse openly complained that "they shouldn't have even coded him the last time he came in." When patients have an illness that will never improve and when their continued existence seems unwarranted in the doctors' eyes, either the doctor will note in the chart that the patient should not be resuscitated, or word will get passed informally around the staff that the patient should not again be coded the next time he gets into a life-threatening situation.

There was some feeling in the hospital that Freddy Grazzo had already been granted or burdened with too many codes, but he was still to survive this twenty-third admission. As the interns leisurely carried out the resuscitation like a familiar routine and inserted intravenous lines for his drugs, they argued about which floor of the hospital Freddy should be admitted to because no one wanted to do the work-up examination. It was late at night, and when Dr. Jenkins (a physician covering for Dr. Rosen, who was the regular doctor on the case) arrived in the Emergency Room, the charge nurse asked why he had bothered to come in. Jenkins replied that a decision might have to be made that night about keeping the patient alive. (As he put it: "In case something brews tonight a decision should be made.") Although Freddy Grazzo survived this admission, it was not long after that he was one day declared dead on arrival in the Emergency Room.

But even after his death Freddy Grazzo's name was still often heard, because toward the end of his life his physician became convinced that this was no ordinary case of geriatric decline, no mere piece of "medical garbage" after all. Dr. Rosen felt that he might just have stumbled across an exciting rare disease in Freddy Grazzo.

When the mortality meeting was held a few weeks later, Rosen seemed pleased that the case would be reviewed. He had indicated that he was convinced that Freddy had been an unsalvageable patient and he was happy to have a chance to show off his unusual diagnosis.

Rosen had first come to the hospital as a specialist in internal medicine twenty years before. In the old days he had been considered one of the more highly trained physicians in the hospital, and he had been given a free hand in treating the whole range of medical cases, including the most esoteric ones. But in the last few years the power in the hospital had progressively shifted to the newer "subspecialists" on the staff. Now the most challenging heart cases were referred to the cardiologists, and not to doctors like Rosen.

Furthermore, all the internists (an internist is a specialist in internal medicine, not to be confused with an intern, who is an untrained doctor fresh out of medical school) like himself were now expected to call in the specialists for consultations and special diagnostic tests whenever they had anything but the most routine cases. This meant that the specialists wound up managing all the interesting cases while Rosen was supposed to be satisfied with what he called the "lumps and bumps."

His reluctance to bow to pressure and invite consultation from the experts was not a matter of resentment, Rosen had argued to the house officers. For he believed that most consultation from these subspecialists was pointless because their recommendations were completely predictable. For example, during the previous week one of his patients had been admitted after being found unconscious with symptoms possibly suggesting a subarachnoid (brain) hemorrhage. This diagnosis could only have been positively confirmed by doing a somewhat risky and uncomfortable procedure, a cerebral arteriogram. The resident assigned to the case had been in favor of having the diagnostic procedure done, and knowing that Rosen was opposed to it, he had tactfully asked Rosen if they could get a specialist's opinion before ruling it out. Rosen had refused and explained why it was pointless: he could tell the resident exactly what the consultants would say without bothering to have them look at the patient. If the hospital neurologist (who was known to be conservative) was consulted, he would say, "Don't do anything." And if instead, they invited the opinion of the neurosurgeon, he would be sure to say, "Let's operate." So, as Rosen had argued to the resident, since it was all an arbitrary choice, it was better made by the doctor who knew something about the patient (and Rosen felt she was a nervous woman who would be upset by the diagnostic procedure) than on the basis of the prejudice of either subspecialist.

But to return to the Grazzo case, Rosen had indicated his confidence in the care the patient had received, and he was looking forward to the Mortality Review. In fact, he had asked the Chief of Medicine to let him use the entire meeting for this case, although it was customary to go through two cases in each meeting. The chief had refused but compromised by curtailing the discussion on the first case, explaining to the group that he wanted to leave more time for "Hal Rosen's masterpiece."

As Rosen came cheerfully tripping down the stairs to the front of the auditorium he conceded that the case was perhaps a "masterpiece with flaws." Proudly pointing to the twelve volumes of the patient's chart, he apologized that because of time constraints they would have to begin their review with the patient's eighteenth hospital admission. The facts were as follows: the patient had suffered recurrent dyspnea (breathlessness) and pulmonary edema, would often faint after eating, and they had long suspected that the cause of the symptoms were pulmonary emboli which were causing the edema. To illustrate the symptoms, Rosen entertained the audience with stories of how Freddy Grazzo would collapse on the street but somehow always get to the hospital in time to be resuscitated. On one occasion, Rosen smiled, Grazzo had suffered a coronary arrest (they believed an embolus had triggered a cardiac arrhythmia) on a street corner in the next town, and he would never have made it to the hospital in time had he not unknowingly reached out and grabbed on to what turned out to be a fire alarm box to steady himself before he collapsed to the ground. A fire truck had arrived within two minutes, and seeing the man collapsed to the ground, the firemen had thrown him on the back of the truck and hauled him into the hospital.

After the laughter subsided Rosen described how they had made their discovery of the suspected rare disease. One day, upon being released from the hospital, Freddy had been waiting in front of the hospital for a taxi to take him home only to collapse, once more, into the arms of Rosen's colleague, Dr. Paul Jenkins, who had been walking by. Grabbing him in his arms, Jenkins had suddenly had the inspiration that the patient might be suffering not from pulmonary emboli but rather from the interesting and unusual central nervous hyperventilation syndrome. And, Rosen concluded with a smile, he concurred.

What followed next was some friendly joking about whether Rosen was only daydreaming to come up with such a diagnosis. Gordon Frank, the Chief of Cardiology, looked annoyed and finally openly expressed his disapproval. Standing up, he interrupted the friendly teasing: "I am deeply disturbed by the levity of this meeting, and I must say it matches the levity with which this patient was admitted every time to the Coronary Care Unit. Each time he came in everyone would giggle 'Guess who's back, ha-ha.' And I think that instead of sending him into our unit each time without knowing what was wrong with him, the patient should have had tests to ascertain what was wrong. The tests might have shown that he had a treatable illness."

As Frank explained, by saying "I don't like the levity with which this case was handled" he was actually saying that he didn't like the way that Rosen had managed the case medically. There had long been tension and disagreement between Rosen and himself. As he described it, Rosen would never come to him for help when he was out of his depth, and so Frank considered Rosen to be a potentially dangerous doctor. But, he admitted, a doctor couldn't come right out at a Mortality Meeting and say that he didn't like the way someone managed a case, so he had criticized the joking. Those who knew how he felt about Rosen would understand the deeper meaning of his remarks, and those who didn't, or who refused to acknowledge the issue, would be spared an unpleasant scene.

At the Mortality Meeting, Rosen met Frank's challenge and defended his refusal to do the diagnostic tests. There would have been no point, he argued, in performing angiography on this patient because even if the test had shown emboli as the cause of edema, the patient would never have consented to corrective surgery anyway. Frank replied, with obvious irritation, that if Rosen had allowed him to perform a diagnostic angiogram, it might have confirmed one of two possible diseases which were treatable even without surgery. He then described some new procedures, unknown to Rosen, which might have allowed them to treat Grazzo's problem without surgery.

The meeting time was coming to an end and so the doctors in the audience called out their final guesses about the true cause of Freddy Grazzo's illness. The intern who had pronounced the patient dead in the Emergency Room placed his bet on aspiration as the cause of death. An older physician in the audience hazarded the guess of atrial myxoma (a tumor in the heart).

The positions having been staked, it was now time for the final verdict. Solemnly, the pathologist stepped to the front of the room to announce what he had found in his autopsy.

To fully appreciate this moment it must be understood that the part of their work that medical doctors enjoy most is the challenging diagnosis. For most surgeons, the excitement and pleasure in the work is in doing a good job in the operating room: it is in the operating room that surgeons get to use their most highly specialized skills. But for medical doctors, the most exciting opportunity in the work is to make a brilliant diagnosis. Surgeons may also enjoy witnessing a dramatic cure as a result of an operation, but a medical doctor is often denied the satisfaction of bringing about a dramatic cure, especially in the treatment of elderly or chronically ill patients. In such cases, the work of internists can only prolong a painful and limited life. Under these circumstances, pleasure and excitement in the work are found, not in what can be done for patients, but rather in being the first one to come up with a brilliant diagnosis. That is why there would be special satisfaction in turning a routine and boring medical case into a good detective story with a surprising turn of events.

The pathologist, who paused before giving the final verdict on the Grazzo case, did not give away the ending all at once. Instead, he eliminated the losing guesses first. Like runners-up at a beauty contest, those who had guessed incorrectly bowed out good-naturedly. No, the death had not been caused by aspiration; the intern who guessed this possibility received the thumbs-down sign from the doctors sitting around him. And no, there had been no myxoma; the older physician who had made that guess shrugged his shoulders in concession. The pathologist turned to Rosen, sympathetically. While there *had* been some reason to suspect central nervous hyperventilation syndrome, not all of the criteria necessary to make that diagnosis were met in this case, and so that rare disorder could not be claimed. Freddy Grazzo had died the most ordinary death after all: his cardiac arrhythmias (irregularities of the heart beat) had been brought on by atherosclerosis (thickening and occlusion of the walls of the coronary arteries), and it was this common condition of the elderly which had triggered the emboli and his pulmonary edema.

As the meeting broke up, several of Rosen's friends patted him on the back for making a valiant effort at finding an exciting disease.

It is difficult to talk about mistakes without thinking about the feelings which mistakes arouse, both in the individual who has made the error and in the others around him. Acknowledging a consequential mistake is a profoundly upsetting experience for many reasons. First, there is the pain of fully knowing that things might have turned out better had one acted the way one should have. Then there is the unbearable self-doubt that follows from admitting to a mistake. The person who has recognized that he is capable of grave errors is suddenly unable to trust his own judgment. Every future act is cast in doubt and every decision agonized over lest it lead to further disaster. Finally, there is the fact, fair or not, that the individual who has made a mistake is somewhat tarnished in the eyes of his associates, and may even be formally punished or sanctioned. There is sad irony here, for the designation "mistake" is meant, at least on the surface, to excuse or pardon the actor. To say "it was just a mistake" signifies that such a wrong act was out of keeping for such an ordinarily trustworthy individual, just a fluke of nature unlikely to happen again. Nevertheless, most people are naturally suspicious of "mistakes," and the reputation of the person who makes them is often permanently stained.

No wonder, then, that most people try to avoid admitting to mistakes and prefer to live with the continued bad consequences of errors than with the distress of admitting to the mistake. But even if an individual is personally prepared to admit to a mistake, those whose lives and fates are tied up with his own are very likely to talk him out of such an admission, for the acknowledgment of a mistake is upsetting for groups as well as for individuals. When one member of a group starts calling attention to mistakes, not only does everyone else become vulnerable to the same exposure, but the entire collective enterprise they have committed themselves to begins to look more and more shabby.

Groups of doctors are not exempt from the upsetting possibility of having mistakes exposed. The works of just one outspoken member are enough to make everyone uncomfortable. The admission of mistakes is especially upsetting in the world of medicine because it is a world that rests and depends upon a faith in science, objectivity and rationality. A mistake in such a world is as disruptive as the commission of a sin in a religious society. It challenges the most cherished beliefs and identities of its members. Furthermore, since self-sufficiency and self-confidence are so highly valued in the medical profession, an admission of uncertainty or error exposes the physician to the kind of self-doubt that is unacceptable among his colleagues. The admission of a mistake is also very difficult in medicine because the stakes are so high. Many doctors, for example, retain disturbing memories for the rest of their lives of how they were responsible for a patient's death when they were residents because they had been too inexperienced to handle a situation properly.

For all of these reasons, it is not surprising that individual doctors are strictly discouraged by their group and their profession from being too willing to point out a mistake, or to openly admit to a feeling of guilt. The likelihood of making a bad mistake is too high and the price of admitting to it too costly to the group to leave the matter open to the discretion and dispositions of individual members. That is why a doctor is carefully taught in training and afterward not to regard as a mistake what most lay people would consider a mistake, and not to make too much of these unfortunate episodes.

A similar point can be made about feelings of guilt in medicine. Given the probability of making a bad mistake sometime in one's career, and given the probability of recognizing that the cynical reality of medical work is dramatically different from the idealistic expectations and self-images that one began with as a young student, the potential for feeling guilty is very high for physicians. That is why there are strong professional and institutional supports for avoiding feelings of guilt. Indeed, if a doctor is still prone to feeling guilty despite all of the supports to the contrary, he will quickly learn to keep his feelings to himself. Nobody wants to hear about a colleague's feelings of guilt, and talking too freely about such feelings with other doctors is considered a very embarrassing faux pas.

So it is that doctors are not likely to dig too deeply into one another's errors nor even to recognize fully the extent to which they collude in covering up each other's mistakes and incompetence. It is easier for them to shift the blame and responsibility for mistakes away from themselves, either to the patient, who becomes discredited in the process, or to surrounding impersonal circumstances such as misleading or unusual evidence in a particular case. Under these circumstances, mistakes are allowed to flourish and be repeated, and incompetence goes unchecked. Clearly it is the patient who pays the highest price in this arrangement for insuring the comfort of physician-colleagues, but some unusually conscientious doctors also pay the smaller price of being left alone with the residual feelings that manage to survive the professional neutralization and justifications.

Note

1. All names in this article are pseudonyms—Eds.

Part Three

Contemporary Critical Debates

U p until this point we have presented our analysis of health and medical care as if all critical analysts were more or less in agreement. But in health care, as in any social and intellectual enterprise, controversies and debates rage over the source of problems and appropriate solutions. In Part Three we present articles illustrative of contemporary debates on four different but related critical issues in the sociology of health and illness.

Medical Services: Nemesis or Nihilism?

UNTIL VERY RECENTLY MOST CRITICS of medical care agreed on one thing: health would be improved if only more medical services were readily available to more people. Ivan Illich (1976), a foremost critic of technologized and professionalized society (e.g., see Illich, 1971), turns this assumption around: he argues that modern medical care is generally ineffective and is now itself a threat to our health, and that people would be better off with *fewer* medical services rather than more. He suggests that our health crisis is built into our present system and calls the system a medical "Nemesis." Illich argues that at the core of our medical Nemesis is *iatrogenic* or harmful consequences of medical care, which are manifested on three levels. Clinical iatrogenesis is the sickness and damage inflicted by doctors in their attempt to cure the patient (in part accounting for so many malpractice suits in the U.S.). Social iatrogenesis is the medicalization of life or, in Illich's terms, the expropriation of health that encourages people to become compulsive consumers of medicine. Cultural iatrogenesis runs deeper and is more subtle. By relying on medical care, "the potential for people to deal with their human weakness, vulnerability, and uniqueness in a personal and autonomous way" is destroyed (Illich, 1976: 33). We can no longer adapt to pain and death nor see them as natural concomitants of life. Illich sees medical Nemesis as irreversible and argues that the only way to "recover health" is to deprofessionalize medicine and encourage the development of self-care so that individuals may recover their autonomous ability to cope. (Illich does note that we might need a few physicians to provide technical services such as setting a broken leg.) Illich's article in this section, "Medical Nemesis," is an early formulation of his ideas, and touches on all of these major themes.

Illich's argument has provoked vigorous response. Some health care analysts have embraced it and argued for the limitation of medical services, on the one hand, and increased self-help and self-care, on the other. But other critics of medicine have been more skeptical. They question whether the effectiveness of medical care can be measured only by "cure" rates, and suggest that medical "care" might be equally important (although more difficult to measure). Some maintain that Illich proposes an idyllic individualism and romanticizes the value of pain and suffering. Others are concerned that his argument provides intellectual support for cutbacks in medical services, especially in times of fiscal retrenchment. While Illich's analysis appears radical, some contend that its ramifications are ultimately conservative (see, for example Navarro, 1975).

Many of Illich's critics agree with at least part of his analysis, but many also disagree with his proposed remedies. Whereas Illich questions the value of medical services, Paul Starr questions the value of abandoning them in "The Politics of Therapeutic Nihilism." To Starr (and others) the issue is not services per se, but what services are delivered to whom and with what effects? The central issue, then, becomes inequality of access to services. As Starr shows, race and class at least partly reduce equality of access. Rather than being nihilistic about all medical services, Starr contends we should discover what services are iatrogenic and why, and what services are helpful. But, most importantly, we must cre-

ate a real equality of access, for without this we will only exacerbate existing inequalities in health.

References

Illich, Ivan. 1971. Deschooling Society. New York: Harper and Row.
    1976. Medical Nemesis. New York: Pantheon.
Navarro, Vicente. 1975. "The industrialization of fetishism or the fetishism of
    industrialization: A critique of Ivan Illich." International Journal of Health
    Services 5 (3).

28

Medical Nemesis

Ivan Illich

Within the last decade medical professional practice has become a major threat to health. Depression, infection, disability, dysfunction, and other specific iatrogenic diseases now cause more suffering than all accidents from traffic or industry. Beyond this, medical practice sponsors sickness by the reinforcement of a morbid society which not only industrially preserves its defectives but breeds the therapist's client in a cybernetic way. Finally, the so-called health-professions have an indirect sickening power—a structurally health-denying effect. I want to focus on this last syndrome, which I designate as medical Nemesis. By transforming pain, illness, and death from a personal challenge into a technical problem, medical practice expropriates the potential of people to deal with their human condition in an autonomous way and becomes the source of a new kind of un-health.

Much suffering has always been man-made: history is the record of enslavement and exploitation. It tells of war, and of the pillage, famine, and pestilence which come in its wake. War between commonwealths and classes has so far been the main planned agency of man-made misery. Thus, man is the only animal whose evolution has been conditioned by adaptation on two fronts. If he did not succumb to the elements, he had to cope with use and abuse by others of his kind. He replaced instincts by character and culture, to be capable of this struggle on two frontiers. A third frontier of possible doom has been recognised since Homer; but common mortals were considered immune to its threat. Nemesis, the Greek name for the awe which loomed from this third direction, was the fate of a few heroes who had fallen prey to the envy of the gods. The common man grew up and perished in a struggle with Nature and neighbor. Only the élite would challenge the thresholds set by Nature for man.

Prometheus was not everyman, but a deviant. Driven by Pleonexia, or radical greed, he trespassed the boundaries of the human condition. In hubris or measureless presumption, he brought fire from heaven, and thereby brought Nemesis on himself. He was put into irons on a Caucasian rock. A vulture preys at his innards, and heartlessly healing gods keep him alive by regrafting his liver each night. The encounter with Nemesis made the classical hero an immortal reminder of inescapable cosmic retaliation. He becomes a subject for epic tragedy, but certainly not a model for everyday aspiration. Now Nemesis has become endemic; it is the backlash of progress. Paradoxically, it has spread as far and as wide as the franchise, schooling, mechanical acceleration, and medical care. Everyman has fallen prey to the envy of the gods. If the species is to survive it can do so only by learning to cope in this third group.

Industrial Nemesis

Most man-made misery is now the byproduct of enterprises which were originally designed to protect the common man in his struggle with the inclemency of the environment and against wanton injustices inflicted by the élite. The main source of pain, disability, and death is now an engineered—albeit non-intentional—harassment. The prevailing ailments, helplessness and injustice, are now the side-effects of strategies for progress. Nemesis is now so prevalent that it is readily mistaken for part of the human condition. The desperate disability of contemporary man to envisage an alternative to the industrial aggression on the human condition is an integral part of the curse from which he suffers. Progress has come with a vengeance which cannot be called a price. The down payment was on the label and can be stated in measurable terms. The instalments accrue under forms of suffering which exceed the notion of "pain".

At some point in the expansion of our major institutions their clients begin to pay a higher price every day for their continued consumption, in spite of the evidence that they will inevitably suffer more. At this point in development the prevalent behavior of society corresponds to that traditionally recognised in addicts. Declining returns pale in comparison with marginally increasing disutilities. *Homo economicus* turns into *Homo religiosus*. His expectations become heroic. The vengeance of economic development not only outweighs the price at which this vengeance was purchased; it also outweighs the compound tort done by Nature and neighbors. Classical Nemesis was punishment for the rash abuse of a privilege. Industrialised Nemesis is retribution for dutiful participation in society.

War and hunger, pestilence and sudden death, torture and madness remain man's companions, but they are now shaped into a new *Gestalt* by the Nemesis overarching them. The greater the economic progress of any community, the greater the part played by industrial Nemesis in the pain, discrimination, and death suffered by its members. Therefore, it seems that the disciplined study of the distinctive character of Nemesis ought to be the key theme for research amongst those who are concerned with health care, healing, and consoling.

Tantalus

Medical Nemesis is but one aspect of the more general "counter-intuitive misadventures" characteristic of industrial society. It is the monstrous outcome of a very specific dream of reason—namely, "tantalising" hubris. Tantalus was a famous king whom the gods invited to Olympus to share one of their meals. He purloined Ambrosia, the divine potion which gave the gods unending life. For punishment, he was made immortal in Hades and condemned to suffer unending thirst and hunger. When he bows towards the river in which he stands, the water recedes, and when he reaches for the fruit above his head the branches move out of his reach. Ethologists might say that Hygienic Nemesis has programed him for compulsory counter-intuitive behavior. Craving for Ambrosia has now spread to the common mortal. Scientific and political optimism have combined to propagate the addiction. To sustain it, the priesthood of Tantalus has organised itself, offering unlimited medical improvement of human health. The members of this guild pass themselves off as disciples of healing Asklepios, while in fact they peddle Ambrosia. People demand of them that life be improved, prolonged, rendered compatible with machines, and capable of surviving all modes of acceleration, distortion, and stress. As a result, health has become scarce to the degree to which the common man makes health depend upon the consumption of Ambrosia.

Culture and Health

Mankind evolved only because each of its individuals came into existence protected by various visible and invisible cocoons. Each one knew the womb from which he had come, and oriented himself by the stars under which he was born. To be human and to become human, the individual of our species has to find his destiny in his unique struggle with Nature and neighbor. He is on his own in the struggle, but the weapons and the rules and the style are given to him by the culture in which he grew up. Each culture is the sum of rules with which the individual could come to terms with pain, sickness, and death—could interpret them and practise compassion amongst others faced by the same threats. Each culture set the myth, the rituals, the taboos, and the ethical standards needed to deal with the fragility of life—to explain the reason for pain, the dignity of the sick, and the role of dying or death.

Cosmopolitan medical civilisation denies the need for man's acceptance of these evils. Medical civilisation is planned and organised to kill pain, to eliminate sickness, and to struggle against death. These are new goals, which have never before been guidelines for social life and which are antithetic to every one of the cultures with which medical civilisation meets when it is dumped on the so-called poor as part and parcel of their economic progress.

The health-denying effect of medical civilisation is thus equally powerful in rich and in poor countries, even though the latter are often spared some of its more sinister sides.

The Killing of Pain

For an experience to be pain in the full sense, it must fit into a culture. Precisely because each culture provides a mode for suffering, culture is a particular form of health. The act of suffering is shaped by culture into a question which can be stated and shared.

Medical civilisation replaces the culturally determined competence in suffering with a growing demand by each individual for the institutional management of his pain. A myriad of different feelings, each expressing some kind of fortitude, are homogenised into the political pressure of anæsthesia consumers. Pain becomes an item on a list of complaints. As a result, a new kind of horror emerges. Conceptually it is still pain, but the impact on our emotions of this valueless, opaque, and impersonal hurt is something quite new.

In this way, pain has come to pose only a technical question for industrial man—what do I need to get in order to have my pain managed or killed? If the pain continues, the fault is not with the universe, God, my sins, or the devil, but with the medical system. Suffering is an expression of consumer demand for increased medical outputs. By becoming unnecessary, pain has become unbearable. With this attitude, it now seems rational to flee pain rather than to face it, even at the cost of addiction. It also seems reasonable to eliminate pain, even at the cost of health. It seems enlightened to deny legitimacy to all non-technical issues which pain raises, even at the cost of disarming the victims of residual pain. For a while it can be argued that the total pain anæsthetised in a society is greater than the totality of pain newly generated. But at some point, rising marginal disutilities set in. The new suffering is not only unmanageable, but it has lost its referential character. It has become meaningless, questionless torture. Only the recovery of the will and ability to suffer can restore health into pain.

The Elimination of Sickness

Medical interventions have not affected total mortality-rates: at best they have shifted survival from one segment of the population to another. Dramatic changes in the nature of disease afflicting Western societies during the last 100 years are well documented. First industrialisation exacerbated infections, which then subsided. Tuberculosis peaked over a 50–75-year period and declined before either the tubercle bacillus had been discovered or antituberculous programes had been initiated. It was replaced in Britain and the U.S. by major malnutrition syndromes—rickets and pellagra—which peaked and declined, to be replaced by disease of early childhood, which in turn gave way to duodenal ulcers in young men. When that declined the modern epidemics took their toll—coronary heart-disease, hypertension, cancer, arthritis, diabetes, and mental disorders. At least in the U.S., death-rates from hypertensive heart-disease seem to be declining. Despite intensive research no connection between these changes in disease patterns can be attributed to the professional practice of medicine.

Neither decline in any of the major epidemics of killing diseases, nor major changes in the age structure of the population, nor falling and rising absenteeism at the workbench have been significantly related to sick care—even to immunisation. Medical services deserve neither credit for longevity nor blame for the threatening population pressure.

Longevity owes much more to the railroad and to the synthesis of fertilisers and insecticides than it owes to new drugs and syringes. Professional practice is both ineffective and increasingly sought out. This technically unwarranted rise of medical prestige can only be explained as a magical ritual for the achievement of goals which are beyond technical and political reach. It can be countered only through legislation and political action which favours the deprofessionalisation of health care.

The overwhelming majority of modern diagnostic and therapeutic interventions which demonstrably do more good than harm have two characteristics: the material resources for them are extremely cheap, and they can be packaged and designed for self-use or application by family members. The price of technology that is significantly health-furthering or curative in Canadian medicine is so low that the resources now squandered in India on modern medicine would suffice to make it available in the entire sub-continent. On the other hand, the skills needed for the application of the most generally used diagnostic and therapeutic aids are so simple that the careful observation of instruction by people who personally care would guarantee more effective and responsible use than medical practice can provide.

The deprofessionalisation of medicine does not imply and should not be read as implying negation of specialised healers, of competence, of mutual criticism, or of public control. It does imply a bias against mystification, against transnational dominance of one orthodox view, against disbarment of healers chosen by their patients but not certified by the guild. The deprofessionalisation of medicine does not mean denial of public funds for curative purposes; it does mean a bias against the disbursement of any such funds under the prescription and control of guild-members, rather than under the control of the consumer. Deprofessionalisation does not mean the elimination of modern medicine, nor obstacles to the invention of new ones, nor necessarily the return to ancient programs, rituals, and devices. It means that no professional shall have the power to lavish on any one of his patients a package of curative resources larger than that which any other could claim on his own. Finally, the deprofessionalisation of medicine does not mean disregard for the special needs which people manifest at special moments of their lives; when they are born, break a leg, marry, give birth, become crippled, or face death. It only means that people have a right to live in an environment which is hospitable to them at such high points of experience.

The Struggle Against Death

The ultimate effect of medical Nemesis is the expropriation of death. In every society the image of death is the culturally conditioned anticipation of an uncertain date. This anticipation determines a series of behavioral norms during life and the structure of certain institutions.

Wherever modern medical civilisation has penetrated a traditional medical culture, a novel cultural ideal of death has been fostered. The new ideal spreads by means of technology and the professional ethos which corresponds to it.

In primitive societies death is always conceived as the intervention of an actor—an enemy, a witch, an ancestor, or a god. The Christian and the Islamic Middle Ages saw in each death the hand of God. Western death had no face until about 1420. The Western ideal of death which comes to all equally from natural causes is of quite recent origin. Only during the autumn of the Middle Ages death appears as a skeleton with power in its own right. Only during the 16th century, as an answer European peoples developed the "arte and crafte to knowe ye Will to Dye." For the next three centuries peasant and noble, priest and whore, prepared themselves throughout life to preside at their own death. Foul death, bitter death, became the end rather than the goal of living. The idea that natural death should come in healthy old age appeared only in the 18th century as a class-specific phenomenon of the bourgeois. The demand that doctors struggle against death and keep valetudinarians healthy has nothing to do with their ability to provide such service: Ariès has shown that the costly attempts to prolong life appear at first only among bankers whose power is compounded by the years they spend at a desk.

We cannot fully understand contemporary social organisation unless we see in it a multi-faceted exorcism of all forms of evil death. Our major institutions constitute a gigantic defense program waged on behalf of "humanity" against all those people who can be associated with what is currently conceived of as death-dealing social injustice. Not only medical agencies, but welfare, international relief, and development programs are enlisted in this struggle. Ideological bureaucracies of all colors join the crusade. Even war has been used to justify the defeat of those who are blamed for wanton tolerance of sickness and death. Producing "natural death" for all men is at the point of becoming an ultimate justification for social control. Under the influence of medical rituals contemporary death is again the rationale for a witch-hunt.

Conclusion

Rising irreparable damage accompanies industrial expansion in all sectors. In medicine these damages appear as iatrogenesis. Iatrogenesis can be direct, when pain, sickness, and death result from medical care; or it can be indirect, when health policies reinforce an industrial organisation which generates ill-health: it can be structural when medically sponsored behavior and delusion restrict the vital autonomy of people by undermining their competence in growing up, caring, aging; or when it nullifies the personal challenge arising from their pain, disability, and anguish.

Most of the remedies proposed to reduce iatrogenesis are engineering interventions. They are therapeutically designed in their approach to the individual, the group, the institution, or the environment. These so-called remedies generate second-order iatrogenic ills by creating a new prejudice against the autonomy of the citizen.

The most profound iatrogenic effects of the medical technostructure result from its non-technical social functions. The sickening technical and non-technical consequences of the institutionalisation of medicine coalesce to generate a new kind of suffering—anæsthetised and solitary survival in a world-wide hospital ward.

Medical Nemesis cannot be operationally verified. Much less can it be measured. The intensity with which it is experienced depends on the independence, vitality, and relatedness of each individual. As a theoretical concept it is one component in a broad theory to explain the anomalies plaguing health-care systems in our day. It is a distinct aspect of an even more general phenomenon which I have called industrial Nemesis, the backlash of institutionally structured industrial hubris. This hubris consists of a disregard for the boundaries within which the human phenomenon remains viable. Current research is overwhelmingly oriented towards unattainable "breakthroughs". What I have called counterfoil research is the disciplined analysis of the levels at which such reverberations must inevitably damage man.

The perception of enveloping Nemesis leads to a social choice. Either the natural boundaries of human endeavor are estimated, recognised, and translated into politically determined limits, or the alternative to extinction is compulsory survival in a planned and engineered Hell.

In several nations the public is ready for a review of its health-care system. The frustrations which have become manifest from private-enterprise systems and from socialised care have come to resemble each other frighteningly. The difference between the annoyances of the Russian, French, Americans, and English have become trivial. There is a serious danger that these evaluations will be performed within the coordinates set by post-cartesian illusions. In rich and poor countries the demand for reform of national health care is dominated by demands for equitable access to the wares of the guild, professional expansion and sub-professionalisation, and for more truth in the advertising of progress and lay-control of the temple of Tantalus. The public discussion of the health crisis could easily be used to channel even more power, prestige, and money to bio-medical engineers and designers.

There is still time in the next few years to avoid a debate which would reinforce a frustrating system. The coming debate can be reoriented by making medical Nemesis the central issue. The explanation of Nemesis requires simultaneous assessment of both the technical and the non-technical side of medicine—and must focus on it as both industry and religion. The indictment of medicine as a form of institutional hubris exposes precisely those personal illusions which make the critic dependent on the health care.

The perception and comprehension of Nemesis has therefore the power of leading us to policies which could break the magic circle of complaints which now reinforce the dependence of the plaintiff on the health engineering and planning agencies whom he sues. Recognition of Nemesis can provide the catharsis to prepare for a non-violent revolution in our attitudes towards evil and pain. The alternative to a war against these ills is the search for the peace of the strong.

Health designates a process of adaptation. It is not the result of instinct, but of autonomous and live reaction to an experienced reality. It designates the ability to adapt to changing environments, to growing up and to aging, to healing when damaged, to suffering and to the peaceful expectation of death. Health embraces the future as well, and therefore includes anguish and the inner resource to live with it.

Man's consciously lived fragility, individuality, and relatedness make the experience of pain, of sickness, and of death an integral part of his life. The ability to cope with this trio in autonomy is fundamental to his health. To the degree to which he becomes dependent on the management of his intimacy he renounces his autonomy and his health *must* decline. The true miracle of modern medicine is diabolical. It consists of making not only individuals but whole populations survive on inhumanly low levels of personal health. That health should decline with increasing health-service delivery is unforeseen only by the health manager, precisely because his strategies are the result of his blindness to the inalienability of health.

The level of public health corresponds to the degree to which the means and responsibility for coping with illness are distributed amongst the total population. This ability to cope can be enhanced but never replaced by medical intervention in the lives of people or the hygienic characteristics of the environment. That society which can reduce professional intervention to the minimum will provide the best conditions for health. The greater the potential for autonomous adaptation to self and to others and to the environment, the less management of adaptation will be needed or tolerated.

The recovery of a health attitude towards sickness is neither Luddite nor Romantic nor Utopian: it is a guiding ideal which will never be fully achieved, which can be achieved with modern devices as never before in history, and which must orient politics to avoid encroaching Nemesis.

Note

This article is abridged from a lecture given in Edinburgh on April 26 and in Nottingham on May 1, 1974. The lecture was based on the book *Medical Nemesis* (published in 1976 in America by Pantheon, N.Y.).

29

The Politics of Therapeutic Nihilism

Paul Starr

For most of this century, indeed until just the past several years, liberals and socialists had a relatively uncomplicated perception of medicine as a political question. There was one fundamental issue: equal access to medical services. No one doubted that medical care was a good thing; the trouble was that poor people were denied attention or went broke trying to pay for it. Some also thought doctors ought to be concerned with "community" medicine, and expand their concerns to include all manner of behavioral and social problems. The advantages of professional competence in medical matters, and the necessity of professional authority, seemed self-evident.

This was not always so. In the nineteenth century, many people, even some leading physicians, believed that most medical practice was completely ineffective, or even harmful. Critics, particularly during the Jacksonian period, attacked professional competence as illusory, denounced medicine as a "privileged monopoly," and sought the democratization of useful medical knowledge, so that every man (as the slogan then went) might be his own physician. Political and medical dissent had a close kinship. In the late nineteenth century, populists and others resisted giving the medical profession licensing powers that would enable it to exclude various forms of unorthodox practice. As earlier radicals had taken an interest in mesmerism or botanic medicine, so the populists had an affinity for faith-healers and other "irregular" practitioners. In the twentieth century the left, like the larger society, repudiated these tendencies. Rather than challenging the actual content of medical practice or the structure of professional authority, socialists and liberals gave their attention almost exclusively to the problem of health insurance—to the financing and rationalizing of institutions whose value was beyond debate.

Old Questions Reopened

However, in the past few years, almost all the questions about medicine that had been closed since the nineteenth century have been reopened. There has been a renewed interest in the democratization of medical knowledge, particularly in the women's movement. Professional authority has again come under attack. So has the actual content of medical practice, especially its technological character. But most important, there is, once more, widespread questioning of the ultimate value and effectiveness of medicine. Medical care, it turns out, may not be an unambiguously good thing. In the nineteenth century, some leading scientists held that virtually all existing drugs and treatments were of no use, and that the sick had no other hope than the healing power of nature. This doctrine was known as therapeutic nihilism. Today disbelief has returned in a new form: now the net effectiveness of the medical system as a whole, rather than particular treatments, is called in question. The most serious critics of the system now doubt that it does much good for our health. Instead of suggesting that medicine expand its concerns into behavioral and social matters, many people think the "medicalization" of experience has gone too far, and that childbirth, sickness, anxiety, aging, and death should be reclaimed from professional hegemony.

This recent attack on medicine seems to have begun in the 1960s with the mounting criticism of psychiatry and psychiatric institutions. The books of Thomas Szasz, R.D. Laing, and Erving Goffman, all widely read in the past decade, have portrayed medicine as an instrument primarily of social control rather than therapeutic assistance. The great recent successes of the play *Equus* and of *One Flew Over the Cuckoo's Nest* as a novel, play, and movie testify to the temper of public sentiment. In both *Equus* and *Cuckoo's Nest,* medicine is the force of oppression and conformity, called upon by society to domesticate the passion and spontaneity of patients caged against their will. One is given to understand, of course, that the settings and characters are symbolic (even allegorical!), but it is significant nonetheless what symbols writers select, at a particular moment in history, of all those that are potentially available.

From psychiatry, doubts and criticism have spread to medicine at large. Students of public health have long observed, without anyone's paying much attention, that the effect of environment and behavior on the health of populations is much greater than that of medical care. Suddenly this point is being treated, in influential circles, as if it were a major discovery. People ask, and none too soon, why medicine commands so much of our resources if it makes so little difference in health and life expectancy. In a book given widespread and serious attention in Europe last year and more recently in the United States, Ivan Illich has suggested that the entire medical system has become counterproductive, and now causes more illness than it relieves.[1] I will go into details of the argument later. One point interests me here. By taking the doubts about medicine to the extreme, Illich has brought out the latent implications of the new criticism of the value of medicine. If the attack is justified, then the traditional concern of the left for equality in medical care no longer makes any sense. To give the lower classes greater access to health services, Illich writes in *Medical Nemesis,* "would only equalize the delivery of professional illusions and torts." In the earlier English edition of his book, he put the point even more bluntly: "Less access to the present health system would, contrary to political rhetoric, *benefit* the poor." (Emphasis added) This is, I believe, an indefensible statement, but it is just as well Illich has laid the issue open, for it underlies a more general problem in contemporary political argument.

The Tensions of Criticism

Two antagonistic impulses now dominate criticism of social policy. The first and more familiar impulse of the left is to argue that the poor and minorities receive inadequate services from schools, hospitals, public welfare agencies, and other institutions. The second, more novel, and in a sense more radical impulse is to call into question the value and efficacy (particularly the long-range effects) of the services themselves. Yet this second impulse undercuts the first. For if the services are worthless or in some way destructive, why worry about the poor—or, for that matter, anyone—not getting enough of them?

This conflict now exists in almost every department of social policy. It has long been familiar in education. From some critics one hears that the poor are short-changed by the schools and consequently left at a permanent social and economic disadvantage. On the contrary, others maintain, it would not make much difference, in terms of long-range effects, if the poor had the best schools in Scarsdale. Still others regard schooling itself as a problem. Similarly, there is one voice on the left that says the poor need more adequate mental health services. At the same time, others claim that mental health programs are totally ineffective, or serve as a means of channeling discontent into self-reproach, or of "labeling deviant behavior," or of providing middle-class psychologists with comfortable incomes.

The poor, argues one camp, need better legal services. What they really need, says another, are laws and courts that are on their side, and a radical simplification of the legal system to make it accessible to ordinary people—less law and less legalism, rather than more lawyers. And again: some critics see a need for more social workers and greater welfare benefits, while others view welfare bureaucracies as an instrument of oppression, and welfare dependency as an evil in itself.

These conflicts can be—indeed, have been—resolved in various ways. Inevitably, people make distinctions between the short and the long term. So, for example, they argue that in a just society in the future, we ought to need fewer welfare and mental health programs, fewer lawyers and fewer social workers. But in the meantime, some people require assistance, and other people need jobs, so we must have more of nearly everything. Or, while the long-run effects of schooling on inequality may be small, the immediate reality is that children spend a large part of their lives in school, and this in itself may justify a large commitment of resources to their education. Perhaps the most disingenuous argument is that by pressing demands for adequate services, say, in the welfare system, we will push the society toward more profound changes precisely because those programs will then collapse. (The evidence is all about us as to how well that clever strategy has worked.) Perhaps the most idly hopeful argument is that by investing more money in the social services, we will eventually learn how to make them effective, by accumulating experience and research.

Distributive justice is a morally compelling concern only when what there is to distribute, or redistribute, is genuinely important and valuable. If it is irrelevant or harmful to human welfare, then the poor would clearly be better off without it. At a time of fiscal austerity, when public services to the poor are frequently in jeopardy, it becomes extremely difficult to resist cutbacks if one simultaneously concedes that schools and hospitals, welfare programs and mental health centers, legal services and employment bureaus don't make much difference in the long run, or are positively damaging to the interests of the poor. The more one questions the ultimate value of the social services, the less urgent, the less vital equal access to them appear; furthermore, the more difficult it becomes to argue persuasively that the government should spend more on domestic needs.

This is precisely the situation that confronts us today. In addition to the current fiscal crisis, the social services are in the midst of an intellectual crisis that has sapped their legitimacy and prepared the ground for retrenchment. Ironically, the left has played a part in the process of de-legitimation. The effect, unintended but no less real, has been to facilitate cutbacks in services that are likely to affect those groups least able to defend themselves politically.

Under these circumstances, those who fault the social services for being ineffective or harmful should at least be careful and deliberate about their claims. They ought to be clear about what the evidence says and what it doesn't say. They ought to be wary of diagnosing failure from fragmentary data that refer only to one of several functions that institutions and programs usefully perform.

I do not propose to deal with these issues in a general fashion here, but only to address the question as it has arisen in medical care. What I would like to do is to review the argument about the effectiveness and dangers of medicine, as well as the evidence regarding inequalities in health and life expectancy and in access to medical services. Does the traditional concern of the left for equality in medical care still make sense, particularly if it is not the way to achieve equality in health?

The Case Against Medicine

Those, like Ivan Illich, who argue that medicine has a negligible or deleterious effect on health typically rest their case on a series of distinct points. The following seem to me to be the most important:

1. *Historical record.* Great advances in health and life expectancy during the past several centuries have come from improvements in the standard of living, particularly in nutrition, and from public health measures, such as improved sanitation. Improvements in the treatment of individual illness do not seem to have been a major factor in decreased rates of mortality.

2. *Geographic variation.* Regional differences in the ratio of doctors or hospital beds to population, or in any other index of health services, seem to have no measurable relation to variations in mortality or life expectancy.

3. *Marginal returns.* In recent decades, national expenditures, measured either absolutely or as a proportion of gross national product, have

increased enormously throughout most of the industrial world, but there has been no corresponding improvement in health. Life expectancy at ages beyond infancy has reached a plateau. In fact, in the United States, mortality rates for adult males at most ages have been increasing rather than declining.

4. *Empirical analysis of health services.* A few careful studies ("randomized controlled trials") of the effectiveness of specific procedures and treatments, such as intensive care, have cast doubt as to whether they have any positive value. The returns in health and extended life from technologically complex services, even when successfully used, are rather small. Typically, the most expensive medical technology, absorbing huge investments, is used to treat patients who have multiple problems and short life expectancies even if cured of the immediate problem at hand.

5. *Excess capacity.* A great deal of evidence suggests that there are too many hospital beds, too many surgeons, and much unnecessary surgery in the United States; that antibiotics, psychoactive drugs and other medications are vastly overprescribed; and that these overuses of medicine lead to adverse, often fatal complications.

6. *Iatrogenic (doctor-caused) injuries.* Good statistics are unavailable, but some studies suggest there may be several million every year. Malpractice suits suggest there may be several million every year. Malpractice suits touch a small fraction of the total.

7. *Medicine as an epidemic.* Illich argues that in addition to *clinical* iatrogenesis, medicine has created even more illness by redefining normal human experience as sickness. This "medicalization" of life he calls *social* iatrogensis. Medical institutions, he suggests, have also helped create illness by weakening individual autonomy and the capacity of people to "suffer their reality." In other words, whereas in simpler times, people steadfastly endured pain, anxiety, and death, now they feel *sick* and expect to be made well. This Illich calls *cultural* iatrogenesis.

What ought we to conclude from these arguments? Is medical care worthless or even, as Illich maintains, destructive of health? Illich sees health as the autonomous ability of an individual organism to cope with its internal experience and external environment, and he argues that we ought to turn away from professionals toward self-care. But on what grounds are we to believe that self-care would be harmless? Especially when sick, people are fully capable of doing great harm to themselves. That is exactly why they seek out professional assistance. Such assistance need not destroy their autonomous ability to cope with the world; it may help them to regain it. Sickness itself creates dependency; medicine often relieves it. The ideal of pure autonomy that Illich offers is a romantic myth as illusory as the omnipotence of science.

Both clinical and social iatrogenesis I take to be serious problems, but one need not conclude they outweigh the positive effects of medicine.

"Among murderous institutional torts," Illich writes, "only modern mal-nutrition injures more people than iatrogenic disease in its various mani-festations." This is typical of Illich's rhetoric, but there is, as far as I know, no evidence that could possibly sustain this assertion.

Still, if it is true, as the historical and empirical data indicate, that medicine has had a relatively small effect on mortality rates and life expec-tancy, why do we bother with it? First of all, we are talking about only the most gross index of the outcome of medical services—mortality rates, which are governed by numerous other variables. Most medical care in-volves the relief of discomfort, disability, and uncertainty. Only a small part makes the difference between life and death (and almost all of that must be used for television melodramas). Most of us at some point have suffered injuries that might have left us disabled or disfigured had it not been for quick medical intervention. The more emotional functions of medicine should also not be slighted. People consult physicians not just for remedies, but also for clarification of the nature and meaning of their internal experience. "Am I sick?" we ask. "Is what I feel significant, or should I ignore it?" The resolution of ambiguity has a value in itself. Medicine, like most institutions, has a variety of legitimate functions, not only for the sick but for their families. Hospitals, for example, have grown in the last century not only because of their advantages for treatment, but because they help reduce the physical and emotional burden confronted by families when one member becomes acutely ill.

I do not wish to minimize the lifesaving aspect of medicine. The statisti-cal effect on overall mortality rates is a poor measure of its psychological and moral importance. Consider the following figures: in the United States, in 1940, nearly 9,000 women died in childbirth. In 1973, with 99 percent of all births occurring in hospitals (compared with about half in 1940), fewer than 500 women died.[2] This decline has had some effect on female mortality rates, which have continued to decline significantly in the last several decades, unlike mortality rates for men. But the real point is the greater sense of security that such diminished risks afford. Illich and others lament the "medicalization" of normal aspects of human develop-ment like childbirth, but it seems quite plausible that women have made an entirely rational decision in seeking out medical attention. People may intelligently conclude that the reduction of risks, even at the margin, is worth the cost and the loss of autonomy they endure from consulting a physician.

The general plateau in mortality rates during the past few decades conceals changes in deaths from specific diseases that have been responsive to medicine. Among Americans aged fifteen to forty-four, for example, there were about 30,000 deaths from tuberculosis in 1940, but in 1973 only 407. Influenza and pneumonia took the lives of 11,600 young adults in 1940; in 1973, only 3,200. It happens, however, these declines have been partially offset, particularly among males, by increasing rates of deaths from violence and accidents. Yet it would be absurd to conclude from such facts that medicine has been ineffective. Had it not been for good medical care, the situation might have been worse.[3]

There is no question but that the medical system in America is overextended in many areas. But along with excess capacity, there are shortages and inadequacies in needed services. There are too many surgeons, but too few "primary care" physicians; too many hospital beds in some communities, but too few neighborhood clinics in others. All this shows is that there are problems in allocating and organizing resources. While the system overproduces facilities and services whose costs can be covered by insurance, it underproduces them where coverage is weak. Recently Aaron Wildavsky wrote that "the marginal value of one, or one billion dollars spent on medical care would be close to zero in improving health." Given the current structure of incentives, this may be so, but it need not be. Large socioeconomic differences remain in diseases and deaths that ought to be therapeutically preventable. Medical care for mothers and young children, for example, has historically had a significant effect in improving their health. Were additional funds spent on maternal, infant, and child care, the marginal returns in improving health might be substantial. By concentrating on children, one might also affect the health of the future adult population. Such considerations have not traditionally governed medical policy. The nation has tended to invest resources in the treatment of diseases for which no effective therapy exists.[4]

Under the cirmcumstances, it should not be surprising that the results of government expenditures have been unimpressive. A critic like Illich argues that because medical care has made no difference in health, we should not be particularly concerned about inequalities of access. He has the point turned around. We will have to be especially concerned about inequalities if we are to make future investments in medical care effective. Precisely because there is excess capacity in the medical system, the persistence of inadequacies in basic services is not merely unjust, but gratuitous.

The Dimensions of Inequality

For reasons that have nothing to do with deliberate social policy, we are probably in a period of increasing equality in health and life expectancy. As Anton Antonovsky has shown in an examination of the history of class differences in average length of life, the most dramatic contrasts appeared in the eighteenth and nineteenth centuries. In the preindustrial era, mortality rates were universally high, and the differences between upper and lower classes seem to have been relatively limited. But with industrialization, a substantial gap opened up: life expectancy increased much faster for the upper than for the lower classes. The ratio in average life span between rich and poor seems to have been on the order of two to one. In the twentieth century, that ratio has declined in industrialized countries to about 1.3 to one, or less, as the lower classes have caught up.[5]

Not all countries have done equally well. While socioeconomic differences in mortality rates are low in Britain, they continue to be relatively high in the United States. Unfortunately, comprehensive, up-to-date figures are unavailable for the United States, but we do have evidence of four kinds: a national study of differential mortality from 1960 data; comparisons of mortality rates in poverty and nonpoverty neighborhoods during 1969–71; socioeconomic data on infant mortality for 1964–66; and statistics on mortality by race and region for 1969–71. The study of 1960 deaths showed that among white males aged twenty-five to sixty-four, mortality rates were 80 percent higher for men in families with less than $2,000 income in 1959 than for men in families with $10,000 or more. Such statistics have the obvious problem that income in the year prior to death may have been affected by serious illness. However, much the same pattern emerges when using another index of socioeconomic status, years of education, which should be unaffected by this reverse causal link. Those men who had fewer than five years of school had mortality rates 64 percent higher than men with at least four years of college.[6] Comparisons of death rates in poverty and nonpoverty areas in major cities yield similar results. Depending on the city, crude death rates were 50 to 100 percent higher in poverty neighborhoods, despite their generally younger population.[7] Rates of infant mortality were also 50 to 100 percent greater in the lowest socioeconomic group than in the middle and upper classes, regardless of whether status was measured by family income or father's or mother's education. Half of the infant deaths in the lowest socioeconomic group were judged preventable.[8] Differences by race and region are striking. A black man born in the District of Columbia, which has a lower average life expectancy than any state in the country, can expect to live eleven fewer years than a white man born in Minnesota, which has one of the highest. Under 1970 mortality rates, the chances of living to age sixty-five were 81 out of 100 for a white female, 66 out of 100 for a white male, and 50 out of 100 for a nonwhite male. Infant mortality among non-whites, according to preliminary estimates for 1974, was 24.6 deaths per thousand; for whites, 14.7. This gap had been widening for the previous fifteen years. The ratio of black and white infant mortality rates now stands at the same level it was in 1950.

Are the poor in worse health than the rich? They certainly seem to think so. In all age groups, people in lower-income families are reported to be less healthy, sometimes dramatically so. (See Table 1.) Among people aged forty-five to sixty-four, 45 percent in low-income families say their health is fair or poor, while only 10 percent do so in upper-income fami-

Table 1.
Assessed Health, 1973

Family Income	Health Status			
	Excellent	*Good*	*Fair*	*Poor*
All ages				
Under $5,000	32.4%	41.3%	17.9%	7.7%
$15,000 and over	60.7	33.2	4.7	0.8
Under 17 years				
Under $5,000	42.4	48.1	7.8	0.9
$15,000 and over	72.1	25.3	1.9	—
17–44 years				
Under $5,000	40.3	42.3	13.0	3.8
$15,000 and over	61.5	33.7	3.8	0.6
45–64 years				
Under $5,000	18.4	35.3	28.1	17.7
$15,000 and over	47.3	41.8	8.7	1.8
65 years and over				
Under $5,000	24.5	38.1	25.3	11.4
$15,000 and over	39.0	41.1	14.7	4.4

SOURCE: *Health: United States, 1975,* pp. 243, 377, 437, 439, 531.

lies. Rates of chronic illness in this same age group show strong socioeconomic differences. The prevalence rates per 1,000 persons for arthritis are 297.8 in low-income families versus 159.8 in upper-income families; for diabetes, 74.1 versus 30.5; for heart conditions, 139.3 versus 66.6; for hypertension, 172.7 versus 105.3; for impairments of the back and spine, 102.8 versus 52.2. According to 1971 statistics, again for ages forty-five to sixty-four, the rate for total loss of teeth was three times as high in families with incomes under $3,000 as in families with $15,000 or more in income. Men in lower-income families report more than three times as many days of restricted activity as their upper-income counterparts. Some of this relationship is explained by the reverse causal linkage—the effect that disability has on income. But we find the association between low income and ill health even among children, and in that case poverty is clearly the independent variable.

How much of this inequality in health could be eliminated by equalizing access to medical care? Probably not much. The last decade has already seen a very significant movement toward equalization in the use of medical services. In fact, the overall rate of physician visits is now higher for the poor than for higher-income families. (See Table 2.) This was not so in 1964, before Medicaid, and it continues not to be true for both

Table 2.
Physician Visits Per Year

Ages	Poor	Not Poor
All ages		
1964	4.3	4.6
1973	5.6	4.9
Ages 1–17		
1964	2.3	4.0
1973	3.8	4.3
Age 65 and over		
1964	6.0	7.3
1973	6.5	6.9

SOURCE: *Health: United States, 1975*, pp. 289, 409, 569. Definition of poor based on family income: under $3,000 in 1964; under $6,000 in 1973. In each case, this represented about one fifth of the population.

children and the aged. At all ages, rates of hospitalization are today higher for the poor, reversing the dominant pattern of a decade ago. (Table 3.)

One must emphasize that these are measures of utilization, not access. Since the poor are less healthy and more prone to chronic illness—indeed, many are poor precisely because they are disabled—they probably require greater medical attention. Genuine equality of access might lead to higher utilization by the poor than is now observed: we have no way of knowing. There is some scattered evidence suggesting that when the poor receive medical attention, they do so at more severe stages of illness. This suggests either less access to care, or less inclination to use it. Because physicians tend to avoid locating their practices in poor communities, they are less directly accessible to the poor. Inequalities persist in the conditions under which health care is received. The poor more often see doctors in emergency rooms and hospital outpatient departments than in private offices. The physical conditions of the public facilities they use is often abysmal. In receiving hospital care, they are more likely to experience a loss of privacy, because of their use as "clinical material" for medical education. Most obviously, they face financial insecurity. The families of low-income workers, particularly in the "secondary" labor force, have less insurance coverage for medical costs. The newly unemployed often have no coverage at all. Families on welfare find their eligibility for Medicaid is constantly changing, because of changes in employment status or new welfare regulations.

Cutbacks in public support for medical care will probably not restrict expensive medical technology of dubious value. Costs of that sort will continue to be absorbed by third-party insurance. Retrenchment will more likely increase financial insecurity among low-income patients, and pro-

Table 3.
Hospital Discharges Per 1,000 Persons Per Year

Ages	Poor	Not Poor
Ages 1–17		
1964	58	70
1973	96	63
Ages 17–44		
1964	181	161
1973	198	148
Ages 45–64		
1964	146	148
1973	225	152
Age 65 and over		
1964	179	202
1973	248	234

SOURCES: *Health: United States, 1975*, pp. 417, 517, 519, 577. Poverty defined as in Table 2.

mote the deterioration of public hospitals and clinics. With inadequate staffing, a declining physical plant, and delays in service, all the iatrogenic aspects of medicine will be magnified. That, in fact, is the irony of Illich's jeremiad. Retrenchment in medical services would almost surely aggravate the very qualities in the system that he deplores.

Rationing Medical Care

The facts seem to support these conclusions:

1. Environment and behavior are the principal determinants of health and life expectancy; medical care plays a relatively small part. The medical services that seem to have the most impact, like vaccinations, tend to be relatively simple. No one familiar with the evidence disagrees with that. If one wishes to equalize health, equalizing medical care is probably not the most effective strategy.

2. On the other hand, the expansion and improvement of medical services probably have had a positive effect on health. The reduction of risks at the margin has enhanced personal security. Had it not been for medical care, mortality rates might be higher. Medicine has useful functions other than saving lives, such as relieving discomfort and disability and making sickness more bearable for patients and their families. Further investments in certain areas of medical care, such as maternal and child health, may continue to yield positive returns.

3. There has been a substantial equalization in the use of physicians' and hospital services during the past decade. In some categories, the poor now appear to have higher rates of utilization than other classes. The enactment of Medicare and Medicaid probably played a major role in this development.

4. Because the poor have higher rates of disability and chronic illness, they probably require more medical services. Equal utilization, therefore, may not prove equal access to services. Furthermore, there are persistent inequalities in the conditions under which treatment is received and in the security and degree of financial coverage.The chief effect of cutbacks in public support would be to exacerbate these problems.

5. The hard and discriminating eye that distinguishes useless from effective practices in medicine, or other fields, need not be unfriendly to the concern for equality. To improve the effectiveness of social services, we will have to be especially attentive to inequalities. It makes no sense to add more where there is already too much.

6. Some means must be found to put firm limits on the funds the medical system absorbs. But while such limits are necessary, the rationing of services under the present medical system would almost certainly be neither just nor efficient, given the incentives that now govern the allocation of resources. If limits are to be placed on the system, this means challenging the authority of physicians and the structure of the medical market.

The recent debate over medicine has failed to address a central issue. Is it the purpose of national medical policy to maximize the health of the country, or is it to underwrite the services that individual physicians believe are warranted for their individual patients? The two are very different. If we continue to follow the second policy, we should not try to measure it by the standard of the first. It will always be found wanting.

The therapeutic nihilism of the nineteenth century had its justification in objective fact. We now know that it was correct: most medical treatment of the day was absolutely useless. Much of it—the bleeding, blistering, and purging of patients—was lethal. By helping to rid medicine of such techniques, therapeutic nihilism contributed to the liberation of medicine from the dead hand of the past. Today, medical institutions are often as ineffective as specific treatments were then. Let us hope that the new therapeutic nihilism, which questions the medical system in its totality, will have the same liberating effect.

References

1. Ivan Illich, *Medical Nemesis: The Expropriation of Health* (London: Calder & Boyars 1975; New York: Pantheon, 1976). The literature of therapeutic nihil-

ism and disenchantment has grown rapidly in the past few years, and varies in political outlook and certainty of judgment. Some observers are more guarded and qualified than others, but there is a common ground of skepticism about the value of medical services. In addition to Illich, some principal examples are Rick J. Carlson, *The End of Medicine* (New York: John Wiley & Sons, 1975); Marc Lalonde, *A New Perspective on the Health of Canadians* (Ottawa: Government of Canada, 1974); A. L. Cochrane, *Effectiveness and Efficiency: Random Reflections on Health Services* (The Nuffield Provincial Hospitals Trust, 1972); Leon R. Kass, "Regarding the End of Medicine and The Pursuit of Health," *The Public Interest,* Summer 1975; Michel Bosquet, "Quand la medicine rend malade." *Le Nouvel Observateur,* Nos. 519 and 520, (1974); Eric J. Cassel, "Disease as a Way of Life," *Commentary,* February 1973; Victor Fuchs, *Who Shall Live?* (New York: Basic Books, 1974), Chapter 2. One of the most eloquent and humane books on the subject remains René Dubos' *Mirage of Health* (New York: Harper & Row, 1959). See also the excellent paper by Lewis Thomas, "Aspects of Biomedical Science Policy," an address to the Institute of Medicine, Fall Meeting. Nov. 9, 1972, Washington, D.C. A new issue of *Daedalus* edited by John Knowles is to treat the same themes: see especially the contribution by Aaron Wildavsky. An international conference last year on "The Limits to Medicine," held in Davos, Switzerland, brought together a wide array of speakers from various countries around the same theme. I am grateful to the Program in Law, Science and Medicine at Yale Law School, which enabled me to attend that conference.

2. These statistics and others not otherwise footnoted are drawn from *Health: United States, 1975* (Rockville, Md.: U.S. Department of Health, Education and Welfare, 1976).

3. Because of improved medical care and faster transportation, 81 percent of soldiers wounded in Vietnam survived, compared with 74 percent of the wounded in Korea and 71 percent in World War II. At World War II rates, an additional 30,000 men would have died in Southeast Asia. See my book *The Discarded Army: Veterans After Vietnam* (New York: Charterhouse, 1974), p. 54.

4. A good case in point: President Johnson's regional medical program, which in the mid-1960s established centers for the treatment of heart disease, cancer, and stroke. Elizabeth Drew, writing in *The Atlantic* in 1967, raised the questions that ought to have been asked before the program was enacted: "If the federal government is going to provide centers for certain diseases, would it be better to provide them for diseases which can be cured or for those which cannot yet be cured? Similarly, if such a departure is to be made, should it focus on diseases which affect primarily the elderly, as these do, or on diseases which affect primarily the young? These kinds of policy considerations should have preceded a decision to initiate a program of centers for heart disease, cancer and stroke, but they did not."

5. Anton Antonovsky, "Social Class, Life Expectancy, and Overall Mortality," *Milbank Memorial Fund Quarterly,* 45 (April 1967), 31–73.

6. Evelyn M. Kitagawa and Philip M. Hauser. *Differential Mortality in the United States: A Study in Socioeconomic Epidemiology* (Cambridge, Mass.: Harvard University Press, 1973), pp. 11, 152.

7. U.S. Public Health Service, *Selected Vital and Health Statistics in Poverty and Nonpoverty Areas of 19 Large Cities, United States, 1969–71, Series 21, No. 26, p. 7.* Age-standardized rates were not computed.

8. U.S. Public Health Service, *Infant Mortality Rates: Socioeconomic Factors,* Series 22, No. 14, p. 1.

Individual Responsibility for Health

WITH GROWING RECOGNITION OF THE limitations of medical care and the environmental and behavioral components of much of modern disease, a debate has emerged as to who is responsible for individual health. For many years, the medical model conceptualized disease as one of those things, like earthquakes or tornados, over which humans simply had no control. When critics began to articulate the relationships among society, behavior, and sickness however, it became clear that disease is socially patterned, is connected with the values of society, and, importantly, much of it can be prevented.

A series of articles in *The New York Times* (2/3/80–2/5/80) recently presented information about " . . . petrochemical companies [which] have quietly tested thousands of American workers to determine if any of the genes they were born with are what industry doctors call 'defective,' making the employees especially vulnerable to certain chemicals in the workplace. The process is called genetic screening." An enormous controversy surrounds genetic screening; some workers, scientists, and union leaders claim that such testing is in fact a "Brave New World nightmare, an Orwellian stew in which the victims of toxic chemicals will be blamed for having faulty genes." These critics " . . . want industry to place the emphasis on cleaning up the workplace, not deciding which workers ought to be removed from conditions that could ultimately be bad for all."

Central to the controversy surrounding genetic screening (and the topic of the articles in this section) is the issue of who is responsible for an individual's health. Specifically, to what extent are we, as individuals, responsible for preventing disease and maintaining our own health? One of the most articulate spokespersons for the argument that individuals are ultimately responsible for their own health is John Knowles, former Director of Massachusetts General Hospital and past President of the Rockefeller Foundation. In "The Responsibility of the Individual" Knowles argues that people are born healthy and made sick by personal "misbehavior" and environmental conditions. While acknowledging the role of the environment in creating disease, his emphasis is on the "bad habits" of individuals, which he sees as the cause of much of our current state of unhealthiness. These bad habits include " . . . overeating, too much drinking, taking pills, staying up at night, engaging in promiscuous sex, driving too fast, and smoking cigarettes. . . ." According to this view, these behaviors are encouraged because our society has subordinated individual responsibility to "individual rights." Solutions to health problems should by and large focus on changing the behaviors of people, who are themselves simultaneously victims and victimizers, via education, rewards and punishments, etc., thus allowing them to improve their health through their own efforts. Preservation of health should be a public duty. Knowles rejects what he terms the "liberal" ideology which stresses societal responsibility for the ills of humanity, and, in fact, he blames this ideology for eroding individual responsibility in the first place.

Knowles makes a good case for the importance of individual change and self-improvement. There is little doubt that better health could be promoted and much disease prevented if only we could adopt healthier lifestyles and relinquish some of our "bad habits." There are, however, several problems with his argument. Knowles condemns " . . . sloth, gluttony, alcoholic intemperance, reckless driving, sexual frenzy, and smoking . . . " in essentially moralistic terms. He does not address the problem of pain and suffering, which has its roots in flawed institutions and environments over which, at least as individuals, people have little or no control. He ignores the obvious efforts—the spending of huge sums of money for medical help, the hours spent waiting to see physicians, etc.—that people *do* make in an attempt to make or keep themselves healthy. If these efforts are misdirected, then we must ask why people believe in them. Nor does Knowles address the problem of the very limited power people have to effect changes over those social organizations and institutions that produce the toxic chemicals, the noise, the stress, etc. which lead so many to seek relief through such unhealthy means as alcohol, cigarettes, and licit or illicit mood-altering drugs.

Robert Crawford's article "Individual Responsibility and Health Politics" explores the problems of seeing individual responsibility for health in the context of what he sees as a "victim-blaming" ideology. As Crawford notes, focusing attention on the victims of problems (such as environmental pollution or stress-induced alcohol or cigarette addiction) ignores and thereby masks the role of the particular social arrangements that may be disease-producing and the inability of individuals to prevent or cure those diseases themselves. He also argues that the ideology of individual responsibility helps "justify shifting the burden of costs back to users" and legitimate a retrenchment from social responsibility. The moralism of much of the writing of those advocating individual responsibility for health, as Crawford observes, is a moralism that ultimately blames ill health on those with the least power and resources to effect change for the better.

The social scientist must ask who gains and who "pays" in these differing views of the relative responsibility of individuals for their own health—that is, what are the social consequences of each perspective? For those who advocate individual responsibility, the broad social arrangements which exist (the status quo) are not to be challenged. Rather, strategies of *adaptation* should be developed for individuals who, from the "liberal" perspective, are the victims of those very social arrangments to which they're being encouraged to adapt.

No one, of course, claims that the individual has absolutely no power to effect changes in life style that will promote health and well being. It can be argued, however, that these efforts need not be limited to individual adjustment, but can involve collective efforts at community change and social reform, in addition to individual self-help. The balance ultimately struck between the opposing views expressed in the Knowles and Crawford articles is likely to be a crucial determinant of the future course of medical care efforts in the United States.

30

The Responsibility of the Individual

John H. Knowles

· ·

More than half the reduction in mortality rates over the past three centuries occurred before 1900 and was due in nearly equal measure to improved nutrition and reduced exposure to air- and water-borne infection. The provision of safe water and milk supplies, the improvement in both personal and food hygiene, and the efficient disposal of sewage all helped to reduce the incidence of infectious disease. Vaccination further reduced mortality rates from smallpox in the nineteenth century and from diphtheria, pertussis, tetanus, poliomyelitis, measles, and tuberculosis in the twentieth century, although the contribution of vaccinations to the overall reduction in mortality rates over the past hundred years is small (perhaps as small as 10 percent) as contrasted with that due to improved nutrition and reduction in the transmission of infectious disease.[1] An even smaller contribution has been made by the introduction of medical and surgical therapy, namely antibiotics and the excision of tumors, in the twentieth century.

Over the past 100 years, infanticide has declined in the developed countries as changes in reproductive practice, such as the use of contraceptives, have been introduced to contain family size and reduce national growth rates of population, thus sustaining the improvement in health and standards of living. The population of England and Wales trebled between 1700 and 1850 without any significant importation of food. If the birth rate had been maintained, the population by now would be some 140 million instead of the 46 million it actually is. Changes in reproductive behavior maintained a rough balance between food production and population growth and allowed standards of living to rise. A similarly remarkable change in reproductive behavior occurred in Ireland following the potato famines of the eighteen-forties, and birth rates have been sustained voluntarily at a low level to this day in that largely Catholic country.

Improvement in health resulted from changes in personal behavior (hygiene, reproductive practices) and in environmental conditions (food supplies, provision of safe milk and water, and sewage disposal). Cartesian rationalism, Baconian empiricism, and the results of the Industrial Revolution led the medical profession into scientific and technical approaches to disease. The engineering approach to the human machine was strengthened by the germ theory of disease which followed the work of Pasteur and Koch in the late nineteenth century. The idea was simple, unitary, and compelling: one germ—one disease—one therapy. Population factors, personal behavior, and environmental conditions were neglected in such a pure model or paradigm of approach and were picked up by elements less powerful and perceived increasingly as marginal to health, i.e., politicians, state departments, and schools of public health. The medical profession hitched its wagon to the rising stars of science and technology. The results have been spectacular for some individuals in terms of cure, containment of disease, and alleviation of suffering; as spectacular in terms of the horrendous costs compounding now at a rate of 15 percent annually; and even more spectacular to some because allocation of more and more men and women, money, and machines has affected mortality and morbidity rates only marginally. The problem of diminishing returns, if current trends continue, will loom as large and pregnant to the American people in the future as the mushrooming atomic cloud does today.

I will not berate the medical profession, its practitioners and its professors—they reflect our culture, its values, beliefs, rites, and symbols. Central to the culture is faith in progress through science, technology, and industrial growth; increasingly peripheral to it is the idea, vis-à-vis health, that over 99 percent of us are born healthy and made sick as a result of personal misbehavior and environmental conditions. The solution to the problems of ill health in modern American society involves individual responsibility, in the first instance, and social responsibility through public legislative and private voluntary efforts, in the second instance. Alas, the medical profession isn't interested, because the intellectual, emotional, and financial rewards of the present system are too great and because there is no incentive and very little demand to change. But the problems of rising costs; the allocation of scarce national resources among competing claims for improving life; diminishing returns on health from the system of acute, curative, high-cost, hospital-based medicine; and increasing evidence that personal behavior, food, and the nature of the environment around us are the prime determinants of health and disease will present us with critical choices and will inevitably force change.

Most individuals do not worry about their health until they lose it. Uncertain attempts at healthy living may be thwarted by the temptations of a culture whose economy depends on high production and high consumption. Asceticism is reserved for hair-shirted clerics and constipated cranks, and everytime one of them dies at the age of 50, the hedonist smiles, inhales deeply, and takes another drink. Everyone is a gambler and knows someone who has lived it up and hit 90 years, so bad nurture doesn't necessarily spell doom. For others, a genetic fatalism takes hold: Nature—your parents' genes—will decide your fate no matter what you do. For those who remain undecided, there is always the reassuring story—and we all know it—of someone with living parents who has led a temperate, viceless life and died of a heart attack at the age of 45. As for stress, how about Winston Churchill at the age of 90! And he drank brandy, smoked cigars, never exercised, and was grossly overweight! Facing the insufferable insult of extinction with the years, and knowing how we might improve our health, we still don't do much about it. The reasons for this peculiar behavior may include: (1) a denial of death and disease coupled with the demand for instant gratification and the orientation of most people in most cultures to living day by day; (2) the feeling that nature, including death and disease, can be conquered through scientific and technologic advance or overcome by personal will; (3) the dispiriting conditions of old people leads to a decision by some that they don't want infirmities and unhappiness and would just as soon die early; (4) chronic depression in some individuals to the extent that they wish consciously or unconsciously for death and have no desire to take care of themselves; and (5) the disinterest of the one person to whom we ascribe the ultimate wisdom about health—the physician.

Prevention of disease means forsaking the bad habits which many people enjoy—overeating, too much drinking, taking pills, staying up at night, engaging in promiscuous sex, driving too fast, and smoking cigarettes—or, put another way, it means doing things which require special effort—exercising regularly, going to the dentist, practicing contraception, ensuring harmonious family life, submitting to screening examinations. The idea of individual responsibility flies in the face of American history which has seen a people steadfastly sanctifying individual freedom while progressively narrowing it through the development of the beneficent state. On the one hand, Social Darwinism maintains its hold on the American mind despite the best intentions of the neo-liberals. Those who aren't supine before the Federal Leviathan proclaim the survival of the fittest. On the other, the idea of individual responsibility has been submerged to individual rights—rights, or demands, to be guaranteed by government and delivered by public and private institutions. The cost of sloth, gluttony, alcoholic intemperance, reckless driving, sexual frenzy, and smoking is now a national, and not an individual, responsibility. This is justified as individual freedom—but one man's freedom in health is another man's shackle in taxes and insurance premiums. I believe the idea of a "right" to health should be replaced by the idea of an individual moral obligation to preserve one's own health—a public duty if you will. The individual then has the "right" to expect help with information, accessible services of good quality, and minimal financial barriers. Meanwhile, the people have been led to believe that national health insurance, more doctors, and greater use of high-cost, hospital-based technologies will improve health. Unfortunately none of them will.

More and more the artificer of the possible is "society"—not the individual; he thereby becomes more dependent on things external and less on his own inner resources. The paranoid style of consumer groups demands a fight against something, usually a Big Bureaucracy. In the case of health, it is the hospitals, the doctors, the medical schools, the Medicaid-Medicare combine, the government. Nader's Raiders have yet to allow that the next major advances in the health of the American people will come from the assumption of individual responsibility for one's own health and a necessary change in habits for the majority of Americans. We do spend over $30 billion annually for cigarettes and whiskey.

The behavior of Americans might be changed if there were adequate programs of health education in primary and secondary schools and even colleges—but there aren't. School health programs are abysmal at best, confining themselves to preemptory sick calls and posters on brushing teeth and eating three meals a day; there are no examinations to determine if anything's been learned. Awareness of danger to body and mind isn't acquired until the mid-twenties in our culture, and by then patterns of behavior are set which are hard to change. Children tire of "scrub your teeth," "don't eat that junk," "leave your dingy alone," "go to bed," and "get some exercise." By the time they are sixteen, society says they shall have cars, drink beer, smoke, eat junk at drive-ins, and have a go at fornication. If they demur, they are sissies or queer or both. The pressure of the peer group to do wrong is hardly balanced by the limp protestations of permissive parents, nervously keeping up with the Joneses in suburban ranch houses crammed with snacks and mobile bars.

The barriers to the assumption of individual responsibility for one's own health are lack of knowledge (implicating the inadequacies of formal education, the all-too-powerful force of advertising, and of the informal systems of continuing education), lack of sufficient interest in, and knowledge about, what is preventable and the "cost-to-benefit" ratios of nationwide health programs (thereby implicating all the powerful interests in the health establishment, which couldn't be less interested, and calling for a much larger investment in fundamental and applied research), and a culture which has progressively eroded the idea of individual responsibility while stressing individual rights, the responsibility of society-at-large, and the steady growth of production and consumption ("We have met the enemy and it is us!"). Changing human behavior involves sustaining and repeating an intelligible message, reinforcing it through peer pressure and approval, and establishing clearly perceived rewards which materialize in as short a time as possible. Advertising agencies know this, but it is easier to sell deodorants, pantyhose, and automobiles than it is health.

What is the problem? During the nineteenth and early twentieth centuries, communicable disease was the major health problem in the United States. In 1900, the average life expectancy at birth was 49.2 years. By 1966, it had increased to 70.1 years, due mainly to marked reduction in infant and child mortality (between birth and age 15). By mid-century, accidents were by far the leading cause of death in youngsters, and the majority of accidents were related to excessive use of alcohol by their parents, by adults generally, and even occasionally by themselves. While 21 years were added to life expectancy at birth, only 2.7 years were added to it at age 65—the remaining life expectancy at age 65 being 11.9 years in 1900 and 14.6 in 1966. The marked increase in life expectancy at birth was due to the control and eradication of infectious disease, directly through improved nutrition and personal hygiene, and environmental changes, namely, the provision for safe water and milk supplies and for sewage disposal.

Today, the major health problems in the United States are the chronic diseases of middle and later age, mainly heart disease, cancer, and strokes. Death and disability in middle age is premature and potentially preventable. For those under 44 years, the leading causes of death are accidents, heart disease, cancer, homicide, and suicide. For those under 25 years, accidents are by far the most common cause of death, with homicide and suicide the next leading causes. Of the roughly 2 million deaths in the United States in 1969, 50 percent were due to heart disease (40%) and strokes (10%); 16 percent to cancer; and 8 percent to accidents (6%), homicide (1%), and suicide (1%). But death statistics tell only a small part of the story. For every successful suicide, an estimated ten others, or 200,000 people, have made the attempt. For every death due to accidents, hundreds of others are injured, and many of those are permanently disabled. Over 17 percent, or 36 million people, have serious disabilities limiting their activities.

Premature death and disability are far too common. For the 178,000 people between the ages of 45 and 64 years who died of heart disease in 1969, 1.2 million (or 3 percent of the 40.5 million people in this age group) were chronically disabled because of heart disease.[2] For the over 30,000 people who died of cirrhosis of the liver in 1969—a disease related directly to excessive ingestion of alcohol together with poor nutrition—as many as 10 million people suffer from alcoholism and varying degrees of malnutrition. Twenty-six million Americans, 11 million of whom receive no federal food assistance, live below the federally defined poverty level, a level which does not support an adequate diet.

The control of communicable disease depended as much (or even more) on broad changes in the environment attendant upon economic development (improved housing and nutrition, sanitary engineering for safe water supplies, and sewage disposal) as it did on the individual's knowledge and behavior (need for immunization, personal hygiene, and cooperation with case finding). However, control of the present major health problems in the United States depends directly on modification of the individual's behavior and habits of living. The need for improved nutrition remains unchanged. The knowledge required to persuade the individual to change his habits is far more complex, far less dramatic in its results, far more difficult to organize and convey—in short, far less appealing and compelling than the need for immunization, getting rid of sewage, and drinking safe water. Even the problems of immunizing the population in contemporary America are difficult, however—witness the failure to eradicate measles ten years after the technical means became available.

Studies by Breslow and Belloc[3] of nearly 7,000 adults followed for five and one-half years showed that life expectancy and health are significantly related to the following basic health habits:

1) three meals a day at regular times and no snacking;
2) breakfast every day;
3) moderate exercise two or three times a week;
4) adequate sleep (7 or 8 hours a night);
5) no smoking;
6) moderate weight;
7) no alcohol or only in moderation.

A 45-year-old man who practiced 0–3 of these habits has a remaining life expectancy of 21.6 years (to age 67), while one with 6–7 of these habits has a life expectancy of 33.1 years (to age 78). In other words, 11 years could be added to life expectancy by relatively simple changes in habits of living, recalling that only 2.7 years were added to the life expectancy at age 65 between 1900 and 1966. Breslow also found that the health status of those who practiced all seven habits was similar to those 30 years younger who observed none.

A large percentage of deaths (estimates up to 80 percent) due to cardiovascular disease and cancer are "premature," that is, occur in relatively young individuals and are related to the individual's bad habits. Heart disease and strokes are related to dietary factors, cigarette smoking, potentially treatable but undetected hypertension, and lack of exercise. Cancer is related to smoking (oral, buccal, lung, and bladder cancer) and probably to diets rich in fat and refined foodstuffs and low in residue (gastrointestinal and perhaps breast and prostatic cancer) and to the ingestion of food additives and certain drugs, or the inhalation of a wide variety of noxious agents. Certain occupational exposures and personal hygienic factors account for a small but important fraction of the total deaths due to cancer. Theoretically, all deaths due to accidents, homicide, and suicide are preventable.

Stress appears to play a critical role in disease. The stress of adjusting to change may generate a wide variety of diseases, and change is the hallmark of modern society. It is known that the death rate for widows and widowers is 10 times higher in the first year of bereavement than it is for others of comparable age; in the year following divorce the divorced persons have 12 times the incidence of disease that married persons have. People living in primitive societies insulated from change have low blood pressures and blood cholesterol levels which do not vary from youth to old age. Blood pressure and cholesterol tend to rise with age in our culture and are thought to be a prime cause of heart attacks and strokes. Studies indicate that up to 80 percent of serious physical illnesses seem to develop at a time when the individual feels helpless or hopeless. Studies on cancer patients have revealed lives marked by chronic anxiety, depression, or hostility and a lack of close emotional ties with parents—significantly greater than in a control group.

Despite the well-known hazards of smoking, per-capita consumption of cigarettes is expected to increase in 1975–76 after having been relatively stable between 1963—when the Surgeon General sounded the warning against smoking—and 1973, at 211 packs annually per person over 18 years. Some 15 percent of boys and girls under 18 years smoke cigarettes. Cigarette production is increasing at about 3.5 percent per year due to population growth and to a marked increase in smoking in teenage girls, which has risen from 8 to 15 percent in the past several years. If cigarette smoking were to be eliminated entirely, a 20 percent reduction in deaths due to cancer would result (based on the assumption that 85 percent of lung cancer is causally related to cigarette smoking). If all contributing environmental factors and personal bad health habits were eliminated, it is possible that cancer could be virtually eliminated as a cause of death. This would increase the average life expectancy at birth by 6 to 7 years, and at age 65 by 1.4 years for men and 2.1 years for women. The use of averages gives an erroneous impression, however, for one out of six people die of cancer. The elimination of cancer would mean that one out of six people would live 10.8 years longer.

Bad nutritional status (of the too-much-fat-intake-resulting-in-obesity type) can predispose the individual to heart attacks, strokes, cancer of the gastrointestinal tract, diabetes, liver and gall-bladder disease, degenerative arthritis of the hips, knees, and ankles, and injuries. It is estimated that 16 percent of Americans under the age of 30 years are obese, while 40 percent of the total population, or 80 million Americans, are 20 or more pounds above the ideal weight for their height, sex, and age. Over 30 percent of all men between 50 and 59 years are 20 percent overweight and 60 percent are at least 10 percent overweight.

Excessive use of alcohol is directly related to accidents and to liver disease (cirrhosis) as well as to a wide variety of other disorders, including vitamin deficiencies, inflammation of the pancreas, esophagus, and stomach, and muscular and neurologic diseases. Alcohol is a strong "risk factor" in cancer of the mouth, pharynx, larynx, and esophagus. More than 50 percent and probably nearer to 75 percent of all deaths and injuries due to automobile accidents are associated with the excessive use of alcohol. Alcoholism in one or both parents is significantly associated with home injuries to children (more than 50 percent in some studies). The prevalence of "heavy-escape" drinkers in the United States has been estimated at 6.5 million people (5.4 percent of total adult population), and the figures for those who use alcohol chronically and excessively range up to 10 million adults. Teenage drinking is now nearly universal. A study of high school students revealed that 36 percent reported getting drunk at least four times a year (remember, 15 percent smoke!). An increased frequency of cancer of the mouth, pharynx, larynx, and esophagus is seen in those who both smoke and drink and is less frequent, but still significantly higher than normal, in those who only smoke or only drink.

Dietary factors play a major role in cardiovascular disease and cancer. The major variable, as deduced from studies of migrant populations, seems to be fat content. For example, cancer of the large bowel as well as that of the breast and prostate is much more common in the United States than in Japan, and seems to be related to the difference in fat intake. The American derives 40 to 45 percent of his calories from fat, whereas the Japanese obtains only 15 to 20 percent of his calories from that source. Japanese descendants living in the United States have an incidence of bowel cancer similar to that seen in native Americans. Although the mechanism has not been established, it would appear that high fat intake (usually with resultant obesity) predisposes the American to both cancer and cardiovascular disease. Data from a long-term study of cardiovascular disease in Framingham, Massachusetts, indicate that each 10 percent reduction in weight in men 35–55 years old would result in a 20 percent decrease in the incidence of coronary disease. A 10 percent increase in weight would result in a 30 percent increase in coronary disease.[4]

The incidence of cancer of the colon and rectum in Americans both white and black is 10 times the incidence estimated for rural Africans. The removal of dietary fiber and a high intake of refined carbohydrates typical of diets in developed countries such as the United States result in a slowed transit time of food through the intestines. This is thought to facilitate the development of cancer, along with such diseases as diverticulitis, appendicitis, and even hemorrhoids. Prudence would dictate a reduction in fat and refined carbohydrates (and therefore increased fiber content) in the American diet. High-carbohydrate diets typical in the American culture also lead to dental caries, and may, over time, increase the risk of acquiring diabetes.

Knowledge of cancer and evidence for its multiple causes have increased to the point where the statement can be made with confidence that over 80 percent of human neoplasms depend either directly or indirectly on environmental factors. The term "environmental factors" includes cancer-provoking substances or carcinogens in the food and the drugs we ingest, the air we breathe, the water we drink, the occupations we pursue, and the habits we indulge. There are three major groups at high risk of cancer: (1) those with known host factors such as genetic and other congenital defects and immunologic-deficiency diseases; (2) those with exposure to environmental contaminants known to produce cancer; and (3) those with certain demographic characteristics which reflect as yet unknown carcinogenic factors such as place of residence or migration.[5]

The familial occurrence of cancer is a well-known phenomenon. A significant two to four times excess occurrence in relatives of patients has been noted in cancer of the stomach, breast, large intestine, uterus, and lung. Increased familial incidence has also been noted in leukemia, brain tumors in children, and sarcomas. Individuals with hereditary deficiencies of the immune system of the body develop malignant diseases of the blood vessels and lymphatic system. Acquired immunodeficiency also leads to the development of cancer. When patients with kidney transplants are given drugs over a long time to suppress the immune system in order to prevent rejection of the grafted kidney, cancer of the lymphatic system (lymphoma of the reticulum-cell-sarcoma type), frequently confined to the brain, and cancer of the skin develop in a significant proportion of the patients. Women who have had genital herpes (herpes simplex virus 2) have an increased incidence of cancer of the cervix of the uterus and constitute a high-risk population. People with pernicious anemia with associated gastritis develop cancer of the stomach at five times the rate of the normal population. Cirrhosis is associated with an increased incidence of cancer of the liver. Patients with diabetes have two times the incidence of cancer of the pancreas as normal individuals. The presence of gallstones and kidney stones increases the risk of developing cancer in the respective organs. Single episodes of trauma have been implicated in cancer of the bone, breast, and testicles. Chronic irritation of a skin mole may lead to cancerous degeneration, called malignant melanoma.

Environmental factors include tobacco, alcohol, radiation, occupation, drugs, air pollutants, diet, viruses, and other organisms, and sexual factors. The evidence on cigarette smoking is incontrovertible. It greatly increases the risk of lung cancer as well as cancer of the mouth, pharynx, larynx, esophagus, and urinary bladder. The incidence of cancer in cigarette smokers is higher in urban than rural dwellers, suggesting that air pollutants are additional major causative factors. Occupational exposure to asbestos fibers results in lung cancer, but here again the incidence is higher in those who smoke. Alcohol as a carcinogenic agent in malignancy of the mouth, larynx, esophagus, and liver (in association with cirrhosis) has been noted. A major long-term effect of radiation is cancer. Radiologists are ten times more likely to die of leukemia than are physicians not exposed to x-rays.

The list of drugs known or thought to be carcinogenic also continues to expand. Studies have shown that post-menopausal women given estrogens (so-called "replacement therapy" to diminish menopausal complaints and advertised to "keep women feminine") are five to fourteen times more likely to develop cancer of the uterus (endometrial cancer) than post-menopausal women not given the drug. (Other factors known to be associated with uterine cancer such as obesity, high blood pressure, never having borne a child, and age were not significant variables in these studies.) The risk increased with dosage size and duration of estrogen therapy. Other studies have shown beyond a doubt that the daughters of women given diethylstilbestrol (DES) during pregnancy are at higher risk of developing a rare form of cancer of the vagina. Despite this knowledge, DES is still being given to pregnant women to prevent spontaneous abortion. Most astounding has been the discovery of over 100 cases of liver tumors in women taking oral contraceptive pills. Most of the tumors were benign, but some showed cancerous degeneration and others ruptured with hemorrhage into the abdomen. Many carcinogenic agents incite the disease only many years after the initial exposure (e.g., atomic-bomb radiation) or after prolonged use, so it is not known whether an epidemic of liver tumors will ultimately develop in oral-contraceptive users. (The "pill" also causes a small but significant risk for heart attacks in users.) Long-term epidemiologic research is needed to establish knowledge necessary for control programs, but there is sufficient knowledge now to suggest that we should sharply restrict use of many drugs.

Sexual factors (both hormonal and behavioral) play a role in the causation of cancer of the breast and uterus (cervix and body of the uterus), penis, prostate, and testis. Cancer of the cervix occurs much more frequently in women who have had many sexual partners beginning at an early age, who come from a lower socioeconomic status, and who have had infection with Herpes simplex virus type 2, which is transmitted venereally. Celibate women are at very low risk, although they are at high risk for cancer of the breast. Cancer of the penis occurs in those who have poor penile hygiene and are uncircumcised in infancy (circumcision after the age of two years does not protect against the disease).

Attempts to prevent disease and improve and maintain health involve multifaceted strategies and expertise from many disciplines. Fundamental to any and all such attempts is sufficient empirical knowledge, i.e., knowledge gained through observation and trial-and-error experimentation that allows the advocate to convey his information with sufficient conviction to change the behavior of his audience. Although a great deal of information is available, the whole field of preventive medicine and health education needs far more fundamental research and long-term field experimentation. The biological and epidemiological effects of a wide variety of pollutants, the cost-benefit ratios of many available screening services, the influence of financial sanctions on changing health behavior, the use of the mass media and their effect on cognition and behavior, the long-term effects of various therapeutic regimens on the morbidity and mortality of individuals with asymptomatic high blood pressure, the long-term effects of marked reduction of fat in the diet on the incidence of cancer and heart disease, the influence of personal income on the development of cancer and coronary disease (the death rate from both lung cancer and coronary disease is significantly lower for the affluent than for the poor) are all examples of problems that need study. These problems demand for their solution the participation and integration of the disciplines of the biological sciences, the behavioral and social sciences (psychology, economics, cultural anthropology, political science), and public health (epidemiology and biostatistics).

It is a sad fact that of a total annual national expenditure on health of $120 billion, only 2 to 2.5 percent is spent on disease prevention and control measures, and only 0.5 percent each for health education and for improving the organization and delivery of health services. The national (federal) outlay for environmental-health research is around 0.25 percent of total health expenditures. These relatively meagre expenditures speak for the lack of interest in fields that rationally demand a much heavier commitment. The support of fundamental biomedical research has also flagged alarmingly in the past several years. The basic biological mechanisms of most of the common diseases are still not well enough known to give clear direction to preventive measures.

Strategies for improving health must include the incorporation of preventive measures into personal health services and into the environment, and individual and mass educational efforts.[6] For example, in dealing with the health problem of heart attacks, preventive measures would include screening for high-risk factors (high blood pressure, elevated blood cholesterol and fat levels, overweight, cigarette smoking, stress, and family history) and making available emergency services and measures for rapid transit to hospital-based coronary-care units; environmental measures would include altering food supply to reduce the intake of fat (i.e., those substances that raise blood cholesterol) and encouraging experiments in reducing work-related stress; and individual and mass educational efforts would include encouraging the use of screening examinations, the cessation of smoking, the maintenance of optimal weight with a balanced, low-fat diet, and obtaining regular exercise. Carrying out such a strategy involves many variables—convincing the doctor to play his pivotal role (and most medical educators and physicians are singularly uninterested in prevention), altering financing mechanisms to provide incentives to use preventive services (and most health insurance is, in fact, "disease insurance" which does not cover health education and preventive measures), and stimulating public as well as private efforts to exercise restraint on advertising and to exert positive sanctions for dissemination of health information through the mass media.

The health catastrophe related to automobile accidents presents a different type of problem. Here, personal-health services include availability of rapid transportation and first aid, emergency medical services, and definitive acute-care services in regional general hospitals; environmental measures would relate to road and highway construction (including lighting, warning signs, speed limits, safety rails), and the design and construction of automobiles for safety; and educational measures would include driver training, relicensing with eye examination, avoidance of alcohol and other drugs before driving, and reduction of speed. Which of these efforts will produce the most benefit at least cost? An interesting answer was provided during the oil-embargo energy crisis which necessitated reductions in speed limits and in the use of vehicles. The result in California was a 40 percent reduction in death rates from automobile accidents during the month of February, 1974, as contrasted with the previous February. Accidents on the New Jersey Turnpike dropped by one-fifth from 1973 to 1974, and fatalities were down by almost one-half, the lowest figure since 1966. Meanwhile, many people won't change their habits and wear seat belts, stop drinking, or reduce speed—and are annoyed with the restrictions on their freedom when someone tries to make them.

Dental health involves the personal services of the dentist and dental hygienist, the environmental measures of fluoridation of water supplies and the dietary restriction of refined carbohydrates, and the educational measures of prudent dietary habits, brushing the teeth, and visiting the dentist regularly. Where is the greatest benefit-cost ratio to be found? There is unequivocal evidence that fluoridation of water supplies will reduce dental caries by as much as 60 percent. It is safe and inexpensive, costing only 20 cents a year per person to prevent dental decay in children. Fluoridation of water supplies began about 1950. By 1967 over 3,000 communities with some 60 million people had adopted fluoridation. But the pace of change has slowed considerably, and the majority of people still lack fluoridated water due to fears of poisoning and resistance to what is perceived as an encroachment on their freedom. This highest benefit-cost dental-health program is still unavailable to the majority of Americans. Personal dental services are unavailable to large segments of our population and qualify as a luxury item.

. . . .

But what is the responsibility of the individual in matters pertaining to health? The United States now spends more on health in absolute terms and as a percentage of the gross national product than any other nation in the world—from $39 billion or 5.9 percent of the GNP in 1965 to $120 billion or 8.3 percent of the GNP in 1975 (over $550 per person per year). No one—but no one—can deny the fact that billions of dollars could be saved directly—and billions more indirectly (in terms of family suffering, time lost, and the erosion of human capital)—if our present knowledge of health and disease could be utilized in programs of primary, secondary, and tertiary prevention. The greatest portion of our national expenditure goes for the caring of the major causes of premature, and therefore preventable, death and/or disability in the United States, i.e., heart disease, cancer, strokes, accidents, bronchitis and emphysema, cirrhosis of the liver, mental illness and retardation, dental caries, suicide and homicide, venereal disease, and other infections. If no one smoked cigarettes or consumed alcohol and everyone exercised regularly, maintained optimal weight on a low fat, low refined-carbohydrate, high fiber-content diet, reduced stress by simplifying their lives, obtained adequate rest and recreation, understood the needs of infants and children for the proper nutrition and nurturing of their intellectual and affective development, had available to them, and would use, genetic counseling and selective abortion, drank fluoridated water, followed the doctor's orders for medications and self-care once disease was detected, used available health services at the appropriate time for screening examinations and health education-preventive medicine programs, the savings to the country would be mammoth in terms of billions of dollars, a vast reduction in human misery, and an attendant marked improvement in the quality of life. Our country would be strengthened immeasurably, and we could divert our energies—human and financial—to other pressing issues of national and international concern.

But so much conspires against this rational ideal: our historic emphasis on rugged individualism, social Darwinism, and unrestricted freedom together with our recent emphasis on individual rights as contrasted with responsibilities; a neo-liberal ideology which has stressed societal responsibility and the obligations of the beneficent state, resulting in an erosion of individual responsibility and initiative; a credit-minded culture which does it now and pays for it later, whether in drinking and eating or in buying cars and houses; an economy which depends on profligate production and consumption regardless of the results to individual health, or to the public health in terms of a wide variety of environmental pollutants; ignorance (and therefore a lack of conviction and commitment) on the part of both producers and consumers as to exact costs and benefits of many preventive and health-education measures, a reflection of the sparse national commitment to research in these areas: the failure, conceptually, to view health holistically, i.e., its interdependence with educational attainment, poverty, the availability of work, housing and the density of populations, degree of environmental pollution (air, water, noise, mass-media offerings), and levels of stress in work, play, and love; and finally, the values and habits of the health establishment itself. One cannot hope to develop a rational health system if the parts of the whole that bear on health are moving in irrational ways.

Within the health system, medical educators and the teaching hospitals display only acute curative, after-the-fact medicine. The rewards—intellectually, financially, and emotionally—for specialist care far outweight those for the low-status generalist (primary-care physician) or public health worker. The specialty organizations (surgeons, internists, radiologists, for example), the American Medical Association, the Association of American Medical Colleges, the American Hospital Association, the "disease-insurance" companies, as well as governmental insurance programs (Medicare-Medicaid), pay lip service or no service to reordering priorities and sanctions to the needs of the people for prevention and health education. Present plans for national health insurance do not contend with the issues of preventive medicine and health education. Over 65 percent of the 4.5 million workers in the health system are employed in hospitals, and their interests demand more expenditures and an even higher priority for acute, curative, after-the-fact medicine and the care of those with chronic disease. There is one health educator for every 17,000 people, while there is one physician for every 650 and one nurse for every 280 people.

Research priorities stress biological and not epidemiological, social, and environmental research. Even here, we should be willing to take decisive action when inferential evidence, e.g., the production of cancer in animals by drugs, is available, unacceptable as this may be to scientists. I cannot believe that man was meant to ingest drugs and artificial-food substances, breathe polluted air, or have his ears banged mercilessly by the uproar of industrial society. Those who do work in the field of prevention and health education have too often stressed social control (some have called them "health fascists") rather than social change and have become curiously indifferent to the needs and aspirations of families, communities, and particularly minority groups. Those places where benefit-cost ratios are potentially most favorable for programs of health education and prevention— and where long-range research could be conducted—have been neglected: the schools and universities, places of work, hospitals and clinics, and, obviously, doctors' offices. Very little is known about how television functions as a cognitive medium; little sophistication is shown by interested experts in developing sanctions, i.e., financial or other incentives, to modify bad habits of living. Those in the health professions play a minimal role in supporting the needs of minority groups for better housing and jobs, higher income, and improved transportation—not realizing that the fulfillment of these needs will reduce stress and anxiety and therefore improve health by reducing susceptibility to disease or to the disease-provoking habits of smoking and drinking.

If the health establishment isn't interested and the consumers don't want or demand health education and preventive medicine, what is to be done? First of all we should look at a few concrete changes in behavior which, through a variety of mechanisms, have improved health:

1) When the Surgeon General issued his report on the hazards of smoking in 1964, 52 percent of the male population smoked cigarettes. Through massive public educational programs and restrictions on advertising, the percentage was reduced over a 10-year period to roughly 42 percent. (This desirable change has been accompanied, however, by an equally undesirable increase in teen-age smoking, particularly among females, and no change in the 41 percent of 17-to-25-year-olds who smoke.)

2) During World War I, the United Kingdom increased taxes on alcohol, reduced the amount of alcohol available for consumption, and restricted the hours of sale. Consumption of alcohol fell and, with it, deaths from cirrhosis of the liver—from 10.3 per 100,000 people in 1914 to 4.5 in 1920. Following the war, the regulations governing the amount of alcohol allowed for consumption and the hours of its sale were relaxed, but taxes on alcoholic beverages were continually increased. By 1936, the death rate due to cirrhosis was down to 3.1 per 100,000, and it has remained at this level in that country. In the United States, wartime prohibition also reduced the cirrhosis death rate, from 11.8 per 100,000 in 1916 to 7.1 per 100,000 in 1920; it was still 7.2 in 1932, the year before prohibition was ended. But following the repeal of prohibition, the death rate from cirrhosis climbed steadily to an all-time high of 16.0 deaths per 100,000 in 1973, five times the rate in Great Britain. These results suggest a national strategy for the United States of (a) steadily increasing taxes on alcoholic beverages, (b) a massive public education program on the hazards of alcohol plus restrictions on all advertising, (c) aid to farmers and companies to help them shift to other crops and products. Increased tax income should temporarily help to defray the costs of public health education. The same strategy should be applied to cigarettes.

3) The marked reduction in auto fatalities and injuries during the oil crisis suggests that a permanent reduction of speed limits combined with sanctions to limit the use of automobiles would more than justify the cost of enforcing such a program.

4) A program to improve the self-care of patients with diabetes (tertiary prevention) at the University of Southern California resulted in a 50 percent reduction in emergency-ward visits, a decrease in the number of patients with diabetic coma from 300 to 100 over a two-year period, and the avoidance of 2,300 visits for medications. The theme was, "You must take responsibility for your own health." Savings were estimated at $1.7 million. In other studies involving the care and education of diabetics, hemophiliacs, and others, hospital readmissions decreased by over 50 percent. These efforts resulted in tremendous savings of time and money and reflected vastly improved self-care in cases of chronic disease.

5) A heart-disease-prevention program run by Stanford University

similarly demonstrated that an intensive program of health education and preventive medicine—utilizing personal instructions, television spots, and printed material—resulted in a markedly higher level of information about the disease by the community and a marked improvement in dietary habits and in the reduction of smoking among those at high risk.

· ·

I began by saying that the health of human beings is determined by their behavior, their food, and the nature of their environment. Over 99 percent of us are born healthy and suffer premature death and disability only as a result of personal misbehavior and environmental conditions. The sociocultural effects of urban industrial life are profound in terms of stress, an unnatural sedentary existence, bad habits, and unhealthy environmental influences.[7] The individual has the power—indeed, the moral responsibility—to maintain his own health by the observance of simple, prudent rules of behavior relating to sleep, exercise, diet and weight, alcohol, and smoking. In addition, he should avoid where possible the long-term use of drugs. He should be aware of the dangers of stress and the need for precautionary measures during periods of sudden change, such as bereavement, divorce, or new employment. He should submit to selective medical examination and screening procedures.

These simple rules can be understood and observed by the majority of Americans, namely the white, well-educated, and affluent middle class. But how do individuals in minority groups follow these rules, when their members include disproportionately large numbers of the impoverished and the illiterate, among whom fear, ignorance, desperation, and superstition conspire against even the desire to remain healthy? Here we must rely on social policies *first,* in order to improve education, employment, civil rights, and economic levels, along with efforts to develop accessible health services.

Beyond these measures, the individual is powerless to control disease-provoking environmental contaminants, be they drugs, air and water pollutants, or food additives, except as he becomes knowledgeable enough to participate in public debate and in support of governmental controls. Here, we must depend on the wisdom of experts, the results of research, and the national will to legislate controls for our protection, as damaging as they may be, in the short run, to our national economy.

When all is said and done, let us not forget that he who hates sin, hates humanity. Life is meant to be enjoyed, and each one of us in the end is still able in our own country to steer his vessel to his own port of desire. But the costs of individual irresponsibility in health have now become prohibitive. The choice is individual responsibility or social failure. Responsibility and duty must gain some degree of parity with right and freedom.

References

1. T. McKeown, *The Modern Rise of Population* (London, 1976), pp. 152–63.
2. M. Susser, ed., *Prevention and Health Maintenance Revisited (Bulletin of the New York Academy of Medicine.* 51[January, 1975], pp. 5–243), p. 96.
3. N. B. Belloc and L. Breslow, "The Relation of Physical Health Status and Health Practices," *Preventive Medicine,* 1(August, 1972), pp. 409–21; see also "Relationship of Health Practices and Mortality." *Preventive Medicine,* 2(1973), pp. 67–81.
4. F. W. Ashley, Jr., and W. B. Kannel, "Relation of Weight Change to Changes in Atherogenic Traits: The Framingham Study," *Journal of Chronic Diseases,* 27(March, 1974), pp. 103–14.
5. J. F. Fraumeni, ed., *Persons at High Risk of Cancer: An Approach to Cancer Etiology and Control* (New York, 1975), p. 526.
6. L. Breslow, "Research in Strategy for Health Improvement," *International Journal of Health Services.* 3(1973), pp. 7–16.
7. J. H. Knowles, *Health in America. Health Service Prospects: An International Survey* (London, 1973). pp. 307–34.

31

Individual Responsibility and Health Politics

Robert Crawford

. . . .

. . . The contention . . . is . . . that although health is a complex matter and therefore requires several kinds of efforts, individual responsibility is the key ingredient. In place of admittedly expensive and ineffective medical services, it is said, individual change must be the focus of the nation's efforts to promote and maintain health. People should use the medical system less and instead adopt healthy lifestyles: or, as it was declared by one pundit, "living a long life is essentially a do-it-yourself proposition." These assertions perform the function of *blaming the victim*. They avert any serious discussion of social or environmental factors and instead locate the problem of poor health and its solution in the individual. Further, they imply, sometimes explicitly, that since people's own misbehavior is the heart of the problem of health and illness, people should *demand less* medical care. Rights and entitlements for access to medical services are almost by definition now considered inappropriate. Thus, in becoming a premise for public policy, these pronouncements are providing the material for a new public philosophy by which problems are defined and answers proposed.

Similar ideologies of individual responsibility have always been popular among providers and academics trying to justify inequality in the utilization of medical services. During the period of rapid expansion in the health sector, higher morbidity and mortality rates for the poor and minorities were explained by emphasizing their lifestyle habits, especially their health and utilization behavior. These "culture of poverty" explanations emphasized delay in seeking medical help, resistance to medical authority, and reliance on unprofessional folk healers or advisors. As Catherine Riessman summarizes:

> According to these researchers, the poor have undergone multiple negative experiences with organizational systems, leading to avoidance behavior, lack of trust, and hence a disinclination to seek care and follow medical regimens except in dire need.[1]

Now, in a period of fiscal crisis and cost control, the same higher morbidity rates and demands for more access through comprehensive national health insurance are met with a barrage of statements about the limits of medicine and the lack of appropriate health behavior. Several commentators now link overuse by the poor with their faulty health habits. Again, education is seen as the solution. Previously the poor were blamed for not using medical services enough, for relying too much on their own resources, for undue suspicion of modern medicine. Now they are blamed for relying too much on medical services and not enough on their own resources. In both cases, of course, structural factors are rarely mentioned; but structural factors are behind this ideological shift.

The Crisis of Costs

The cost crisis is transforming the entire political landscape in the health sector. What makes inflation in the health sector so critical in the 1970s is not only its spectacular rate but also its concurrence with wider economic and fiscal crises. We now face a situation in which inflation and expenditures for human services have become the primary targets of a strategy aimed at restoring "optimal conditions" for investment and growth in the corporate sector. The costs of medical services to government have aggravated a fiscal crisis in which the direction of public spending is the issue and raising taxes is considered inimical to corporate priorities. Further, high medical costs have become a direct threat to the corporate sector in two important ways: first, by adding significantly to the costs of production through increases in health benefit settlements with labor; and, second, by diverting consumer expenditures from other corporate products. The fact that large corporations have extensively invested in medical and health-related products does not significantly alter this picture.

The costs of production for corporations are being dramatically affected by increases in benefit settlements. General Motors claims it spent more money with Blue Cross and Blue Shield in 1975 than it did with U.S. Steel, its principal supplier of metal. Standard Oil of Indiana announced that employee health costs for the corporation had tripled over the past seven years.[2] Chrysler estimates that in 1976 it paid $1,500 per employee for medical benefits or a total of $205 million in the United States. "Unlike most other labor costs that can and do vary with the level of production," the corporation complains, "medical costs continue to rise in good times as well as bad."[3] The implications for consumer costs are obvious. General Motors added $175 to the price of every car and truck by passing on its employee medical benefit costs. In a period in which consumption and investment are stalled, while foreign competition adds an additional barrier to raising prices, such figures are startling. Corporate and union leaders are expressing in every possible forum their concern over the impact of rising medical costs upon prices, wages, and profits.

Thus, substantial political pressures are being mobilized to cut the direct costs to corporations and to cut the indirect costs of social programs generally. The politics of growth that dominated the previous period are giving way to the politics of curbing that growth in the present period. Just a few years ago the political emphasis was on increasing utilization. Now it is on reducing utilization. Besides regulatory measures, the strategies being adopted include cutbacks in public programs, especially Medicaid, and public hospitals and a shifting of the burden of costs back to employees, old people, and consumers in general.[4] In addition, corporations, often with the participation of unions, are adopting new internal strategies aimed at curbing costs.[5]

Most important is the growing consensus among corporate and governmental leaders that comprehensive national health insurance is unacceptable at current cost levels. In his campaign for the presidency, Jimmy Carter, aware of its popular appeal and importance to organized labor, committed himself to a comprehensive insurance program; but, in reminding the nation in April 1977 that balancing the budget by 1981 is his paramount domestic goal, Carter warned that the costs of such a program would be prohibitive. Secretary of Health, Education, and Welfare, Joseph Califano, more explicitly argued that cost control is a necessary precondition for national health insurance or "some other system."[6] These and numerous other signs indicating that the prospects for comprehensive insurance are receding behind a shield of rhetoric and a language of gradualism.

Popular Demand for the Extension of Rights and Entitlements

In order to understand the importance of a new ideology that tells people they must rely less on the medical system and more on themselves, the cost crisis must be viewed in the context of the legacy of the preceding period, a time in which popular expectations of medicine and political demands for unhindered access to medical services reached their highest levels. Growth reinforced those expectations, as did years of propaganda by a medical and research establishment strengthened by occasional but spectacular medical successes. Medicine was promoted in almost religious terms, a promise of deliverance from pain and illness even a "death of death."

For years people were conditioned to believe in the value of consuming high levels of medical services and products. At a time when these beliefs became celebrated cultural values, large numbers of people continued to experience difficulty in obtaining regular access to primary care services and faced financial disaster for unusual medical expenses. Access came to be considered an essential component of family and personal security and an integral part of the wage bargain for organized labor. The idea of medical care as a right became widely accepted in a period in which rights were forced onto the political agenda of the nation. By the early 1970s popular pressures for national health insurance began to swell. As benefits shrink in the face of uncontrollable inflation, the sentiment for a comprehensive program continues to build.

Now, however, just at the point when medical care has become broadly viewed as a right and there is a growing demand for the extension of entitlements, people are suddenly being pressured to use the system less. If people are to modify their expectations, if their demands for guaranteed access are to be sidetracked, and if legislators and other policymakers are to be convinced of the necessity for retrenchment, a new ideology must be developed to replace the unquestioned power of medicine and to break the link between the provision of services and popular political demands. People will not relinquish their expectations unless their belief in medicine as a panacea is broken and the value of access is replaced with a new preoccupation with boot-strapping activities aimed at controlling at-risk behaviors. In a political climate of fiscal, energy, and cost crises, self-sacrifice and self-discipline emerge as popular themes. In lieu of rights and entitlements, individual responsibility, self-help and holistic health move to the center of discussion.[7]

The Politics of Retrenchment

The flavor of the ideology is evident in the comments of some of its more explicit proponents. Both direct policy proposals and indirect policy implications are abundant. With an implied attack on social programs, for example, Victor Fuchs, a noted health economist, writes: "Some future historian, in reviewing mid-twentieth century social reform literature may note . . . a 'resolute refusal' to admit that individuals have any responsibility for their own stress."[8] Robert Whalen, Commissioner of the New York Department of Health, more explicitly makes the tie with high medical costs: "Unless we assume such individual and moral responsibility for our own health, we will soon learn what a cruel and expensive hoax we have worked upon ourselves through our belief that more money spent on health care is the way to better health."[9]

As do many advocates of individual responsibility, Walter McNerney, president of the Blue Cross Association, incorporates elements of both the Illichian and radical critiques of technology-heavy, distorted, and iatrogenic medicine: "We must stop throwing an array of technological processes and systems at lifestyle problems and stop equating more health services with better health. . . . People must have the capability and the will to take greater responsibility for their own health."[10] John Knowles, the late president of the Rockefeller Foundation, spoke more directly to the problem of expectations: "The only thing we've heard about national health insurance from everybody is that it won't solve the problems. It will inflate expectations and demands and cause more frustrations."[11] Knowles argued that the "primary critical choice" facing the individual is "to change his personal bad habits or stop complaining. He can either remain the problem or become the solution to it: Beneficient Government cannot—indeed, should not—do it for him or to him.[12]

The attack on rights is explicit. Leon Kass, writing in *The Public Interest,* states that "it no more makes sense to claim a right to health than a right to health care."[13] "How can we go talking about a right to health," Robert Morrison asks, "without some balancing talk about an individual's responsibility to keep healthy."[14] Again, Knowles offers a clear articulation:

> The idea of individual responsibility has been submerged in individual rights—rights or demands to be guaranteed by Big Brother and delivered by public and private institutions. The cost of sloth, gluttony, alcoholic intemperance, reckless driving, sexual frenzy and smoking have now become a national, not an individual, responsibility, and all justified as individual freedom. But one man's or woman's freedom in health is now another man's shackle in taxes and insurance premiums.[15]

What Knowles is suggesting by national responsibility is public policy aimed at changing individual behavior—and using economic or other sanctions to do it. Economic sanctions on individuals, such as higher taxation on the consumption of cigarettes and alcohol, or higher insurance premiums to those engaging in at-risk behaviors are becoming a popular theme. A guest editorial appeared last year in *The New York Times,* for example, introducing the idea of "Your Fault Insurance."[16] More extreme sanctions are proposed by Leon Kass:

> All the proposals for National Health Insurance embrace, without qualification, the no-fault principle. They therefore choose to ignore, or to treat as irrelevant, the importance of personal responsibility for the state of one's own health. As a result, they pass up an opportunity to build both positive and negative inducements into the insurance payment plan, by measures such as *refusing or reducing benefits for chronic respiratory disease care to persons who continue to smoke* (emphasis added).[17]

These sanctions may be justified under the rubric of "lack of motivation," "unsuitability for treatment," or "inability to profit from therapy."[18] Why waste money, after all, on people whose lifestyle contravenes good therapeutic results, or, as Morrison put it, on a "system which taxes the virtuous to send the improvident to the hospital."[19] In the new system the pariahs of the medical world and larger numbers of people in general could be diagnosed as lifestyle problems, referred to a health counselor, and sent home. At the very least, the victim-blaming ideology will help justify shifting the burden of costs back to users. A person who is responsible for his or her illness should be responsible for the bill as well.[20]

The Social Causation of Disease

If the victim-blaming ideology serves as a legitimization for the retrenchment from rights and entitlements, in relation to the social causation of disease it functions as a colossal masquerade. The complexities of social causation are only beginning to be explored. The ideology of individual responsibility, however, inhibits that understanding and substitutes instead an unrealistic behavioral model. It both ignores what is known about human behavior and minimizes the importance of evidence about the environmental assault on health. It instructs people to be individually responsible at a time when they are becoming less capable as individuals of controlling their total health environment.[21] Although environmental factors are often recognized as "also relevant," the implication is that little can be done about an ineluctable, technological, and industrial society.

A certain portion of illness is, at some level, undoubtedly associated with individual behavior, and if that behavior were altered, it could lead to improved health. Health education efforts aimed at changing individual behavior should be an important part of any health strategy. Offered in a vacuum, however, such efforts will achieve only marginal results. Sociologist John McKinlay has argued convincingly that the frequent failure of health education programs is attributable to the failure to address the social context. He concludes that:

> Certain at-risk behaviors have become so inextricably intertwined with our dominant cultural system (perhaps even symbolic of it) that the routine display of such behavior almost signified membership in this society.... To request people to change or alter these behaviors is more or less to request the abandonment of dominant culture.[22]

What must be questioned is both the effectiveness and the political uses of a focus on lifestyles and on changing individual behavior without changing social structure and processes. Just as the Horatio Alger myth was based on the fact that just enough individuals achieve mobility to make the possibility believable, so too significant health gains might be realized by some of those able to resist the incredible array of social forces aligned against healthy behavior. The vast majority, however, will remain unaffected.

The crisis of social causation is characterized by a growing awareness and politicization of environmental and occupational sources of disease in the face of the failure of medicine to have a significant impact on the modern epidemics, especially cancer. In just the last few years the American people have been inundated with scientific and popular critiques of the environmental and occupational sources of cancer. These revelations have been accompanied by a constant flow of warnings about environmental dangers: air pollution, contamination of drinking supplies, food additive carcinogens, PCB, asbestos, kepone, vinyl chlorides, pesticides, nuclear power plants, saccharine, and even more. The Environmental Protection Agency, the Occupational Safety and Health Administration, and the Food and Drug Administration have been among the most embattled government agencies in recent years.

While there is considerable debate over threshold-limit values, the validity of animal research applications to humans, and specific policy decisions by the above agencies, awareness is growing that the public is being exposed to a multitude of environmental and work place carcinogens. Although many people still cling to the "it won't happen to me" response, the fear of cancer is becoming more widespread. A recent Gallup Poll found that cancer is by far the disease most feared by Americans, almost three times its nearest competitor.[23] The fear is not unwarranted. Cancer is a disease of epidemic proportions. Samuel Epstein, a noted cancer expert, claims that "more than 53 million people in the U.S. (over a quarter of the population) will develop some form of cancer in their lifetimes, and approximately 20 percent will die of it."[24]

Pressure on industrial corporations has been building for years. An occupational health and safety movement from within industry is gaining momentum. Many unions are developing programs and confronting corporate management on health and safety issues. Although suffering from severe setbacks, the environmental movement still poses a serious challenge as environmental consciousness is reinforced by the politicization of public health issues. Government agencies and the courts have never been so assertive, despite the repeated attempts by industry to undermine these efforts. The political constraints on the growth of the nuclear power industry and governmental pressures on steel are not lost on other industries.

The threat to corporate autonomy is clear. One reads almost daily of the economic blackmail threatened by corporations if regulations are imposed, whether production shutdowns, plant closings, or investment strikes. Corporations move their plants to more tractable communities or countries. Advertising campaigns promoting the image of public-spirited corporate activities attempt to counter the threat that the decision to subordinate people's health to profits will become yet more apparent. In short, the "manufacturers of illness" are on the defensive. They must seek new ways to blunt the efforts of the new health activists and to shift the burden of responsibility for health away from their doorstep.

The Politics of Diversion

Victim-blaming ideology offers a perfect opportunity. "For once we cannot blame the environment as much as we have to blame ourselves," says Ernst Wynder, president of the American Health Foundation. "The problem is now the inability of man to take care of himself."[25] Or as New York Health Commissioner Whalen writes: "Many of our most difficult contemporary health problems, such as cancer, heart disease and accidental injury, have a built-in behavioral component. . . . *If they are to be solved at all,* we must change our style of living" (emphasis added).[26] Alternatively, Leon Kass, fearing the consequences of a focus on social causation, warns of "excessive preoccupations, as when cancer phobia leads to government regulations that unreasonably restrict industrial activity."[27]

One after another, the lifestyle proponents admit to the environmental and occupational factors that affect health, but then go on to assert their pragmatism. Victor Fuchs, for example, while recognizing environmental factors as "also relevant," asserts that "the greatest potential for reducing coronary disease, cancer, and other major killers still lies in altering personal behavior." He philosophizes that "emphasizing social responsibility can increase security, but it may be the security of the 'zoo'—purchased at the expense of freedom."[28] Carlson recognizes that social causation "raises some difficult political problems, because if we find the carcinogens in certain places in our environment, we run into institutional forces which will oppose dealing with them." Thus, "we may have to intervene at other levels here."[29] The practical focus of health efforts, in other words, should not be on the massive, expensive, politically difficult, or even politically dangerous task of overhauling our work and community environments. Instead, the focus must be on changing individuals who live and work within those settings. In the name of pragmatism, efficacy is thus ignored.

There are several other expressions of the ideology that should be noted. The diffusion of a psychological world view often reinforces the masking of social causation. Even though the psychiatric model substitutes social for natural explanations, problems still tend to be seen as amenable to change through personal transformation, with or without therapy. And, with or without therapy, individuals are ultimately held responsible for their own psychological well-being. Usually no one has to blame us for some psychological failure; we blame ourselves. Thus, psychological impairment can be just as effective as moral failing or genetic inferiority in blaming the victims and reinforcing dominant social relations.[30] People are alienated, unhappy, dropouts, criminals, angry, and activists, after all, because of maladjustment to one or another psychological norm.

The ideology of individual responsibility for health lends itself to this form of psychological obfuscation. Susceptibility to at-risk behaviors, if not a moral failing, is at least a psychological failing. New evidence relating psychological state to resistance or susceptibility to disease and accidents can and will be used to shift more responsibility to the individual. Industrial psychologists have long been employed with the intention that intervention at the individual level is the best way to reduce plant accidents in lieu of costly production changes. The implication is that people make themselves sick, not only mentally but physically. If job satisfaction is important to health, people should seek more rewarding employment. Cancer is a state of mind.

In another vein, many accounts of the current disease structure in the United States link disease with affluence. The affluent society and the lifestyles it has wrought, it is suggested, are the sources of the individual's degeneration and adoption of at-risk behaviors. Michael Halberstam, for example, writes that "most Americans die of excess rather than neglect or poverty."[31] Knowles's warnings about "sloth, gluttony, alcoholic intemperance, reckless driving, sexual frenzy and smoking," and later about "social failure," are reminiscent of a popularized conception of decaying Rome.[32] Thus, even though some may complain about environmental hazards, people are really suffering from overindulgence of the good society; it is overindulgence that must be checked. Further, by pointing to lifestyles, which are usually presented as if they reflect the problems of homogenized, affluent society, this aspect of the ideology tends to obscure the reality of class and the impact of social inequality of health. It is compatible with the conception that people are free agents. Social structure and constraints recede amid the abundance.

Of course, several diseases do stem from the lifestyles of the more affluent. Discretionary income usually allows for excessive consumption of unhealthy products; and, as Joseph Eyer argues, everyone suffers in variable and specific ways from the nature of work and the conditioning of lifestyles in advanced capitalist society.[33] But are the well-established relationships between low income and high infant mortality, diseases related to poor diet and malnutrition, stress, cancer, mental illness, traumas of various kinds, and other pathologies now to be ignored or relegated to a residual factor?[34] While long-term inequality in morbidity and mortality is declining, for almost every disease and for every indicator of morbidity, incidence increases as income falls.[35] In some specific cases the health gap appears to be widening.[36] Nonetheless, health economist Anne Somers reassures that contemporary society is tending in the direction of homogeneity:

> If poverty seems so widespread, it is at least partly because our definition of poverty is so much more generous than in the past—a generosity made possible only by the pervasive affluence and the impressive technological base upon which it rests. . . . This point—that the current crisis is the result of progress rather than retrogression or decay—is vitally important not only as a historical fact but as a guide to problem solving in the health field as elsewhere.[37]

Finally, by focusing on the individual, the ideology performs the classical role of individualist ideologies in obscuring the class structure of work and the worker's lack of control over working conditions. The failure to maintain health in the work place is attributed to some personal flaw. The more than 2.5 million people disabled by occupational accidents and diseases each year and the 114,000 killed are not explained by the hazards or pace of work as much as by the lack of sufficient caution by workers, laziness about wearing respirators or other protective equipment, psychological maladjustment, including an inability to minimize stress, and even by the worker's genetic susceptibility. Correspondingly, the overworked, overstressed worker is offered transcendental meditation, biofeedback, psychological counseling, or some other holistic approach to healthy behavior change, leaving intact the structure of employer incentives and sanctions that reward the retention of work place hazards and health-denying behavior.

Moreover, corporate management appears to be integrating victim-blaming themes into personnel policies as health becomes an important rubric for traditional managerial strategies aimed at controlling the work force. Holding individual workers responsible for their susceptibility to illness or for their psychological state is not only a response to growing pressures over occupational hazards but it also complements management attempts to control absenteeism and enhance productivity. Job dissatisfaction and job-induced stress (in both their psychological and physical manifestations), principal sources of absenteeism and low productivity, will more and more become identified as lifestyle problems of the worker. Workers found to be "irresponsible" in maintaining their health or psychological stability, as manifest in attendance and productivity records, will face sanctions, dismissals or early retirement, rationalized as stemming from employee health problems. Already the attack on sick-day benefits is well underway. The push toward corporate health maintenance organizations will further reinforce managerial use of health criteria for control purposes.

One such control mechanism is pre-employment and periodic health screening, which is now in regular use in large industry. New businesses are selling employee risk evaluations, called by one firm "health hazard appraisals." Among the specific advantages cited for health screening by the Conference Board, a business research organization, is the selection "of those judged to present the least risk of unstable attendance, costly illness, poor productivity, or short tenure."[38] Screening also holds out the possibility of cost savings from reduced insurance rates and compensation claims. It also raises, however, the possibility of a large and growing category of "high-risk" workers who become permanently unemployable—not only because of existing, incapacitating illnesses but because of their *potential* for becoming ill.

In a period in which we have become accustomed to ozone watches in which "vulnerable" people are warned to reduce activity, workers are being screened for susceptibility to job hazards. Even though they alert individuals to their higher risks, these programs do not address the hazardous conditions that to some degree affect all workers. Thus, all workers may be penalized *to the extent* that such programs function to divert attention from causative conditions. To the degree that the causative agent remains, the more susceptible workers are also penalized in that they must shoulder the burden of the hazardous conditions either by looking for another, perhaps nonexistent, job; or, if it is permitted, by taking a risk in remaining. At a United Auto Workers conference on lead, the union's president summed up industry's tactics as "fix the worker, not the workplace." He further criticized the "exclusion of so-called 'sensitive' groups of workers, the use of dangerous chemical agents to artificially lower workers' blood lead levels, the transfer of workers in and out of high lead areas, and the forced use of personal respirators instead of engineering controls to clean the air in the workplace."[39] These struggles to place responsibility are bound to intensify.

. . . .

Note

For helpful comments and editorial suggestions, mostly on an earlier draft, thanks to Evan Stark, Susan Reverby, John McKnight, Nancy Hartsock, Sol Levine, Cathy Stepanek, Isaac Balbus, and participants in the East Coast Health Discussion Group. I am especially indebted to Lauren Crawford who provided many hours in discussion and in preparation of this manuscript.

References

1. "The Use of Health Services by the Poor," *Social Policy* 5, 1 (1974): 42.
2. *Chicago Sun-Times,* 16 March 1976.
3. "Inflation of Health Care Costs, 1976," hearings before the Sub-Committee on Health of the Committee on Labor and Public Welfare, United States Senate, 94th Congress (Washington, D.C.: U.S. Government Printing Office, 1976), pp. 656–60.
4. Daniel Fox and Robert Crawford, "Health Politics in the United States," in *Handbook of Medical Sociology,* edited by H. E. Freeman, S. Levine, and L. Reeder, (Englewood Cliffs, N.J.: Prentice-Hall 3rd ed., 1979); Ronda Kotel-chuck, "Government Cost Control Strategies," *Health-PAC Bulletin,* no. 75, March–April 1977, pp. 1–6.
5. *The Complex Puzzle of Rising Health Costs: Can the Private Sector Fit It Together?* (Washington, D.C.: Council on Wage and Price Stability, December 1976).
6. *New York Times,* 26 April 1977.
7. The ideology of individual responsibility threatens to incorporate and use the self-help movement for its own purposes. Self-help initially developed as a political response to the oppressive character of professional and male domination in medicine. As such, the self-help movement embodies some of the best strands of grassroots, autonomous action, of people attempting at some level to regain control over their lives, and a response to the overmedicalization of American life. However, because the movement has focused on individual behavior and only rarely addressed the social and physical environment, and because it has not built a movement that goes beyond self-care to demanding the medical and environmental prerequisites for maintaing health, it lends itself to the purposes of victim-blaming. Just as the language of helping obscured the unequal power relationships of a growing therapeutic state (in other words, masking political behavior by calling it therapeutic) the language of self-help obscures the power relations underlying the social causation of disease and the dominant interests that now seek to reorder popular expectations of rights and entitlements for access to medical services.
8. Fuchs, *Who Shall Live?* (New York: Basic Books, 1974), p. 27.
9. *New York Times,* 17 April 1977.
10. *Conference on Future Directions in Health Care,* pp. 4–5.
11. Ibid., pp. 28–29.
12. "The Responsibility of the Individual," in *Doing Better and Feeling Worse: Health in the United States,* ed. by John Knowles (New York: Norton and Co., 1977), p. 78.
13. L. Kass "Regarding the End of Medicine and the Pursuit of Health," *Public Interest* 40 (Summer 1975): 38–39.

14. Quoted in ibid., p. 42.
15. *Conference in Future Directions in Health Care,* pp. 2–3.
16. 14 October 1976.
17. Kass, p. 71.
18. William Ryan, *Blaming the Victim* (New York: Vintage Books, 1971).
19. Quoted in Kass, p. 42.
20. These remarks are in no way intended to imply that access to more services, regardless of their utility for improved health status, is a progressive position. Medical services as a means to maintain health have been grossly oversold. As Paul Starr comments [in "The Politics of Therapeutic Nihilism," reprinted in this book], "a critic like Illich argues that because medical care has made no difference in health, we should not be particularly concerned about access. He has turned the point around. We will have to be especially concerned about inequalities if we are to make future investments in medical care effective" (p. 52). The argument here is that medical expenditures are presently distorted toward unnecessary and ineffective activities that serve to maximize income for providers and suppliers. Political conditions favoring an effective and just reallocation of expenditures are more likely to develop in the context of a publicly accountable system that must allocate services within statutory constraints and a politically determined budget. In such a system political struggles against special interests, misallocation, or underfunding will obviously continue, as will efforts to achieve effectiveness and responsiveness. The concept and definition of need will move to the center of policy discussions. With all the perils and ideological manipulations that process will entail, it is better that such a debate take place in public than be determined by the private market.

    Further, viable programs of cost control must be formulated, first as an alternative to the cutback strategy and, second, as the necessary adjunct to establishing effective and relevant services. Technology-intensive and over-use-related sources of inflationary costs are directly related to the problem of ineffectiveness as well as to iatrogenesis.
21. "Special Issue on the Economy, Medicine and Health," ed. by Joseph Eyer, *International Journal of Health Services 7,* 1(January 1977); "The Social Etiology of Disease, Part I," *HMO-Network for Marxist Studies in Health,* no. 2, January 1977.
22. "A Case for Refocusing Upstream—The Political Economy of Illness" (Boston University, unpublished paper, 1974). Reprinted in this book.
23. *Chicago Sun-Times,* 6 February 1977.
24. "The Political and Economic Basis of Cancer," *Technology Review 78,* 8(1976): 1.
25. *Conference on Future Directions in Health Care,* p. 52.
26. *New York Times,* 17 April 1977.
27. Kass, p. 42.
28. Fuchs, pp. 26, 46.
29. *Conference on Future Directions in Health Care,* p. 116.
30. Thomas Szasz, *Ideology and Insanity: Essays on the Psychiatric Dehumanization of Man* (Garden City, N.Y.: Doubleday-Anchor Press, 1970).

31. Quoted in Anne Somers, *Health Care in Transition: Directions for the Future* (Chicago: Hospital Research and Educational Trust, 1971), p. 32.

32. See note 15, above.

33. "Prosperity as a Cause of Disease," *International Journal of Health Services 7*, 9(January 1977) 125–50.

34. R. Hurley, "The Health Crisis of the Poor," in *The Social Organization of Health*, ed. by H. P. Dreitzel (New York: Macmillan, 1971), pp. 83–122; *Infant Mortality Rates: Socioeconomic Factors*, Washington, D.C.: U.S. Public Health Service, series 22, no. 14, 1972; *Selected Vital and Health Statistics in Poverty and Nonpoverty Areas of 19 Large Cities, U.S., 1969–71*, Washington, D.C.: U.S. Public Health Service, series 21, no. 26, 1975; E. Kitagaw and P. Hauser, *Differential Mortality in the U.S.: A Study of Socioeconomic Epidemiology* (Cambridge: Harvard University Press, 1973); Hila Sherer, "Hypertension," *HMO* no. 2, January 1977.

35. *Preventive Medicine USA* (New York: Prodist Press, 1976), pp. 620–21; A. Antonovsky, "Social Class, Life Expectancy and Overall Mortality," *Milbank Memorial Fund Quarterly 5, 45*, no. 2-part 1(1967): 31–73.

36. C. D. Jenkins, "Recent Evidence Supporting Psychologic and Social Risk Factors for Coronary Heart Diseases," *New England Journal of Medicine 294*, 18(1976). 987–94; and 294, 19(1976): 1,003–38, J. Eyer and P. Sterling, "Stress Related Mortality and Social Organization," *Review of Radical Political Economy*, Summer 1977.

37. Somers, p. 77.

38. S. Lusterman, *Industry Roles in Health Care* (New York: National Industrial Conference Board, 1974) p. 31.

39. *Dollars and Sense*, April 1977, p. 15.

National Health Insurance

We are the world's only industrialized nation without a universal health-insurance program; yet no country on earth spends as much per capita as do we on health care. (Richard J. Margolis, "National Health Insurance—The Dream Whose Time Has Come?")

The idea of national health insurance is certainly not a new one in this country—a health insurance plank was included in Theodore Roosevelt's Progressive Party platform in 1912 (Lander, 1975: 1). From 1912 to 1920 the American Association for Labor Legislation waged a major campaign for enactment of government-sponsored health insurance. This effort ended in the face of concentrated opposition from American business interests, the American Medical Association (AMA), and the insurance companies (Falk, 1977: 163).

As part of his New Deal reforms, President Franklin Roosevelt succeeded in passing the Social Security Act in 1935, which provided very limited medical care support for certain segments of the population as well as the first "permanent authorization to the Public Health Service" for grants to states for public health research and programs. In 1946, the Hill-Burton program was enacted by the federal government to support hospital construction, and in 1965 Medicare and Medicaid legislation was passed. Although various programs for national health insurance have been proposed over the years, primarily by labor unions and political progressives, the continuous opposition of the powerful AMA defeated them all (Harris, 1969).

This section explores what national health insurance (NHI) could mean to Americans, the specific plans recently before Congress, and the debate about whether any national health insurance plan can solve the problems of the American medical care system.

Why do we need a national health insurance plan? Those who support national health insurance point primarily to the maldistribution of available medical services, the skyrocketing costs of medical care, and the lack of insurance coverage for a large segment of the American population. For example, " . . . as of 1975, approximately 25 percent of the poor and near poor were not covered by either Medicaid or Medicare. An estimate that includes 1978 statistics indicates that less than half of the [total] population is protected against catastrophic illness expenses" (Mauksch, 1978: 1323). Medical costs remain the leading cause of personal bankruptcy in the United States. In addition, even when people do have some form of insurance coverage, these policies almost never cover all services or all costs.

Before turning to the debate over NHI, we should note the important difference between all national health *insurance* plans and what has been termed a "national health *service*," or a "national health *system*." Generally speaking, in NHI plans, taxes are used to pay the cost of medical insurance premiums. Although early proposals for insurance programs in the United States eliminated the private health-insurance industry, all current NHI proposals include them as intermediaries.[1] As has been well documented, health-insurance companies under our present system have made enormous profits from premiums and contributed directly to the spiraling costs of medical care.

> Massive national experience shows that the insurance industry adds billions of dollars in cost and distorts sensible patterns of services and expenditure, while contributing little in administration and even less in quality and cost control. (Falk, 1977: 182).

A national health service plan would fund and organize medical care differently. One proposal for a national health service was introduced in Congress by Representative Ronald Dellums in 1977 as "The Health Service Act" (*Congressional Record,* May 4, 1977). While NHI is essentially a form of financing medical care, a national health service reorganizes medical services in addition to having the federal government pay for those services directly. Under the plan of the Health Service Act, for example, medical care would essentially be nationalized, eliminating the making of profit at any point in the health care process. Health services would in large measure be controlled by local community boards made up of consumers (two-thirds) and health care providers (one-third). These local boards would develop and implement plans to meet the needs of the particular communities they serve, and would also set up a non-profit corporation which would coordinate health services, employ all health workers (including physicians), and set standards of quality for all medical services. The mainstay of such a program is that it is designed to be controlled by communities of consumers and workers in the health care system. It would be primarily oriented to *preventive* health maintenance, including public health services. Such a system clearly differs from the provider-dominated, curative system we now have and which would, essentially, remain unchanged under NHI plans before Congress.

In "National Health Insurance—A Dream Whose Time Has Come?" Richard Margolis provides an excellent summary and review of recent NHI proposals before Congress. The costs and benefits of these plans vary, but all involve establishment of rules and procedures for payment of premiums, coverage of medical services, and mechanisms for controlling costs, as well as spelling out the role of the private sector and establishing the relative authority of federal, state, and local governments in the program. Some NHI plans are essentially expanded versions of the current system of piecemeal insurance coverage, while others make a significant effort to design a uniform insurance plan for all. The past decade has seen significant shifts, however, in the type of plans proposed. There has been a narrowing of the coverage in some plans, from comprehensive health care to the payment for catastrophic disease only (Myer, 1976). Margolis gives us a good idea of the range of and differences in proposed NHI plans, and notes that an adequate national health insurance plan is widely perceived as a critical national need.[2]

The second article in this debate, "National Health Insurance: The Great Leap Sideways," is by John Ehrenreich and Oliver Fein. They acknowledge that national health insurance will be a "useful reform for many Americans," as was Medicaid and Medicare before it. However, they argue, any national health insurance plan will fail to solve the problems of financing medical care, and will be ineffective in changing the maldistribution, inaccessibility, and inadequacy of health care which many critics agree plague our current medical care system.

Notes

1. Although all the proposals for NHI currently before Congress include private insurance companies as intermediaries, the original NHI plan submitted by

Senator Ted Kennedy omitted private insurance companies by substituting a public form of financing. That bill, supported by national labor organizations, was stalled in Senator Wilbur Mills' Ways and Means Committee—as a result of heavy lobbying by the insurance industry—until Kennedy changed the plan to include the private insurance carriers.

2. Although some of the current NHI proposals differ in title and content, they essentially mirror the six Margolis discusses.

References

Bodenheimer, Thomas, Steven Cummings and Elizabeth Harding. 1974. "Capitalizing on illness: The health insurance industry." International Journal of Health Services. 4, 4.

Congressional Record. 1977. House of Representatives, Vol. 123, No. 75, May 4.

Falk, I.S. 1977. "Proposals for national health insurance in the U.S.A.: Origins, and evolution, and some perceptions for the future." Milbank Memorial Fund Quarterly, Health and Society. Spring: 161–191.

Harris, Richard. 1969. A Sacred Trust. Baltimore, Maryland: Penguin Books Inc.

Lander, Louise. 1975. National Health Insurance. Health/PAC in cooperation with The Institute for Policy Studies. (Available from Health/PAC, 17 Murray St., New York NY 10007).

Mauksch, Ingeborg G. 1978. "On national health insurance." American Journal of Nursing. August: 1323–1327.

Meyer, Michael F. 1976. "The national health insurance debate: Shifts toward reality?" Journal of Health Politics, Policy and Law. Vol. 1, No. 1, Spring: 13–17.

32

National Health Insurance— The Dream Whose Time Has Come?

Richard J. Margolis

The socialization of medicine is coming. . . . The time now is here for the medical profession to acknowledge that it is tired of the eternal struggle for advantage over one's neighbor.—THE A.M.A. JOURNAL (1914).

During the next four years, Jimmy Carter and the Congress will probably decide whether universal national health insurance—a dream so long deferred that scholars call it "the lost reform"—shall at last be deemed an idea whose time has come, or whether it shall remain an idea that is merely long overdue. Something more than our health appears to be at stake: as with other tough social dilemmas (segregation, for example), this one raises questions about the resources and capacities of our political institutions. In particular, it tests our abilities to overcome the great weight of health-care inertia, a weight that seems to be composed in roughly equal parts of history, bureaucracy, and avarice.

The opinion polls suggest that a sizable majority of Americans is now ready for fundamental changes in health care, and the President appears publicly committed to such changes. The 1976 Democratic platform, largely a Carter creation, calls for "a comprehensive national health-insurance system with universal and mandatory coverage"—meaning a program that goes about as far as it can go: all of the people insured all of the time for all of their care.

Nothing could be simpler; nor, if the past turns out to be prologue, more difficult to achieve. The fact is, we have been here before. The history of national health insurance in this country is strewn with predictions about its imminent arrival.

Part of the trouble may arise from the complexity of our burgeoning medical system, which defies instant rehabilitation, and from the apparently high price we must pay for its reform. Many of the recently tried solutions, notably Medicare and Medicaid, have themselves become part of the problem, encouraging waste and driving up costs. Thus far, at least, reform has played handmaiden to inflation. Nowadays, we spend 8.6 percent of our gross national product on health care, about double the portion two decades ago.

The new Congress and the new President will have to confront this general paradox of social progress, in which measures designed to lighten the burden of some may end by increasing the burden of all. As regards the medical-care paradox, it is not as if there have not been efforts to resolve it. Ever since that A.M.A. Journal editor 62 years ago urged doctors to quit "the eternal struggle for advantage over one's neighbor," reformers have been plumping for national health insurance (without, however, any further encouragement from the A.M.A., which soon changed both its mind and its leadership). Franklin D. Roosevelt came within an ace of combining health insurance with Social Security in 1935, only to be dissuaded by the A.M.A., notably by Dr. Harvey Cushing, author, brain surgeon and father-in-law of young James Roosevelt.

Whatever recommendations FDR might decide to make, Cushing wrote to the President, "no legislation can be effective without the good will of the American Medical Association, which has the organization to put it to work." In the politics of health reform, Cushing's comment remains the heart of the matter; and nowadays politicians must seek the cooperation not only of the A.M.A. but also of other health interest groups that have grown up in the interim. Over the decades our health-care system has invented a potpourri of patchwork schemes as substitutes for "the lost reform," and each new expedient, Blue Cross, for example, in the 30s and 40s, has given rise to a new organization in Washington. Like all newcomers, these organizations have become instantly suspicious of change and broadly committed to things as they are. If Cushing were alive today, he could cite at least four other groups whose goodwill may now be required: the "Blues," the private insurance industry, the hospitals and the medical schools.

The battle did not end with the New Deal. Harry S. Truman took up the cudgels, to secure passage of the Murray-Wagner-Dingell bill, a measure the A.M.A. dismissed as "Marxist medicine." It never reached the floor of Congress, but it has since seen several reincarnations.

Considering the discouraging record, it wasn't any wonder that both John F. Kennedy and Lyndon B. Johnson chose to fight on narrower ground. Each came to the White House prepared to settle for something less than "the lost reform." With the passage of Medicare and Medicaid in 1965, the Congress conferred the blessings of free or low-cost medical care upon both the elderly and the poor. The new programs enlarged the public's sense of possibilities. If we are closer now to the Promised Land, it is because the events of 1965 showed us a way out of the wilderness.

No sooner, it seemed, had the bills been signed into law than news of yet another "health care crisis"—it was really the same old one—spread throughout the land. LBJ called on Congress to do something about "the soaring cost of medical care," and also about "the inexcusably high rate of infant mortality in the United States." (Seventeen countries still have rates below ours.) A few years later Richard M. Nixon sounded the familiar alarm: "We face a massive crisis in health care, and unless action is taken . . . we will have a breakdown in our medical care system."

The Congress began to consider new measures, a fresh generation of legislative proposals that would extend the protection of health insurance to some or all of the remaining population. Such proposals have grown more numerous of late. In the last Congress, the 94th, no less than 18 different bills were submitted, each alleging to offer the most practical solutions. These plans are Jimmy Carter's health reform legacy.

If the titles sound maddeningly alike, their contents exhibit some real differences. By and large, they reflect the contradictory hopes of people and organizations who have something to gain or lose from the redistribution of health care in America—doctors, hospitals, insurers, medical schools and patients. As consumers and taxpayers, one can try to test the merits of the proposals by keeping close to two familiar touchstones: the benefits offered and the costs incurred. In addition, one can examine any bill for its reform potential, meaning the extent to which it can be expected to reorganize health care along lines that make sense.

Of the 18 now before Congress a half-dozen perhaps can be considered "major," either because of the power and celebrity of their Congressional sponsors or because of the influence of their outside backers. Like the lobbies that support them, these six are a mixed bag. All but one would make health insurance compulsory. They range from a modest proposal that would extend benefits to citizens who have incurred unusually high medical costs—the so-called "Catastrophic Health Insurance and Medical Assistance Reform Act," introduced by Democratic Senators Russell Long of Louisiana and Abraham Ribicoff of Connecticut—to the sweeping "Health Security" measure that Senator Edward M. Kennedy has been promoting since 1969.

Taken together, the six proposals offer a fair sampling of what the experts are thinking, what the health care industry is demanding as ransom and what the public is wishing. What we see is what we may get. Before we pursue this pharmacopeia—an all-Democratic drugstore, no less—it may be well to glance at one object of great attention, what commentators are pleased to call "the national health-care delivery system." In truth, it is less a system than a collection of medical sins and services, a network that appears to be ever-expanding and ever more remote from the patient. Most of us have sensed the new remoteness, both in the reckonings we get and in the services we do not.

We are the world's only industrialized nation without a universal health-insurance program; yet no country on earth spends as much per capita as do we on health care. In a single generation, the total price has soared from $12 billion (in 1950) to $133 billion (in fiscal 1976), making health care America's third largest industry, just behind agriculture and construction. Some of the increase reflects genuine improvements in medicine, and some can be attributed to a wider distribution of services; but much of it must be chalked up to medical inflation pure and simple. Hospital charges, for instance, have risen four times as fast during the past decade as the Consumer Price Index itself.

Health care inflation is not a new problem; it has long been a fixture on the medical landscape. "Everywhere," lamented the health demographer Louis I. Dublin in 1927, "there is a feeling that something is wrong with the economics of medicine. Large numbers of middle-class families . . . chafe under what they generally consider the unjustifiably heavy cost." With the passage of Medicare and Medicaid, however, inflation took a quantum leap: Costs more than tripled, while annual per capita expenditures shot up 250 percent. In 1965, the average American spent $198 for health care; last fiscal year the sum was more than $500. The alarming spiral seems to have a life of its own; it has proved confoundedly resistant to voluntary self-controls and to Congressional tinkering, like the introduction two years ago of "peer review" for all treatments paid for by the federal government.

The dismal history of the medical dollar has made many wary of starting another round of reform. Yet there seems nothing mysterious or inevitable about medical inflation; in theory, at least, it can be controlled. Richard Nixon came close to doing just that with his 1971–74 price freeze, when health-care prices climbed at about one-third their usual rate. What seems chiefly at fault is Medicare's and Medicaid's peculiar method of reimbursement, whereby they pay whatever the doctor or the hospital claims to be "reasonable" and "customary." In effect, the Congress has handed a blank check to the health care industry, with predictable results. Not only has the industry jacked up prices for unimproved services, in many instances it has submitted bills for services never rendered. Fraud begets inflation.

It is true that only about one-third of the national health care bill is charged directly to consumers. The rest is paid for by the Federal Government, the states and the private insurance companies. But the citizen ultimately pays those bills, too, in higher taxes and stiffer premiums. Medicare premiums have been hiked a half dozen times since the program's inception; during the same period, Blue Cross rates in some areas have risen fourfold.

Although four-fifths of the population is covered by some kind of health insurance, the protection afforded is often skimpy and unreliable. In last year's recession an estimated 27 million workers and their families were deprived of coverage because of layoffs. Many of the policies still in force, moreover, fail to protect patients against the costs of home care or visits to the doctor's office. Close to half the people who file pleas for bankruptcies each year do so because of medical debts.

Americans might bear these medical burdens more cheerfully were they getting their money's worth; but if the price of health care isn't right, neither is the product. As nearly everyone knows by now, the medical network suffers from several strains of maldistribution, both professional and geographic. Chief among these is a surplus of specialists, particularly of surgeons, and a shortage of primary care physicians—internists, pediatricians and general practitioners.

Officially certified specialties have been part of the health care scene since 1917, when eye doctors founded the American Board of Ophthalmology. Since then physicians have created more than 20 board-recognized specialties along with some 200 subspecialties, and each year they have attracted a larger proportion of medical school graduates. In 1931, only 17 percent of the nation's doctors were specialists: today the figure is 72 percent.

The imbalance has tended to drive up costs still more (specialists usually charge more than G.P.s) and to reduce patients to the status of machines with broken parts; it is another symptom of medical remoteness. In surgery, according to more than one Congressional committee, the surplus of specialists has created a greater "demand" for operations, which is to say that some surgeons examine their bank accounts before they examine their patients. At least two million of the operations performed each year are said to be unnecessary, and these lead to some 15,000 preventable deaths.

The geography of health care seems equally unjust, but for the contrary reason: too few doctors, in some places, rather than too many. Because most of the nation's 378,000 physicians locate their practices within easy reach of the affluent, the residents of urban ghettos and rural areas frequently find themselves shortchanged; they are medical orphans. To cite one of the many available statistics, the state of Mississippi, relatively poor and rural, has only 82 doctors for every 100,000 citizens, while in suburban Westchester County, N.Y., the comparable ratio is 260 per 100,000. At last count some 5000 towns in 135 counties in the United States had no doctor at all: One of them was Webster County, Ga., the county next door to Jimmy Carter's.

The desperate shortage of health care personnel in some areas works to strengthen local medical oligopolies, inviting its practitioners to profit at the patient's expense. I came across an instance of how this can occur, and the misery it can cause, when I interviewed a woman who lives in the hills of eastern Kentucky. One day, she told me, her 4-year-old son, Danny, complained of a pain in his stomach.

"I didn't have much money, but Danny was in awful pain, so I paid somebody to ride me into Prestonsburg. The doctor, he looked at Danny. He said the boy had to be operated before his appendix ruptured, but first I had to work things out with the hospital director. Me and Danny went to the director. He told me it would cost $350 and I would have to give a $100 down payment. I said I didn't have no $100. He said, 'Well, when you get it come back, and we'll fix your boy up.' My Danny was vomiting right there in the director's office. He was real sick. I went and borrowed the money from a cousin, and I came back with the money. The director, he says, 'you have to show you got an income so as you can pay the debt.' I said all I ever get is a check every month from the Veterans for $57. He said that would be just fine. Then he made me sign a paper promising to turn over the check to him each month till the bill was paid. I couldn't fight him. My Danny had to be operated."

One story does not make a pattern, but the hearing rooms of Congress over the past few years have resonated with hundreds of such tales. The impression one gets overall is that something has gone sour in American health care and that money has had a lot to do with it—which may be why more patients are writing their Congressmen nowadays.

Overlaid upon all these headaches is the increasingly widespread suspicion that the health care network, having run amok, is now beyond political reach and therefore beyond redemption. Its phenomenal growth in recent years has been unruly and unplanned, and that is a major part of the problem. But in the political arena the industry, for all its disunity and competing claims, has presented a single face to the public. It is the face of an institution that does not suffer reform gladly.

So: back to the pharmacopeia.

Besides Kennedy-Corman and Long-Ribicoff, four proposals seem worth considering, listed here in a sequence that runs from the relatively broad and generous to the relatively narrow and penny-pinching:

The "Comprehensive Health Insurance Plan" (CHIP), introduced by Kentucky Democratic Representative Lee Carter—no relation. It has been called a "block off the old CHIP" because it closely resembles a bill of the same name that the Nixon Administration submitted to the Congress in 1973. A nearly identical plan, moreover, in 1974 almost got past Wilbur Mills' House Ways and Means Committee, the historic gatekeeper of health reform.

A complex proposal submitted by Representative Al Ullman, an Oregon Democrat, who succeeded Mills as Ways and Means chairman; it is called the "National Health Care Services Reorganization and Financing Act," quite a mouthful, and it has the official blessings of the American Hospital Association.

The A.M.A.'s latest entry, "The Comprehensive Health Care Insurance Act," sponsored by Representative Richard Fulton, a Tennessee Democrat.

And "The National Health Care Act," a favorite of the Health Insurance Association of America (HIAA). It was introduced by two conservative Democrats, Senator Thomas McIntyre of New Hampshire and Representative Omar Burleson of Texas.

As might be expected, not all of the bills confront all of the problems; by and large they concentrate on ways of defraying patient costs and of spreading patient benefits, with the unspoken hope that the rest will take care of itself. Still, with the exception of Long-Ribicoff—which continues Medicare's blank-check system of reimbursement—the proposals do make an effort to curb inflation. The chief restraining device envisioned in these bills entails an annual round of negotiations, with doctors and hospitals, on all fees and rates; an attempt to commit the health care industry each year to an immutable schedule of charges. In all but the Kennedy-Corman measure, the responsibility for negotiating these schedules is assigned to the individual states; only Kennedy-Corman, which we shall consider first, sees the federal government as prime negotiator.

The Kennedy-Corman Health Security bill calls for a compulsory federalized system of health care managed within HEW by a five-member health-security board, and financed chiefly through a half-and-half combination of payroll taxes and general revenues. As is the case with most of the other bills, the payroll taxes are shared by employers and employees. The benefits offered by Kennedy-Corman are broad, generous, and virtually free of the kinds of restrictions one finds in the other proposals. But the benefits are not the whole story; what distinguishes this bill from all others is its unique approach to budgeting, an approach that makes private enterprise an instrument of public policy.

Health Security stops short of nationalizing the health care system, but it does nationalize the health care budget. Every dollar spent—whether for construction of a new hospital or for purchase of a new tongue depressor—becomes a federal dollar. The budgeting process is supposed to begin at the local levels where groups of consumers and professionals annually assess their health care needs and estimate the costs. These estimates filter up through a regionalized system and eventually land in Washington on the health-security board's desk, becoming part of the year's national health care budget.

Cost controls under Kennedy-Corman turn traditional procedures upside-down: The bill stipulates that the annual health care budget cannot exceed expected revenues, thereby tying the medical budget to the fortunes of the general economy. If the economy should slip, the federal government would have to negotiate a reduced budget, and the bill's supporters insist that the burden of such a reduction would be assumed not by the patient but by the health care providers. In other words, rather than curtailing services, Kennedy-Corman would curtail the fees and rates paid to doctors and hospitals. The proposal thus jeopardizes the industry's time-honored privilege of controlling fees and services, one reason for the measure's bad reputation among medical practitioners. On the other hand, it enjoys sustained support from both the AFL-CIO and the United Auto Workers, as well as from a coalition of church groups and liberal-leaning organizations like Common Cause and the Urban League. It is the only proposal thus far to have attracted substantial consumer backing.

The Long-Ribicoff proposal is a "major-medical" plan to insure patients against costly illness. Its benefits, presumably, begin about the time a patient has run out of money: after he has spent $2,000 for medical services or has been in the hospital for 60 days. An employer can buy this insurance for his employee either from the government, in which case he pays a one percent payroll tax, or he can choose a government-approved private plan—Blue Cross, for instance. (As with nearly all the bills, this one makes special provision for both the self-employed and the poor.)

Compared with Kennedy's Health Security proposal, Long-Ribicoff seems both paltry and narrow. It leaves the gears and levers of the health care enterprise untouched, and the benefits it provides, while they may save some families from bankruptcy, are far from dazzling. Still, the measure has a certain appeal. It is simple and can be immediately "put into place," as the health analysts like to say, whereas most of the other plans would take years to become fully effective. It is also inexpensive, at least from the standpoint of federal budgeting; and it can be seen not as the Grand Solution but as merely a first step toward eventual enactment of "the lost reform."

Finally, the bill gives the health-insurance industry a piece of the action, an idea that may or may not have merit, but which in any case can be seen to make some tactical sense. It will come as no surprise that the private insurance companies are said to have bestowed their tacit approval upon this modest measure—in fact, to have taken a hand in its drafting. A Kennedy-Corman aficionado claims last year to have seen "at least a dozen of the insurance boys from Hartford in the back of the hearing room, just before the hearing started, making last-minute changes in the bill." The Ribicoff aides I have talked to say this is news to them; but it is true that an earlier version of the Long-Ribicoff bill provided for *federal insurance only,* leaving no room for participation by private companies.

In any event, because Senator Long is chairman of the Finance Committee, the womb from which any successful Senate bill must issue, the proposal has not lacked for a public platform.

Nor has CHIP, the Nixon bill that never dies. Benefits under CHIP are in some respects as far-reaching as those under Kennedy-Corman, but they include a $150 deductible for each person and also a 25 percent "coinsurance" requirement; that is, the family must pay either one-fourth of its health care charges or $1,500, whichever is less during a given year. All this is to be financed not by taxes but by premiums paid directly to private insurance companies by employees and their employers; the latter group pays the larger share.

Unlike the other two bills, CHIP leaves virtually all of the program's management to insurance firms and to the individual states, with the federal government playing a small, regulatory role. Each state makes its own reimbursement policy, deciding how much money doctors and other providers should be paid for their services. The formula is similar to that now being used under Medicaid, and given that program's record, it is not a promising one. Nevertheless, CHIP has impressed some Congressmen as a workable compromise between "the two extremes" of catastrophic insurance and Health Security. It offers citizens more than the first and it costs the government less than the second.

The remaining three proposals, like CHIP, give citizens a chance to buy private health insurance at modest cost, entitling them to a variety of benefits, but the benefits are hedged with coinsurance charges and other limits, and they, too, are essentially devoid of cost controls, with all administrative responsibility ceded to the states. What makes these proposals interesting is not the substance of their ideas but the nature of their support. Each is officially backed by a different lobby, and each can tell us something about the aspirations of the health care network.

Al Ullman's bill, backed by the American Hospital Association, may be the most Byzantine. Besides the insurance and financing provisions, the act mandates creation in every locale of health care corporations to which citizens may subscribe in advance of services. Apparently, these corporations would function as health-maintenance organizations (HMOs), which is what medical commentators now call groups that offer services on a prepaid basis. The doctors working for HMOs earn salaries, or else are paid capitation fees—so much per member-patient. Either way, they are cut loose from standard fee-for-service arrangements and thus from temptations to overcharge or overtreat. Studies have shown that in HMOs the incidence of needless surgery is far less than it is in fee-for-service practice.

All of which sounds promising—but it is not clear from the bill how these local health care corporations would operate or whether, in fact, an employer or employee could not skirt the corporation entirely and buy his health care from other sources. What does seem clear is that hospitals would play a central role in the new system, since in most places they are the only institutions extant that are capable of developing and managing so complex a plan.

The A.M.A.'s bill is less generous than CHIP and less ambitious than Ullman's. It would leave fee-for-service practice and private-insurance precedents unscathed, with the federal government content to mandate the size of the premiums the subscribers would pay and to let the system lurch ahead on its own. To the self-employed wishing to buy insurance, the bill offers a few tax advantages; to the poor it provides "subsidy certificates" they can cash in at their local insurance company. As inadequate as this seems, it represents the furthest A.M.A. members have yet traveled down the road to "Marxist medicine." An earlier, and less-liberal, A.M.A.-backed measure, Medi-credit, had to be discarded after the post-Watergate elections of 1974, when 55 of its Congressional sponsors were defeated. (The AFL-CIO ran a nationwide campaign to unseat these enemies of Health Security, using the slogan "Your Congressman may be dangerous to your health.")

Finally, there is the "National Health Care Act," the darling of the HIAA. It has the distinction of being the only plan among the six that permits employers to dismiss it—which is to say that the program is strictly voluntary. If an employer chooses not to buy in, his employees are out of luck. In consequence, the bill has been given short shrift everywhere but in the executive suites of insurance companies. As a labor lobbyist remarked recently, "When you get a proposal that offers less than the A.M.A. does, what have you got? . . . Nothing."

We can pay our money, then, and take our choice, though it is not at all certain just how much money we shall have to pay. A recent HEW study indicates that all six programs are costly—some are more costly than others, but the differences may not be all that great.

The man who conducted the study is Gordon R. Trapnell, a consulting actuary. According to Trapnell, if we enact no new health care programs during the rest of the decade and continue spending at the present rate, medical costs will rise to $180.2 billion by 1980–a gain of about 30 percent over this year's tab. From that empyrean base, Trapnell calculated the additional costs that might be incurred by each of the six plans, concluding that the three cheapest were Long-Ribicoff, CHIP and the HIAA's voluntary plan. Each would cost at least an extra $10 billion annually. The other three proposals would each run more than twice that amount—an additional $20 billion in the case of the A.M.A.'s program, and an extra $25 billion for Ullman or Kennedy-Corman.

Trapnell's estimates suggest that health care inflation will remain part of the picture regardless of which program the Congress enacts. Any new plan, he notes, will increase administrative expenses and encourage wider use of medical services, especially among the poor. Yet supporters of Kennedy-Corman continue to insist that their proposal is more or less inflation-proof—in part, because it subsidizes *preventive* medicine and, in part, because its budget is linked to national productivity. "We have the only measure with built-in controls," says Max Fine, who directs the Committee for National Health Insurance, a labor-financed lobby.

Many remain skeptical, among them HEW's Saul Waldman, whose detailed 210-page summary of all 18 health-insurance bills is the bible of analysts and lobbyists alike. "Nobody really knows whether Health Security could keep the lid on," he says. "True, there's a ceiling on the budget,

The Six Key Health-Insurance Plans

Bill	National Support	Estimated Cost by 1980	Administration
Kennedy-Corman	AFL-CIO, Committee for National Health Insurance.	$24.8 billion	Special board within HEW; regional and local offices will operate program.
CHIP	No formal support.	$11.3 billion	Insurance through private carriers: states to supervise under federal regulations.
Ullman	American Hospital Association.	$25.1 billion	Private insurance carriers under state supervision, according to federal guidelines.

Financing	Benefits
Half to come from federal general revenues, half from special taxes; 1 percent of payroll for employees, 2.5 percent for employers and self-employed.	Institutional services: hospital care, skilled nursing facilities up to 120 days. Diagnosis and treatment: physicians' services, lab and X-ray, home health services, prescription drugs (for chronic illnesses), medical supplies and appliances. Other services: physical checkups, well-child care, maternity, family planning, dental care (up to age 25), vision care and eyeglasses, hearing care and hearing aids. Patient cost-sharing: none.
Employer-employee premium payments, with employer paying 75 percent (65 percent first three years); special provisions for small employers and those with high increases in payroll costs.	Institutional services: hospital care, skilled nursing facilities up to 100 days. Diagnosis and treatment: physicians' services, lab and X-ray, home health services (up to 100 visits), prescription drugs, medical supplies and appliances. Other services: well-child care, maternity, family planning, dental care (under age 13), hearing care and hearing aids (under age 13). Patient cost-sharing: annual deductible* of $150 per person; 25 percent coinsurance,** with annual ceiling of $1,500 per family.
Employer-employee premium payments, with employer paying at least 75 percent; Federal subsidy for low-income workers and certain small employers; patients enrolling in health-care corporation get 10 percent subsidy.	Institutional services: hospital care up to 90 days, skilled nursing facilities (30 days), health-related custodial nursing home care (90 days.) Diagnosis and treatment: physicians' services up to 10 visits, lab and X-ray, home health services (100 days), prescription drugs limited to specified conditions, medical supplies and appliances. Other services: physical checkups, well-child care, maternity, dental care (under age 13), vision care and eyeglasses (under age 13). Patient cost-sharing: coinsurance (20 percent) or co-payments*** (up to $5) on most items; special "catastrophic" provisions become effective when patient's out-of-pocket expenses reach a specified amount.

*Deductible: Patient's share of annual medical costs before insurance coverage begins.
**Coinsurance: the percentage of a given bill that is charged to the patient.
***Copayment: a flat rate charged to the insured patient on specific items (such as $2 per office visit).

The Six Key Health-Insurance Plans (cont'd)

Bill	National Support	Estimated Cost by 1980	Administration
Fulton	American Medical Association	$20.3 billion	Private carriers provide insurance under state supervision; regulations issued by a new federal board.
Burleson-McIntyre	Health Insurance Association of America.	$11 billion	Insurance administered by private carriers under state supervision; plan is voluntary.
Long-Ribicoff	No formal support	$9.8 billion	Employers and employees have two choices: to join Federal insurance program administered by HEW, or to buy private insurance from federally approved carriers, under HEW supervision.

Financing	Benefits
Employer-employee premium payments, with employer paying at least 65 percent; small employers get Federal help as do all employers with unusual payroll cost increases; self-employed pay own premiums but are assisted by income-tax credits computed on a sliding scale (the lower the income, the higher the credits).	Institutional services: hospital care, skilled nursing facilities up to 100 days. Diagnosis and treatment: physicians' services, lab and X-ray, home health services, medical supplies and equipment. Other services: physical checkups, well-child care, maternity, family planning, dental care (under age 18). Patient cost-sharing: 20 percent coinsurance, with an annual maximum of $1,500 per person and $2,000 per family.
Employer-employee premium payments, the ratios to be negotiated between them; low-income workers pay less; self-employed pay entire premium; all participants eligible for special tax deductions.	Institutional services: hospital care, skilled nursing facilities up to 180 days. Diagnosis and treatment: physicians' services, lab and X-ray, home health care (270 days), prescription drugs, medical supplies and appliances. Other services: well-child care, maternity, family planning, dental care (under age 13, one visit), vision care (under age 13, one visit). Patient cost-sharing: annual deductible of $100 per person; 20 percent coinsurance on all items, with annual family limit of $1,000.
Employers pay one percent payroll tax and are allowed similar provisions for self-employed.	Institutional services: hospital care, skilled nursing facilities up to 100 days. Diagnosis and treatment: physicians' services, lab and X-ray, home health services, medical supplies and appliances. Other services: None. Patient cost-sharing: first 60 days of hospitalization not covered; first $2,000 in family medical expenses not covered.

but there's also a clause in the bill that says Congress can be asked for supplemental funds in case of emergencies. The emergency wouldn't necessarily have to be medical, like an epidemic; it could be an *economic* emergency."

On balance, though, the Kennedy-Corman bill does appear to encourage a fiscal climate in which health care prices will rise no faster than prices over-all. The probability under Kennedy-Corman is one of controlled inflation, something we haven't seen in health care circles since the Nixon price freeze; it would amount to a mild revolution within the health care industry—a revolution of reimbursements.

But the revolution that Health Security invites us all to join goes beyond fiscal policy. At bottom, it represents a major shift of power and responsibility within the health care network, a shift away from state governments and private insurance companies toward HEW and the federal bureaucracy. All other plans cede administrative control to the states (under federal guidelines) and commercial control to the private insurers. In opposing Kennedy-Corman, the health-insurance industry is fighting for its very existence. The stakes are high. Last year the industry collected nearly $30 billion in premiums.

Dr. Cushing's law writ large is that no legislation can be effective without the goodwill of health care interest groups. In assessing the various alternatives, Congress and the President will have to ask themselves whether the superior efficiency and the more generous benefits claimed by Kennedy-Corman are worth the wrench. The other bills' sponsors have already answered the question. "Health Security is too risky," notes Dr. Susan Irving, a health economist who works for Senator Ribicoff. "You can't simply dismantle the insurance industry and expect no consequences. Besides, who said the HEW could run the program efficiently? Its record with Medicare suggests the opposite." Ned Helms, a health specialist on Senator McIntyre's staff, says, "There are 500,000 people working in private health insurance. Are we supposed to fire them or turn them into federal bureaucrats in the name of health reform?"

The public could make a difference by agitating for one or another approach, but in matters of health reform the public has always been remarkably passive. Even in recent years, with all those bills floating around Congress, citizen interest has seemed anything but keen. The health reform debate of the past eight years owes less to public pressures than it does to presidential politics. Because, until recently, Senator Kennedy was viewed as a prime presidential threat, his introduction of Health Security in 1969 acted as an enzyme in the chemistry of health reform. Richard Nixon responded by announcing his own Family Insurance Plan (FIP), a measure he never got around to submitting. A few years later, with Kennedy again a presidential possibility, FIP gave way to

CHIP, a plan Nixon at one point insisted was $47 billion cheaper than Kennedy's.

In 1974, Gerald Ford was in the White House; Wilbur Mills was still presiding over Ways and Means, and CHIP came close to winning that committee's approval. It did so because Ford, looking to 1976, needed an answer to Health Security, and Mills needed a bill that would buttress his rickety reputation. And the measure failed, largely because most Americans were not aware that it existed. (It failed, too, because the labor unions withheld support; they were counting on the fall elections to bring them a "veto-proof Congress" ready to fling Health Security in Ford's face.)

"The politicians," recalls Paul Rettig, counsel for the Ways and Means health subcommittee, "did not perceive national health insurance as a deeply felt public issue." In the end, and without much fear of public complaint, Ford pulled out, personally telling one of Mills's deputies that CHIP no longer had presidential backing. "After that," says Rettig, "we were just dancing."

The dance goes on, while lobbyists mark up their bills and patients await "the lost reform" or a reasonable facsimile thereof. "Political life," observed the late Hannah Arendt, "is based on the assumption that we can produce equality through organization." If, in the case of national health insurance, that cheerful supposition seems shaky, it may be because there is so much to organize and so little equality to start with. Perhaps Jimmy Carter, a passionate reorganizer, will be able to make sense of it all; perhaps he can come up with a plan that pleases everyone, even the health care industry. Thus far, he has kept his own counsel. The few utterances he has made on the subject have been tactful but contradictory. He has, on various occasions, emphasized his belief in "compulsory health insurance," "voluntarism," "immediate action," "a phased-in approach," "universal and comprehensive benefits," "inflation controls," " a federal role" and "local initiative." No wonder every Congressman I talked to thought his particular health bill had Carter's secret support. They were blind legislators feeling different parts of the Carter elephant (or donkey).

Nevertheless, after the rhetoric of transition has settled, Carter will have to face up to the hard choices. The best guess is that he will appoint a health task force similar to the Committee on Economic Security that FDR created in 1934. The task force will make recommendations; more important, it will give Carter time to do what Presidents before him have had to do: negotiate. The upshot, to continue the guess may well be a CHIP-type program (Nixon's legacy) that offers a slice of the pie to everyone—doctors, hospitals, insurers, and patients. Such a prospect is both scary and pleasing: all that money, all those benefits. But no one can predict anything for certain about the future of health reform.

33

National Health Insurance: The Great Leap Sideways

John Ehrenreich and Oliver Fein

. . . .

Proposals for National Health Insurance are nothing new in the nation's health history. What is new in the 1970 situation is the army of political forces forming to push for some form of National Health Insurance. On the one flank is the public, led on by the mass media to expect ever-greater miracles from the medical magicians, but increasingly frustrated in their ability to obtain even ordinary nostrums. On the other flank is labor, management, the hospitals, Blue Cross, the companies that manufacture and sell hospital supplies, and local and state governments, each faced with an increasingly serious set of problems growing out of the horse-and-buggy methods of financing medical services, each coming to one or another brand of National Health Insurance as a possible solution to its own special health care crisis.

"Labor's number one legislative goal . . . is National Health Insurance," declared AFL-CIO President George Meany, "and the AFL-CIO believes it can—and must—be enacted." Labor needs National Health Insurance to eliminate the hassle at the bargaining table over health fringe benefits, which have taken increasingly larger bites out of the wage package. In 1965, for example, in the steel industry, 19 cents an hour, or 4 percent of the average steel workers' total wages and benefits, went for health and life insurance. Today, because medical prices have gone up two to three times as fast as prices in general, as much as 8 percent to 10 percent of any new wage and benefit package must go to health and life insurance, just to maintain the existing health benefits. At a time when the real disposable income of American workers has stopped growing for the first time in 35 years (due largely to inflation and increased taxes because of the Vietnam war), labor is desperate to find ways to augment workers' wages. Relegating health insurance to the government leaves more dollars and cents for wage increases.

Increasingly, elements of management, particularly in big business, are also flirting with National Health Insurance. For these businessmen, health insurance premiums have become a significant and rapidly rising component of their overall labor costs. Businesses would like to stabilize the contribution they make for their employees' health care: predictability of costs permits planning for larger profits. In addition, National Health Insurance may shift part of management's labor costs (i.e., the health insurance component) onto government, leading to greater profits. This shift of labor costs from management to government would be limited to those large industrial employers whom labor has already compelled to make substantial contributions to health insurance. The marginal, small shop and agricultural employer who now makes little or no contribution to health insurance for his employees, may find National Health Insurance increases his labor costs. While management is not unified on the issue of National Health Insurance, those that count (big business and industry) are increasingly for one or another form of such insurance.

Of the medical-industrial complex—the hospital supply and equipment companies, the medical electronics and computer companies, and at least those drug companies who are diversified into hospital supplies—all would benefit from National Health Insurance. Their experience with Medicare and Medicaid has been profitable. National Health Insurance, like Medicare before it, would provide the dollars to guarantee the demand, and thereby still the lingering doubts that many companies have about the advisability of government involvement in health.

For the voluntary (private, nonprofit) hospitals, almost any program of National Health Insurance would be better than the present Medicaid program. Eligibility has become so restricted under Medicaid that many patients are no longer covered. That leaves the hospitals stuck with the bills of patients who are too rich for Medicaid but too poor to pay. A National Health Insurance program allows the possibility of universal coverage without eligibility restrictions. Equally important, National Health Insurance would stabilize hospital income by guaranteeing a certain level of reimbursement. Government will be reluctant to cut a program that affects a large cross-section of Americans. Of course, the voluntaries would prefer a National Health Insurance plan which merely subsidized their operations with minimal interference from government. But almost any form of National Health Insurance would be better than none.

Blue Cross/Blue Shield, the most important non-governmental health financer, while certainly not wild about any government take-over of the health insurance business, would settle for a brand of National Health Insurance that would expand Blue Cross hegemony over the health insurance market. Although Blue Cross enrollment has flowered over the last decades, its percentage of the health insurance market has been declining. In 1945, Blue Cross insured 61 percent of the hospital insurance market compared to 33 percent by the commercial insurance companies. Today, that figure is reversed for the population under age 65, with Blue Cross garnering only 34 percent of the hospital insurance market compared to 60 percent by the commercial insurance companies. However, Medicare and Medicaid represented a big boost to Blue Cross since virtually every state turned over administration of their programs to Blue Cross. It is just such a relationship to National Health Insurance that Blue Cross wishes to foster. Parenthetically, even the commercial insurance companies are not total in their opposition to all varieties of National Health Insurance. For example, the president of Aetna has said, "A program for universal health insurance . . . could be structured to retain the advantages of competition and the profit incentive. . . . I have full confidence in our ability to work successfully in partnership with government."

Finally, local and state governments see rising costs for their health programs (state and city hospitals, Medicaid, etc.) as an unlimited drain on already scarce funds. Any program that shifts parts of the burden off their backs is welcome. As a result, even the most ardent states' righters voted enthusiastically to support New York Governor Nelson Rockefeller's National Health Insurance proposals at the 1969 National Governors' Conference.

Labor, big business, parts of the medical-industrial complex, the voluntary hospitals, Blue Cross, and local governments—all are attracted by some form of National Health Insurance. The growing consensus on the need for a National Health *Insurance* program will increase pressure . . . [on the federal government] to respond with more than minor "reforms." In any event, it is certain that each "interest" group will try to shape National Health Insurance to its perception of THE crisis in health.

Consumer Crisis vs. Provider Crisis

In fact, however, THE crisis in health is not just one crisis but two: the crisis felt by the consumers of health services, on the one hand, and the crisis experienced by the providers of health services, on the other. For the consumer, the crisis is the failure of the present system to deliver adequate health care at any price. Though not limited to poor people, black and Puerto Rican communities have been the most articulate in their criticisms. Medical care, they say, is fragmented and isolated from the social, economic, and environmental causes of pathology. People are experimented on and used as teaching material. The doctor's priorities come first. And the patient's needs run a poor second. Doctors and hospitals are totally unaccountable and unresponsive to the needs of the users of service. Increasingly, middle-class people are raising the same criticisms. They too experience long waits in overcrowded doctors' waiting rooms, constantly increasing bills, and the growing awareness that despite the wonders of heart transplants, it is increasingly difficult to find a doctor to treat ordinary ills.

Those who provide and pay for health care face a different crisis—the breakdown of the old systems of financing. The hospitals find themselves near collapse as costs skyrocket and financing fails to keep up. This threatens not only the institutions themselves, but also the multibillion-dollar drug and hospital supply companies who depend on the hospitals as a retail outlet for their products. At the same time that the hospitals weep because of "inadequate" funds, the providers of funds groan under the weight of the hospitals. Blue Cross is forced to raise its rates and face its enraged subscribers. The trade unions find themselves allocating an ever-increasing portion of wage hikes merely to maintain their present level of health benefits. Employee health plans cut an ever bigger bite out of corporate profits. Even the government feels the pinch as Medicare and Medicaid costs knock the budget for a loop.

Since the providers and financiers of medical care feel only part of the crisis—the part concerning the financing of medical care—it is little wonder that their solution to the "crisis" concerns only that. The various plans for health insurance being discussed are all primarily programs to put the financing of medical care on a sounder basis. The issues which are debated—coverage, benefits, sources of financing, administrative mechanisms, etc.—all attempt to answer the question of how to finance existing health services. None of the proposals confronts other parts of the crisis— the basic issues of the organization of delivery systems, the relationship between the providers and recipients of care, power in the health delivery system or priorities in the system.

Insurance Won't Work

National Health *Insurance,* to be sure, may well be a useful reform for many Americans. It may help a few people pay for medical services which they otherwise would not get. It may shore up a few hospitals in low income areas whose total collapse would be a tragedy for the people of the community. It is hard to oppose a measure which, in however limited a way, may help a few people, at least, to have greater access to badly needed health services. But National Health *Insurance,* in the end, (1) won't work, and (2) will have regressive effects as well as progressive ones.

The problem is that National Health Insurance will be a mechanism to funnel money out of the pockets of workers and taxpayers into the hands of the people who now run (and mis-run) the health service delivery system—the doctors, the hospital administrators, and the medical-industrial complex which fattens off people's illness. It will thus strengthen those forces that insist that all health care must center on the doctor and the hospital, rather than the forces who wish to totally reorganize the delivery of health care.

At the same time, National Health Insurance will throw a cloud over what is really happening. To liberals, for whom National Health Insurance has long been a goal, it will appear that the problems of the medical system are being solved. Middle-class doubts as to the organization of care may quiet down temporarily if part of the bill is paid by someone else. The accelerating movement for more fundamental reorganization of the medical care system will be de-fused, at least for a while.

Meanwhile, National Health Insurance will solve nothing. First, it is unlikely that any of the proposed plans will be very effective in meeting people's health needs. For this we have the evidence of Medicaid and Medicare. Medicaid, for example, clearly showed that giving the poor an unlimited credit card for medical service did not end the two-class system of medicine. There are other stumbling blocks: institutional inaccessibility, the relationship between doctor and patient, the control by the doctors of priorities for allocating funds, time, and equipment among research, teaching, and patient care, and the unaccountability of the hospital to the medical needs of the community. Medical care is sold in a monopolistic, not a free, marketplace. The effect of National Health Insurance, as with Medicaid and Medicare, may well be a sizeable number of individuals who are enabled to pay for better care. But it will not create and make accessible high-quality medical services for the great majority of poor and middle-class people.

Second, the hopes of some of the insurance plan advocates that the medical-care system can be reorganized through incentives linked to the insurance scheme's repayment system will almost certainly be dashed. For example, there has been much talk of giving doctors and hospitals incentives to operate efficiently. This might save money, but at best, it would have no effect on the patterns of care in the institutions, on the relations of the institution to the community, on the quality of care, etc. In fact, unless very stringent controls by the consumer were introduced, the likely result would be that the hospital would cut down on service in order to save money and pick up its incentive reward. For another thing, economic incentives can at best only conquer economic obstacles to change. They have no power over the other pillars of the two-class medical system. For example, economic incentives may encourage a hospital to be more economical, but they are unlikely to persuade a hospital to accept community control, or to convince $50,000-a-year doctors to put care of the indigent ahead of prestigious research. Finally, incentives are slow. We can't wait 20 or 30 years just to get doctors into group practices.

The third way in which National Health Insurance will fail will be economically. We have seen in the past few years how Medicaid and Medicare fed galloping medical inflation. The mechanisms are clear: the medical establishment which commanded the use of the funds, used them for their own priorities—prestigious and expensive and "interesting" medical technology and high salaries for doctors and administrators. As a result, costs soared, while patient care improved only slightly, if at all. There is no reason to think the same thing would not be repeated under National Health Insurance. No workable cost-control law has yet been devised, and, in any case, the impulse of hospital administrators is to cut costs at the expense of patients and hospital workers. It is entirely conceivable that in 1975, under National Health Insurance, the nation will be spending $90 billion a year instead of the present $60 billion for health services, and $200 a day for a hospital bed without any significant improvement in the quality of care for the average citizen.

NHI Evades Basic Questions

National Health Insurance will fail because it fails to face the fundamental questions about our health system—control, accountability, accessibility, priorities, responsibility to the community. And it fails this test precisely because it is National Health *Insurance*. Under an *insurance* mechanism, no matter how liberal, the private delivery system performs a certain service and the public funding (insurance) system pays for it. The public insurers may try to persuade the controllers of the private delivery system to change the system, but no attempt is made to take the power to control away from them. The key issues about the health system are thus removed from the discussion, right from the start. To this dead end, we can only propose the fundamental alternative: The only way to fundamentally change the health system so that it provides adequate, dignified care for all is to take power over health care away from the people who now control it. Not merely the funding of the health system, but the system itself must be public. It then becomes possible to face such questions as how we decentralize the "National Health Care *System*" to make it responsible to the community and accountable to it, how we ensure that patient care is the primary priority of the system, how we ensure equal access to health institutions and to practitioners, and so on.

Many people have suggested that National Health Insurance might be a step toward such a national health system. Others argue it will be retrogressive: by providing financing, it will stave off the collapse of the present system for a few short years and will strengthen some of the enemies of such a system. At the same time, though, it will establish the necessity for the government to guarantee the right to health care for all, and it will arouse ever greater expectations of adequate health care. Thus National Health Insurance is not clearly either a step towards or a step away from a national health care system . . . it's more of a shuffle sideways.

Note

Adapted from an editorial in the Health/PAC *Bulletin,* January, 1970, and reprinted in Chapter XII of *The American Health Empire* (New York: Vintage Books, 1971).

Contemporary Critical Debates   509

The Medicalization of American Society

ONLY IN THE TWENTIETH CENTURY did medicine become the dominant and prestigious profession we know today. The germ theory
of disease, which achieved dominance after about 1870, provided
medicine with a powerful explanatory tool and some of its greatest
clinical achievements. It proved to be the key that unlocked the
mystery of infectious disease and it came to provide the major
paradigm by which physicians viewed sickness. The claimed success of medicine in controlling infectious disease, coupled with
consolidation and monopolization of medical practice, enabled
medicine to achieve a position of social and professional dominance. Medicine, both in direct and indirect ways, was called upon
to repeat its "miracles" with other human problems. At the same
time, certain segments of the medical profession were intent on
expanding medicine's jurisdiction over societal problems.

By mid-century the domain of medicine had enlarged considerably: childbirth, sexuality, death as well as old age, anxiety,
obesity, child development, alcoholism, addiction, homosexuality,
amongst other human experiences, were being defined and treated
as medical problems. Sociologists began to examine the process
and consequences of this *medicalization of society* (e.g., Freidson,
1970; Zola, 1972) and most especially the medicalization of deviance (Conrad and Schneider, 1980a). It was clear that the medical
model—focusing on individual organic pathology and positing
physiological etiologies and biomedical interventions—was being
applied to a wide range of human phenomena. Human life, some
critics observed, was increasingly seen as a sickness-wellness continuum, with significant (if not obvious) social consequences (Zola,
1972; Conrad, 1975).

Other sociologists, however, argue that although some expansion of medical jurisdiction has occurred, the medicalization problem is overstated. They contend that we recently have witnessed a
considerable *de*medicalization. Strong (1979), for instance, points
out that there are numerous factors constraining and limiting

medicalization, including restrictions on the number of physicians, the cost of medical care, doctor's primary interests in manifestly organic problems, and the bourgeois value of individual liberty.

Recently, Conrad and Schneider (1980b) attempted to clarify the debate by suggesting that medicalization occurs on three levels: (1) the conceptual level, at which a medical vocabulary is used to define a problem; (2) the institutional level, at which medical personnel (usually physicians) are supervisors of treatment organizations or gatekeepers to state benefits; and (3) the interactional level, at which physicians actually treat patients' difficulties as medical problems. While there has been considerable discussion about the types and consequences of medicalization, there has thus far been little research on the actual extent of medicalization and its effects on patients' and other peoples' lives.

In "Medicine as an Institution of Social Control," Irving Kenneth Zola presents the medicalization thesis in terms of the expansion of medicine's social control functions. Renée Fox in "The Medicalization and Demedicalization of American Society" contends that a substantial demedicalization has occurred in American society, and that the concerns of critics of medicalization are overdrawn.

References

Conrad, Peter. 1975. "The discovery of hyperkinesis: Notes on the medicalization of deviant behavior." Social Problems 23 (1): 12–21.

Conrad, Peter and Joseph W. Schneider. 1980a. Deviance and Medicalization: From Badness to Sickness. St. Louis: C.V. Mosby.

1980b. "Looking at levels of medicalization: A comment on Strong's critique of the thesis of medical imperialism." Social Science and Medicine 14A (1): 75–79.

Freidson, Eliot. 1970. Profession of Medicine. New York: Dodd, Mead.

Strong, P.M. 1979. "Sociological imperialism and the profession of medicine: A critical examination of the thesis of medical imperialism." Social Science and Medicine 13A (2): 199–215.

Zola, Irving Kenneth. 1972. "Medicine as an institution of social control." Sociological Review 20 (November): 487–504.

34

Medicine as an Institution of Social Control

Irving Kenneth Zola

The theme of this essay is that medicine is becoming a major institution of social control, nudging aside, if not incorporating, the more traditional institutions of religion and law. It is becoming the new repository of truth, the place where absolute and often final judgments are made by supposedly morally neutral and objective experts. And these judgments are made, not in the name of virtue or legitimacy, but in the name of health. Moreover, this is not occurring through the political power physicians hold or can influence, but is largely an insidious and often undramatic phenomenon accomplished by "medicalizing" much of daily living, by making medicine and the labels "healthy" and "ill" *relevant* to an ever increasing part of human existence.

Although many have noted aspects of this process, by confining their concern to the field of psychiatry, these criticisms have been misplaced.[1] For psychiatry has by no means distorted the mandate of medicine, but indeed, though perhaps at a pace faster than other medical specialties, is following instead some of the basic claims and directions of that profession. Nor is this extension into society the result of any professional "imperialism," for this leads us to think of the issue in terms of misguided human efforts or motives. If we search for the "why" of this phenomenon, we will see instead that it is rooted in our increasingly complex technological and bureaucratic system—a system which has led us down the path of the reluctant reliance on the expert.[2]

Quite frankly, what is presented in the following pages is not a definitive argument but rather a case in progress. As such it draws heavily on observations made in the United States, though similar murmurings have long been echoed elsewhere.[3]

An Historical Perspective

The involvement of medicine in the management of society is not new. It did not appear full-blown one day in the mid-twentieth century. As Sigerist[4] has aptly claimed, medicine at base was always not only a social science but an occupation whose very practice was inextricably interwoven into society. This interdependence is perhaps best seen in two branches of medicine which have had a built-in social emphasis from the very start—psychiatry[5] and public health/preventive medicine.[6] Public health was always committed to changing social aspects of life—from sanitary to housing to working conditions—and often used the arm of the state (i.e. through laws and legal power) to gain its ends (e.g. quarantines, vaccinations). Psychiatry's involvement in society is a bit more difficult to trace, but taking the histories of psychiatry as data, then one notes the almost universal reference to one of the early pioneers, a physician named Johan Weyer. His, and thus psychiatry's involvement in social problems lay in the objection that witches ought not to be burned; for they were not possessed by the devil, but rather bedeviled by their problems—namely they were insane. From its early concern with the issue of insanity as a defense in criminal proceedings, psychiatry has grown to become the most dominant rehabilitative perspective in dealing with society's "legal" deviants. Psychiatry, like public health, has also used the legal powers of the state in the accomplishment of its goals (i.e. the cure of the patient through the legal proceedings of involuntary commitment and its concomitant removal of certain rights and privileges).

This is not to say, however, that the rest of medicine has been "socially" uninvolved. For a rereading of history makes it seem a matter of degree. Medicine has long had both a *de jure* and a *de facto* relation to institutions of social control. The *de jure* relationship is seen in the idea of reportable diseases, wherein, if certain phenomena occur in his practice, the physician is required to report them to the appropriate authorities. While this seems somewhat straightforward and even functional where certain highly contagious diseases are concerned, it is less clear where the possible spread of infection is not the primary issue (e.g. with gunshot wounds, attempted suicide, drug use and what is now called child abuse). The *de facto* relation to social control can be argued through a brief look at the disruptions of the last two or three American Medical Association Conventions. For there the American Medical Association members—and really all ancillary health professions—were accused of practicing social control (the term used by the accusers was genocide) in first, *whom* they have traditionally treated with *what*—giving *better* treatment to more favored clientele; and secondly, *what* they have treated—a more subtle form of discrimination in that, with limited resources, by focusing on some diseases others are neglected. Here the accusation was that medicine has focused on the diseases of the rich and the established—cancer, heart disease, stroke—and ignored the diseases of the poor, such as malnutrition and still high infant mortality.

The Myth of Accountability

Even if we acknowledge such a growing medical involvement, it is easy to regard it as primarily a "good" one—which involves the steady destigmatization of many human and social problems. Thus Barbara Wootton was able to conclude:

> Without question . . . in the contemporary attitude toward antisocial behaviour, psychiatry and humanitarianism have marched hand in hand. Just because it is so much in keeping with the mental atmosphere of a scientifically-minded age, the medical treatment of social deviants has been a most powerful, perhaps even the most powerful, reinforcement of humanitarian impulses; for today the prestige of humane proposals is immensely enhanced if these are expressed in the idiom of medical science.[7]

The assumption is thus readily made that such medical involvement in social problems leads to their removal from religious and legal scrutiny and thus from moral and punitive consequences. In turn the problems are placed under medical and scientific scrutiny and thus in objective and therapeutic circumstances.

The fact that we cling to such a hope is at least partly due to two cultural-historical blindspots—one regarding our notion of punishment and the other our notion of moral responsibility. Regarding the first, if there is one insight into human behavior that the twentieth century should have firmly implanted, it is that punishment cannot be seen in merely physical terms, nor only from the perspective of the giver. Granted that capital offenses are on the decrease, that whipping and torture seem to be disappearing, as is the use of chains and other physical restraints, yet our ability if not willingness to inflict human anguish on one another does not seem similarly on the wane. The most effective forms of brain-washing deny any physical contact and the concept of relativism tells much about the psychological costs of even relative deprivation of tangible and intangible wants. Thus, when an individual because of his "disease" and its treatment is forbidden to have intercourse with fellow human beings, is confined until cured, is forced to undergo certain medical procedures for his own good, perhaps deprived forever of the right to have sexual relations and/or produce children, *then* it is difficult for that patient *not* to view what is happening to him as punishment. This does not mean that medicine is the latest form of twentieth century torture, but merely that pain and suffering take many forms, and that the removal of a despicable inhumane procedure by current standards does not necessarily mean that its replacement will be all that beneficial. In part, the satisfaction in seeing the chains cast off by Pinel may have allowed us for far too long to neglect examining with what they had been replaced.

It is the second issue, that of responsibility, which requires more elaboration, for it is argued here that the medical model has had its greatest impact in the lifting of moral condemnation from the individual. While some sceptics note that while the individual is no longer condemned his disease still *is,* they do not go far enough. Most analysts have tried to make a distinction between illness and crime on the issue of personal responsibility.[8] The criminal is thought to be responsible and therefore accountable (or punishable) for his act, while the sick person is not. While the distinction does exist, it seems to be more a quantitative one rather than a qualitative one, with moral judgments but a pinprick below the surface. For instance, while it is probably true that individuals are no longer directly condemned for being sick, it does seem that much of this condemnation is merely displaced. Though his immoral character is not demonstrated in his having a disease, it becomes evident in what he does about it. Without seeming ludicrous, if one listed the traits of people who break appointments, fail to follow treatment regimen, or even delay in seeking medical aid, one finds a long list of "personal flaws." Such people seem to be ever ignorant of the consequences of certain diseases, inaccurate as to symptomatology, unable to plan ahead or find time, burdened with shame, guilt, neurotic tendencies, haunted with traumatic medical experiences or members of some lower status minority group—religious, ethnic, racial or socio-economic. In short, they appear to be a sorely troubled if not disreputable group of people.

The argument need not rest at this level of analysis, for it is not clear that the issues of morality and individual responsibility have been fully banished from the etiological scene itself. At the same time as the label "illness" is being used to attribute "diminished responsibility" to a whole host of phenomena, the issue of "personal responsibility" seems to be re-emerging within medicine itself. Regardless of the truth and insights of the concepts of stress and the perspective of psychosomatics, whatever else they do, they bring man, *not* bacteria to the center of the stage and lead thereby to a re-examination of the individual's role in his own demise, disability and even recovery.

The case, however, need not be confined to professional concepts and their degree of acceptance, for we can look at the beliefs of the man in the street. As most surveys have reported, when an individual is asked what caused his diabetes, heart disease, upper respiratory infection, etc., we may be comforted by the scientific terminology if not the accuracy of his answers. Yet if we follow this questioning with the probe: "Why did you get X now?", or "Of all the people in your community, family, etc. who were exposed to X, why did you get . . . ?", then the rational scientific veneer is pierced and the concern with personal and moral responsibility emerges quite strikingly. Indeed the issue "why me?" becomes of great concern and is generally expressed in quite moral terms of what they did wrong. It is possible to argue that here we are seeing a residue and that it will surely be different in the new generation. A recent experiment I conducted should cast some doubt on this. I asked a class of forty undergraduates, mostly aged seventeen, eighteen and nineteen, to recall the last time they were sick, disabled, or hurt and then to record how they did or would have communicated this experience to a child under the age of five. The purpose of the assignment had nothing to do with the issue of responsibility and it is worth noting that there was no difference in the nature of the response between those who had or had not actually encountered children during their "illness." The responses speak for themselves.

> The opening words of the sick, injured person to the query of the child were:
> "I feel bad"
> "I feel bad all over"
> "I have a bad leg"
> "I have a bad eye"
> "I have a bad stomach ache"
> "I have a bad pain"
> "I have a bad cold"

The reply of the child was inevitable:
"What did you do wrong?"
The "ill person" in no case corrected the child's perspective but rather joined it at that level.
On bacteria
> "There are good germs and bad germs and sometimes the bad germs . . ."
On catching a cold
> "Well you know sometimes when your mother says, 'Wrap up or be careful or you'll catch a cold,' well I . . ."
On an eye sore
> "When you use certain kinds of things (mascara) near your eye you must be very careful and I was not . . ."
On a leg injury
> "You've always got to watch where you're going and I . . ."

Finally to the treatment phase:
On how drugs work
> "You take this medicine and it attacks the bad parts . . ."
On how wounds are healed
> "Within our body there are good forces and bad ones and when there is an injury, all the good ones . . ."
On pus
> "That's the way the body gets rid of all its bad things . . ."
On general recovery
> "If you are good and do all the things the doctor and your mother tell you, you will get better."

In short, on nearly every level, from getting sick to recovering, a moral battle raged. This seems more than the mere anthropomorphising of a phenomenon to communicate it more simply to children. Frankly it seems hard to believe that the English language is so poor that a *moral* rhetoric is needed to describe a supposedly amoral phenomenon—illness.

In short, despite hopes to the contrary, the rhetoric of illness by itself seems to provide no absolution from individual responsibility, accountability and moral judgment.

The Medicalizing of Society

Perhaps it is possible that medicine is not devoid of a potential for moralizing and social control. The first question becomes: "what means are available to exercise it?" Freidson has stated a major aspect of the process most succinctly:

> The medical profession has first claim to jurisdiction over the label of illness and *anything* to which it may be attached, irrespective of its capacity to deal with it effectively.[9]

For illustrative purposes this "attaching" process may be categorized in four concrete ways: first, through the expansion of what in life is deemed relevant to the good practice of medicine; secondly, through the retention of absolute control over certain technical procedures; thirdly, through the retention of near absolute access to certain "taboo" areas; and finally, through the expansion of what in medicine is deemed relevant to the good practice of life.

1. The Expansion of What in Life Is Deemed Relevant to the Good Practice of Medicine

The change of medicine's commitment from a specific etiological model of disease to a multi-causal one and the greater acceptance of the concepts of comprehensive medicine, psychosomatics, etc., have enormously expanded that which is or can be relevant to the understanding, treatment and even prevention of disease. Thus it is no longer necessary for the patient merely to divulge the symptoms of his body, but also the symptoms of daily living, his habits and his worries. Part of this is greatly facilitated in the "age of the computer," for what might be too embarrassing, or take too long, or be inefficient in a face-to-face encounter can now be asked and analyzed impersonally by the machine, and moreover be done before the patient ever sees the physician. With the advent of the computer a certain guarantee of privacy is necessarily lost, for while many physicians might have probed similar issues, the only place where the data were stored was in the mind of the doctor, and only rarely in the medical record. The computer, on the other hand, has a retrievable, transmittable and almost inexhaustible memory.

It is not merely, however, the nature of the data needed to make more accurate diagnoses and treatments, but the perspective which accompanies it—a perspective which pushes the physician far beyond his office and the exercise of technical skills. To rehabilitate or at least alleviate many of the ravages of chronic disease, it has become increasingly necessary to intervene to change permanently the habits of a patient's lifetime—be it of working, sleeping, playing or eating. In prevention the "extension into life" becomes even deeper, since the very idea of primary prevention means getting there *before* the disease process starts. The physician must not only seek out his clientele but once found must often convince them that they must do something *now* and perhaps at a time when the potential patient feels well or not especially troubled. If this in itself does not get the prevention-oriented physician involved in the workings of society, then the nature of "effective" mechanisms for intervention surely does, as illustrated by the statement of a physician trying to deal with health problems in the ghetto:

> Any effort to improve the health of ghetto residents cannot be separated from equal and simultaneous efforts to remove the multiple social, political and economic restraints currently imposed on inner city residents.[10]

Certain forms of social intervention and control emerge even when medicine comes to grips with some of its more traditional problems like heart disease and cancer. An increasing number of physicians feel that a change in diet may be the most effective deterrent to a number of cardiovascular complications. They are, however, so perplexed as to how to get the general population to follow their recommendations that a leading article in a national magazine was entitled "To Save the Heart: Diet by Decree?"[11] It is obvious that there is an increasing pressure for more explicit sanctions against the tobacco companies and against high users to force both to desist. And what will be the implications of even stronger evidence which links age at parity, frequency of sexual intercourse, or the lack of male circumcision to the incidence of cervical cancer, can be left to our imagination!

2. Through the Retention of Absolute Control over Certain Technical Procedures

In particular this refers to skills which in certain jurisdictions are the very operational and legal definition of the practice of medicine—the right to do surgery and prescribe drugs. Both of these take medicine far beyond concern with ordinary organic disease.

In surgery this is seen in several different sub-specialties. The plastic surgeon has at least participated in, if not helped perpetuate, certain aesthetic standards. What once was a practice confined to restoration has now expanded beyond the correction of certain traumatic or even congenital deformities to the creation of new physical properties, from size of nose to size of breast, as well as dealing with certain phenomena—wrinkles, sagging, etc.—formerly associated with the "natural" process of aging. Alterations in sexual and reproductive functioning have long been a medical concern. Yet today the frequency of hysterectomies seems not so highly correlated as one might think with the presence of organic disease. (What avenues the very possibility of sex change will open is anyone's guess.) Transplantations, despite their still relative infrequency, have had a tremendous effect on our very notions of death and dying. And at the other end of life's continuum, since abortion is still essentially a surgical procedure, it is to the physician-surgeon that society is turning (and the physician-surgeon accepting) for criteria and guidelines.

In the exclusive right to prescribe and thus pronounce on and regulate drugs, the power of the physician is even more awesome. Forgetting for the moment our obsession with youth's "illegal" use of drugs, any observer can see, judging by sales alone, that the greatest increase in drug use over the last ten years has not been in the realm of treating any organic disease but in treating a large number of psychosocial states. Thus we have drugs for nearly every mood:

> to help us sleep or keep us awake
> to enhance our appetite or decrease it
> to tone down our energy level or to increase it
> to relieve our depression or stimulate our interest.

Recently the newspapers and more popular magazines, including some medical and scientific ones, have carried articles about drugs which may be effective peace pills or anti-aggression tablets, enhance our memory, our perception, our intelligence and our vision (spiritually or otherwise). This led to the easy prediction:

> We will see new drugs, more targeted, more specific and more potent than anything we have. . . . And many of these would be for people we would call healthy.[12]

This statement incidentally was made not by a visionary science fiction writer but by a former commissioner of the United States Food and Drug Administration.

3. Through the Retention of Near Absolute Access to Certain "Taboo" Areas

These "taboo" areas refer to medicine's almost exclusive license to examine and treat that most personal of individual possessions—the inner workings of our bodies and minds. My contention is that if anything can be shown in some way to affect the workings of the body and to a lesser extent the mind, then it can be labelled an "illness" itself or jurisdictionally "a medical problem." In a sheer statistical sense the import of this is especially great if we look at only four such problems—aging, drug addiction, alcoholism and pregnancy. The first and last were once regarded as normal natural processes and the middle two as human foibles and weaknesses. Now this has changed and to some extent medical specialties have emerged to meet these new needs. Numerically this expands medicine's involvement not only in a longer span of human existence, but it opens the possibility of medicine's services to millions if not billions of people. In the United States at least, the implication of declaring alcoholism a disease (the possible import of a pending Supreme Court decision as well as laws currently being introduced into several state legislatures) would reduce arrests in many jurisdictions by 10 to 50 percent and transfer such "offenders" when "discovered" directly to a medical facility. It is pregnancy, however, which produces the most illuminating illustration. For, again in the United States, it was barely seventy years ago that virtually all births and the concomitants of birth occurred outside the hospital as well as outside medical supervision. I do not frankly have a documentary history, but as this medical claim was solidified, so too was medicine's claim to a whole host of related processes: not only to birth but to prenatal, postnatal, and pediatric care; not only to conception but to infertility; not only to the process of reproduction but to the process and problems of sexual activity itself; not only when life begins (in the issue of abortion) but whether it should be allowed to begin at all (e.g. in genetic counselling).

Partly through this foothold in the "taboo" areas and partly through the simple reduction of other resources, the physician is increasingly becoming the choice for help for many with personal and social problems. Thus a recent British study reported that within a five year period there had been a notable increase (from 25 to 41 percent) in the proportion of the population willing to consult the physician with a personal problem.[13]

4. Through the Expansion of What in Medicine Is Deemed Relevant to the Good Practice of Life

Though in some ways this is the most powerful of all "the medicalizing of society" processes, the point can be made simply. Here we refer to the use of medical rhetoric and evidence in the arguments to advance any cause. For what Wootton attributed to psychiatry is no less true of medicine. To paraphrase her, today the prestige of *any* proposal is immensely enhanced, if not justified, when it is expressed in the idiom of medical science. To say that many who use such labels are not professionals only begs the issue, for the public is only taking its cues from professionals who increasingly have been extending their expertise into the social sphere or have called for such an extension.[14] In politics one hears of the healthy or unhealthy economy or state. More concretely, the physical and mental health of American presidential candidates has been an issue in the last four elections and a recent book claimed to link faulty political decisions with faulty health.[15] For years we knew that the environment was unattractive, polluted, noisy and in certain ways dying, but now we learn that its death may not be unrelated to our own demise. To end with a rather mundane if depressing example, there has always been a constant battle between school authorities and their charges on the basis of dress and such habits as smoking, but recently the issue was happily resolved for a local school administration when they declared that such restrictions were necessary for reasons of health.

The Potential and Consequences of Medical Control

The list of daily activities to which health can be related is ever growing and with the current operating perspective of medicine it seems infinitely expandable. The reasons are manifold. It is not merely that medicine has extended its jurisdiction to cover new problems,[16] or that doctors are professionally committed to finding disease,[17] nor even that society keeps creating disease.[18] For if none of these obtained today we would still find medicine exerting an enormous influence on society. The most powerful empirical stimulus for this is the realization of how much everyone has or believes he has something organically wrong with him, or put more positively, how much can be done to make one feel, look or function better.

The rates of "clinical entities" found on surveys or by periodic health examinations range upwards from 50 to 80 percent of the population studied.[19] The Peckham study found that only 9 percent of their study group were free from clinical disorder. Moreover, they were even wary of this figure and noted in a footnote that, first, some of these 9 percent had subsequently died of a heart attack, and, secondly, that the majority of those without disorder were under the age of five.[20] We used to rationalize that this high level of prevalence did not, however, translate itself into action since not only are rates of medical utilization not astonishingly high but they also have not gone up appreciably. Some recent studies, however, indicate that we may have been looking in the wrong place for this medical action. It has been noted in the United States and the United Kingdom that within a given twenty-four to thirty-six hour period, from 50 to 80 percent of the adult population have taken one or more "medical" drugs.[21]

The belief in the omnipresence of disorder is further enhanced by a reading of the scientific, pharmacological and medical literature, for there one finds a growing litany of indictments of "unhealthy" life activities. From sex to food, from aspirins to clothes, from driving your car to riding the surf, it seems that under certain conditions, or in combination with certain other substances or activities or if done too much or too little, virtually anything can lead to certain medical problems. In short, I at least have finally been convinced that living is injurious to health. This remark is not meant as facetiously as it may sound. But rather every aspect of our daily life has in it elements of risk to health.

These facts take on particular importance not only when health becomes a paramount value in society, but also a phenomenon whose diagnosis and treatment has been restricted to a certain group. For this means that that group, perhaps unwittingly, is in a position to exercise great control and influence about what we should and should not do to attain that "paramount value."

Freidson in his recent book *Profession of Medicine* has very cogently analyzed why the expert in general and the medical expert in particular should be granted a certain autonomy in his researches, his diagnosis and his recommended treatments.[22] On the other hand, when it comes to constraining or directing human behavior *because* of the data of his researches, diagnosis and treatment, a different situation obtains. For in these kinds of decisions it seems that too often the physician is guided not by his technical knowledge but by his values, or values latent in his very techniques.

Perhaps this issue of values can be clarified by reference to some not so randomly chosen medical problems: drug safety, genetic counselling and automated multiphasic testing.

The issue of drug safety should seem straightforward, but both words in that phrase apparently can have some interesting flexibility—namely what is a drug and what is safe. During Prohibition in the United States alcohol was medically regarded as a drug and was often prescribed as a medicine. Yet in recent years, when the issue of dangerous substances and drugs has come up for discussion in medical circles, alcohol has been officially excluded from the debate. As for safety, many have applauded the A.M.A.'s judicious position in declaring the need for much more extensive, longitudinal research on marihuana and their unwillingness to back legalization until much more data are in. This applause might be muted if the public read the 1970 Food and Drug Administration's "Blue Ribbon" Committee Report on the safety, quality and efficacy of *all* medical drugs commercially and legally on the market since 1938.[23] Though appalled at the lack and quality of evidence of any sort, few recommendations were made for the withdrawal of drugs from the market. Moreover there are no recorded cases of anyone dying from an overdose or of extensive adverse side effects from marihuana use, but the literature on the adverse effects of a whole host of "medical drugs" on the market today is legion.

It would seem that the value positions of those on both sides of the abortion issue needs little documenting, but let us pause briefly at a field where "harder" scientists are at work—genetics. The issue of genetic counselling, or whether life should be allowed to begin at all, can only be an ever increasing one. As we learn more and more about congenital, inherited disorders or predispositions, and as the population size for whatever reason becomes more limited, then, inevitably, there will follow an attempt to improve the quality of the population which shall be produced. At a conference on the more limited concern of what to do when there is a documented probability of the offspring of certain unions being damaged, a position was taken that it was not necessary to pass laws or bar marriages that might produce such offspring. Recognizing the power and influence of medicine and the doctor, one of those present argued:

> There is no reason why sensible people could not be dissuaded from marrying if they know that one out of four of their children is likely to inherit a disease.[24]

There are in this statement certain values on marriage and what it is or could be that, while they may be popular, are not necessarily shared by all. Thus, in addition to presenting the argument against marriage, it would seem that the doctor should—if he were to engage in the issue at all—present at the same time some of the other alternatives:

> Some "parents" could be willing to live with the risk that out of four children, three may turn out fine.
> Depending on the diagnostic procedures available they could take the risk and if indications were negative abort.
> If this risk were too great but the desire to bear children was there, and depending on the type of problem, artificial insemination might be a possibility.
> Barring all these and not wanting to take any risk, they could adopt children.
> Finally, there is the option of being married without having any children.

It is perhaps appropriate to end with a seemingly innocuous and technical advance in medicine, automatic multiphasic testing. It has been a procedure hailed as a boon to aid the doctor if not replace him. While some have questioned the validity of all those test-results and still others fear that it will lead to second class medicine for already underprivileged populations, it is apparent that its major use to date and in the future may not be in promoting health or detecting disease to prevent it. Thus three large institutions are now or are planning to make use of this method, not to treat people, but to "deselect" them. The armed services use it to weed out the physically and mentally unfit, insurance companies to reject "uninsurables" and large industrial firms to point out "high risks." At a recent conference representatives of these same institutions were asked what responsibility they did or would recognize to those whom they have just informed that they have been "rejected" because of some physical or mental anomaly. They calmly and universally stated: none—neither to provide them with any appropriate aid nor even to ensure that they get or be put in touch with any help.

Conclusion

C. S. Lewis warned us more than a quarter of a century ago that "man's power over Nature is really the power of some men over other men, with Nature as their instrument." The same could be said regarding man's power over health and illness, for the labels health and illness are remarkable "depoliticizers" of an issue. By locating the source and the treatment of problems in an individual, other levels of intervention are effectively closed. By the very acceptance of a specific behavior as an "illness" and the definition of illness as an undesirable state, the issue becomes not whether to deal with a particular problem, but *how* and *when*.[25] Thus the debate over homosexuality, drugs or abortion becomes focused on the degree of sickness attached to the phenomenon in question or the extent of the health risk involved. And the more principled, more perplexing, or even moral issue, of *what* freedom should an individual have over his or her own body is shunted aside.

As stated in the very beginning this "medicalizing of society" is as much a result of medicine's potential as it is of society's wish for medicine to use that potential. Why then has the focus been more on the medical potential than on the social desire? In part it is a function of space, but also of political expediency. For the time rapidly may be approaching when recourse to the populace's wishes may be impossible. Let me illustrate this with the statements of two medical scientists who, if they read this essay, would probably dismiss all my fears as groundless. The first was commenting on the ethical, moral, and legal procedures of the sex change operation:

> Physicians generally consider it unethical to destroy or alter tissue except in the presence of disease or deformity. The interference with a person's natural procreative function entails definite moral tenets, by which not only physicians but also the general public are influenced. The administration of physical harm as treatment for mental or behavioral problems—as corporal punishment, lobotomy for unmanageable psychotics and sterilization of criminals—is abhorrent in our society.[26]

Here he states, as almost an absolute condition of human nature, something which is at best a recent phenomenon. He seems to forget that there were laws promulgating just such procedures through much of the twentieth century, that within the past few years at least one Californian jurist ordered the sterilization of an unwed mother as a condition of probation, and that such procedures were done by Nazi scientists and physicians as part of a series of medical experiments. More recently, there is the misguided patriotism of the cancer researchers under contract to the United States Department of Defense who allowed their dying patients to be exposed to massive doses of radiation to analyze the psychological and physical results of simulated nuclear fall-out. True, the experiments were stopped, but not until they had been going on for *eleven* years.

The second statement is by Francis Crick at a conference on the implications of certain genetic findings:

> Some of the wild genetic proposals will never be adopted because the people will simply not stand for them.[27]

Note where his emphasis is: on the people not the scientist. In order, however, for the people to be concerned, to act and to protest, they must first be aware of what is going on. Yet in the very privatized nature of medical practice, plus the continued emphasis that certain expert judgments must be free from public scrutiny, there are certain processes which will prevent the public from ever knowing what has taken place and thus from doing something about it. Let me cite two examples.

> Recently, in a European country, I overheard the following conversation in a kidney dialysis unit. The chief was being questioned about whether or not there were self-help groups among his patients. "No" he almost shouted "that is the last thing we want. Already the patients are sharing too much knowledge while they sit in the waiting room, thus making our task increasingly difficult. We are working now on a procedure to prevent them from even meeting with one another."

The second example removes certain information even further from public view.

> The issue of fluoridation in the U.S. has been for many years a hot political one. It was in the political arena because, in order to fluoridate local water supplies, the decision in many jurisdictions had to be put to a popular referendum. And when it was, it was often defeated. A solution was found and a series of state laws were passed to make fluoridation a public health decision and to be treated, as all other public health decisions, by the medical officers best qualified to decide questions of such a technical, scientific and medical nature.

Thus the issue at base here is the question of what factors are actually of a solely technical, scientific and medical nature.

To return to our opening caution, this paper is not an attack on medicine so much as on a situation in which we find ourselves in the latter part of the twentieth century; for the medical area is the arena or the example *par excellence* of today's identity crisis—what is or will become of man. It is the battleground, not because there are visible threats and oppressors, but because they are almost invisible; not because the perspective, tools and practitioners of medicine and the other helping professions are evil, but because they are not. It is so frightening because there are elements here of the banality of evil so uncomfortably written about by Hannah Arendt.[28] But here the danger is greater, for not only is the process masked as a technical, scientific, objective one, but one done for our own good. A few years ago a physician speculated on what, based on current knowledge, would be the composite picture of an individual with a low risk of developing atherosclerosis or coronary-artery disease. He would be:

> ... an effeminate municipal worker or embalmer completely lacking in physical or mental alertness and without drive, ambition, or competitive spirit; who has never attempted to meet a deadline of any kind; a man with poor appetite, subsisting on fruits and vegetables laced with corn and whale oil, detesting tobacco, spurning ownership of radio, television, or motorcar, with full head of hair but scrawny and unathletic appearance, yet constantly straining his puny muscles by exercise. Low in income, blood pressure, blood sugar, uric acid and cholesterol, he has been taking nicotinic acid, pyridoxine, and long term antocoagulant therapy ever since his prophylactic castration.[29]

Thus I fear with Freidson:

> A profession and a society which are so concerned with physical and functional wellbeing as to sacrifice civil liberty and moral integrity must inevitably press for a "scientific" environment similar to that provided laying hens on progressive chicken farms—hens who produce eggs industriously and have no disease or other cares.[30]

Nor does it really matter that if, instead of the above depressing picture, we were guaranteed six more inches in height, thirty more years of life, or drugs to expand our potentialities and potencies; we should still be able to ask: what do six more inches matter, in what kind of environment will the thirty additional years be spent, or who will decide what potentialities and potencies will be expanded and what curbed.

I must confess that given the road down which so much expertise has taken us, I am willing to live with some of the frustrations and even mistakes that will follow when the authority for many decisions becomes shared with those whose lives and activities are involved. For I am convinced that patients have so much to teach to their doctors as do students their professors and children their parents.

Note

This paper was written while the author was a consultant in residence at the Netherlands Institute for Preventive Medicine, Leiden. For their general encouragement and the opportunity to pursue this topic I will always be grateful.

It was presented at the Medical Sociology Conference of the British Sociological Association at Weston-Super-Mare in November 1971. My special thanks for their extensive editorial and substantive comments go to Egon Bittner, Mara Sanadi, Alwyn Smith, and Bruce Wheaton.

References

1. T. Szasz: *The Myth of Mental Illness,* Harper and Row, New York, 1961; and R. Leifer: *In the Name of Mental Health,* Science House, New York, 1969.
2. E.g. A. Toffler: *Future Shock,* Random House, New York, 1970; and P. E. Slater: *The Pursuit of Loneliness,* Beacon Press, Boston, 1970.
3. Such as B. Wootton: *Social Science and Social Pathology,* Allen and Unwin, London, 1959.
4. H. Sigerist: *Civilization and Disease,* Cornell University Press, New York, 1943.
5. M. Foucault: *Madness and Civilization,* Pantheon, New York, 1965; and Szasz: *op. cit.*
6. G. Rosen: *A History of Public Health,* MD Publications, New York, 1955; and G. Rosen: "The Evolution of Social Medicine", in H. E. Freeman, S. Levine and L. G. Reeder (eds.): *Handbook of Medical Sociology,* Prentice-Hall, Englewood Cliffs, N.J., 1963, pp. 17–61.
7. Wootton: *op. cit.,* p. 206.
8. Two excellent discussions are found in V. Aubert and S. Messinger: "The Criminal and the Sick", *Inquiry,* Vol. 1, 1958, pp. 137–160; and E. Freidson: *Profession of Medicine,* Dodd-Mead, New York, 1970, pp. 205–277.
9. Freidson: *op. cit.,* p. 251.
10. J. C. Norman: "Medicine in the Ghetto", *New Engl. J. Med.,* Vol. 281, 1969, p. 1271.
11. "To Save the Heart; Diet by Decree?" *Time Magazine,* 10th January, 1968, p. 42.
12. J. L. Goddard quoted in the *Boston Globe,* August 7th, 1966.
13. K. Dunnell and A. Cartwright: *Medicine Takers, Prescribers and Hoarders,* in press.
14. E.g. S. Alinsky: "The Poor and the Powerful", in *Poverty and Mental Health,* Psychiat. Res. Rep. No. 21 of the Amer. Psychiat. Ass., January 1967; and B. Wedge: "Psychiatry and International Affairs", *Science,* Vol. 157, 1961, pp. 281–285.
15. H. L'Etang: *The Pathology of Leadership,* Hawthorne Books, New York, 1970.
16. Szasz: *op. cit.,* and Leifer: *op. cit.*
17. Freidson: *op. cit.;* and T. Scheff: "Preferred Errors in Diagnoses", *Medical Care,* Vol. 2, 1964, pp. 166–172.
18. R. Dubos: *The Mirage of Health,* Doubleday, Garden City, N.Y., 1959; and R. Dubos: *Man Adapting,* Yale University Press, 1965.
19. E.g. the general summaries of J. W. Meigs: "Occupational Medicine", *New Eng. J. Med.,* Vol. 264, 1961, pp. 861–867; and G. S. Siegel: *Periodic Health Examinations—Abstracts from the Literature,* Publ. Hlth. Serv. Publ. No. 1010, U.S. Government Printing Office, Washington D.C., 1963.
20. I. H. Pearse and L. H. Crocker: *Biologists in Search of Material,* Faber and Faber, London, 1938; and I. H. Pearse and L. H Crocker: *The Peckham Experiment,* Allen and Unwin, London, 1949.

21. Dunnell and Cartwright: *op. cit.;* and K. White, A. Andjelkovic, R. J. C. Pearson, J. H. Mabry, A. Ross and O. K. Sagan: "International Comparisons of Medical Care Utilization", *New Engl. J. of Med.,* Vol. 277, 1967, pp. 516–522.
22. Freidson: *op. cit.*
23. *Drug Efficiency Study—Final Report to the Commissioner of Food and Drugs,* Food and Drug Adm. Med. Nat. Res. Council, Nat. Acad. Sci., Washington D.C., 1969.
24. Reported in L. Eisenberg: "Genetics and the Survival of the Unfit", *Harper's Magazine,* Vol. 232, 1966, p. 57.
25. This general case is argued more specifically in I. K. Zola: *Medicine, Morality, and Social Problems—Some Implications of the Label Mental Illness,* Paper presented at the Amer. Ortho-Psychiat. Ass., March 20–23, 1968.
26. D. H. Russell: "The Sex Conversion Controversy", *New Engl. J. Med.,* Vol. 279, 1968, p. 536.
27. F. Crick reported in *Time Magazine,* April 19th, 1971.
28. H. Arendt: *Eichmann in Jerusalem—A Report on the Banality of Evil,* Viking Press, New York, 1963.
29. G. S. Myers quoted in L. Losagna: *Life, Death and the Doctor,* Alfred Knopf, New York, 1968, pp. 215–216.
30. Freidson: *op. cit.,* p. 354.

35

The Medicalization and Demedicalization of American Society

Renée C. Fox

. . . .

Along with progressive medicalization, a process of demedicalization seems also to be taking place in the society. To some extent the signs of demedicalization are reactions to what is felt by various individuals and groups to be a state of "*over*-medicalization." One of the most significant manifestations of this counter-trend is the mounting concern over implications that have arisen from the continuously expanding conception of "sickness" in the society. Commentators on this process would not necessarily agree with Peter Sedgwick that it will continue to "the point where everybody has become so luxuriantly ill" that perhaps sickness will no longer be "in" and a "backlash" will be set in motion;[1] they may not envision such an engulfing state of societally defined illness. But many observers from diverse professional backgrounds have published works in which they express concern about the "coercive" aspects of the "label" illness and the treatment of illness by medical professionals in medical institutions.[2] The admonitory perspectives on the enlarged domain of illness and medicine that these works of social science and social criticism represent appear to have gained the attention of young physicians- and nurses-in-training interested in change, and various consumer and civil-rights groups interested in health care.

This emerging view emphasizes the degree to which what is defined as health and illness, normality and abnormality, sanity and insanity varies from one society, culture, and historical period to another. Thus, it is contended, medical diagnostic categories such as "sick," "abnormal," and "insane" are not universal, objective, or necessarily reliable. Rather, they are culture-, class-, and time-bound, often ethnocentric, and as much artifacts of the preconceptions of socially biased observers as they are valid summaries of the characteristics of the observed. In this view, illness (especially mental illness) is largely a mythical construct, created and enforced by the society. The hospitals to which seriously ill persons are confined are portrayed as "total institutions": segregated, encompassing, depersonalizing organizations, "dominated" by physicians who are disinclined to convey information to patients about their conditions, or to encourage paramedical personnel to do so. These "oppressive" and "counter-therapeutic" attributes of the hospital environment are seen as emanating from the professional ideology of physicians and the kind of hierarchical relationships that they establish with patients and other medical professionals partly as a consequence of this ideology, as well as from the bureaucratic and technological features of the hospital itself. Whatever their source, the argument continues, the characteristics of the hospital and of the doctor-patient relationship increase the "powerlessness" of the sick person, "maintain his uncertainty," and systematically "mortify" and "curtail" the "self" with which he enters the sick role and arrives at the hospital door.

This critical perspective links the labeling of illness, the "imperialist" outlook and capitalist behavior of physicians, the "stigmatizing" and "dehumanizing" experiences of patients, and the problems of the health-care system more generally to imperfections and injustices in the society as a whole. Thus, for example, the various forms of social inequality, prejudice, discrimination, and acquisitive self-interest that persist in capitalistic American society are held responsible for causing illness, as well as for contributing to the undesirable attitudes and actions of physicians and other medical professionals. Casting persons in the sick role is regarded as a powerful, latent way for the society to exact conformity and maintain the status quo. For it allows a semi-approved form of deviance to occur which siphons off potential for insurgent protest and which can be controlled through the supervision or, in some cases, the "enforced therapy" of the medical profession. Thus, however permissive and merciful it may be to expand the category of illness, these observers point out, there is always the danger that the society will become a "therapeutic state" that excessively restricts the "right to be different" and the right to dissent. They feel that this danger may already have reached serious proportions in this society through its progressive medicalization.

The criticism of medicalization and the advocacy of demedicalization have not been confined to rhetoric. Concrete steps have been taken to declassify certain conditions as illness. Most notable among these is the American Psychiatric Association's decision to remove homosexuality from its official catalogue ("Nomenclature") of mental disorders. In addition, serious efforts have been made to heighten physicians' awareness of the fact that because they share certain prejudiced, often unconscious assumptions about women, they tend to over-attribute psychological conditions to their female patients. Thus, for example, distinguished medical publications such as the *New England Journal of Medicine* have featured articles and editorials on the excessive readiness with which medical specialists and textbook authors accept the undocumented belief that dysmenorrhea, nausea of pregnancy, pain in labor, and infantile colic are all psychogenic disorders, caused or aggravated by women's emotional problems. Another related development is feminist protest against what is felt to be a too great tendency to define pregnancy as an illness, and childbirth as a "technologized" medical-surgical event, prevailed over by the obstetrician-gynecologist. These sentiments have contributed to the preference that many middle-class couples have shown for natural childbirth in recent years, and to the revival of midwifery. The last example also illustrates an allied movement, namely a growing tendency to shift some responsibility for medical care and authority over it from the physician, the medical team, and hospital to the patient, the family, and the home.

A number of attempts to "destratify" the doctor's relationships with patients and with other medical professionals and to make them more open and egalitarian have developed. "Patients' rights" are being asserted and codified, and, in some states, drafted into law. Greater emphasis is being placed, for example, on the patient's "right to treatment," right to information (relevant to diagnosis, therapy, prognosis, or to the giving of knowledgeable consent for any procedure), right to privacy and confidentiality, and right to be "allowed to die," rather than being "kept alive by artificial means or heroic measures . . . if the situation should arise in which there is no reasonable expectation of . . . recovery from physical or mental disability."[3]

In some medical milieux (for example, community health centers and health maintenance organizations), and in critical and self-consciously progressive writings about medicine, the term "client" or "consumer" is being substituted for "patient." This change in terminology is intended to underline the importance of preventing illness while stressing the desirability of a non-supine, non-subordinate relationship for those who seek care to those who provide it. The emergence of nurse-practitioners and physician's assistants on the American scene is perhaps the most significant sign that some blurring of the physician's supremacy vis-à-vis other medical professionals may also be taking place. For some of the responsibilities for diagnosis, treatment, and patient management that were formerly prerogatives of physicians have been incorporated into these new, essentially marginal roles.[4]

Enjoinders to patients to care for themselves rather than to rely so heavily on the services of medical professionals and institutions are more frequently heard. Much attention is being given to studies such as the one conducted by Lester Breslow and his colleagues at the University of California at Los Angeles which suggest that good health and longevity are as much related to a self-enforced regimen of sufficient sleep, regular, well-balanced meals, moderate exercise and weight, no smoking, and little or no drinking, as they are to professionally administered medical care. Groups such as those involved in the Women's Liberation Movement are advocating the social and psychic as well as the medical value of knowing, examining, and caring for one's own body. Self-therapy techniques and programs have been developed for conditions as complicated and grave as terminal renal disease and hemophilia A and B. Proponents of such regimens affirm that many aspects of managing even serious chronic illnesses can be handled safely at home by the patient and his family, who will, in turn, benefit both financially and emotionally. In addition, they claim that in many cases the biomedical results obtained seem superior to those of the traditional physician-administered, health-care-delivery system.

The underlying assumption in these instances is that, if self-care is collectivized and reinforced by mutual aid, not only will persons with a medical problem be freed from some of the exigencies of the sick role, but both personal and public health will thereby improve, all with considerable savings in cost. This point of view is based on the moral supposition that greater autonomy from the medical profession coupled with greater responsibility for self and others in the realm of health and illness is an ethically and societally superior state.

> We have the medicine we deserve. We freely choose to live the way we do.
> We choose to live recklessly, to abuse our bodies with what we consume, to

expose ourselves to environmental insults, to rush frantically from place to place, and to sit on our spreading bottoms and watch paid professionals exercise for us. . . . Today few patients have the confidence to care for themselves. The inexorable professionalization of medicine, together with reverence for the scientific method, have invested practitioners with sacrosanct powers, and correspondingly vitiated the responsibility of the rest of us for health. . . . What is tragic is not what has happened to the revered professions, but what has happened to us as a result of professional dominance. In times of inordinate complexity and stress we have been made a profoundly dependent people. Most of us have lost the ability to care for ourselves. . . . I have tried to demonstrate three propositions. First, medical care has less impact on health than is generally assumed. Second, medical care has less impact on health than have social and environmental factors. And third, given the way in which society is evolving and the evolutionary imperatives of the medical care system, medical care in the future will have even less impact on health than it has now. . . . We have not understood what health is. . . . But in the next few decades our understanding will deepen. The pursuit of health and of well-being will then be possible, but only if our environment is made safe for us to live in and our social order is transformed to foster health, rather than suppress joy. If not, we shall remain a sick and dependent people. . . . The end of medicine is not the end of health but the beginning. . . .[5]

The foregoing passage (excerpted from Rick Carlson's book, *The End of Medicine*) touches upon many of the demedicalization themes that have been discussed. It proclaims the desirability of demedicalizing American society, predicting that, if we do so, we can overcome the "harm" that excessive medicalization has brought in its wake and progress beyond the "limits" that it has set. Like most critics of medicalization on the American scene, Carlson inveighs against the way that medical care is currently organized and implemented, but he attaches exceptional importance to the health-illness-medical sector of the society. In common with other commentators, he views health, illness, and medicine as inextricably associated with values and beliefs of American tradition that are both critical and desirable. It is primarily for this reason that in spite of the numerous signs that certain *structural* changes in the delivery of care will have occurred by the time we reach the year 2000, American society is not likely to undergo a significant process of *cultural* demedicalization.

Dissatisfaction with the distribution of professional medical care in the United States, its costs, and its accessibility has become sufficiently acute and generalized to make the enactment of a national health-insurance system in the foreseeable future likely. Exactly what form that system should take still evokes heated debate about free enterprise and socialism, public and private regulation, national and local government, tax rates, deductibles and co-insurance, the right to health care, the equality principle, and the principle of distributive justice. But the institutionalization of a national system that will provide more extensive and equitable health-insurance protection now seems necessary as well as inevitable even to those who do not approve of it.

There is still another change in the health-illness-medicine area of the society that seems to be forthcoming and that, like national health insurance, would alter the structure within which care is delivered. This is the movement toward effecting greater equality, collegiality, and accountability in the relationship of physicians to patients and their families, to other medical professionals, and to the lay public. Attempts to reduce the hierarchical dimension in the physician's role, as well as the increased insistence on patient's rights, self-therapy, mutual medical aid, community medical services and care by non-physician health professionals, and the growth of legislative and judicial participation in health and medicine by both federal and local government are all part of this movement. There is reason to believe that, as a consequence of pressure from both outside and inside the medical profession, the doctor will become less "dominant" and "autonomous," and will be subject to more controls.

This evolution in the direction of greater egalitarianism and regulation notwithstanding, it seems unlikely that all elements of hierarchy and autonomy will, or even can, be eliminated from the physician's role. For that to occur, the medical knowledge, skill, experience, and responsibility of patients and paramedical professionals would have to equal, if not replicate, the physician's. In addition, the social and psychic meaning of health and illness would have to become trivial in order to remove all vestiges of institutionalized charisma from the physician's role. Health, illness, and medicine have never been viewed casually in any society and, as indicated, they seem to be gaining rather than losing importance in American society.

It is significant that often the discussions and developments relevant to the destratification and control of the physician's role and to the enactment of national health insurance are accompanied by reaffirmations of traditional American values: equality, independence, self-reliance, universalism, distributive justice, solidarity, reciprocity, and individual and community responsibility. What seems to be involved here is not so much a change in values as the initiation of action intended to modify certain structural features of American medicine, so that it will more fully realize long-standing societal values.

In contrast, the new emphasis on health as a right, along with the emerging perspective on illness as medically and socially engendered, seems to entail major conceptual rather than structural shifts in the health-illness-medical matrix of the society. These shifts are indicative of a less fatalistic and individualistic attitude toward illness, increased personal and communal espousal of health, and a spreading conviction that health is as much a consequence of the good life and the good society as it is of professional medical care. The strongest impetus for demedicalization comes from this altered point of view. It will probably contribute to the decategorization of certain conditions as illness, greater appreciation and utilization of non-physician medical professionals, the institutionalization of more preventive medicine and personal and public health measures, and, perhaps, to the undertaking of non-medical reforms (such as full employment, improved transportation, or adequate recreation) in the name of the ultimate goal of health.

However, none of these trends implies that what we have called *cultural* demedicalization will take place. The shifts in emphasis from illness to health, from therapeutic to preventive medicine, and from the dominance and autonomy of the doctor to patient's rights and greater control of the medical profession do not alter the fact that health, illness, and medicine are central preoccupations in the society which have diffuse symbolic as well as practical meaning. All signs suggest that they will maintain the social, ethical, and existential significance they have acquired, even though by the year 2000 some structural aspects of the way that medicine and care are organized and delivered may have changed. In fact, if the issues now being considered under the rubric of bioethics are predictive of what lies ahead, we can expect that in the future, health, illness, and medicine will acquire even greater importance as one of the primary symbolic media through which American society will grapple with fundamental questions of value and belief. What social mechanisms we will develop to come to terms with these "collective conscience" issues, and exactly what role physicians, health professionals, biologists, jurists, politicians, philosophers, theologians, social scientists, and the public at large will play in their resolution remains to be seen. But it is a distinctive characteristic of an advanced modern society like our own that scientific, technical, clinical, social, ethical, and religious concerns should be joined in this way.

References

1. Sedgwick, "Illness—Mental and Otherwise," *The Hastings Center Studies,* 1:3(1973), p. 37.
2. In addition to Illich, *Medical Nemesis,* and Kittrie, *The Right To Be Different,* see, for example, Rick J. Carlson, *The End of Medicine* (New York, 1975); Michael Foucault, *Madness and Civilization* (New York, 1967); Eliot Freidson, *Professional Dominance* (Chicago, 1970); Erving Goffman, *Asylums* (New York, 1961); R. D. Laing, *The Politics of Experience* (New York, 1967); Thomas J. Scheff, *Being Mentally Ill* (Chicago, 1966); Thomas S. Szasz, *The Myth of Mental Illness* (New York, 1961); and Howard D. Waitzkin and Barbara Waterman, *The Exploitation of Illness in Capitalist Society* (Indianapolis, 1974).

3. This particular way of requesting that one be allowed to die is excerpted from the "Living Will'" (revised April, 1974 version), prepared and promoted by the Euthanasia Educational Council.
4. See the article by David Rogers, "The Challenge of Primary Care," in *Daedalus,* 106, Winter, 1977:81–103.
5. Carlson, *The End of Medicine,* pp. 44, 141, and 203–31.

Toward Alternatives in Health Care

As part of a critical sociological examination of American health and medical care, it is important that we explore what can be done to create alternatives to improve health in our society. In so doing, we look beyond the "medical model" and the current organization and delivery of medical services. We can differentiate two types of possible change or alternatives: (1) *community* or local alternatives; and (2) *societal* (sometimes called systemic) alternatives. In the first section of Part Four we examine various community alternatives to existing medical services and discuss their problems and limitations, as well as their potential for improving health care. In the second section we look at the potential of broader, societal changes by reconceptualizing prevention and considering alternatives presented by other medical care systems. Neither we nor the writers of the articles included here claim to have *the* answer to our "health crisis." The editors of this volume do contend, however, that the answers to our health problems will ultimately be found by searching in the directions pointed out in this final section.

Community Alternatives

SEVERAL ISSUES EMERGE WHEN WE examine and evaluate community-level efforts to improve medical care. The first such issue pertains to inherent limitations of such efforts. It is widely argued that the possibilities for change within the existing societal and medical care system are inherently limited. Although some of the most exciting and interesting health innovations have occurred through local efforts on the community level—e.g., women's self-help clinics, neighborhood health centers—these efforts are constantly being shaped and limited by the societal context in which they emerge and in which, often, they must struggle to survive. The realities of the present system (e.g. the professional dominance of physicians, the control of medical payments by the insurance industry and medical care providers, and the limitations imposed by existing medical organizations on access to their services) constitute systemic boundaries to the power of community alternative health care organizations to effect real change. Some critics even contend that these societal-level constraints will, in the very nature of things, always undermine the progressive potential of alternative services: the medical establishment will either coopt their successes or use their unavoidable difficulties as evidence of their failure (Taylor, 1979; Kronenfeld, 1979).

Another issue raised by discussions of community alternatives concerns the underlying conceptualizations and purposes of local projects. Two approaches to community level projects represent different although related perspectives on the problems of and solutions to current medical care. John Ehrenreich (1978) terms these two perspectives the "political economic" and the "cultural."

The first approach, the "political economic," "challenges the poor distribution of an otherwise admirable service" and generates efforts to extend existing medical services to particular underserved populations, such as the poor and elderly. The second approach challenges the idea that Western-style medical care is the humane, effective, and desirable solution to health problems that its supporters and even some of its critics believe it to be. Those community projects which adopt this "cultural" perspective seek to develop truly alternative organizations and approaches to health care, such as, for example, women's self-help clinics.

Each approach has its advantages and disadvantages in the face of the limitations inherent in developing local alternatives. Ehrenreich suggests that a synthesis of these perspectives provides a vision of medical and health care whereby new and equitably distributed forms of services would be available to and controlled by the community that they serve. In Ehrenreich's words, the question raised by this vision becomes, "How, then, do we reconcile notions of individual freedom [vs. dependency] and dignity with a rational and social approach to healing technology?" (Ehrenreich,

1978: 31). The answer to this question necessarily involves addressing the broader, societal structure within which such a healing technology would develop.

A further issue related to this entire discussion of community alternatives is the idea of medical "self-help." The 1970s saw a widespread and increasing interest in self-help or self-care. Self-help groups and other indigenous initiatives in health care emerged as adjuncts and alternatives to medical care. Self-help and mutual aid have a long history in Western society (Katz and Bender, 1976). While critics like Ivan Illich (1976) see self-help as a panacea for our medical ills, most view it as having a more limited role. Self-help groups can provide assistance, encouragement, and needed services to people with chronic and disabling conditions that involve emotional and social problems not provided for by traditional medical care (Gussow and Tracy, 1976). They can also create alternative services, as in the women's health movement. Equally important, self-help groups can aid in demystifying medicine, build a sense of community among people with similar problems, and provide consumer control of, and low-cost, services.

While the idea of self-help is really not a new notion, it appears on today's medical scene as a somewhat radical departure from the traditional medical notion of a compliant patient and an expert physician. Self-help organizations such as Alcoholics Anonymous (AA) predate the current self-help wave and have apparently successfully demonstrated the possibility of people helping themselves and one another to better health. Often taken as a model for other groups, AA focuses upon behavior, symptoms, and a perception of alcoholism as a chronic and individual problem. It also insists that alcoholics need the continuous social support of other nondrinking alcoholics to maintain their sobriety. A number of analysts (e.g., Kronenfeld, 1979: 263) have noted that AA and other self-help programs modeled on it are somewhat authoritarian in their structure. AA, for example, does not question existing societal and cultural arrangements which may have contributed to the drinking problems of its members.

In part as a response to the recognition of the limitations of modern medicine and in reaction to frustrations with existing medical care options, self-help groups and the ideology of self-help have become increasingly popular, not only among former patients of the existing system, but also among professional critics of

American medical care (see for example, Illich, 1976; Levin, Katz and Holst, 1976; Carlson, 1975). There is, however, a tendency in these approaches to focus on individual responsibility for change without stressing simultaneously the difficulties of individual change within existing social arrangements. This has led several critics to note the potential for victim-blaming in recommendations for self-help (Kronenfeld, 1979; Ehrenreich, 1978) and the limitations of self-help approaches for many of the health problems of various, especially non-middle-class populations in the United States.

It is nonetheless clear that the idea of self-help is an exciting prospect and one would certainly not want to see the energy and excitement contained within it diminished. The self-help movement has given rise to a range of important criticisms of existing medical care and to a number of significant discoveries for improved health. Self-help approaches envision the possibility of people taking control over their own lives as well as of demystifying traditional medical care. However, unless self-help incorporates a strategy for community *and* societal change, it is likely to reduce this potential vision to the simplistic contention that people are responsible for their own stresses and diseases. Although providing mutual support and encouraging individuals to alter their "unhealthy" behaviors, self-help programs only rarely confront the real options of what people can do as individuals. What is needed, then, is a linking together of self-help movements with struggles for community and social change—in essence, a politicization of self-help.

Both the promise and the reality of self-help and community alternatives are evident in each of the articles in this section. The first, "Improving the Use of Health Services by the Poor" by Catherine Kohler Riessman, reviews a number of medical care experiments designed to bring medical services to underserved populations in the United States. From a "political economic" perspective, Riessman assesses how well these experiments increased utilization of medical services among groups defined as "underutilizers." Each of the projects demonstrated that when structural barriers were reduced and comprehensive medical care was made readily available to the poor, the "underutilizers" did indeed use the medical services they needed. While careful to point out that she is not assessing the effectiveness of those services in improving the community's general health, Riessman offers evidence that when structural changes are made, people respond by using medical services.

The other two articles in this section reflect primarily the "cultural" perspective of medical care and provide quite different examples of people reassessing their own health needs and developing alternative health care services through collective, community efforts. The first article, "Politicizing Health Care" by John McKnight, describes a fascinating and innovative community effort to assess health needs and design local medical care alternatives aimed at improving health in the community. In this project, people discovered a number of important things, including: (1) many "medical" problems had little to do with disease, and could more accurately be termed "social problems"; (2) they could, as a community, take collective action to make real changes in their own health; (3) they could build alternative organizations for meeting their health and social needs and in the process include heretofore ignored groups (e.g., the elderly) as productive contributors to the community's health; and (4) they could develop new "tools" of production which would remain under their own control and which would serve their own particular needs. Despite these marvelous lessons, McKnight acknowledges the limitations of local efforts to change the basic maldistribution of resources and services and notes the need for self-help efforts to come to grips with "external" authorities and structures.

In the last selection, Sheryl Ruzek describes the alternative forms of health care developed in the past decade by "The Women's Self-Help Health Movement." Probably the most widespread and successful self-help movement in recent years, the women's health movement is a product of the Women's Liberation Movement. It emerged from women's growing recognition of the role of medicine in their oppression and of the medical establishment's contribution to women's relative ignorance about their own bodies and health. In self-help clinics all across America, women discovered the joy of learning about their own bodies in a mutual-help atmosphere free of the connotations of a doctor-patient relationship. They learned, too, the liberating effect of having informed options regarding such issues as contraception or childbirth. The women's health movement has not only helped those directly involved in it. It has also been active in political efforts to eliminate dangerous medicines and medical devices prescribed by physicians (e.g., DES, the Dalcon Shield) and to alert women to the potential risks of using widely accepted medical techniques (e.g., birth control pills, fetal monitoring machines, minor tranquilizers). As with other community efforts, there have been struggles. The women's self-help movement has been faced with conflicts arising from its crossing over onto traditional medicine's "legitimate" turf (there have even been some arrests of women for "practicing medicine" without a license). It continually has problems in financing its alternative services, particularly for poor women who must rely on public funds and other third-party payments for their medical services. The women's health movement has sometimes imposed limitations on itself by rejecting much of what traditional medicine has to offer.

Probably the most significant consequence of the women's self-help movement has been the reconceptualization of "gynecology," women's health needs, and the position of women vis-à-vis traditional medical care. Assessing the effectiveness of this and all community alternatives, however, is often difficult since traditional measures of "quality of care" tend to include the very ideas of medical care these community groups are struggling to change.

References

Carlson, R.J. 1975. The End of Medicine. New York: John Wiley.

Ehrenreich, John. 1978. "Introduction: The cultural crisis of modern medicine." Pp. 1–35 in John Ehrenreich [Ed.] The Cultural Crisis of Modern Medicine. New York: Monthly Review Press.

Gussow, Zachary and George Z. Tracy. 1976. "The role of self-help clubs in the adaptation to chronic illness and disability." Social Science and Medicine 10 (7/8): 407–414.

Illich, Ivan. 1976. Medical Nemesis: The Expropriation of Health. New York: Pantheon Books.

Katz, A.H. and E.I. Bender. 1976. "Self-help groups in Western society." Journal of Applied Behavioral Science 12: 265–282.

Kronenfeld, Jennie J. 1979. "Self care as a panacea for the ills of the health care system: An assessment." Social Science and Medicine 13A: 263–267.

Levin, L., A. Katz and E. Holst. 1976. Self-Care: Lay Initiatives in Health. New York: Prodist.

Taylor, Rosemary C.R. 1979. "Alternative services: The case of free clinics." International Journal of Health Services 9, 2: 227–253.

36

Improving the Use of Health Services by the Poor

Catherine Kohler Riessman

Research over the past several decades has documented the lower utilization of health services by the poor. Use of both preventive and treatment services has been explored in numerous health surveys, and data have emerged regarding the underutilizaiton of medical and dental services by lower social-economic groups, especially Blacks. Even though there has been a steady reduction of class differentials in the use made of physicians over time, overall class differences appear to persist.[1]

More precisely, . . . National Health Survey (1966–67) [data] reveal that race, income, and education are the best predictors of utilization. Those families where the head of household had some college had a significantly higher number of visits to a doctor per year than those with less education; this difference becomes most striking with respect to services to children (immunizations, routine pediatric exams, etc., during the early years when preventive care is considered to be especially important) and young adolescents under age 15.[2]

Differential utilization by color is especially marked, with whites exceeding nonwhites by 50 percent, except in the ages 25–34 (presumably due to childbirth and the higher rate of injury of Black males in this age group).[3] Again, number of visits of children and adolescents shows the sharpest differentials by color, illustrating the historic underutilization of preventive pediatric services by Blacks.

For the rest of the population, however, income is a crucial variable determining utilization. Anderson and Anderson found in 1963 that 56 percent of those with incomes under $4,000 saw a physician during the year, compared to 71 percent with incomes of $7,000 and above.[4] Income differentials in relation to dental care are also pronounced, although it is worth stressing that irrespective of social class and prepayment dental services are underutilized generally (42 percent of those with incomes over $10,000 did not consult a dentist in 1963, in spite of the high prevalence of dental disease demonstrated in many studies).[5]

Use of medical specialists increases with education and income, with urban whites being the primary users. Nonmedical practitioners (such as chiropractors) account for 15.6 visits per 100 individuals per year, the primary users here being those with less than college education.[6] The greater use of marginal and quasi-practitioners (including druggists) by the poor has contributed to the formulation that they are more "parochial" and less "cosmopolitan" in their health orientation.[7]

Classic studies in the sociomedical field have explored the relationship between social class and use of such preventive and screening services as immunizations, chest X-rays, Pap smears, prenatal exams, and asymptomatic checkups.[8] Participation in these health programs has been found to be associated with sex, age, educational level, income, and color.

Two major explanations of the above phenomena have been suggested by medical sociologists: one is psychocultural, embodying the "culture of poverty thesis" originally formulated by Oscar Lewis in 1959, in which poverty is defined as a "way of life" or a "culture" comprising a body of interrelated social, economic, and psychological traits (including dependence, violence, easy sex, inability to delay gratification) that are transmitted from generation to generation.

On the other end of the continuum are writers who have emphasized economic and sociostructural influences on health behavior. Economic factors that have been shown to greatly influence the utilization of health services include price of services, the presence or absence of health insurance, and family income.[9] Rather than emphasizing subjective factors such as the extent of need or the predisposition to seek care, this approach stresses the potential user's structural position and hence his access to medical services. As Anderson states, "The economic model stresses means through which people can obtain services or translate their perceived need into economic demand for medical care."[10]

The "Culture of Poverty" View

In the field of health, theorists and researchers favoring the culture-of-poverty thesis have emphasized the psychological and attitudinal dimensions influencing health behavior, as well as the degree of alienation and anomie. Thus Moody and Gray find "social integration" to be antecedent to oral polio vaccine acceptance.[11]

Health and illness behavior are seen as a function of personal characteristics: motivation, a constellation of health beliefs, and medical orientation.[12] As lower-class individuals allegedly accord greater priority to immediate rewards than to long-term goals, medical care is sought in emergency situations or in times of severe illness, and often after considerable delay. Immunizations, routine dental and prenatal care, asymptomatic checkups, and the following of medical regimens occur with significantly less frequency in poor groups because a "psychological readiness" and future orientation supposedly do not exist. The poor constitute a "core of resistance and nonparticipation to many of the more advanced medical and educational programs," according to Suchman.[13]

According to the culture-of-poverty proponents, the poor have also used preventive services less and are less knowledgeable about appropriate health behavior because they possess a culture which does not place a high value on health. Experiencing a sense of helplessness and resignation in coping with their environment, the poor do not exhibit the active, individually responsible, and disciplined behavior necessary in seeking appropriate medical care. As Rosenblatt and Suchman have noted:

> The body can be seen as simply another class of object to be worn out but not repaired. Thus teeth are left without dental care. . . . Corrective eye examinations, even for those who wear glasses, are often neglected. . . . It is as though . . . blue collar groups think of the body as having a limited span of utility, to be enjoyed in youth and then to suffer with and to endure stoically with age and decrepitude.[14]

By definition this "culture" is fixed; it is passed from generation and creates a self-propelling cycle of poverty and poor health. Efforts to intervene and change patterns of behavior will be largely fruitless given the values and traditions deeply embedded in the "culture."[15] Rosenstock summarizes this point of view:

> The culture of poverty may originally have been based on a history of economic deprivation, but it seems to be a culture exhibiting its own rationale, and structure, and reflecting a way of life that is transmitted to new generations. It is therefore suggested that while financial costs may serve as barriers to obtaining health services, their removal would probably not have the effect of creating widespread changes in health behavior of the poor, at least not in the foreseeable future.[16]

The Sociostructural View

While being sensitive to the "lifestyle" differences patients bring with them, Anselm Strauss draws attention to the professional and organizational "culture" which leads to inadequate clinic operations: the long waits, impersonality, and bureaucratic procedures to which the patient must adapt. Changing professional practice and improving clinic experiences are stressed, rather than changing the client.[17] Further, Coe and Wesson suggest that certain conditions imposed by the contemporary practice of medicine may influence utilization: the extreme impersonality of the encounter between physician and patient, and the inability to achieve a relationship may account for some of the resistance to seeking service.[18]

Richardson cites data showing higher rates of morbidity yet lower utilization of ambulatory services by the poor, and concludes that economic and geographic availability plus the generally unfavorable nature of the way services are offered account for these class differentials.[19] Indeed other studies have attempted to measure the relationship of geographic proximity of a service to its utilization. Lerner, for example, found that a two-mile "threshold" exists beyond which utilization decreases markedly.[20]

Duff and Hollinshead have documented the second-class and highly discriminatory care offered the poor.[21] Freidson has described the professional attitudes and patterns of interaction operating in medical practice which may be especially alien to patients from lower socioeconomic groups.[22]

Sol Levine and others have stated that the "culture of medicine" rather than the limitations in the culture of the patient represents the major impediment to the improvement of health: the accretion of habits, customs, and expectations of health professionals and the needs of bureaucratic organizations.[23] The social relationship between user and provider is seen as a crucial variable influencing utilization, with social distance, medical jargon and lack of effective communication,[24] and prejudicial attitudes on the part of health professionals the prime deterrents to greater utilization.

According to these researchers, the poor have undergone multiple negative experiences with organizational systems, leading to avoidance behavior, lack of trust, and hence a disinclination to seek care and follow medical regimens except in dire need. The assumption is that "good" experiences will result in behavior change: the lack of appropriate utilization of health care by lower socioeconomic groups is not deeply culture bound, but can be modified given changes in the professional and the organization of medical care.

Unfortunately, relatively few empirical studies of health utilization have focused on these structural elements as independent variables. Rather, the majority of research concerns intrapersonal and cultural variables (health beliefs, and attitudes, knowledge about health, alienation, cultural and demographic factors). A cursory analysis of a bibliography of indices and correlates of utilization of health services reveals that only a small fraction of the existing studies relates to cost of care, distance, patient-physician interaction, and other similar variables as correlates of utilization; the sociodemographic and social psychological are significantly more prevalent.[25] Perhaps unwittingly, this research emphasis has subtly encouraged the cultural hypotheses (lower utilization equals lower motivation). And yet, Martin Rein found a marked increase in utilization of both physician and hospital services by the lower classes, with the poorest groups eventually exceeding the middle class, following the introduction of national health insurance in Great Britain.[26] What does the American experience reveal with less radical innovations in health care delivery? In this perspective, then, it seems important to review recent experiments in health care delivery which suggest answers to the question: Does utilization by the poor change when the context of care is altered?

Recent Data on Utilization

Within the last decade several experiments have been attempted in the delivery of health care to lower socioeconomic groups. Experimental programs sponsored by the OEO and others made comprehensive medical care genuinely available, structural barriers were reduced, and utilization was encouraged. By a close examination of these programs, we can begin to assess alternative explanations for the historic class differentials in utilization. These experimental projects cover a wide area and thus do not represent one "solution," or one model, for more equitable care. A university-affiliated demonstration project, a prepaid group practice plan, research emanating from the neighborhood health centers and decentralized family planning programs will be reviewed. All have attempted to deal with the structural variables outlined before, which my thesis contends have been primary in deterring higher utilization by lower socioeconomic groups. None of the programs I will describe have had as their major thrust the changing of cultural values and attitudes regarding health. Yet all have markedly affected behavior. Utilization by the poor of both preventive and curative services has consistently increased in these varied programs. The rapid speed at which change in health behavior was achieved is especially worth noting.

New York Hospital-Cornell Project

This demonstration project, carried on between 1960 and 1965, compared utilization in two systems of medical care: the existing fragmented and haphazard "system" used by welfare recipients in New York City and a model demonstration project for another group of welfare families set up at New York Hospital. Subjects for the experimental and control groups were randomly selected from a local welfare district. (Total N=2,500 persons.) The experimental group was offered complete medical, pediatric, casework, and public health nursing services at New York Hospital, with each patient assigned to a personal staff physician. Emergency, inpatient, home care, and other services were also provided or coordinated by the project. Bilingual staffing was stressed. Half of the experimental group was given an appointment for a physical with the letter of invitation to join the project; the other half was merely told to contact the project (demand group). Those in the control group were sent nothing and utilized their usual source of care through the two years of the project.

The offering of an appointment was found to markedly affect utilization. Of the welfare cases offered an appointment, 74 percent came to the project for care, compared to 51 percent in the demand group.[27] Many of the patients had to travel considerable distances to reach New York Hospital (from the lower East Side and East Harlem, for example); thus the barriers of travel time and cost remained, although one structural variable, the availability of high quality comprehensive care, was manipulated in the experiment.

An initial and two followup interviews were conducted for the experimental and control groups. It was found that the experimental groups had higher utilization: 8.1 visits per person per year for the appointment group, 7.1 visits for the demand group, and 6.5 visits for the control group.[28] The rates for the experimental groups declined somewhat during the second year, presumably due to better health status. Inpatient utilization was highest in the experimental group the first year and then dropped markedly in the second.[29]

Patient satisfaction with the service was high in the experimental groups, a variable which is perhaps not unrelated to high utilization. All indications are that the experimental groups made appropriate and continuous use of the project-services and "shopping" for medical care elsewhere was nonexistent. The use of preventive services increased markedly, with mothers in the experimental group using postpartum and well-baby care in greater numbers than the control group.

The authors conclude that the barriers to greater utilization of health services by poverty families did not lie in the clients but rather in the existing organization of medical care, specifically the eligibility requirements and districting rules of New York City hospitals.

Thus structural changes in the way health care was offered in this experimental project radically altered health utilization behavior of a sample of welfare recipients in a two-year period.

Low-Income Families in a Prepaid Group Practice

Another project had similar results using prepaid group practice. OEO sponsored a total of 3,000 families in four prepaid plans (Kaiser at Fontana, California; Kaiser at Portland, Oregon; Group Health of Puget Sound, Washington; and HIP of New York at Suffolk County). Those selected for sponsorship had low incomes, large families, and were considered "high risk" (had a current illness or a recent pregnancy).[30] Individuals 65 and over were excluded, and 50 percent of the enrollees were under 15 years. Data were then collected from medical records on utilization rates of regular plan members and on those enrolled in each project through OEO sponsorship. In Fontana, the physician utilization rate of the OEO group exceeded significantly that of the regular members; at Puget Sound and Portland, the rates were almost identical for the two groups;

only at Suffolk County did the OEO group utilize less. In addition to physician utilization, rates for visits to mid-level practitioners (nurses, home health aides, etc.) were calculated, which brought the total medical utilization rates for the OEO group above the regular rates in every case. Utilization was highest during the first year, when medical needs were greatest, with a modest downward drift and then stabilization the following year.[31]

Rates for inpatient utilization demonstrate the effects of comprehensive outpatient care coupled with reasonable gatekeeping functions over hospital bed use. Prepaid group practices generally have lower hospitalization rates than traditional fee-for-service systems.[32] Comparing data from the OEO-sponsored groups and regular members, admissions for the low-income group were slightly higher, though below the national average for low-income persons under 65. Number of inpatient days per 1,000 persons were comparable between the two groups, with the OEO-sponsored members experiencing a 50 percent reduction over national rates for low-income groups in length of stay.[33]

Patient transportation was provided for the OEO group, as were outreach and home health and mental health services. Sparer and Anderson feel that the provision of these services was crucial to the success of the project: "Scant anecdotal data suggest that not even minimal utilization would occur without the support services."[34] How much service and for how long it would be needed clearly needs to be assessed in future research.

These data strongly suggest that the traditionally lower utilization by poor families of health services can be turned around within a short period of time. The provision of a quality service, the availability of patient transportation, and community and outreach services increased utilization of the poor group to middle-class levels. Changes in attitudes and health beliefs apparently were not necessary in order to increase utilization; rather structural barriers were removed and features were included to facilitate access.

Neighborhood Health Centers

Data are now beginning to emerge from the approximately 80 health service projects funded by the OEO in the late 1960s, 50 of which are neighborhood health centers. These centers are designed to provide comprehensive services, with emphasis on prevention and early treatment, to urban and rural areas having high concentrations of poverty and previously inadequate health services. The guidelines spell out the intent of the program.

> The project must contain provisions to assure that services will be provided in such ways and in such circumstances as to be both accessible and acceptable to

the people being served. The project must include mechanisms which will eliminate the problems that have plagued other health service institutions for the poor, including unpleasant physical surroundings, crowding, long waits and depersonalization. The project must be able to deal effectively with barriers to medical care usually encountered by the poor, including problems of costs, distance, transportation, hours during which services are available, and cumbersome intake and ineligibility procedures.[35]

Thus the neighborhood health centers have attempted to correct or minimize the structural impediments to quality health care for low-income families, and therefore data on utilization are important to examine in light of my hypothesis.

In a recent study of patterns of utilization in 21 of the oldest centers, user families and comparable nonuser families in each service area were compared with a control group of similar families in nearby comparison areas. Probability sampling techniques were used to select participants for the study (total N=9,500 families). Regarding utilization, an average of 66 percent of all eligible individuals have used the centers (range equals 33–97 percent). Furthermore appropriate utilization has been characteristic of the users.

> NHC users seek treatment for their most limiting conditions more often, receive immunizations and examinations more often, have had a more recent dental check, and use weekend and emergency care less than either the nonusers or the control groups.[36]

Characteristics of the neighborhood health center users are worth noting: user families were significantly younger and larger than nonusers, had a lower per capita income, and were more likely to be receiving Medicaid and other welfare benefits. Regarding racial differences, in 8 of the 21 neighborhood health center areas, the proportion of Blacks using center services was significantly higher than the percentage of Blacks in the area. Moreover in no case was the percentage of Blacks higher among the nonusers than in the areas as a whole.[37] This is a striking finding when contrasted with the 1966–67 National Health Survey findings cited earlier: Blacks nationally made 50 percent fewer physician visits than did whites. Perhaps this is related to the fact that NHC services were offered with fewer structural impediments, without discrimination, and preserving the dignity of patients.

Strauss and Sparer intensively studied eight OEO-funded comprehensive health service projects, five of which were neighborhood health centers. They found relatively higher physician-nurse utilization by "users" and "active registrants."[38] All projects showed an initial surge of use (when health needs are greatest and when many baseline exams are performed). Then the rates appear to taper off and approximate national averages. Rural projects had rates similar to urban projects,[39] a finding that contradicts the previous patterns of lower utilization in rural areas noted in the National Health Survey of 1966–67.

Children under 15 account for one-third to one-half of the registrants using physician-provided services in neighborhood health centers,[40] in contrast to past national health surveys which revealed the aged to be the group with the highest utilization rate.[41] Thus aside from apparently increasing utilization by lower socioeconomic groups generally, these projects appear to be reaching children and young adolescents in poor families, the age group that previously had the largest differentials by class.

These preliminary data seem to suggest a high utilization by low-income persons of these programs especially designed for them, in numbers comparable to middle-class patterns, particularly when one considers all providers (public health nurses, paraprofessionals, etc.) and not just physician-registrant encounters. According to OEO, nonphysician encounters account for 25 percent of the total,[42] and it appears that many of these mid-level practitioners are providing many preventive and social services.

According to recent estimates, 6,000 community residents are employed in the 50 neighborhood health centers (50 percent of the staffs of all centers). A large portion of these are home health aides, community-outreach and family workers, and other paraprofessionals. Gartner has cited the numerous studies demonstrating how these workers markedly affect utilization.[43] In the Denver Maternal and Infant Care Project, 42 percent higher attendance occurred in disadvantaged areas using "neighborhood representatives." These workers accounted for 60 percent of the new referrals, and a 20 percent hike in unwed mothers applying for service was noted. In neighborhoods where representatives were employed for six months or more, 50 percent of the pregnant patients were being seen in their first or second trimester, compared to 32 percent in unserved neighborhoods.[44] In another study of an Oklahoma immunization project cited by Gartner, seven paraprofessionals brought in ten times the number of persons as did three public health nurses.[45] The well-trained indigenous paraprofessional can eclipse the usual social distance between health professional and low-income consumer. She/he relates as a peer and as a model, and her/his presence lessens the likelihood of miscommunication between provider and consumer. The greater utilization of neighborhood health centers by the poor may be due in part to these new workers and the cultural understanding that their presence insures.

Family Planning

A particularly critical example of preventive service has long been family planning. Many researchers and theorists have historically argued that of all preventive services, family planning would be especially resisted by the poor because of the "culture of poverty," and the supposed inability of the poor to plan for the future and defer gratification.[46]

As early as 1960, experimental programs were initiated in an attempt to encourage contraceptive use among lower socioeconomic groups. A pilot project in Mecklenburg County, North Carolina, made oral contraceptives available to 264 women volunteers (married, previously married, and single parous women) who were public welfare clients. Ninety percent were Black, 10 percent white. Their mean age was 29, mean grade in high school completed was 9, mean number of children was 4.8. Of the women working, 89 percent held unskilled positions, largely as domestics. The majority lived in overcrowded, depressed-area housing. After two years, 223 of these women were still active in the program. But perhaps more significant, other women in the county virtually began knocking the doors down to be referred to the "pill clinic."[47]

The Chicago Planned Parenthood conducted a study involving more than 14,000 patients using oral contraceptives: 83 percent of the patients were nonwhite, slightly less than half had not completed high school, and one out of six was a welfare recipient. It was found that between 70 and 83 percent continued to take the pills in the required manner for 30 months after they came to the clinic.[48] As Jaffe states, "This is an astonishingly high retention rate for any procedure requiring continuous self-administration of medication and says something about the readiness of the poor to respond to well-conceived, energetically delivered voluntary programs employing coitus-independent methods."[49]

Current nationwide data on family planning programs reveal unparalleled utilization by poor women. A recent study found that 3.2 million women (52 percent of all poverty-level women) were being served, the vast majority in organized programs rather than by private physicians. In just a few years (large-scale federal funding for these programs commenced in 1969–70), the program has passed its halfway mark in reaching all financially needy women.[50] Moreover a study comparing a sample of low- and middle-income women using the pill found little difference between the two groups in the continuation rate. In fact the low-income women slightly exceeded the middle-income group in effective use of contraception.[51]

In sharp contrast, recent studies of physicians reveal their lack of confidence in poor women's ability to use the pill effectively. Many of the doctors sampled felt the poor did not have the "intelligence" or motivation to take the pill dependably.[52] In light of this, it is worth noting that 73 percent of the 3.2 million low-income women currently using family planning services chose the oral contraceptive[53]—the method requiring the most planning and future time orientation.

Comparison of a 1970 survey of a probability sample of 5,884 married women under 45 years of age with a similar survey in 1965 reveals a 36 percent decline in the rate of unwanted childbearing. The largest declines were registered for Blacks (56 percent) and Catholics (45 percent), particularly those of low education.[54]

Columbia Point Neighborhood Health Center

Columbia Point was the first OEO-funded neighborhood health center (it opened its doors in December 1965). It is situated in a low-income, public housing community in the Dorchester area of Boston, Massachusetts. I will examine this particular center more closely since the passage of time and a heavy research emphasis have produced especially valuable data on utilization.

The volume of use of this center has been high from the outset. Data from medical records revealed that 75 percent of the total population of Columbia Point visited the center for care at least once during the third year of operation. Surveys revealed that the health center was the regular source of care for about 97 percent of the children (versus 71 percent of the adults).[55]

A baseline survey prior to the center's opening provided data on previous sources of care, patterns of utilization, health beliefs, and other variables. Of the original randomly selected respondents, 86 percent were successfully reinterviewed two years after the opening of the center.[56] The findings regarding use of preventive services are particularly noteworthy.

Yearly asymptomatic general health exams increased from 17 to 59 percent (p<.001). Prior to the health center's opening only 57 percent of the adult respondents and 78 percent of their youngest children had received polio immunization. Eighteen months later the percentage of adult immunization was unchanged (57 percent), but increased to 92 percent among children (p<.01). Before the center's opening 23 percent acknowledged that they or someone in their family had put off seeking care in the previous six-month period; two years later this figure declined to 10 percent (p<.001).[57] Thus in the area of preventive care, where the poor have historically underutilized services, dramatic changes were effected in a two-year period.

Data were also collected on "health beliefs," and major changes occurred here as well. At the time of the initial survey, 47 percent disagreed with the statement that "There is no need to see a doctor regularly if you are not sick." Two years later this figure was 62 percent (p<.001). A checklist of conditions for which a doctor should be seen was presented to respondents and significant changes occurred in attitudes toward the majority of items. Regarding conditions felt to be serious by health professionals, between 77 and 92 percent of the sample rated the symptoms as needing medical attention,[58] a finding that is in sharp contrast to Koos's finding that the poor had a "marked indifference" to most signals of serious medical problems.[59]

The situational or structural determinants of health behavior were directly addressed in the Columbia Point study. Previous to the opening of the health center, respondents cited cost of care, transportation cost, time lost, and lack of babysitter as reasons for delaying medical care. Previous to the opening 84 percent of the respondents stated they spent two hours or more door-to-door when they sought care; 14 percent reported spending five hours and longer per physician visit. Two years later only 17 percent reported two or more hours.[60] Patient satisfaction with the health facilities was also measured; it increased 67 percent between 1965 and 1967 (p<.001)[61]

Hospital records were used to calculate inpatient use before and after the center opened; an 84 percent drop in admissions occurred after the second year the center was in operation. Only neurological and psychiatric admissions rose slightly.

Number of total hospital bed days also dropped markedly in the second year. No similar decline occurred with patients from other areas. The investigators feel that preventing conditions from becoming serious enough to require hospitalization accounts for the difference.[62]

Again there is evidence to suggest that the poor appropriately use preventive and curative services when these services are made available and structural barriers are removed or minimized. Moreover, by enabling behavior to change (through the provision of health services), attitude change quickly followed.

Conclusion

Data from a university-sponsored demonstration project, a prepaid group practice plan, neighborhood health centers, and nationwide family planning programs all suggest that the health behavior of the poor can be radically altered, and within a relatively short period of time, by introducing structural changes in the way the services are offered.[63] Too often, as Gibson states, "it is the individual patient (or potential patient) that is blamed and the system ignored in the search for causes and rationales for change."[64]

I have intentionally avoided the issue of the effectiveness of these experimental programs in improving the health status of the populations they serve. The poor may very well continue to be sicker than their middle-class counterparts due to a variety of factors. My focus has been solely on utilization rates and how these may be affected by changes in the delivery system. Measuring the quality of care provided by these programs and their ultimate impact on the high chronic disease morbidity characteristic of lower socioeconomic groups awaits further research. Also needed are cost-benefit analyses and evaluation research based on outcome variables such as decreased mortality and morbidity. Patient satisfaction and increased utilization, while important, should not be the ultimate indicators of a successful health strategy.

Future research will need to explore rigorously the relationship of a large array of structural variables to utilization. The possible contribution of attitudinal and subjective dimensions can only be fully evaluated when structural barriers are removed and access to a quality service is equally available irrespective of class.

References

1. R. Anderson, R. Greely, J. Kravitz, O. Anderson, *Health Service Use: National Trends and Variations*, U.S. Dept. of Health Education, and Welfare, Health Services and Mental Health Administration, DHEW Pub. No 73-3004, October 1972. A recent study found no class differences in certain types of health-seeking behavior. See William C. Richardson, "Ambulatory Use of Physicians' Services in Response to Illness Episodes in a Low Income Neighborhood," Research Series 29, Univ. of Chicago, Center for Health Administration Studies, 1971.
2. National Center for Health Statistics, Vital and Health Statistics, *Volume of Physician Visits, U.S., July 1966–1967*, U.S. Public Health Service Pub. No. 1000—Series No. 49 (Washington, D.C.: U.S. Government Printing Office, November 1968).
3. Ibid.
4. R. Anderson and O. Anderson, *A Decade of Health Services: Social Survey Trends in Use and Expenditures* (Chicago: Univ. of Chicago Press, 1967).
5. Ibid., Table 25, p. 47. See also M.K. Nikias, "Social Class and the Use of Dental Care under Prepayment," *Medical Care* 6 (1968), pp. 381–393.
6. National Center for Health Statistics, Vital and Health Statistics, *Family Use of Health Services, U.S., July 1963–June 1964*, PHS Pub. No. 100—Series 10, No. 55 (Washington, D.C.: U.S. Government Printing Office, July 1969).
7. Edward A. Suchman, "Social Patterns of Illness and Medical Care," in *Patients, Physicians and Illness*, E.G. Jaco, ed. (N.Y.: The Free Press, 1972), pp. 262–279.
8. Stephen S. Kegeles et al., "Survey of Beliefs about Cancer Detection and Taking Papanicolaou Tests," *Public Health Reports* 80 (September 1965), pp. 815–824. Don P. Haefner et al., "Preventive Actions in Dental Disease, TB and Cancer," *Public Health Reports* 82 (May 1967), pp. 451–460. Godfrey N. Hochbaum, *Public Participation in Medical Screening Programs*, U.S. Public Health Service Pub. No. 572 (Washington, D.C.: U.S. Government Printing Office, 1958). Leila C. Deasy, "Socioeconomic Status and Participation in the Poliomyelitis Vaccine Trial," in *Sociological Studies of Health and Sickness*, Dorrian Apple, ed. (N.Y.: McGraw-Hill, 1960), pp. 15–25.

9. H. Klarman, *The Economics of Health* (N.Y.: Columbia Univ. Press, 1965), pp. 20–40. T.W. Bice and R.L. Eichhorn, "Socioeconomic Status and Use of Physicians' Services: A Reconsideration," *Medical Care* 12 (1972), pp. 261–271. L.A. Aday, "Dimensions of Family's Social Status and Their Relationships to Children's Utilization of Health Services," unpublished manuscript, Johns Hopkins University, Dept. of Medical Care and Hospitals, 1971.

10. R. Anderson, op. cit., p. 11.

11. P. Moody and R. Gray, "Social Class, Social Integration, and the Use of Preventive Health Services," in E.G. Jaco, ed. op. cit., pp. 250–261.

12. E. Suchman, op. cit.; S. Kegeles et al., op cit.; G. Hochbaum, op. cit.; L. Deasy, op cit.; I.M. Rosenstock, "Prevention of Illness and Maintenance of Health," in *Poverty and Health: A Sociological Analysis,* Kosa et al., eds. (Cambridge, Mass.: Harvard Univ. Press, 1969); Earl L. Koos, *The Health of Regionville* (N.Y.: Columbia Univ. Press, 1954).

13. E. Suchman, op. cit., p. 279.

14. D. Rosenblatt and E. Suchman, "Blue Collar Attitudes and Information toward Health and Illness," in *Blue Collar World,* Shostak and Gomberg, eds. (Englewood Cliffs, N.J.: Prentice-Hall, 1964), pp. 341–349.

15. The concept of a culture of poverty has been widely criticized for many years. See Jack L. Roach and O.R. Gursslin, "An Evaluation of the Concept 'Culture of Poverty,'" *Social Forces* 45 (1967), pp. 383–392; S.M. Miller and F. Riessman, "The Culture of Poverty: A Critique," in *Social Class and Social Policy* (N.Y.: Basic Books, 1968), pp. 52–66; William Ryan, *Blaming the Victim* (N.Y.: Pantheon Books, 1971); Charles A. Valentine, *Culture and Poverty: Critique and Counterproposals* (Chicago: Univ. of Chicago Press, 1968); Eleanor B. Leacock, ed., *The Culture of Poverty: A Critique* (N.Y.: Simon & Schuster, 1971).

16. I.M. Rosenstock, op. cit., p. 188.

17. A. Strauss, "Medical Ghettos," in E.G. Jaco, ed., op. cit., pp. 381–388.

18. R.M. Coe and A. Wesson, "Social-psychological Factors Influencing the Use of Community Health Resources," *American Journal of Public Health* 55 (1965), pp. 1,024–1,031.

19. William C. Richardson, "Poverty, Illness and the Use of Health Services in the U.S.," in the E.G. Jaco, ed., op. cit., pp. 240–249.

20. R. Lerner, C. Kicher, and E. Dieckman, *Data on Social Backgrounds, Medical Care Utilization and Attitudes of Outpatients by Hospital,* N.Y.C. Municipal General Hospital Outpatient Population Study (N.Y.: Columbia Univ. School of Public Health, 1968). J.E. Weiss and M.R. Greenlick, "Determinants of Medical Care Utilization: The Effect of Social Class and Distance on Contacts with the Medical Care System," *Medical Care* 8 (1970), pp. 456–462. G.W. Shannon et al., "The Concept of Distance as a Factor in Accessibility and Utilization of Health Care," *Medical Care Review* 26 (1969), pp. 143–161. P.J. Jehlik and R.L. McNamara, "The Relation of Distance to the Differential Use of Certain Health Personnel and Facilities and the Extent of Bad Illness," *Rural Sociology* 17 (1952), pp. 261–265.

21. Raymond S. Duff and August B. Hollingshead, *Sickness and Society* (N.Y.: Harper & Row, 1968).

22. Eliot Freidson, *Profession of Medicine* (N.Y.: Dodd, Mead & Co., 1971), pp. 302–331; "Dilemmas in the Doctor-Patient Relationship," in *Patients View Their Medical Practice* (N.Y.: Russell Sage, 1961), pp. 171–191.
23. S. Levine, N. Scotch, and G. Vlasak, "Unraveling Technology—Culture in Public Health," *American Journal of Public Health* 59 (1969), pp. 237–244.
24. B. Korsch and V. Negrete, "Doctor-Patient Communication," *Scientific American* 227 (1972).
25. National Center for Health Services Research and Development, *The Utilization of Health Services: Indices and Correlates; A Research Bibliography,* DHEW Pub. No. 73-3003, 1972.
26. M. Rein, "Social Class and the Health Service," *New Society* 20 (1969), pp. 807–810.
27. C. Goodrich, M. Olendski, and G. Reader, *Welfare Medical Care: An Experiment* (Cambridge, Mass.: Harvard Univ., Press, 1970), p. 208. Self-selection factors may bias the findings, for 26 percent of the appointment group and 49 percent of the demand group did not choose to participate and thus their characteristics are not included in the analysis. No attempt was apparently made in the study to sample them and not any differences. The levels of statistical significance in all of these comparisons are unfortunately omitted by the authors.
28. Ibid., p. 137.
29. Ibid., pp. 150–156.
30. Sparer and Anderson do not specify in sufficient detail the selection procedures used for OEO families, so it is impossible to rule out self-selection as a source of invalidity. Ideally, randomization should be used, with active recruiting and intensive study of any subjects reluctant to take part.
31. G. Sparer and A. Anderson, "Utilization and Cost Experience of Low Income Families in Four Prepaid Group Practice Plans, 1970–1971," paper presented at annual conference of American Public Health Association, Atlantic City, N.J., November 1972.
32. O. Anderson, "Patterns of Use of Health Services," in *Handbook of Medical Sociology,* H. Freeman, S. Levine, and L. Reader, eds. (Englewood Cliffs, N.J.: Prentice-Hall, 1972), p. 400.
33. Sparer and Anderson, op. cit., pp. 16–18.
34. Ibid., p. 23.
35. U.S. Office of Economic Opportunity, *The Comprehensive Neighborhood Health Services Program Guidelines: Health Services* (Washington, D.C., 1970), p. 5.
36. Office of Planning, Research and Evaluation, U.S. Office of Economic Opportunity, *An Evaluation of the Neighborhood Health Center Program: Summary of Results and Methodology,* May 1972.
37. Ibid., p. 17.
38. The authors attempt to deal with the difficult issue of defining a denominator for any utilization rate. Many registration rosters of centers may be inflated with "nominal registrants" (i.e., those who do not use the center as their primary source of care, those who have moved from the service area or otherwise ineligible), resulting in inflated denominators and therefore unduly low

rates. The authors utilize the concept of any "active registrant" (person is eligible and has used service at least once during 18 months) and a "user" (registered patient with one MD-RN encounter in one-year period) as the basis for their calculations. See Strauss and Sparer, pp. 38–41. Although useful conceptually, calculating rates in this manner makes it difficult to compare utilization in centers with national averages of utilization of other types of health delivery systems. The standardization of calculating procedures for utilization rates is clearly needed to further research and comparative studies in this area.

39. M. Strauss and G. Sparer, "Basic Utilization Experience of OEO Comprehensive Health Services Projects," *Inquiry* 8 (December 1971), pp. 36–49.
40. U.S. Office of Economic Opportunity, Comprehensive Health Services Projects, *Summary Report,* second quarter 1972.
41. National Center for Health Statistics, *Volume of Physician Visits, U.S., July 1966–June 1967,* op. cit.
42. OEO, *Summary Report,* op. cit., p. 2.
43. Alan Gartner, *Paraprofessionals and Their Performance: A Survey of Education, Health and Social Service Programs* (N.Y.: Praeger, 1971).
44. Ibid., p. 72.
45. Ibid., p. 73.
46. F. Lorimer, "Issues in Population Policy," in *The Population Dilemma,* P. Hauser, ed., (Englewood Cliffs, N.J.: Prentice-Hall, 1963), pp. 148–149; B. Bollough, "Poverty Ethnic Identification, and Preventive Health Care," *Journal of Health and Social Behavior* 13 (1972), pp. 347–359.
47. W. Kuralt, "Mecklenberg County: A Pilot Pill Project for Welfare Recipients," in *Birth Control Services in Tax-Supported Hospitals, Health Departments, and Welfare Agencies,* Planned Parenthood-World Population New York, pp. 38–39.
48. R. Frank and C. Rietz, "Acceptance of an Oral Contraceptive Program in a Large Metropolitan Area," *American Journal of Obstetrics and Gynecology* 93 (1965).
49. F. Jaffe, "Family Planning, Public Policy and Intervention Strategy," *Journal of Social Issues* 13 (1967), pp. 159–160.
50. Center for Family Planning Program Development, "Data and Analyses for 1973 Revision of DHEW Five-Year Plan for Family Planning Services" (N.Y.: Planned Parenthood, 1973), pp. 25–26.
51. J.G. Feldman, S. Ogra, J. Lippes et al., "Patterns and Purposes of Oral Contraceptive Use by Economic Status," *American Journal of Public Health* 61 (1971), p. 1,089.
52. A.R. Measham, R.A. Hatcher, C.B. Arnold, "Physicians and Contraception: A Study of Perceptions and Practices in an Urban South-eastern U.S. Community," *Southern Medical Journal* 64 (1971), p. 499. M. Silver, "Survey of Private Physicians—Summary of Initial Findings," paper presented at 99th annual meeting, American Public Health Association, Minneapolis, Minnesota, October 11, 1971.
53. "Data and Analysis for 1973 Revision of DHEW Five-Year Plan for Family Planning Services," op. cit., p. 33.

54. N. Ryder and C. Westoff, "National Fertility Study," Princeton University, Office of Population Research, 1970.
55. S. Bellin and H.J. Geiger, "Actual Public Acceptance of the Neighborhood Health Center by the Urban Poor," *Journal of American Medical Association* 214 (1970), pp. 2,147–2,153.
56. Additional randomly selected respondents were added to the time 2 sample.
57. S. Bellin and H.J. Geiger, "The Impact of a Neighborhood Health Center on Patient's Behavior and Attitudes Relating to Health Care: A Study of a Low Income Housing Project," *Medical Care* 10 (1972), pp. 224–239.
58. Ibid., pp. 229–230.
59. Koos, op. cit.
60. Bellin and Geiger, "The Impact of a Neighborhood Health Center," op. cit., p. 236.
61. Ibid., pp. 231–235.
62. S. Bellin, H.J. Geiger, and C.D. Gibson, "Impact of Ambulatory Health Care Services on the Demand for Hospital Beds," *New England Journal of Medicine* 280 (April 1969), pp. 808–812.
63. It could be that middle-class levels of utilization would rise if they were given these supportive services, thus maintaining the class differentials. Or it could be argued that these groups are utilizing at close to saturation levels already, and are therefore less needful of support services to facilitate physician use.
64. G. Gibson, "Explanatory Models and Strategies for Social Change in Health Care Behavior," *Social Science and Medicine* 6 (1971), pp. 636–637.

37
Politicizing Health Care

John McKnight

Is it possible that out of the contradictions of medicine one can develop the possibilities of politics? The example I want to describe is not going to create a new social order. It is, however, the beginning of an effort to free people from medical clienthood, so that they can perceive the possibility of being citizens engaged in political action.

The example involves a community of about 60,000 people on the west side of Chicago. The people are poor and Black, and the majority are dependent on welfare payments. They have a voluntary community organization which encompasses an area in which there are two hospitals.

The neighborhood was originally all white. During the 1960s it went through a racial transition and over a period of a few years, it became largely populated with Black people.

The two hospitals continued to serve the white people who had lived in the neighborhood before transition, leaving the Black people, struggling to gain access to the hospitals' services.

This became a political struggle and the community organization finally "captured" the two hospitals. The boards of directors of the hospitals then accepted people from the neighborhood, employed Black people on their staffs, and treated members of the neighborhood rather than the previous white clients.

After several years, the community organization felt that it was time to stand back and look at the health status of their community. As a result of their analysis, they found that, although they had "captured" the hospitals, there was no significant evidence that the health of the people had changed since they had gained control of the medical services.

The organization then contacted the Center for Urban Affairs where I work. They asked us to assist in finding out why, if the people controlled the two hospitals, their health was not any better.

It was agreed that the Center would do a study of the hospitals' medical records to see why people were receiving medical care. We took a sample of the emergency room medical records to determine the frequency of the various problems that brought the people into the hospitals.

We found that the seven most common reasons for hospitalization, in order of frequency, were:

1. Automobile accidents.
2. Interpersonal attacks.
3. Accidents (non-auto).
4. Bronchial ailments.
5. Alcoholism.
6. Drug-related problems (medically administered and nonmedically administered).
7. Dog bites.

The people from the organization were startled by these findings. The language of medicine is focused upon disease—yet the problems we identified have very little to do with disease. The medicalization of health had led them to believe that "disease" was the problem which hospitals were addressing, but they discovered instead that the hospitals were dealing with many problems which were not disease. It was an important step in increasing consciousness to recognize that modern medical systems are usually dealing with maladies—social problems—rather than disease. Maladies and social problems are the domain of citizens and their community organizations.

A Strategy For Health

Having seen the list of maladies, the people from the organization considered what they ought to do, or could do, about them. First of all, as good political strategists, they decided to tackle a problem which they felt they could win. They didn't want to start out and immediately lose. So they went down the list and picked dog bites, which caused about four percent of the emergency room visits at an average hospital cost of $185.

How could this problem best be approached? It interested me to see the people in the organization thinking about that problem. The city government has employees who are paid to be "dog-catchers," but the organization did not choose to contact the city. Instead, they said: "Let us see what we can do ourselves." They decided to take a small part of their money and use it for "dog bounties." Through their block clubs they let it be known that for a period of one month, in an area of about a square mile, they would pay a bounty of five dollars for every stray dog that was brought in to the organization or had its location identified so that they could go and capture it.

There were packs of wild dogs in the neighborhood that had frightened many people. The children of the neighborhood, on the other hand, thought that catching dogs was a wonderful idea—so they helped to identify them. In one month, 160 of these dogs were captured and cases of dog bites brought to the hospitals decreased.

Two things happened as a result of this success. The people began to learn that their action, rather than the hospital, determines their health. They were also building their organization by involving the children as community activists.

The second course of action was to deal with something more difficult—automobile accidents. "How can we do anything if we don't understand where these accidents are taking place?" the people said. They asked us to try to get information which would help to deal with the accident problem, but we found it extremely difficult to find information regarding when, where, and how an accident took place.

We considered going back to the hospitals and looking at the medical records to determine the nature of the accident that brought each injured person to the hospital. If medicine was thought of as a system that was related to the possibilities of community action, it should have been possible. It was not. The medical record did not say, "This person has a malady because she was hit by an automobile at six o'clock in the evening on January 3rd at the corner of Madison and Kedzie." Sometimes the record did not even say that the cause was an automobile accident. Instead, the record simply tells you that the person has a "broken tibia." It is a record system that obscures the community nature of the problem, by focusing on the therapeutic to the exclusion of the primary cause.

We began, therefore, a search of the data systems of macroplanners. Finally we found one macroplanning group that had data regarding the nature of auto accidents in the city. It was data on a complex, computerized system, to be used in macroplanning to facilitate automobile traffic! We persuaded the planners to do a printout that could be used by the neighborhood people for their own action purposes. This had never occurred to them as a use for their information.

The printouts were so complex, however, that the organization could not comprehend them. So we took the numbers and transposed them onto a neighborhood map showing where the accidents took place. Where people were injured, we put a blue X. Where people were killed, we put a red X.

We did this for all accidents for a period of three months. There are 60,000 residents living in the neighborhood. In that area, in three months, there were more than 1,000 accidents. From the map the people could see, for example, that within three months six people had been injured, and one person killed, in an area 60 feet wide. They immediately identified this place as the entrance to a parking lot for a department store. They were then ready to act, rather than be treated, by dealing with the store owner because information had been "liberated" from its medical and macroplanning captivity.

The experience with the map had two consequences. One, it was an opportunity to invent several different ways to deal with a health problem that the community could understand. The community organization could negotiate with the department store owner and force a change in its entrance.

Two, it became very clear that there were accident problems that the community organization could not handle directly. For example, one of the main reasons for many of the accidents was the fact that higher authorities had decided to make several of the streets through the neighborhood major throughways for automobiles going from the heart of the city out to the affluent suburbs. Those who made this trip were a primary cause of injury to the local people. Dealing with this problem is not within the control of people at the neighborhood level—but they understood the necessity of getting other community organizations involved in a similar process, so that together they could assemble enough power to force the authorities to change the policies that serve the interests of those who use the neighborhoods as their freeway.

The third community action activity developed when the people focused on "bronchial problems." They learned that good nutrition was a factor in these problems, and concluded that they did not have enough fresh fruit and vegetables for good nutrition. In the city, particularly in the winter, these foods were too expensive. So could they grow fresh fruit and vegetables themselves? They looked around, but it seemed difficult in the heart of the city. Then several people pointed out that most of their houses were two story apartments with flat roofs. "Supposing we could build a greenhouse on the roof, couldn't we grow our own fruit and vegetables?" So they built a greenhouse on one of the roofs as an experiment. Then, a fascinating thing began to happen.

Originally, the greenhouse was built to deal with a health problem—inadequate nutrition. The greenhouse was a tool, appropriate to the environment, that people could make and use to improve health. Quickly, however, people began to see that the greenhouse was also an economic development tool. It increased their income because they now produced a commodity to use and also to sell.

Then, another use for the greenhouse appeared. In the United States, energy costs are extremely high and a great burden for poor people. One of the main places where people lose (waste) energy is from the rooftops of their houses—so the greenhouse on top of the roof converted the energy loss into an asset. The energy that did escape from the house went into the greenhouse where heat was needed. The greenhouse, therefore, was an energy conservation tool.

Another use for the greenhouse developed by chance. The community organization owned a retirement home for elderly people, and one day one of the elderly people discovered the greenhouse. She went to work there, and told the other old people and they started coming to the greenhouse every day to help care for the plants. The administrator of the old people's home noticed that the attitude of the older people changed. They were excited. They had found a function. The greenhouse became a tool to empower older people—to allow discarded people to be productive.

Multility vs. Unitility

The people began to see something about technology that they had not realized before. Here was a simple tool—a greenhouse. It could be built locally, used locally and among its "outputs" were health, economic development, energy conservation and enabling older people to be productive. A simple tool requiring a minimum "inputs" produced multiple "outputs" with few negative side effects. We called the greenhouse a "multility."

Most tools in a modernized consumer-oriented society are the reverse of the greenhouse. They are systems requiring a complex organization with multiple inputs that produce only a single output. Let me give you an example. If you get bauxite from Jamaica, copper from Chile, rubber from Indonesia, oil from Saudi Arabia, lumber from Canada, and labor from all these countries, and process these resources in an American corporation that uses American labor and professional skills to manufacture a commodity, you can produce an electric toothbrush. This tool is what we call a "unitility." It has multiple inputs and one output. However, if a tool is basically a labor-saving device, then the electric toothbrush is an anti-tool. If you added up all the labor put into producing it, its sum is infinitely more than the labor saved by its use.

The electric toothbrush and the systems for its production are the essence of the technological mistake. The greenhouse is the essence of the technological possibility. The toothbrush (unitility) is a tool that disables capacity and maximizes exploitation. The greenhouse (multility) is a tool that minimizes exploitation and enables community action.

Similarly, the greenhouse is a health tool that creates citizen action and improves health. The hospitalized focus on health disables community capacity by concentrating on therapeutic tools and techniques requiring tremendous inputs, with limited outputs in terms of standard health measures.

Conclusions

Let me draw several conclusions from the health work of the community organization.

First, out of all this activity, it is most important that the health action process has strengthened a community organization. Health is a political issue. To convert a medical problem into a political issue is central to health improvement. Therefore, as our action has developed the organization's vitality and power, we have begun the critical health development. Health action must lead away from dependence on professional tools and techniques, towards community building and citizen action. Effective health action must convert a professional-technical problem into a political, communal issue.

Second, effective health action identifies what you can do at the local level with local resources. It must also identify those external authorities and structures that control the limits of the community to act in the interest of its health.

Third, health action develops tools for the people's use, under their own control. To develop these tools may require us to diminish the resources consumed by the medical system. As the community organization's health activity becomes more effective, the swollen balloon of medicine should shrink. For example, after the dogs were captured, the hospital lost clients. Nonetheless, we cannot expect that this action will stop the medical balloon from growing. The medical system will make new claims for resources and power, but our action will intensify the contradictions of medicalized definitions of health. We can now see people saying: "Look, we may have saved $185 in hospital care for many of the 160 dogs that will not now bite people. That's a lot of money! But it still stays with that hospital. We want our $185! We want to begin to trade in an economy in which you don't exchange our action for more medical service. We need income, not therapy. If we are to act in our health interest, we will need the resources medicine claims for its therapeutic purposes in order to diminish our therapeutic need."

These three principles of community health action suggest that improved health is basically about moving away from being "medical consumers."

The experience I have described suggests that the sickness which we face is the captivity of tools, resources, power, and consciousness by medical "unitilities" that create consumers.

Health is a political question. It requires citizens and communities. The health action process can enable "another health development" by translating medically defined problems and resources into politically actionable community problems.

38

The Women's Self-Help
Health Movement

Sheryl K. Ruzek

Women use many gynecological and obstetrical services when they are "well" rather than "sick," for women are generally in good health when they seek routine gynecological examinations, contraceptives, abortions, and obstetrical care. They are rarely in life-threatening situations or incapacitated. Yet typically, women must seek care for these routine needs in institutions organized around a medical model based on serious illness. In this model of interaction the physician's autonomy and authority are necessitated by the incapacity and incompetence of the patient. While such a model may be appropriate for emergency surgery or the treatment of acute disease, it is not appropriate to routine care situations.

During the past five years women in the health movement have voiced dissatisfaction with this model of health care. They are particularly irate at the way they are treated by gynecologists. These women dislike being denied the right to participate fully in decisions about their bodies. They are particularly bitter that they are ignorant and incompetent to do this because doctors make it difficult for them to acquire the information they need to make competent decisions for themselves. Women also feel that their relationships with physicians often perpetuate stereotypical sex-roles by expecting the male professional to be active, instrumental and authoritative and the female patient to be passive and dependent.

The Self-Help Approach

Women in the health movement are dissatisfied with this type of health care, and have developed a wide range of strategies for restructuring routine care. One of the most innovative approaches is self-help gynecology. Women involved in self-help attempt to take routine care out of the hands of professionals who typically operate on the medical model appropriate to acute illness. These women want to re-establish routine care as the legitimate domain of women themselves. They aim to utilize their own shared knowledge and expertise on themselves and each other rather than rely exclusively on the advice and ministrations of professionals.

Self-help gynecology is not simply "do-it-yourself doctoring." It involves conceptualizing health and illness in a fundamentally different manner. Typically health and health care are conceptualized as commodities which can be delivered to consumers by individual and institutional providers. In this scheme providers and consumers meet and exchange specific services, supplies and advice for cash. While the professional provider is expected to learn and gain incremental knowledge through years of practice and experience, the patient is not really expected to increase her stock of knowledge about her body or her health from these encounters. In fact, patients who do acquire knowledge and expertise and attempt to utilize this knowledge are often viewed as troublemakers.

In contrast, women involved in self-help conceptualize routine health care as an ongoing process which eliminates or minimizes distinctions between providers and receivers, experts and lay persons. The split between subject and object inherent in traditional conceptualizations of health care is replaced by a holistic perspective which encourages all participants to share in observing, advising, treating and being treated. The role or status of "patient" is replaced with the person as participant. In this mode of interaction individuals fluidly move from asking to answering questions, from observing self to observing others, from presenting symptoms to proffering therapeutic advice. Over time, all participants gain increasing knowledge and expertise about their own bodies and health and that of other women. In doing this women come to view routine care as extending beyond the amelioration of clinical conditions or securing desired drugs and devices. They begin to conceptualize and experience health as a state of being—social, psychological, and political.

This paper will describe how women practice self-help gynecology and then turn to the issue of what type of women find this approach desirable and why. It will then discuss some of the difficulties involved in researching such emerging forms of health care and analyzing the effectiveness of gynecological self-help.

It is difficult to compare self-help gynecology with traditional gynecology because of some basic underlying differences which must be understood clearly. They are difficult to understand because they violate taken-for-granted assumptions about ourselves both as persons and professionals. Self-help advocates believe that regardless of the quality of care in traditional settings, regardless of the competency or humaneness of physicians—male or female—routine care is simply performed in the wrong place by the wrong people. It is defined, controlled and supervised by professional experts rather than by women themselves. Some argue that it is even inaccurate to use the phrase "care for routine gynecological problems" for they believe that women's health is problematic only because the medical profession has denied women access to the tools and technology they need to care for themselves. Professionals invoke the power of the state to restrict practice, restrict access to drugs and devices and maintain decision making about all such matters in their own hands. Thus, on a social-psychological level women are discouraged from learning to care for themselves.

Moreover, common socialization practices forbid women to look at or touch their own bodies—both of which are essential for self-care. Women are also socialized to depend on male professionals and submit to their authority without question. Indeed, the mere act of questioning is often taken as evidence of emotional disturbance. Consequently, when women question physicians or challenge their authority, they are labeled troublemakers or neurotics. Self-help advocates decry this state of affairs and aim to re-establish women's ability and inclination to care for themselves and make their own decisions about their bodies.

Self-Help Groups

The core of self-help is the self-help group where women discuss their mutual health concerns and learn about their bodies in a safe, supportive setting. With the guidance of experienced self-helpers, women learn to perform pelvic examinations on themselves and each other. Using a hand mirror, lamp and speculum women do their own pelvic examinations and recognize early signs of vaginal infections, syphilis and pregnancy, and check the placement of IUD's. Women also study basic anatomy and physiology and consider the importance of nutrition and preventive care. Breast self-examination is learned and some advanced groups undertake pregnancy testing and laboratory work. Commonly prescribed drugs and alternative home remedies are discussed. (Self-help groups and clinics vary greatly in their emphasis on drugs, home remedies, and non-drug contraceptive techniques. Some rely heavily on home remedies and resort to drugs only after considering non-drug methods. Others utilize drugs routinely but fully inform women of the possible hazards and side effects and respect the decision of individuals to refuse drugs.) Contraceptives are considered in detail, and women have the opportunity to express their concerns over the various methods without any pressure to choose a particular type. In these groups women freely ask questions, express fears, and relate problems without fear of being judged ignorant, treated with condescension, or coerced into using particular modes of treatment.

Proponents of self-help point to the many benefits. Women who learn more about their bodies can recognize problems early when they can be most easily treated. These women are better able to seek appropriate medical attention and can be actively involved in their own care. Most important, women learn to look to themselves rather than to professionals to maintain their own health. They learn to utilize their own resources and become active participants in their own care.

Self-Help Clinics

Of course technical medical expertise is needed at times. To integrate self-help philosophy and practice with needed technical expertise, women have established their own lay-controlled gynecology and obstetrics clinics. (A few groups have expanded their services to general primary care including pediatrics.) Some are organized around group care; others follow the more traditional one-to-one client-practitioner relationship. Regardless of which approach is taken, these clinics encourage maximum participation of lay persons.

Let us first consider one form of group care which integrates the self-help approach with the need for technical expertise. In California, the Feminist Women's Health Centers offer an innovative program called the participatory gynecology clinic. Women who need routine examinations—Pap smears, breast exams, venereal disease testing, lab work for vaginal and urinary tract infections, sickle cell testing and standard contraceptives—meet in groups. Six to eight women meet for two hours with self-help workers and a female physician or nurse-practitioner. The atmosphere is relaxed, supportive and informal. Everyone, including the professionals, is on a first-name basis. Medical "herstories" are discussed and women share both their medical concerns and the medical knowledge they each have acquired in various ways. Breast and cervical self-examinations are shared so that women learn to recognize their own normal physiology. They also have the opportunity to observe specific symptoms and pathological conditions in themselves and others. Lab tests and physical exams are largely done by the women themselves with the assistance of the professional and self-help workers. Diaphragms and IUD's are fitted and inserted in the group setting, and questions and explanations are jointly considered. Similar clinics are also conducted for pregnancy screening and prenatal care.

Proponents of participatory clinics believe that this type of care allows women to ask questions, share knowledge, and learn about their own bodies. They also believe that it is superior to waiting for hours to see a hurried gynecologist for ten minutes at the most. Professionals benefit as well. All too often they only get partial information from fearful, intimidated patients. Under such circumstances diagnosis and treatment are difficult. The full participation of women in the clinic provides professionals with complete information and the immediate feedback promotes the development of sensitive clinical skills. In addition, professionals learn to accept the active participation of women and become accustomed to lay observation and evaluation of their performance, a step crucial for the development of meaningful systems of professional accountability.

Clinics in which women are seen individually also attempt to maintain maximum participation and decision making for women themselves. Much of the appointment typically is carried on between the individual women and self-help workers rather than a physician or nurse practitioner. Professionals only perform tasks restricted by law such as inserting IUD's or prescribing drugs. Essentially the professional is utilized as a consultant who proffers specific advice and services only on request.

. . . .

Who Uses Self-Help?

As is apparent thus far, self-help is an approach to health with a strong social, psychological and political message: people have within themselves the potential for meeting their basic health needs and assuming responsibility for making decisions about their own bodies. To whom does such a philosophy appeal?

First, women involved in self-help are staunch feminists. As feminists they want to assume full responsibility for every aspect of their lives including their health. They also believe that controlling their bodies is *essential* to controlling their lives. Thus, these women are highly motivated to care for themselves. But what of their other characteristics?

Self-help appeals to women from divergent backgrounds at all stages of the life cycle. Some ongoing self-help groups consist largely of women in their twenties and thirties. Others draw more mature women. There are self-help groups specifically for menopausal women. Others are organized for lesbians. However, many groups include women spanning a wide range of age and interest.

In the United States there are self-help groups and women's gynecology clinics in nearly every major metropolitan area and in many smaller communities as well. Thirty menstrual extraction groups are currently active. Feminist gynecology groups have also been established in Canada, Mexico, England, France, Germany, Italy, Northern Ireland, Belgium, Denmark, West Berlin, and New Zealand. . . .

Although there are no statistics available, a disproportionate number of participants are young, mostly under thirty. This may be due in part to the preponderance of reproductive problems encountered by women in this age group and the appeal of feminism to younger women. Nonetheless, self-help was originated by women in their middle years, women with considerable personal experience in obstetrics and gynecology.

While women from all races and classes practice self-help in the United States and Canada, white middle-class women predominate. This may be related to their high level of education and propensity to put their knowledge into practice. Also, middle-class childrearing practices which encourage women to be independent and express themselves may predispose these women to participate actively in maintaining their own health.

Efforts to introduce self-help formally into women's clinics in the United States which serve predominately Asian and Latin-American women have been largely unsuccessful. Adherents believe that self-care is difficult to promote in these settings because the women's cultural values and morals strongly prohibit them from publicly exposing or touching their bodies in the presence of other women.

. . . .

How Effective Is Self-Help Gynecology?

Self-help proponents claim that they can and do meet their routine gynecological needs. And they will continue to do so despite the threat of arrest and harassment. However, there are few systematic data available on effectiveness. Most studies of self-help are descriptive and anecdotal and do not systematically analyze effectiveness. The problem is complex, for we do not have clear, shared standards for what constitutes "effective" self-care. Doing nose-counts in doctors' offices will not yield much insight.

Let me elaborate on the problem of analysis. If we want to determine whether or not self-help participants in fact stay "healthier" or freer from disease or require less medical attention, we must be cautious when selecting measures or indicators. For example, if we interview self-help participants they may report *more* symptoms than non-participating women. But this tells us little about the relative "healthiness" of these women. Similarly, number of physician visits per year is difficult to interpret. Self-help participants may be so skilled at caring for themselves that they rarely consult professionals. On the other hand, they may become so knowledgeable that they seek professional help more readily. Furthermore, individuals' perceptions of health and illness and experienced need for medical attention vary greatly. While these perceptions and expectations are shaped by cultural factors, it is difficult to unravel which grow out of the self-help experience and which come from other cultural and subcultural groups in which some participate. Thus knowledge of women's cultural background, depth of involvement in and identification with self-help must be considered to meaningfully analyze the effectiveness of self-help for individual women.

To answer crucial questions about effectiveness, we must, as has already been indicated here, enter into women's subjective experience of their own well-being. We must not only ask how many vaginal infections women get each year or how many physician visits they log. We must ask how self-help participants experience vaginal infections or pregnancies, abortions, or contraceptive decisions after assuming the self-help approach. Do these women feel threatened, overwhelmed, or powerless when they need medical care? Or does their knowledge and experience in self-help promote competence and the ability to manage these states of being? Are self-help participants' perceptions of their ability to maintain their own health significantly different after engaging in self-help gynecology, and are they different from those of women who have not had the self-help experience? These are the crucial questions.

However, to investigate the effectiveness of self-help we must put aside many preconceived notions about who has the right and ability to utilize technical expertise and give up taken-for-granted assumptions about what practices are most desirable or cost-effective. For example, we generally accept physicians seeing patients privately as most desirable. Given this assumption we structure routine examinations as hurried affairs to keep physician costs down. Self-help advocates approach routine care quite differently. Beginning with the premise that women possess considerable knowledge and expertise themselves, routine care is structured to provide women access to each others' expertise. Professionals' participation in group settings is economically feasible and even more cost effective when lower paid nurse-practitioners and women's health care specialists are utilized. Routine care organized on the self-help model clearly offers women greater opportunity to learn to care for themselves. Of course to see the benefits of such an approach one must value increasing the competence of lay persons and reconsider notions of what is most appropriately done in private or in groups.

In short, we must approach self-help as free as possible of preconceived ideas about how routine care can best be undertaken. We cannot simply accept standard professional practices as the most appropriate or desirable model for promoting well-being. We must seriously consider alternative perspectives if we are to find new ways of ensuring women optimal health. It seems most sensible to look to women themselves to discover how routine needs might best be met.

Societal Alternatives

COMMUNITY EFFORTS AT HEALTH CARE change are limited by societal-level priorities and structures. In the long run, significant improvements in health and medical care must involve a societal-level change.

There is little doubt that if we are serious about reorienting our approach to health from "cure" to prevention of illness, medicine must become more of a "social science." Illness and disease are socially as well as biophysiologically produced. For over a century, under the reign of the germ-theory "medical model," medical research searched for specific etiologies (e.g., germs or viruses) of specific diseases. With the present predominance of chronic disease in American society, the limitations of this viewpoint are becoming apparent. If we push our etiological analysis far enough, as often as not we come to sociological factors as primary causes. We must investigate environments, lifestyles, and social structures in our search for etiological factors of disease with the same commitment and zeal we investigate bodily systems and begin to conceptualize preventive measures on the societal level as well as the biophysical. This is not to say that we should ignore or jettison established biomedical knowledge; rather, we need to focus on the production of disease in the interaction of social environments and human physiology.

The Surgeon General's report on disease prevention and health promotion titled *Healthy People* (1979) took steps in this direction. The report recognizes the "limitations of modern medicine" and highlights the importance of behavioral and social factors for health. It deemphasizes the role of physicians in controlling health activities and argues persuasively for the need to turn from "sick care" to prevention. Most significantly, the report officially legitimatizes the centrality of social and behavioral factors in caring for our health. It argues that people must take responsibility for changing disease-producing conditions and take positive steps toward good health. In some circles, *Healthy People* was deemed a revolutionary report, more significant even than the 1964 Surgeon General's report on smoking. The fact, however, that most people

Table 1.
Conceptualization of Prevention

Level of Prevention	Type of Intervention	Place of Intervention	Examples of Intervention
Medical	Biophysiological	Individual's body	Vaccinations; early diagnosis; medical intervention.
Behavioral	Psychological (and Social Psychological)	Individual's behavior and lifestyle	Change habits or behavior (e.g., eat better, stop smoking, exercise, wear seat belts); learn appropriate coping mechanisms (e.g., meditation).
Structural	Sociological (social and political)	Social structure, systems, environments	Legislate controls on nutritional values of food; change work environment; reduce pollution; floridate water supplies.

have not yet heard about this 1979 report, much less are familiar with what it says, raises some questions about its potential impact on health behavior.

Yet from a sociological perspective the report was also something of a disappointment. While social and behavioral factors are depicted as central in causation and prevention of ill health, a close reading shows that most of these factors are little more than "healthy habits." The report exhorts people to adopt better diets, with more whole grains and less red meat, sugar, and salt; to stop smoking; to exercise regularly; to keep weight down; to seek proper prenatal and postnatal care; and so forth. While these things are surely important to prevention of illness, we must today conceptualize prevention more broadly and as involving at least three levels: medical, behavioral, and structural (see Table 1). Simply, medical prevention is directed at the individual's body; behavioral prevention is directed at changing people's behavior; and structural prevention is directed at changing the society or environments in which people work and live.

Healthy People urges us to prevent disease on a behavioral level. While this is undoubtedly a useful level of prevention, some problems remain. For example, social scientists have very little knowledge about *how* to change people's (healthy or unhealthy) habits. The report encourages patient and health education as a solution, but clearly this is not sufficient. Most people are aware of the health risks of smoking or not wearing seat belts, yet roughly 30 percent of Americans smoke and 80 percent don't regularly use their seat belts. Sometimes individual habits are responses to complex social situations, such as smoking as a coping response to stressful and alienating work environments. Behavioral approaches focus on the individual and place the entire burden of change on the individual. Individuals who do not or cannot change their unhealthy habits are often seen merely as "at risk" or noncompliant patients, another form of the blame-the-victim response to health problems. *Healthy People* rarely discusses the structural level of causation and intervention. It hardly touches on significant social structural variables such as gender, race, and class and is strangely silent about the corporate aspects of prevention (Conrad and Schlesinger, 1980).

When we seek alternatives to our own medical care organization, we do well to look to other societies for comparison and guidance, especially to societies that have similar health problems or have developed innovative organizational solutions. While no medical system is without problems and none is completely transferable to the United States, there are lessons to be learned in considering alternative models to our own.

One model for health service delivery is Britain's National Health Service (NHS). In 1948 Great Britain reorganized its medical system to create a national health service. (See Stevens, 1966, for an account of NHS's formation and early development.) The NHS is a public system of medicine: hospitals, clinics, physicians, and other medical personnel work under the auspices and control of the Ministry of Health of the British Government. The fee-for-service system has all but been eliminated: the NHS is financed by tax revenues (through "progressive taxation"), with essentially no cost to the patient at the time of services, and physicians paid stipulated yearly salaries. This system has reduced the "profit motive" in medicine. For example, it is well known that Great Britain has about half the amount of surgery per capita as does the United States. The incomes of physicians are relatively low by American standards (or, perhaps more correctly, American physicians' incomes are astronomical by international standards). There exist two levels of physicians in the NHS, the community-based GP and the hospital-based consultant. Until recently the higher status and incomes of the hospital consultants were a source of dissatisfaction to GPs. While the rigid two-tier system still exists, some of the inequities have been reduced.

During its thirty-year development, the NHS has managed admirable accomplishments, including: (1) eliminating financial barriers to access; (2) making the system more rational and equitable; (3) providing care on a community level with community-based primary physicians; (4) maintaining a high level of medical-care quality; and (5) controlling costs. This final point deserves elaboration.

The NHS seems to be a more cost efficient method of delivering health care than the largely private American system. Great Britain spends about 6 percent of its gross national product on health, whereas America spends nearly 10 percent. Specifically, the British government spent only about $300 per citizen per year in 1978 for health care, compared to $863 per person for all public and private health care in the United States that same year (Malone, 1979: 22). And by most measures the health status of the populations are roughly equal. Further, there is evidence that the NHS delivers medical care more equitably. The British have controlled costs by "rationing" medical services. While all necessary medical services are more or less readily available, patients who wish elective services must "queue up" for them. There are, in fact, two- and three-year waiting lists for some elective medical care. There is little doubt that we as a nation cannot afford all the medical services we are scientifically capable of providing (Fuchs, 1975), so it is likely we too will have to adopt some type of rationing. It is undoubtedly more humane and just when medical services are rationed on the basis of need rather than on the ability to pay.

The NHS is by no means a medical utopia (Turshen, 1977). As it is a public service, it must compete with other services (e.g., education) for funding and thus by some accounts is perpetually underfinanced. While inequities of services have lessened, they have not disappeared. The high status of the hospital consultant is a continuing problem and reinforces NHS emphasis on "sick care" rather than prevention. In the final analysis, however, the NHS delivers better care to more parts of the population at less cost (and with no discernible difference in "health" status) than is accomplished in the United States and cannot be ignored as a possible alternative model for medical care delivery in American society.

In "A National Health Service: Principles and Practice," Derek Gill comments on the basic principles of the British NHS—universality, equity, and public accountability—and gives a detailed account of how the system operates. He reviews some persistent dilemmas as well as the successes of the NHS. Gill is particularly astute in his presentation of ways to increase the public accountability of medicine and to further protect patients' interests and control rising costs. He argues that central to increasing accountability is a reduction in the functional autonomy of the medical profession and an increase in the public's participation in health-care decisions. He concludes with some thoughts on how the principles of the NHS might some day be applied to the American medical system.

If the British NHS may serve as a model for industrialized societies, medical care in China can serve as an example to developing nations. There is probably no society that has improved the health status of its population so quickly as have the Chinese since the establishment of the People's Republic in 1949. From being one of the literally sickest societies on earth, the Chinese have eliminated or controlled most infectious diseases, made significant advances in surgery and medicine, established massive prevention programs, and organized medical-care delivery to reach even the remotest rural hinterland. The keys to China's medical success have been its recognition of the manifest connection of medical care with the social and political organization of society and the encouragement of a "serve-the-people" ethic (Sidel and Sidel, 1973; Horn, 1969). The innovation of peasant doctors ("barefoot doctors" who are neither barefoot nor doctors), the blend of traditional and Western medicine, and the involvement of the local community have created a system that delivers good basic primary care at very little cost. In the second article in this section, "The Delivery of Medical Care in China," Victor W. Sidel and Ruth Sidel describe the emergence and functioning of medicine in China, and show how improved medical care and health are intimately related to social and political change.

John McKinlay, in our final article, "A Case for Refocussing

Upstream: The Political Economy of Illness," argues that we need to change the way we think about prevention and start to "refocus upstream," beyond healthy habits to the structure of society. He suggests we should concentrate on and investigate political-economic aspects of disease causation and prevention, and in particular "the manufacturers of illness." McKinlay singles out the food industry as a major manufacturer of illness. However, the major contribution of his article is to go beyond the conventional view of prevention as a biomedical or lifestyle problem to a conceptualization of prevention as a socio-economic issue.

References

Conrad, Peter and Lynn Schlesinger. 1980. "Beyond healthy habits: Society and the pursuit of health." Unpublished manuscript.

Fuchs, Victor. 1974. Who Shall Live? New York: Basic Books.

Horn, Joshua. 1969. Away with All Pests. New York: Monthly Review Press.

Malone, Patrick. 1979. "British medicine/American medicine: Leaning closer but still an ocean apart." New Physician 28 (December): 20–24.

Sidel, Victor W. and Ruth Sidel. 1973. Serve the People. Boston: Beacon Press.

Stevens, Rosemary. 1966. Medical Practice in Modern England. New Haven: Yale University Press.

Turshen, Meredith. 1977. The British National Health Services: Its Achievements and Lessons for the United States. Washington D.C.: Health Service Action.

U. S. Department of Health, Education and Welfare. 1979. Healthy People: The Surgeon General's Report on Health Promotion and Disease Prevention. Washington D.C.: U. S. Government Printing Office.

39

A National Health Service: Principles and Practice

Derek Gill

It seems reasonable to assume that some restructuring of the American health care delivery system is likely in the not too distant future.[1] This is not the place to discuss the history of attempts to change the American health care system, but it is perhaps worth noting that as early as the decade preceding World War I, suggestions were emerging in American society for the introduction of the principle of health insurance established earlier by Bismarck in Germany and subsequently in Great Britain in 1911. In the Depression some political and social pressure developed to consider national health insurance for American health care delivery, but the movement had little impact. During World War II, many unions were able to bargain effectively for fringe benefits which included a variety of schemes to provide health insurance for the work force, particularly in the automobile industry. Subsequent to World War II, pressure slowly began to build up to reduce the plight of the poor and the elderly by doing something to remove the financial barrier between the poor and the elderly and medical care services. Hence, in 1965 Medicare and Medicaid were introduced to deal with the glaringly obvious problems that medical care costs presented to the elderly, the deprived, and the underprivileged.

Since 1965, there has been a growing public and political awareness of the need to alter the American medical care delivery system in order to protect the population from the often financially disastrous consequences of illness and disease. In 1973, what was basically the first form of catastrophic health insurance was introduced on a national basis. In that year the United States government made itself responsible for assuming, in large part, fiscal immunity for the cost of treatment to sufferers of end-stage renal disease. The two basic treatments for end-stage renal disease, hemodialysis and kidney transplantation, are both horrendously expensive. Persons suffering from these conditions might have to meet medical bills of up to $30,000 in any one financial year. Such enormous costs dramatically demonstrated the need for government involvement in the care of citizens suffering from this particular illness.

Although other medical treatments are comparatively less expensive, the fifteen years since the introduction of Medicare and Medicaid have been accompanied by vast increases in the cost of medical services in general. Although figures on medical costs are difficult to generate, it seems reasonable to suppose that the current average cost of an uncomplicated delivery is somewhere between $1,000 and $1,500. Hence, for example, the birth of a baby could absorb approximately 10 percent of the annual income of an American average wage earner without health insurance. It is, therefore, not surprising that both Republican and Democratic administrations have recently accepted the need to sponsor measures to ameliorate the financial burden placed on the American public by the increasing costs of medical care services.

While general agreement exists on the need for such measures, the mode of financing medical and related services generates considerable dispute. The range of solutions proposed is considerable, with most Republican legislators, and the American Medical Association, recommending an expansion of private health insurance schemes, under systems which would leave the basic structure of medical service provision in this country relatively intact. Liberal Democrats, on the other hand, including Senator Edward Kennedy and his supporters, have advocated the development of what might be described as a full-fledged national health service. Kennedy, for example, has expressed admiration for the British National Health Service. But, of course, the British system is the product of a long process of socio-historical development which reflects ideological developments and social change more or less peculiar to the British Isles and is thus not directly or wholly exportable.

Principles of a National Health Service

The concept of a *national* health service clearly implies the ideal of delivery of medical and health care services uniformly to all members of society. The concept of a national health service also implies that the quality of medical care available should be uniform across the nation. This second implication of a national health service relates to the principle of equity and further implies that medical care services should be provided in such a way that no one is barred from access to them. In general, this means the delivery of services at zero cost at point of delivery. If medical services are not "free" at point of delivery, those least able or unable to bear the cost of such services are denied equity. These principles of uniform distribution of uniform quality medical services can become truly viable only under the overarching principle of public accountability. The principle that distinguishes a national health service from all other forms of medical and health care delivery is that it is a delivery system accountable, through the body politic, to the population it serves. In practice, the degree of public accountability of a national health service may be limited, as indeed is the case in Great Britain, in relation to the profession of medicine. Nevertheless, once the principles underlying a national health service have been accepted, the functional and professional autonomy of the medical-care industry is limited, to a greater or lesser degree, by the government.

The principles of health-service universality, equity, and accountability are in a sense sequels to a political principle developed very much further in British and Continental political systems than has been the case in the United States: greater emphasis upon collectivism than upon individualism. The nations of Europe have seen the emergence of powerful collectivist Communist and socialist political parties which have had an obvious impact upon the political ideologies and social realities of European society. The establishments, the power elites in these societies, have had to respond to collectivist pressures stemming from left-wing ideologies and to come to terms with a shift towards a collectivist ethic and away from the historically dominant individualistic ideologies of the eighteenth and nineteenth centuries. The development of national health services and other reformist medical care delivery systems are the natural consequence of the gradual development of a collectivist ideology. Of course, collectivist principles do not have to predominate to influence change. Once significant components of the social, educational, economic, and political infrastructure of the social system provide at least partial support for a collectivist social philosophy, the introduction of a medical care delivery system based on the principles of universality, equity, and public accountability is more or less inevitable. The British National Health Service is only one example of this more or less "national" phenomenon. It is also evident in Scandinavia, the East European Bloc countries, and to a lesser extent, in the medical care systems of the Low Countries, France and Germany.

The British National Health Service in Principle and in Practice

In countries characterized by the Western liberal-democratic tradition of representative democracy, the simplest way to achieve health-care public accountability, universality, and equity is to place in public ownership all forms of medical service provision. Once medical resources are publicly owned, they become open to public control. Given the predominance of the hospital in modern Western medical care, it is particularly important that the hospital sector be nationalized, and this is what the British government did in 1948.

Nevertheless, medicine is a powerful profession and highly effective as a political pressure group, so the extent of public control and public accountability, although theoretically absolute once medical care resources have been nationalized, is limited by the extent to which the profession and other groups and interests in the medical care industry are able to influence the body politic. Thus, although the British hospital sector was nationalized in 1948, the elite of British medicine (hospital consultants and surgeons) were permitted a limited degree of private practice. Senior hospital physicians could elect full- or part-time commitment to the National Health Service and continue taking care of private patients, and, indeed, they were permitted to utilize some beds within the National Health Service to accommodate private patients. In this sense, a private sector still persists within the British National Health Service (NHS) and insurance companies have sprung up, notably the British United Provident Association, to provide financial coverage for those who choose to pay premiums and receive part of their medical care within the private sector. The major advantage to the patient of the private sector in Britain seems to be the opportunity "to jump the queue." In parts of the country where waiting lists for elective surgery may be very long, the private patient can enter hospital for surgical care at times convenient to the consumer rather than wait upon the convenience of the system. As one might expect, the private sector in the United Kingdom is relatively small, affecting perhaps five to seven million people, but, nevertheless, it breaches the principle of equity. Those who can afford private care can be treated at their convenience and are thus able to sidestep one of the most unpleasant characteristics of the system, waiting time. Moreover, senior hospital staff have continued to do comparatively well in terms of salary and service conditions compared with physicians in the local authority health services and general practitioners.[2]

Nevertheless the state has been able to impose a measure of control upon the medical profession. Studies of the Emergency Medical Service established during World War II revealed that many hospitals up and down the country were desperately short of consultant staffs and surgeons. The National Health Service was able to redistribute senior hospital staff by preventing the teaching hospitals and other highly prestigious secondary and tertiary care institutions from recruiting additional staff and by restricting senior appointments to hospitals in those parts of the country which had a shortage of consultant obstetricians/gynecologists, surgeons, internal medicine specialists, and so on. Some degree of control was also imposed upon the primary care sector by steps taken to influence the distribution of new recruits to general practice. The distribution of general practitioners in the National Health Service was gradually affected by a negative (as opposed to a positive) system of control. Physicians were never directed to where they might practice (positive control). Rather variations in general practitioner/population ratios in different parts of the country were assessed in such a say as to provide at least some positive incentives for general practitioners who were prepared to set up practice in under-doctored areas, as well as to limit or, indeed, even to eliminate employment possibilities in areas of the country considered adequately served or over-doctored. This latter scheme had some degree of success in improving the overall general practitioner/population ratios across the country, but its effectiveness was limited by the fact that most of the increase in the output from medical schools that occurred during the first twenty-five years of the NHS was absorbed into the shortage areas in the *hospital* sector. Hence there were fewer general practitioners available to be affected by the system of negative control in the primary care sector (1,2).

When Britain's National Health Service was first introduced, it was assumed that, while initially the expense of the service would increase, expenditure would eventually level off as the backlog of hitherto untreated disabilities was gradually eradicated. Expenditure on health care, it was felt, would soon peak, and perhaps in the long term decline as the population became more healthy. The removal of the financial barrier between doctor and patient did lead to an increase in the utilization of health services and, presumably, to higher standards of health in the population, but the costs of the NHS continued to accelerate. Today most authorities believe that the demand for health care services is virtually insatiable. Indeed the pressure of rising demand upon health care resources is becoming so great, both in terms of the increasing proportion of the gross national product allocated to the health industry and the increasing manpower demands to meet the increased use of health care services, that many national health care systems are now not only attempting to improve the efficiency of health care delivery, but also to ration the supply.

Any attempt to assess the impact of the National Health Service upon the health status of the British population is necessarily fraught with difficulty. The major improvements in the health status of the British population in the period 1850 through the early part of the twentieth century were almost certainly the consequence of improved standards of living and improved hygienic conditions stemming from public health measures of the nineteenth century, rather than the result of improvement in the medical treatment of illness and disease. In more recent years, however, biomedical knowledge and the management and treatment of a whole range of illness and disease conditions have improved dramatically. The question necessarily becomes: Has the National Health Service, whose basic systemic change was the removal of the financial barrier between the doctor and patient, been successful in enabling the general population to derive benefit from these advances in medical knowledge and technique?

The death rate per 1,000 of population in England and Wales shows very little variation between 1949 and 1971–1973, although the expectation of life for males at birth was increased from 66.3 years for the period 1948–1950 to 69.2 years for the period 1971–1973 and for females from

71.0 to 75.2 years respectively (data from Department of Health and Social Security, 1974). The mortality statistics related to reproduction show a fairly significant decline. This decline has been accompanied by an increasing proportion of hospital confinements, until, today, virtually all women who choose to do so can be delivered in a hospital. There is no doubt that declines in perinatal and maternal mortality are due in part to the better supervision and management of pregnancy and parturition made possible because well over 90 percent of maternity cases are now delivered in the hospital. On the other hand, one cannot ignore the possibility that part of the improvement is due to a rise in the "biological efficiency" consequent upon continuing improvements in standards of living of the generations of women born during or after World War II.

There is no doubt that the standard of eye care has improved tremendously since the inception of the National Health Service. When spectacles first became available on the NHS, demand completely outstripped supply. Many people, previously unable to afford eye testing and prescriptions for spectacles, were able to receive diagnosis and treatment through the NHS.

Cartwright's representative sampling of the population indicated that the British people are very satisfied with the treatment and the care they receive in hospitals and with the services provided by their general practitioners (3,4). It is notoriously difficult, however, to interpret patients' expression of satisfaction with the services they receive since, in most instances, when they present themselves for treatment they are often under considerable stress and fearful, and alleviation of this stress and fear is itself likely to generate high levels of satisfaction. Moreover, as Stimson and Webb (5) have shown, when patients are encouraged to talk about their experiences in general practice outside the surgery setting, either in groups or individually with the research workers, they are more forthcoming with critical comments. The "stories" the patients present to the research workers often depict the doctor/patient interaction in such a way as to cast a more favorable light on the patient in terms of his or her involvement in the interaction. In a sense, the patients "rewrite" the consultation episode, depicting themselves in a more active role than was actually the case, thus compensating, perhaps, for what they perceived as an imbalance of power in the doctor/patient relationship. Nevertheless, the general popularity and sense of satisfaction with the NHS are such that neither political party has attempted either to abolish or even significantly alter the basic structure of the system, and any attempt to do so would probably mean political suicide for the party involved.

In general the NHS has turned out to be a fairly successful mechanism for the provision of health care services to the British population at zero cost at point of delivery. No one in Britain need be without medical care because of financial barriers; no one has to face complete financial disaster as a result of an illness. While sickness benefits and disability pensions do not provide for a standard of living commensurate with that most fully employed people enjoy from wages or salaries, they nevertheless afford a considerable cushion against extreme impoverishment as a result of illness.

The NHS absorbs less than 6 percent of the gross national product. This is much less than either America or Canada spends on health care and is below the level of expenditure in most European countries as well. The relatively low cost of the British National Health Service is partly due to a continued maldistribution of health care resources across the country and, therefore, an inequitable inconsistency of medical care standards. Moreover, certain forms of elective surgical intervention are rationed by means of the waiting list. Even the most prestigious and powerful element of the medical profession, the hospital doctors, have had to get used to operating with limited financial resources. Even though the hospital sector absorbs the vast majority of financial resources devoted to health care, this sum is still much less than the specialists and consultants would prefer to have available. Yet, despite the apparent power and political influence of the elite of the medical profession, the state's intervention in the health care sector has continued to limit the overall cost of health care provision against the constant clamor of the leaders of the profession for more and more resources to be devoted to health care in general and to the hospital sector in particular.

This is not to say that the community and primary care services have received an adequate or even an appropriate portion of health care expenditure. These less prestigious and powerful sections of the profession have consistently been underfinanced because the state has used funds that might have been available to them to appease the leaders of the profession. Indeed, all sections of the health care professions, general practitioners, junior hospital doctors, senior consultants and surgeons, nursing staff, and support workers, from orderlies to secretaries and janitors, have complained bitterly about the rationing of financial resources to the health care sector. That a covert system of rationing of health care expenditure should have been introduced and maintained despite constant pressure from these various health care interest groups is in itself surprising.

The state's intervention into health care has in various ways limited the functional autonomy of the profession of medicine. This state of affairs owes much to the emergence of the reformist tradition in British politics in the nineteenth century, the gradual institutionalization of radicalism in the latter part of the nineteenth century and the early part of the twentieth century, and the emergence of the Labour Party as a powerful force on the British political scene. Socialism has as one of its central tenets the need to distribute scarce resources equitably and with due regard to competing social and humanitarian priorities. Medicine, therefore, has had to accept, albeit most reluctantly, the fact of competition from other forms of social expenditure aimed at improving the quality of life for the less privileged and to acknowledge that the state has the right and the duty to monitor the allocation of resources to education, welfare, transport and communication, housing—to all forms of public expenditure aimed at improving the standard of living of the population.

In recent years the financial problems of the NHS have been exacerbated by the need to pay higher salaries and wages to nursing staff, hospital ancillary workers, and junior hospital doctors. In the past, nurses were subjected to a high degree of social control both during training and subsequently. Trainees were expected to live in and were paid hardly enough to provide them with pocket money. Even after completing training, nurses were expected to live frugal lives dedicated only to duty. Hospital ancillary workers, while not subjected to similarly rigid social controls, were also poorly paid. Semiskilled and unskilled manual workers, particularly in service industries where the units of production are relatively small (in this case hospitals), tended to lag behind in the development of an effective trade union structure, thus placing themselves in a poor bargaining position during wage negotiations with employers. However, nurses and hospital ancillary workers have, in recent years, organized much more effectively, and this has led to the generation of substantial wage and salary increases. (Junior hospital doctors have been similarly successful in extracting considerable salary increases from the NHS. Nurses and junior hospital doctors have, in short, discovered the advantages to be gained by injecting an element of traditional "trade unionism" into their professional organizations.)

These wage and salary increases have had to be paid for in overall economic circumstances in which the resources allocated to the medical sectors of society have risen only very slowly or remained static. The impact of such increases can be quite dramatic. East Anglia, for example, has been poorly provided with medical resources for many years. In 1976–1977 the region was awarded an increased annual budget in the form of development funds to improve service provision. A large portion of the funds—in the Cambridgeshire area over 50 percent—was absorbed by an increase in salaries to junior hospital doctors (6).

Recent changes in the allocation of funds across regional and area health authorities have created considerable anxiety in the ranks of the medical profession, particularly those who work in the better-endowed sectors. The elite of the profession, the senior staff of the university teaching hospitals, had become accustomed to annual budget increases. Generally speaking, funds were previously allocated on the previous year's budget, plus a little extra, depending upon the government's overall generosity towards the NHS. Consequently, the richer regions tended to maintain or even increase their share of the financial cake while the poorer regions, in real terms, had to make do with minimal-growth budgets. The Resource Allocation Working Party has now begun to change this situation. Rich regions will receive no or very limited budget increases, whereas the poorer regions will receive slightly more generous allocations. However, the pace of these changes has been very slow and is likely to remain slow in the foreseeable future.

Under these circumstances, it is not surprising that the medical profession should look to alternative sources of income for the NHS. The British Medical Association (BMA) in its evidence to the Royal Commission on the NHS (7) has advocated the reintroduction of a fee-for-service system of payment for medical services. Patients would pay physicians directly and subsequently be reimbursed by the NHS. The BMA also advocated the introduction of "hotel" charges for hospitalized patients and substantial increases in prescription charges. The assumption of the BMA is that revenues available to the NHS would be substantially increased by these proposals. However, as the Radical Statistics Health Group (8) makes clear, and as the Labour Party argues in its document, "The Right to Health" (9), these mechanisms would be administratively wasteful as well as socially expensive. If precedent is any guide and the principle of at least minimal social justice is to be preserved, exceptions would have to be introduced for the elderly, the chronically sick, children, nursing mothers, the unemployed, physically and mentally handicapped persons, etc. The administrative costs of such a scheme would clearly absorb a large proportion of the revenue so generated. Moreover, the scheme would have to be buttressed by the hateful apparatus of the means test.[3] Ample evidence already exists of the low rate of take-up of benefits and/or exemptions when both medical and social services are provided under means tests. The end result of such proposals, critics aver, would simply be to penalize the poor for their underprivileged position in society.

Where fee-for-service payment mechanisms are the predominant mode for remunerating medical doctors, the medical marketplace tends to be characterized by high physician income, especially for surgeons. In West Germany and the United States, for example, physicians' incomes may exceed the average industrial wage by a factor of six or seven (10). Some United States physicians enjoy incomes as high as $150,000 per year or higher. There is also increasing evidence from the United States that rates of surgical interventions are increased by fee-for-service payments (11).

Large increases in the NHS budget are unlikely to occur now or in the forseeable future. Public money will continue to be in short supply while the United Kingdom's economy continues to suffer from balance-of-payments problems. Increasing revenue by increasing charges to patients, if appropriate safeguards were introduced to protect the less well-off, would generate very little additional income. In the immediate future the best mechanism for increasing the resources available to the NHS is probably increased efficiency within the service, which might make available some monies for both current and capital expenditure. Attempts to improve the efficiency of the NHS will, however, almost certainly impinge upon the profession's functional autonomy, so jealously guarded by the medical establishment, if not by all physicians.

Our discussion thus far leads to the inescapable conclusion that public accountability of the profession of medicine in Britain both will and ought to increase in the future. Leading commentators such as Rudolph Klein and Margaret Stacey have been severely critical of the complaint procedures available to patients in the British National Health Service. They both feel that mechanisms for increasing the public accountability of the profession of medicine are necessary if patients' concerns over treatment and their sense of satisfaction or dissatisfaction with the health service are to be taken seriously. Klein proposes the establishment of a Council of Professions, which would operate in a manner similar to that of the Press Council. Stacey considers the possibility of establishing a government inspectorate to oversee the operation of the NHS (but assumes that this would be totally unacceptable to the profession).

The major problem, however (characteristic of the complaints procedures in both the hospital and primary care sectors), is that the persons who hear and pass judgment on complaints are not independent of the branch of the service which employs them. (This is not the case with the Health Service Commissioner, but he is specifically excluded from hearing complaints which may occur in the practice of medicine.) It seems reasonable to suggest that the public should have the right to expose errors to independent arbitrators, if for no other reason than to ensure that the same mistake is not made again. Marx long ago and Dahrendorf (12) more recently, demonstrated that conflict, either open or institutionalized, is endemic in industrialized capitalist social systems. This being so, the wisest course would seem to be to simply recognize potential conflict situations in the NHS and introduce truly effective mechanisms to handle such disagreements—regardless of whether or not these mechanisms are seen by the medical profession as threats to its autonomy.

When a conflict does emerge between a doctor and a patient, the imbalance of power in the doctor/patient relationship places the patient at a disadvantage. A complaints procedure, if it is to be equitable, must address this problem. Community health councils may help reduce this imbalance of power by providing the patient with a knowledgeable advocate to help the patient make his complaint.

To whom should the complaint be addressed? The Health Service Commissioner (HSC), as noted above, is independent of the NHS, and a simple extension of his jurisdiction to complaints arising from clinical practice might, at first sight, seem attractive. However, the HSC and his staff are relatively remote from everyday medical practice. His staff would have to travel to the complaint area, collect evidence, hear the complaint, and make recommendations. A more efficient alternative might be to appoint tribunals in each region, chaired by a senior lawyer and including lay persons as well as physicians, but not physicians from the area in which the complaint originated. The tribunals would, of course, be independent of the NHS structure and thus ensure for both doctor and patient a fair hearing. This system would have the additional merit of being relatively familiar to the British public, since tribunals of a very similar kind exist to deal with, for example, complaints concerning allocations made by the public officials who supervise welfare supplementary benefits.

One further change needs to be introduced at the primary care level if the patients' interests are to be protected. At present, general practitioners can remove patients from their lists without having to give reason for such action. A patient who wishes to make a complaint against his doctor may be hesitant to do so if he is aware of this proviso. It seems reasonable to suggest that a general practitioner should not be allowed to remove a patient from his list without demonstrating just cause. The arbitrator in such cases might, again, be the tribunals described above.

While the changes suggested above may improve the procedures for handling complaints, they are unlikely to prove beneficial in the area of cost. On the contrary, in the short term the implementation of such a system would undoubtedly impose an additional drain on NHS funds. In the long term, however, economies of scale might be generated if experience shows that one tribunal could deal with complaints concerning both hospital and general practioner's services. At present, two separate mechanisms are in place to deal with such complaints.

Although Stacey is pessimistic concerning her suggestion that a government inspectorate might be established for the NHS, the rudiments of a medical inspection system are to be found in the monitoring of prescription charges to which general pracititoners are subjected. Tricker's proposal for improving the efficiency and capability of the Prescription Pricing Authority (PPA) by computerizing its day-to-day operation could make this monitoring system even more effective: more accurate and up-to-date information could be provided on general practitioners' prescribing habits, the rate of utilization of new drugs, etc. If these objectives were realized, then the PPA might be capable of undertaking a wider set of responsibilities.

Such additional responsibilties might introduce a higher degree of rationality into prescribing patterns by expanding even further the data base of the PPA. The lists of medicines commonly prescribed by general practitioners could be extracted from the PPA files and submitted to a panel of experts, as was done in the Sainsbury Committee's inquiry into the pharmaceuticcal industry and the NHS (13). The panel could be asked to identify those drugs for which there was no evidence of therapeutic effectiveness, to define minimum effective dosages, etc. This information could then be passed on to general practitioners, together with a computerized breakdown of their own prescribing habits. GPs who persisted in irrational prescribing behavior might then have remuneration withheld for that part of their medical practice. Alternatively, a restricted list of medicines available from prescriptions by GPs might be developed, and drugs prescribed that were not on this list might be made available only when the GP stated his reasons in writing. The PPA might also be required to provide GPs with a list of generic rather than brand names commonly prescribed drugs. The local pharmacist could then fill the prescription utilizing the cheapest available generic drug in his stock. If the GP felt that a particular brand-name drug was necessary for a particular patient, he or she could so indicate on the prescription form. Experiments on the lines suggested above could be introduced for large numbers of GPs and the results analyzed by the computerized PPA system, the data assessed, and the procedure made routine for all primary care practitioners if the results were successful.

An even greater cost saving might be introduced if the rate of admissions to hospital medical wards for adverse drug reactions could be reduced from its present level of 5 percent. The feasibility of computer-based information systems providing guidance on drug-drug interactions, contraindications for particular drugs used in combination, and other serious side effects has already been demonstrated, although physicians may be reluctant to utilize such systems if the procedures to be followed at the computer terminal are complicated or involve much waiting time (14). The cost of introducing computer terminals into every GP's office would probably be prohibitive, but developments in the field of mini-computers and micro-processors may eventually overcome this economic problem. A centrally located drug information system might be established, the responsibility of which would be to update on a monthly basis information derived from the pharmaceutical manufacturers, the medical journals, etc., on drug characteristics, dosages, adverse reactions, etc. If such a system were linked to a restricted list of available medications, this information could be mailed to general practitioners initially perhaps in the form of printed sheets, but ultimately in an electronic form which the GP would insert into his desk micro-processor. This suggestion may seem rather fanciful at this stage, but the rate of development in the electronics industry is so fast that such a process may soon be economically feasible.

In the large hospitals, a computer-based drug information system would be both effective and economical. Both patients and staff are concentrated in a relatively small area, and access to suitably placed terminals should not present a problem. The staff of the pharmacy could also be charged with the responsibility of making random spot checks on the medications of patients, and this information could be fed back into the computer or sent directly to the patient's physician. Physicians would then have, routinely, advice from pharmacologists about side effects, drug interactions, etc., available to them in addition to the information supplied by the computer system. Such a system might also enable hospitals to econo-mize on drug expenses on a large scale. Recently, a California hospital experimented with such a system and reported a 10 percent drop in medi-cation costs over a three month period (however, this report still awaits validation).

Apart from the public health movement, the practice of medicine has generally been a matter of doctor/patient interaction in a relatively isolated situation. Other parties may be present during the interaction—the son or daughter of an aged parent, the mother of a child, a husband, a wife, etc.—but the attending physician alone is responsible for the medical decisions made about the patient, even if another physician is called in as a consultant. When the body of knowledge concerning illness and disease available to the profession was limited, the fact that most medical deci-sions were made in relative isolation probably did not matter very much. Today the circumstances are very different. There has been a vast expan-sion in medico-scientific knowledge in this century, particularly since World War II. In these circumstances, physicians are less able to make informed clinical decisions based on their own isolated clinical experience and selective recall of previous cases. Currently the half-life of medical knowledge is said to be about seven years. Most modern medical care systems are beginning to introduce continuing education programs for physicians, and some countries are even beginning to establish compulsory relicensure examinations.

If the medical profession continues to insist upon individual functional autonomy—the right of each physician to exercise clinical judgment without referring to his or her peers and without making use of institu-tionalized mechanisms for updating his or her data base—the interests of patients will not be adequately protected. If necessary, a shift from an individualistic to a collectivist orientation must be imposed upon the medical profession.

The British General Medical Act of 1858 assured the profession a virtual monopoly in the treatment of illness and disease. Only today are the full implications of this decision being recognized. The terms of the Act of 1858 also gave responsibility to the profession for monitoring the training, licensure, and conduct of its members. Few safeguards were incorporated to protect the interests of patients. (George Bernard Shaw, reflecting on the potential misuse of the power of professional groups, suggested in the 1890s that "all professions are a conspiracy against the laity.") The intervention of the state in the British medical care system has, it has been argued, done something to redress the imbalance of power characteristic of physician/patient relationships. This is perhaps true, but it is clear that the state must continue to accept responsibility for monitoring the procedures and practices of medical doctors in order to protect the interest of patients.

While the state may be able to act indirectly as the protector of patients' rights and interests, the NHS structure provides few opportunities for the general public to have its say. For example, induction of labor has recently become a routine delivery procedure in certain parts of the country. Induction of labor attracted severe condemnation from various consumer groups and supporters of women's rights. Mrs. Jean Robinson, the chairperson of the Patients' Association, an independent pressure group funded on a shoestring, was almost alone in officially representing the concerns of women who were worried about encouraging further expansion of deliveries by induction. At least, however, certain categories of pregnant women had an advocate prepared to argue their case knowledgeably and forcefully.

In general, the mechanisms available to assist patients or patients' representatives to plead their case are relatively primitive and underdeveloped. The Community Health Councils, particularly through publication of their annual reports, may be able to expose to wider scrutiny new medical practices and procedures as they emerge. Nevertheless, direct representation of the public interest in the structure of organization of the NHS is limited. Involved in this issue are the difficult problems associated with representative v. participatory democracy and the relationship between national and local government.

The NHS has only been moderately successful in equitably redistributing medical resources across the nation. Allocation of scarce resources to the medical system, a responsibility of the central government, must be balanced against the demands of other components of the welfare state—housing, education, social services, etc. In Britain, the political system is reasonably sophisticated, and more or less centrist, with forms of socialism and conservatism competing for votes in national elections. The Parliaments that emerge out of the British political system are, however, recognizably, if marginally, different in their approach to NHS. The Conservatives generally favor the retention of concepts such as self-help, some competition, restriction of public expenditures, retention of private beds, etc. The Labour Party generally favors collective responsibility, cooperation rather than competition with the economic sector, continuing or expanding public expenditure, and the elimination of private beds. In the 1979 General Election, had the Labour Party been reelected, phase-out of private beds would probably have continued, with appropriate directions emanating from the Department of Health and Social Security (D.H.S.S.) being given to the district management teams via the various regional and local health authorities. However, the Conservatives were returned to power, and it is probable that the elimination of private beds from the NHS will be discontinued, and just possible that even more assistance will be made available to the private sector. Thus the different ideological perspectives of the two major poitical parties in Britain influence the day-to-day operational

procedures of the NHS. Policy guidelines are devised in Parliament, opera-
tionalized by the DHSS, and transmitted downwards through the hierarchical administrative structure for implementation at the area and district
levels. These administrative procedures clearly follow the principles of
representative democracy and of centralized direction and control typical
of a nationally organized medical care system.

What of the principles of participatory democracy? Since the Reorganization Act of 1973, some administrative directives have been introduced
which increase the participation of hospital ancillary workers in the omit-
tee structure at area and regional levels (see Figure 1). Porters, domestics,
and technologists are, therefore, slightly better represented than previously. Such changes are clearly appropriate but they do little to increase
general public participation in the NHS. Britain is currently grappling with
proposals for devolution of political and administrative power and the
NHS is unlikely to remain isolated from the growing demand for more
direct participation in matters which directly affect local and regional
circumstances. Consideration needs to be given to the relationships between local government and the NHS. At all three levels, regional, area,
and district, it might be sensible to introduce directly elected committees to
which NHS management would be answerable. The DHSS would continue
to formulate policy, which would, of course, reflect national politics. In
this way, the professionals and the administrators of the NHSS would be
answerable to regional and local elected bodies for the way in which they
interpret and implement national guidelines. Such proposals would introduce an additional level of representative democracy into the NHS, but
because the catchment areas would relate to the administrative units of the
regional and local health authorities, a sense of closer public involvement
in the operation of the NHS might be engendered.

At the district level, further public involvement could be induced by
introducing arrangements which would enable the public to be represented
in the neighborhood health centers. As more and more health and social
work professionals practice out of health centers, some direct public participation on their boards of management would increase the degree of
participation of patients and public representatives. Such arrangement
could also be gradually extended to group practices.

Public representation in NHS and accountability of the medical care
system to the social system could be further improved by greater recognition of the potential benefits to be derived by the institutionalization of
other groups with monitoring responsibilities. The community health
councils, for example, are comprised of an interesting mixture of local-au-
thority representatives, members of voluntary organizations, and state ap-
pointees. These councils might develop a degree of quasi-professional expertise sufficient to generate a different perspective on medical services
than that held by health care professionals and the managers. Measures

Figure 1. *The Reorganized National Health Service*

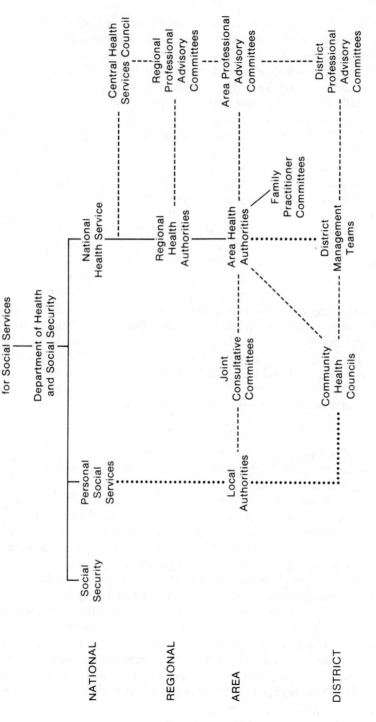

—— Consultation/Advice
••• Other
—— Accountability

SOURCE: **Management Arrangements for the Reorganised National Health Service,** HMSO, 1972.

designed to encourage the development of differing perspectives on the role of medicine and the medical care system in society can only serve to better protect the interests of patients and the public.

Arrangements to increase the public accountability of the profession of medicine and the medical care system take on particular significance when one considers the socio-historical origins and present development of the British health care system. In the late nineteenth and early twentieth centuries, both the political and industrial wings of the working class movement were in their early formative stages. Much more socio-historical research needs to be undertaken before these early stages can be completely understood, but it seems reasonable to hypothesize that the early phases of the development of the socialist movement tended to generate a much more radical political and social atmosphere than that which prevails in Britain today. The early socialists, and also to some degree the early trade unionists, tended in their writings and public statements to challenge more directly the irrationality and exploitative nature of the capitalist infrastructure. The Labour Party today, as Dingwall (15) has suggested, tends to adopt a "social democratic" position in which basic challenges to the capitalist infrastructure of a mixed economy are underplayed. Only industries and services which cannot survive in a mixed economy are nationalized. The profitable private sector is left relatively free and uncontrolled. (As Chamberlain once remarked, "Whoever is in power in Parliament, it is the Conservatives who run the country.") Only the industrial wing of the labor movement occasionally emerges to challenge the dominant ideologies of the establishment. A recent example of this phenomenon is the National Union of Public Employee's campaign against private beds in the NHS. It is to be hoped that the trade union movement will continue to represent the interests of the working class and to continue to challenge the establishment whenever the opportunity arises. Mechanisms which generate the information upon which such challenges can be erected can help ensure that the public interest in the NHS (and elsewhere in the social fabric of British society) is protected.

But the health status of populations is affected by the general social and economic conditions which prevail in a society, even more than it is by devolution of its medical care system. Moreover, it was a professor of medical history (16) who established this fact in the British context, not a clinical specialist. This finding was dependent upon the work of epidemiologists, medical historians, and, to a lesser extent, social scientists. In the light of this new awareness of the importance of social and economic conditions, the responsibility placed upon the new specialty of community medicine which emerged out of the 1974 reorganization is truly awesome. If this specialty is to maintain the investigative tradition of epidemiologists and medical historians it must continue to take into account aspects of the social structure which impinge upon the health status of the population.

Improvements in economic conditions and dietary standards might, for example, be the best method for reducing rates of infant mortality. Community medicine under the 1973 Act is responsible for "determining the health care needs of communities and assessing the extent to which current service provision does or does not meet those needs." Poor-Law medical officers in the nineteenth century found themselves simply prescribing "medical necessities"—decent food and drink—for the sick poor. Community medicine specialties in the last quarter of the twentieth century must monitor the socio-economic conditions which determine the health status of the population—work, patterns of leisure, diet, housing, etc. As Virchow stated long ago, "Medicine is a social science."

Application of National Health Service Principles to Medical Care in the United States

The key element in a national health service is the public ownership of medical care resources, particularly the hospital sector. This objective may seem to be a practical and political impossibility in the United States, but certain characteristics of the current United States medical system make nationalization of the hospital sector not quite so impossible as it might at first glance seem.[4] The Veterans Administration Hospital System operates rather like a small-scale national health service. Each hospital is publicly owned and staffed by public employees. Patients are treated without regard to their ability to pay.

Other similarities exist between the American and the British medical care systems. Departmental regions and the regional officers and the Health Systems Agencies (HSAs) resemble the Regional and Area Health Authorities of the English system. These administrative units are charged with the planning, development, integration, and coordination of medical services. Moreover, the parallelism may become even greater in the future. The English system of centralization, previously dominated by a strong central government authority passing on its directives to the regions, areas, and districts, was modified somewhat by the 1974 reorganization, but central control is still being attacked as too constraining. In addition, the establishment of community health councils was an attempt, however rudimentary, to involve the local public more closely in the affairs of the NHS. The looser federal structure of American government already ensures delegation of authority at the local level. Indeed this would appear to be one of the basic principles underpinning present HSA legislation. All that is required in the United States system is the strengthening of policy making at the central level, which would then set the limits within which the HSAs could adjust medical service provision to reflect the specific circumstances of their constituent communities. In this respect, the situation in America today is more advantageous than that which faced the English in 1948.

Medicare and Medicaid are somewhat remniscent of Lloyd George's Health Insurance Act of 1911. Both introduced a degree of fiscal protection for the medically indigent, if one accepts that the elderly, because they usually live on fixed incomes and have a high rate of utilization of medical services, are actually or potentially indigent. Actually, the 1911 Act was vastly inferior to Medicare and Medicaid in that only lower-paid members of the gainfully employed were covered by Lloyd George's scheme. Medicaid and Medicare cover much wider segments of the population. Medicare and Medicaid also represent a strengthening of the collectivist ethic on the American scene, as did the introduction of what amounted to catastrophic health insurance for the sufferers of end-stage renal disease in 1973. The collectivist ethic is, as noted above, essential to the establishment and development of a national health service.

Nevertheless, it would be unrealistic to end this short essay on too optimistic a note so far as a United States national health service is concerned. The emergence of the National Health Service in Britain owed much to the development of socialist principles in the British political spectrum. While one would not want to argue that socialism and the Labour Party were solely responsible for the introduction of the present British medical care system, the gradual (but occasionally violent) development of working-class movement involving a radical shift towards a collectivist morality undoubtedly played an important part in the genesis of the NHS. Most observers would agree that America has yet to produce a viable working class movement, let alone an effective socialist political party. Perhaps radical reform of the American medical care industry will be impossible until the country's political system can present real ideological alternatives, real choices between left and right, to the electorate.

Notes

1. The medical sociology seminar series of the Departments of Sociology and Family and Community Medicine at the University of Missouri-Columbia provide an opportunity for medical sociologists at the institution to present their work to graduate students and colleagues for critical review. I gratefully acknowledge the comments and suggestions of Sylvester Alubo, Ed Brent, Jim Campbell, Lisbeth Claus, Tim Diamond, Robert Hagemen, Stan Ingman, Phyllis Kultgen, Hans Mauksch, Andrew Twaddle, and Cheryl Tyree on an earlier draft of this essay. Grateful thanks are also due to Peter Conrad for editorial comments and suggestions. Most of the material presented here was originally

presented in D. G. Gill, "The British Health Service: A Sociologist's Perspective," United States Department of Health, Education and Welfare, 1980.

2. In Britain, the separation of general practice and consultant (hospital sector) practice has historically been strict. Consultants have long enjoyed a higher status than practitioners, who have often been refused access to a hospital.

3. In the means test, an individual's income is closely examined by an investigator from the NHS, and specified exemption from charges is made if the income falls below a specified minimum amount.

4. I am grateful to my wife, Lucille Salarno Gill, for suggesting this line of analysis.

References

1. Gill, D. G. *The British National Health Service: A Sociologist's Perspective.* The Fogarty International Center, U.S. Department of Health and Welfare, September, 1980.

2. Butler, J. R. *Family Doctors and Public Policy.* London: Routledge & Kegan Paul, 1973

3. Cartwright, A. *Human Relations and Hospital Care.* London: Routledge & Kegan Paul, 1964.

4. Cartwright, A. *Patients and Their Doctors.* London: Routledge & Kegan Paul, 1967.

5. Stimson, G. and Webb, B. *Going to See the Doctor: The Consultation Process in General Practice.* London: Routledge & Kegan Paul, 1975.

6. Heller, T. *Restructuring the Health Service.* Croom Helm, London, 1978.

7. British Medical Association. Evidence to the Royal Commission on the National Health Service. Chapter VII. Finance. *Brit. Med. J.* 7, 1977.

8. Radical Statistics Health Groups. In Defense of the N.H.S. 9, Poland St., London, 1977.

9. The Labour Party. The Right to Health. Transport House, London, 1977.

10. Reinhardt, V. Health Costs and Expenditures in West Germany and the U.S. Chapter X in *International Health Costs and Expenditures.* Ed., Teh-Wei Hu, John F. Fogarty International Center, D.H.E.W. No. (NIH) 76–1067, 1976.

11. Stroman, D. F. *The Quick Knife: Unnecessary Surgery U.S.A.* Kennikat Press, New York and London, 1979.

12. Dahrendorf, R. *Class and Class Conflict in an Industrial Society.* Routledge & Kegan Paul, London, 1949.

13. H.M.SO. Report of the Committee of Inquiry into the Relationship of the Pharmaceutical Industry with the National Health Service 1965–67. (Sainsbury Committee) Cmnd. 3410, London, 1967.

14. Mullins, P.; Laning, L.; Leonard, M.; Doll, J.; Hadidi, R.; and Raffel, G. Drug Information Services/Systems: An Historical Overview, Current Status, Need for Evaluation and Proposed Evaluation Methodology. Health Services Research Center/Health Care Technology Center, University of Missouri-Columbia, U.S.A., 1978.

15. Dingwall, R. Inequality and the National Health Service. In *Essays on the N.H.S.* Eds., Atkinson, P.; Dingwall, R.; and Mucott, A. Croom Helm, London, 1979.

16. McKeown, T. *The Role of Medicare: Dream, Mirage, or Nemesis.* The Nuffield Provincial Hospital Trust. London, 1976.

40

The Delivery of Medical Care in China

Victor W. Sidel and Ruth Sidel

The health of the Chinese people has changed greatly over the past few decades. The change is apparent in many ways, some that are reflected in the anecdotes that returning visitors tell and others that are evident in the few available statistics. In the second category perhaps the most dramatic is the reported change in the principal causes of death. In China during the 1930s and 1940s the leading causes of death were on the one hand infectious and parasitic diseases and on the other complications of malnutrition (in many cases a euphemism for starvation). Today it appears that the leading causes of death, at least in a large city such as Shanghai, are the same as those in the developed nations of the West: cancer, stroke, and heart disease.

On the surface this change might seem merely to substitute one termination of life for another. Its significance, however, is inescapable: it is evidence that the people of China are dying at progressively higher ages. Other statistics point to the same conclusion. For example, in the 1930's the life expectancy of a newborn child in Shanghai was some 40 years. Data compiled by the city's Bureau of Public Health in 1972 suggest that today the life expectancy is more than 70 years. The data are all the more remarkable when one considers that they are from what is one of the poorer and technologically less developed nations in the world.

In some ways the anecdotal evidence is even more convincing than the statistical, much of which is fragmentary and unconfirmed. Almost all visitors from abroad who travel the urban lanes and country paths they knew 25 years or more ago comment on the change in appearances. Where sick children and ailing adults were once a commonplace sight, today they are rarely seen; both children and adults appear to be in excellent health.

How have the Chinese, with their limited technical resources, managed to do this? The answer is that their revolution of 25 years ago gave rise to many changes in the Chinese way of life, including changes in the methods of delivering health care. To understand the nature of these changes and to see today's pattern of Chinese medical and social services in context, it is necessary to know something about former conditions.

In 1949 the population of China was estimated to be 540 million, some 85 percent of which was rural. With respect to the practice of what the Chinesse call "Western medicine," there were then in China 40,000 Western-style physicians at most and perhaps 90,000 beds in Western-style hospitals. If these medical resources had been evenly distributed, the ratio of physicians to potential patients would have been one to every 13,000 and of beds per patient one to every 6,000. Instead, of course, most of the resources were concentrated in a few cities, and even there most of the population depended on practitioners of traditional Chinese medicine for such care as they received.

Beginning in 1949 China's new government confronted this deficiency in health resources by initiating a dual program. Some of the strategies adopted by the new Ministry of Health were unique to China; others were the same strategies that have been adopted by many other technologically underdeveloped nations. In the first category were innovative efforts to involve the bulk of the population in "mass movements." These were aimed primarily at improving the public health and sanitation. A further innovation was an attempt to enlist the practitioners of traditional medicine in overall health programs.

In the second category were programs that emphasized the training of large numbers of new health workers. The principal efforts to increase the numbers of health personnel were directed on the one hand toward the training of "middle level" health workers and on the other hand toward the establishment of "centers of excellence." These centers were urban training facilities that were expected to pioneer new medical techniques and also to provide a flow of skilled personnel to areas of special need.

Following Russian models, the Ministry of Health set up a number of "middle medical schools." Students who had reached the intermediate level of the secondary school system were sent to middle medical schools for a three-year course that prepared them to work as "assistant doctors." This is a category comparable to the Russian *feldsher,* a physician's assistant who is expected to act as a physician when necessary. At the same time the middle medical schools trained other personnel as nurses, midwives, technicians, and pharmacists.

The Ministry of Health also expanded the existing program of "higher" medical education. Some medical schools were moved from the coastal cities to the interior and some new schools were founded. Here again Russian models were followed. Separate faculties were responsible for pediatrics, for general medicine, for stomatology (dentistry and other treatment of diseases of the mouth), and for public health. The period of study at the higher medical schools was five or six years; the students were recruited from those who had completed the senior level of secondary school. At the pinnacle of this higher-educational system was the China Medical College in Peking. Here an eight-year curriculum was offered, its objective being to train teachers and research personnel.

By 1965 the ambitious program had produced more than 100,000 new physicians and some 170,000 assistant doctors. In the same period, however, China's population had grown from 540 million to about 725 million. Even though the physician-to-patient ratio of one to 5,000 was substantially better than it had been in 1949, it was still far from the ratio of one to 1,000 or better that is typical of richer nations. The progress of the Health Ministry's innovative programs also had been good but large gaps remained. Even though some traditional methods had been adopted, practitioners of traditional medicine were still looked on as second-class physicians. By the same token the mass-movement programs had successfully attacked a number of public health problems, but professional or, as the Chinese say, "expert" health workers continued to dominate Chinese medicine. Perhaps most important of all, the center of gravity of medical care remained in China's urban areas. The inadequate level of health care delivered to the rural Chinese, who are the vast majority of the nation's population, led to criticism of the Ministry of Health. This was climaxed in 1965 by an action that proved to be a forerunner of the "Cultural Revolution" of 1966–1969: publication of what is now known as "Chairman Mao's June 26 Directive." "In medical and health work," the directive ordered, "put the stress on the rural areas."

Both of us work in the field of medical and social services in the U.S. and have studied the delivery of these services in a number of other countries. We thus felt ourselves fortunate to be among the first Americans to be invited to visit China by the Chinese Medical Association soon after the "Ping-Pong breakthrough" of 1971. By then the Cultural Revolution had wound down and we were eager to see what its effects had been. We were able to observe several aspects of contemporary Chinese medicine, including the delivery of medical care, in September and October of 1971 and then again in greater depth in September and October of 1972. We traveled with representatives of the Chinese Medical Association to the nation's two largest cities, Peking and Shanghai, to a number of provincial cities and towns, and to rural areas in both the densely populated coastal regions and the less crowded interior.

A foreigner thinks of Shanghai and Peking as being purely urban areas. In reality, of the almost 11 million Chinese who live in the "independent municipality" of Shanghai five million inhabit the 10 rural counties that surround the city proper. The rural five million are the population of some 200 "communes": self-governing political and economic units that are each divided into between 10 and 30 "production brigades." The production brigades are subdivided into "production teams," each several hundred strong. In all, the rural population of Shanghai incorporates some 2,700 production brigades and nearly 28,000 production teams.

One example of rural health care that we saw in 1971 was provided by the Ma Chiao commune outside Shanghai proper. We visited one brigade of the commune, the Sing Sing brigade, with a total population of 1,850 subdivided into 12 production teams. The brigade health station, where we interviewed the staff, was served by four "barefoot doctors" and a midwife. Each production team in the brigade, we learned, had one to three additional health aides.

It is worth mentioning here that the term *barefoot doctor* is a literal translation of the Chinese appellation *(chijiao yisheng)* that has been given these health workers. We never met a barefoot doctor who was barefoot. Moreover, these workers are not addressed as "doctor" *(yisheng* or, more honorifically, *dafu)* by their patients but are called "comrade" *(tongzhi)*. The barefoot doctors, who generally receive three to six months' initial training, followed by continuing on-the-job education, evidently think of themselves not as "expert" health workers but as peasants who do some medical work.

The eldest of the four barefoot doctors at the brigade health station, Ho Shichang, was 30. Before his medical training his education had consisted of six years of primary school, completed at age 13. Between then and the start of his medical training in 1964 Ho worked as a farmer; in 1971 he still spent about half of his working time farming. The year before Mao's June 26 Directive was issued Ho had been one of 274 students who spent three months at the county hospital receiving basic training from the 13 health workers on the hospital staff. He later spent three additional months at the commune hospital for practical training; he still spends one day a week there as part of his continuing practical education.

Like his colleagues, Ho is responsible for treating the "light diseases" of his fellow brigade members: minor injuries, gastrointestinal illness, colds, and bronchitis. He also administers immunization against diphtheria, tetanus, whooping cough, measles, smallpox, poliomyelitis, Japanese B encephalitis, and meningococcal meningitis. Another of his public health duties is to supervise the collection, treatment, and storage of human excreta for utilization as fertilizer. The actual work may be overseen by the production-team health aides, but the responsibility is his, as are continuing campaigns against pests such as flies, fleas, cockroaches, and snails (the last is the intermediate host of the organism that causes schistosomiasis).

The contents of Ho's medical bag provide a good measure of his capacity to treat various diseases (see Table 1). In the U.S. 39 of these medica-

Table 1.
Medical Supplies at Disposal of "Barefoot Doctors"

Medications

* *Adona (cardiac stimulant) ampules
* **Adrenalin** ampules
* **Aminophyllin** tablets and ampules
* Ammonium chloride tablets and solution
* *Analgin tablets and ampules
* Aspirin-phenacetin-caffeine tablets
* **Atropine** tablets
* **Belladonna** extract tablets
* *Berberine tablets
* **Brown's mixture** tablets and liquid
* **Caffeine sodium benzoate** ampules
* **Chloromycetin** ampules and capsules
* **Chlorpheniramine** maleate tablets
* **Chlorpromazine** tablets and ampules
* *Chlothamine tablets
* *DCT tablets
* **Demerol**
* *DPP in tablets
* **Ephedrine**
* *Furazolidone tablets
* Lactobacillus tablets
* *Lobodura tablets
* **Luminal** tablets
* **Nikethamide** ampules
* **Nitrofurantoin** tablets
* **Penicillin**, crystalline
* **Penicillin**, procaine
* Phenolax tablets
* *8-p-phenylbenzylatropinium bromide tablets
* **Phenylbutazone** tablets
* **Piperazine** citrate tablets
* **Promethazine** tablets
* **Probanthine** tablets
* **Reserpine** tablets
* Sodium bicarbonate tablets
* **Sulfadiazine** tablets and ampules
* **Sulfaguanidine** tablets
* **Sulfamethazine** tablets

Sulfamethoxpyridazine tablets
Sulfathiazole tablets
*Syntomycin capsules
Terramycin tablets
Tetracycline tablets
Valium tablets
Vitamin B1 tablets
Vitamin B2 tablets
Vitamin C tablets
Vitamin K tablets
*Vitamin U tablets
Yeast tablets

Topical agents

Alcohol
Boric acid ointment
Eye drops
Gentian violet
Iodine tincture
Mercurochrome
Nose drops
Sulfa ointment

Equipment

Acupuncture needles
Adhesive tape
Bandages and gauze
Cotton sponges and swabs
Drinking cups
Forceps
Fountain pen
Hypodermic needles
Notebook for records
Paper bag
Rubber tubing
Scissors
Sphygmomanometer
Syringes (2 cc. and 5 cc.)
Thermometers (oral and rectal)

Medical supplies at the disposal of barefoot doctors include 50 medications and 8 topical agents. The names are the most familiar ones; some are proprietary and some generic. Of the 39 medications used in U.S. practice, 30 (bold) are available only by prescription. The items marked with an asterisk are not generally available in the U.S.

tions are in use; only nine of them can be obtained without a physician's prescription. When Ho encounters a problem beyond his scope, he refers the patient to the commune hospital. (The 200 or so commune hospitals in rural Shanghai have an average of 30 beds each.) If the matter is more serious, the patient is referred to the county hospital.

Ho and his colleagues divide their time about equally between farmwork and duty at the brigade health stations. As members of the commune they share in the produce the commune raises. They also share in the commune's cash income, which is divided among the commune's members on the basis of the "work points" each earns. They receive no extra income for their work as barefeet doctors, but their health-station service earns them work points, so that they lose no income either.

At the time of our visit in 1971 Ho was one of 7,700 barefoot doctors working in the communes of rural Shanghai. This represented a new high in the level of health care. In the late 1950s, as part of the initial effort to train health auxiliaries, health teams from the city proper had trained some 3,900 rural residents in health care. During the retrenchment of 1961–1965, however, training was largely discontinued and many rural health aides returned to full-time farmwork. The program that has produced most of the barefoot doctors in China today began only after Mao's June 26 Directive of 1965. By 1968 in the Shanghai area some 4,500 barefoot doctors had been trained, and the new trainees had themselves trained an additional 29,000 health aides to provide part-time health care at the production-team level.

Like Shanghai, Peking has a substantial rural population. The city's nine urban districts have four million residents, but three million more live in the nine counties outside the city proper. During our 1971 visit we found that the delivery of medical care in this rural area differed very little in pattern from the system in rural Shanghai. The commune we visited, the Shuang Chiao commune, had a population of 38,000, subdivided into six production brigades and 77 production teams. The commune hospital had a clinical laboratory and X-ray facilities but had no beds and served outpatients only; any patient requiring hospitalization was referred to the county hospital. At this commune we visited the aid station of one production team, the Shuang Pei team, which was staffed by a single barefoot doctor. Liu Yu-cheng, age 23, had completed the lower level of secondary school. When Mao's June 26 Directive was issued, the other members of the Shuang Pei team nominated Liu for medical training. His basic training had come from a mobile team of physicians who normally worked in Peking proper but were then assigned to the Shuang Chiao commune hospital; the instruction period lasted for three months. Since that time Liu has been given short leaves of absence for further study. Not long before our visit he had spent three months in the city studying traditional Chinese medicine.

During our visit in 1972 we saw one of the commune hospitals in the rural area outside Peking. The hospital had opened in May, 1971. It has 30 beds, and its staff of 48 serves a commune with a total population of 46,000. Seven of the staff members are physicians; five are Western-trained and two are traditional practitioners. All seven are on loan from the staff of a hospital in Peking proper. The balance of the staff consists of 15 nurses, 25 health auxiliaries, 11 technicians and administrators and one cook. In the 17 months between opening day and our visit in October, 1972, some 8,000 members of the commune had received care as outpatients (an average of 500 per month) and 500 more had entered the hospital for treatment (an average of one patient per bed per month).

Medical care in urban China follows the same pattern of decentralization that we observed in the rural areas. In Peking proper, for example, each of the nine urban districts has an average population of about 400,000. The city's municipal medical services include four specialized research hospitals and 23 general hospitals; ten of the general hospitals have more than 500 beds.

Each of the nine districts is subdivided into "neighborhoods." In the West District of Peking, which we visited, there were nine such neighborhoods; the one that was our host, the Fengsheng Neighborhood, has a population of 53,000. One municipal hospital in the West District, the People's Hospital, is where any Fengsheng Neighborhood patients are sent if care at one of the specialized hospitals is not required. Within the neighborhood itself the only hospital-like facility is exclusively for outpatient care. Its staff of 90, however, provides the nucleus of the neighborhood health-care apparatus. The staff includes seven Western-trained physicians and 20 practitioners of traditional medicine, 31 nurses and technicians, 18 administrative and other personnel and 14 trainees. The public-health department is responsible for supervising the urban equivalent of the rural production-team aid stations: a total of 25 health stations operated by Lane Committees.

The Fengsheng Neighborhood has 132 lanes in all, so that each of the 25 Lane Committees represents the residents of five or six lanes, or some 400 families. Each Lane Committee health station is staffed morning and afternoon by local housewives who have the title Red Medical Worker. The daily hours are from 8:00 to 11:00 A.M. and from 1:00 to 5:30 P.M.

The health station we visited was maintained by the Wu Ting Lane Committee. Its plain single room was furnished with an examination couch, a cabinet for medical supplies, and a table and chairs. Three Red Medical Workers were present; we talked at some length to one of the women, Yang Hsio-hua. Yang was 38 years old and had worked at the health station for two years. Married some 20 years ago, she has three children, 19, 15, and 11. She had become a Red Medical Worker by volunteering for a month's basic training at the Fengsheng Neighborhood medical facility. During that time she learned how to take a medical history and how to conduct simple physical examinations, including such routines as measuring blood pressure. She was instructed in the uses of a number of drugs, both Western and traditional, and she had learned the techniques of acupuncture and intramuscular and subcutaneous injection.

A physician from the neighborhood medical facility visited the Wu Ting health sitation as often as three times a week. Yang and her fellow medical workers visited the neighborhood facility when they had questions. She observed that seven to ten patients visited the health station during morning hours and that four or five more might come in the afternoon.

At the health station much of the emphasis is on preventive medicine, in particular immunization against infectious diseases. Most immunization of local children is accomplished at the station. If necessary, one of the medical workers will call for a child at home or even administer an inoculation there. For example, one Lane Committee health-station immunization chart we saw showed that of 160-odd children eligible for immunization against measles in 1971, a total of 154 had received inoculations by the time of our visit. Other charts showed the comparative incidence of infectious diseases from 1958 on. Measles has evidently become uncommon since immunization first began in 1965.

Figure 1.

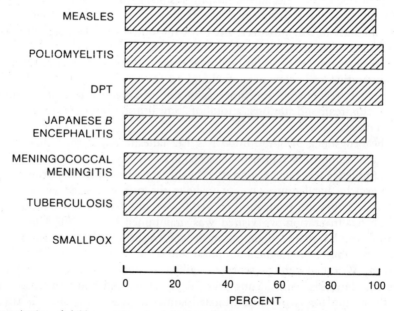

Immunization of children against nine infectious diseases is routine. Bars show the percentage of eligible children immunized in 1971 at one Lane Committee health station.

Figure 2.

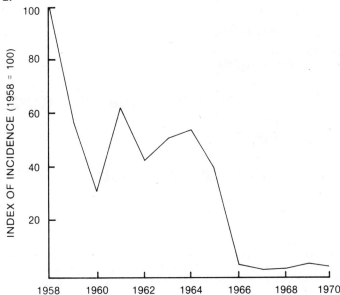

Incidence of measles in one Peking neighborhood has fallen sharply since 1965, the year routine inoculation of children against measles was begun. All immunization is free.

Neighborhood factory workers seldom use the Lane Committee health stations because their own factory medical facility is more convenient. Their dependents, however, do use the Lane Committee stations, and the factory will reimburse half the cost of treatment. The charge is never more than ten *fen* and is usually smaller. (One hundred *fen* make one *yüan* and one *yüan* is equal to about 40 U.S. cents.) Nonetheless, the income from the fees, together with a subsidy that each Lane Committee health station receives from its Neighborhood Committee, allows the Red Medical Workers to receive a monthly stipend of about 15 *yüan*, roughly a third of the wage that a beginning factory worker would be paid.

China has by no means solved its medical problems. For example, both tuberculosis and trachoma are far more prevalent than they are in richer nations. What we have seen of the delivery of medical care in both rural and urban areas, however, convinces us the public health and medical care in China are better than they are in other nations handicapped to a similar degree by technological underdevelopment. One striking instance of this is the success of the Chinese campaign for birth control.

Health workers both in the countryside and in the cities have as one of their main responsibilities a program to make contraception popular. The urban Red Medical Workers make a point of explaining to their patients how a lower birth rate will benefit not only their neighborhood and their

Figure 3.

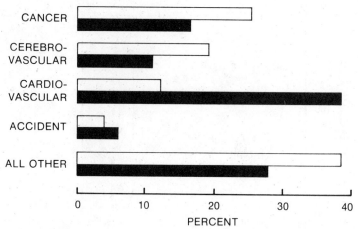

Leading causes of death in Shanghai during the first six months of 1972 *(light)* are contrasted with those in the U.S. *(dark)* as a whole during 1968. In both instances cancer, stroke, and heart disease were responsible for more than 55 percent of all deaths; the parallel indicates that the Chinese are living longer and more of them are dying from diseases of old age.

city but all China. At the same time the medical workers stress the part that birth control plays in the "liberation" of women, a concept that is substantially more radical in tradition-bound China than in Western countries. An example of the effectiveness of the urban effort is provided by the records of one Lane Committee health station in the city of Hangchow. The data represent only a small sample: 369 married couples with wives of childbearing age. Within this group 24 percent of the women and 3 percent of the men had been permanently sterilized. Another 27 percent of the women and 19 percent of the men regularly used contraceptives. Of the 98 wives who reportedly did not use contraceptives, ten were pregnant, seven were newly married, and 16 were still nursing (a period when, it is mistakenly believed by some, a woman cannot conceive). The crude annual birth rate for the population served by the Lane Committee health station is at the remarkably low level of eight per 1,000.

Birth statistics for Shanghai in 1972 are equally remarkable. The reported rate for the city proper is 6.4 per 1,000 and for the entire independent municipality 10.6 per 1,000. By way of comparison, in 1972 the lowest rate in any of the 50 states in the U.S. was 12.6 per 1,000 (in Maryland). In this connection the 1972 crude death rate for Shanghai proper is reported as being 5.6 per 1,000. Assuming that both figures are correct, this means that the city's natural growth rate is less than a tenth of 1 percent (0.8 per 1,000). This is one of the lowest natural growth rates in any urban area in the world.

Birth-control statistics from rural areas are substantially different. For example, one commune in the rural counties outside Peking, with a total population of 46,000, has compiled contraception statistics for 5,777 married couples where the wife is of childbearing age. Only 8 percent of the wives and 2 percent of the husbands have been permanently sterilized. Another 41 percent of the wives use contraceptives, the "pill" being favored over intrauterine devices by 23 percent to 18 percent. Among the husbands 9 percent use the condom, bringing the total of contraceptive users to 50 percent. During 1971 there were 1,181 births in the commune, so that the crude birth rate was slightly less than 24 per 1,000. The 1971 statistics for the 450,000 inhabitants of Shunyi County, a rural district outside Peking, are quite similar. There the married couples where the wife is of childbearing age number 49,297, and 59 percent of them practice contraception. The number of births in the county in 1971 was 9,504, which means a crude birth rate slightly above 21 per 1,000.

The birth rates in both of these rural samples seem high compared with the rates in the urban areas we have cited. Chinese health officials hope to see the national rate eventually fall to about 15 per 1,000. Nonetheless, even the rural rate is substantially below the former rate, which is estimated to have been 45 per 1,000 or higher. (For purposes of comparison the current crude birth rate for Southeast Asia is estimated to be 43 per 1,000.)

One still unresolved medical issue is how to achieve an effective union of Western and traditional medical practices. It will probably never be known exactly how many practitioners of traditional medicine there were in 1949, but they were estimated to number in the hundreds of thousands, and they provided at least some degree of health care to a large and faithful clientele, particularly in the rural areas. Nonetheless, then as now certain difficulties stood in the way of integrating the traditional and the Western-style practitioners.

Traditional Chinese medicine is much more than a collection of empirical remedies. It is based on a large body of theory, accumulated over some 3,000 years, that includes, for example, the concept of "natural" balance between yin and yang. One declared objective of the People's Republic of China, however, is to lead the population away from the "superstitions of feudalism" and toward the practice of "scientific methods."

With eminent practicality Mao dismissed this theoretical conflict early in the 1950s by declaring that traditional Chinese medicine was a "great treasurehouse" and urging that traditional and Western practices be merged. Some progress in this direction was made in the 1950s and early 1960s, but it is only since the Cultural Revolution that emphasis on unifying the two streams has increased significantly. For example, students in the Western-style medical schools now receive more than casual instruction in traditional medicine, and those who study traditional medicine are

Figure 4.

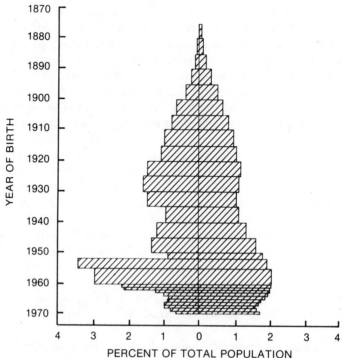

Population profile of the 478,000 inhabitants of the Luwan district of Shanghai in 1971 *(left)* is compared with that of the U.S. as a whole in 1970 *(right)*. The "rectangular" U.S. profile is characteristic of the age distribution found in more developed countries. The "bulge" in the number of Chinese births between 1952 and 1960 may partly reflect the absence of official support for birth control during this period. The "pinch" in Chinese births in the 1963–1970 period, with an eight year total that is scarcely half the U.S. total in the same period, probably reflects a greater use of birth control methods by the urban Chinese.

also taught Western practices. At the same time the years since 1949 have seen the general adoption of certain traditional techniques: the use of herbal preparations, of gymnastic and respiratory exercises, and of two related treatments, moxibustion and acupuncture.

Traditional Chinese pharmacology emphasizes herbal remedies, usually in the form of a broth or tea that the patient drinks. In the countryside today health workers not only gather and prepare wild herbs but also cultivate a number of them. Moreover, the medicine cabinets in rural and urban health stations are stocked with herbal remedies as well as with Western ones. Some herbal remedies are even available as sterile preparations for injection. Medical investigators in China suspect that, just as one traditional herbal remedy, *ma huang,* has been found to contain ephedrine as its active principle, others may prove to contain similar specific phar-

Figure 5.

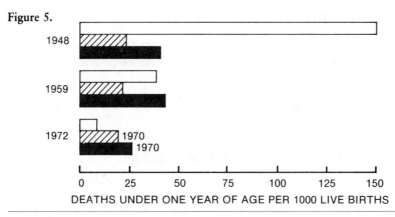

DEATHS UNDER ONE YEAR OF AGE PER 1000 LIVE BIRTHS

Infant deaths in the first year in urban Shanghai *(light)* are compared with the deaths of white *(shaded)* and nonwhite *(dark)* infants in New York City in 1948, in 1959, and in 1972. (The comparable New York figures are for 1970, the latest year for which they are available.) The data for Shanghai are from the Chinese Medical Association; the 1972 rate, less than 1 percent of all live births, is so low that it has met with some skepticism.

macological compounds. A substantial part of current pharmacological research is concerned with examining this possibility.

One tenet of Chinese traditional medicine is that the internal organs of the body are connected to points on the skin by way of channels called *ching lo* that run throughout the body close to the skin. Stimulation of a point along a channel is supposed to affect the internal organ attached to that channel. Although the existence of such channels has never been demonstrated anatomically, it is on their theoretical foundation that moxibustion and acupuncture rest. In moxibustion the stimulus to the skin is produced by heat. The pulverized leaves of an herb, the mugwort, are wrapped in a paper cone, the tip of the cone is ignited, and the smoldering herb is placed on or near the appropriate point.

In acupuncture the stimulus is applied by inserting a needle to a predetermined depth in the patient's skin. Acupuncture can be used both for diagnosis and for treatment. It is even taught in secondary schools in much the same way that first aid is taught in some U.S. school systems. Indeed, health workers whom we met in both rural and urban areas said that as a routine treatment for headache they preferred acupuncture to aspirin.

The Chinese use of acupuncture to produce insensitivity to pain during surgery has attracted much attention in the U.S. The procedure is actually less common in China than widely circulated American accounts might lead one to believe. It is usually called acupuncture anesthesia in English (and in English language publications of Chinese origin). "Anesthesia," of course, implies a general loss of sensation by the patient. It would be more appropriate to use the term analgesia, a loss of pain sensation. In any event the Chinese say that the effect is most successful when the surgical proce-

Figure 6.

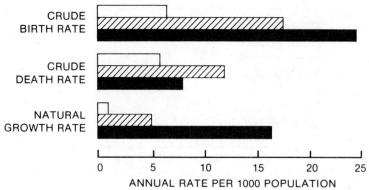

Natural growth rate, the excess of births over deaths is shown for urban Shanghai *(light)* and for the white *(shaded)* and nonwhite *(dark)* population of New York City. The New York data are for 1970; Shanghai data for 1972 suggest a notably low rate.

dure is "above the waist," so that acupuncture for this purpose is largely confined to surgery of the head, the neck, and the thorax. Because the technique is still considered experimental it is applied only with patients who specifically request it and, within this group, only with those who are considered to be "not too anxious" about surgery. Most surgical patients in China receive conventional anesthetics.

With respect to "mass movements" in Chinese health care, the first nation-wide "Patriotic Health Campaigns" were launched in the 1950s. The targets were "four pests": flies, mosquitoes, rats, and the "grain-thieving" sparrow. (The ecologically unjust charge against sparrows was later withdrawn and bedbugs were substituted.)

Similar mass movements continue today, expanded and redirected to include other public-health problems, such as the handling of human excreta, the purity of the water in local wells and streams, methods of food preparation and even the disposal of trash. In the countryside the departments of health in commune and brigade hospitals supervise the campaigns; in the cities district and neighborhood hospital personnel have the same responsibility. In both rural and urban areas the ultimate responsibility rests with the local health workers and the aides they have trained. For example, in Hangchow the Red Medical Workers at one Lane Committee health station set aside three days a month for "cleanup work" with the assistance of their fellow residents. The time is spent removing trash and inspecting potential pest breeding places. Full-scale sessions, however, usually coincide with major festival days and with the state celebrations on May 1 and October 1.

The mass-movement approach has apparently helped the Chinese to dispose of such "social" illnesses as drug addiction and venereal disease.

Figure 7.

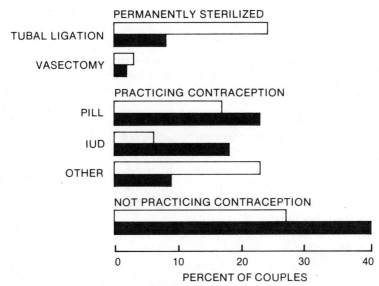

Contraceptive practices in an urban area *(light)* and in a rural area *(dark)* are compared; the urban sample is from a commune outside Peking. Sterilization is nearly three times greater in the urban than in the rural sample and substantially fewer rural males use contraceptives. The bias seems to be reflected in the difference between urban and rural birth rates: below 10 per 1,000 in some urban areas and above 20 per 1,000 in some rural ones.

For example, early in the 1950s checklists of the symptoms of syphilis were posted in every community center. A slogan ("We don't want to take syphilis into Communism") was promulgated, mass surveys were conducted, and social pressure was brought to bear on suspect individuals who failed to seek medical attention. Elimination of prostitutes as carriers of venereal disease was accomplished by giving them the opportunity to engage in "socially constructive" work. As with the birth-control campaign, the Chinese effort to control "social" illnesses seems to have met with greater success than similar efforts in comparably poor nations and even in some technologically advanced ones.

A summary of China's achievements in transforming the delivery of medical care since 1949 shows an interweaving of three main threads: decentralization, demystification, and continuity with the past. Following a pattern that many students of community medicine would be happy to see more widely emulated in Western countries, the delivery of medical care in China begins at the lowest possible level in both the city and the countryside. Initial medical attention is in the hands of health aides who are part of the community they serve. From this initial point of contact a clearly organized system of referral leads level by level up to a plateau of sophisticated medical specialization. (It is worth noting that in some technical areas, such as the treatment of severe burns and the replantation of limbs, Chinese medicine may be ahead of Western medicine.) The patient with a problem that cannot be handled at one level of this decentralized structure moves on to the level above. The system is an efficient, low-cost one. Moreover, it has the advantage of building social cohesion and local self-reliance by emphasizing neighborliness and service for others from the lowest level up.

From the Chinese point of view demystification runs parallel to decentralization. The front-line medical workers are men and women with little in the way of formal education. They work part time and receive their instruction in health care through brief programs that emphasize the practical. They urge participation on the part of the people they look after. For example, each individual is expected, as a patient, to look out for his own health and, as a citizen, to look out for the health of the community. Under these circumstances it is no wonder that much of the mystery medicine so often holds for the layman has been effectively dispelled. Demystification has also been furthered by shortening the term of formal medical education and by assigning urban physicians to periodic tours of duty in the countryside. The two steps express with respect to medicine the determination of Mao and others to eliminate "elitism" in general.

As for continuity with the past, we have already noted the pragmatic adoption of certain traditional Chinese medical practices. What is less commonly appreciated is that the social structure involved in the decentralization process (for example, the pyramidal succession that leads from courtyard to lane, from lane to neighborhood, and from neighborhood to district) preserves, albeit with differences in method and purpose, much of the traditional Chinese social organization. Thus the past is interwoven with the present in many ways. Indeed, in assessing the applicability of Chinese medical methods abroad it is often difficult to judge which methods might be used successfully in other societies and which are so culture-linked as to be uniquely Chinese.

For ourselves, with a concern for the improvement of medical and social services in the U.S., the lessons from China may be more general than specific. Certainly they transcend medical technology and enter the spheres of politics and economics. It seems to us that the Chinese have managed to overcome severe problems, to improve their system of medical care, and to enhance the health of their population only by making medical change an integral part of a change in Chinese society as a whole. We in the U.S. face social and medical problems that, although they are quite different from China's in many ways, are equally difficult. It remains to be seen whether or not we shall meet them in as determined and comprehensive a way as the Chinese have met theirs.

41

A Case for Refocussing Upstream: The Political Economy of Illness

John B. McKinlay

My friend, Irving Zola, relates the story of a physician trying to explain the dilemmas of the modern practice of medicine:

> "You know," he said, "sometimes it feels like this. There I am standing by the shore of a swiftly flowing river and I hear the cry of a drowning man. So I jump into the river, put my arms around him, pull him to shore and apply artificial respiration. Just when he begins to breathe, there is another cry for help. So I jump into the river, reach him, pull him to shore, apply artificial respiration, and then just as he begins to breathe, another cry for help. So back in the river again, reaching, pulling, applying, breathing and then another yell. Again and again, without end, goes the sequence. You know, I am so busy jumping in, pulling them to shore, applying artificial respiration, that I have *no* time to see who the hell is upstream pushing them all in."[1]

I believe this simple story illustrates two important points. *First,* it highlights the fact that a clear majority of our resources and activities in the health field are devoted to what I term "downstream endeavors" in the form of superficial, categorical tinkering in response to almost perennial shifts from one health issue to the next, without really solving anything. I am, of course, not suggesting that such efforts are entirely futile, or that a considerable amount of short-term good is not being accomplished. Clearly, people and groups have important immediate needs which must be recognized and attended to. Nevertheless, one must be wary of the *short-term nature* and *ultimate futility* of such downstream endeavors.

Second, the story indicates that we should somehow cease our preoccupation with this short-term, problem-specific tinkering and begin focussing our attention upstream, where the real problems lie. Such a reorientation would minimally involve an analysis of the means by which various individuals, interest groups, and large-scale, profit-oriented corporations are "pushing people in," and how they subsequently erect, at some point downstream, a health care structure to service the needs which they have had a hand in creating, and for which moral responsibility ought to be assumed.

In this paper two related themes will be developed. *First,* I wish to highlight the activities of the "manufacturers of illness"—those individuals, interest groups, and organizations which, in addition to producing material goods and services, also produce, as an inevitable by-product, widespread morbidity and mortality. Arising out of this, and *second,* I will develop a case for refocussing our attention away from those individuals and groups who are mistakenly held to be responsible for their condition, toward a range of broader upstream political and economic forces.

The task assigned to me for this conference was to review some of the broad social structural factors influencing the onset of heart disease and/or at-risk behavior. Since the issues covered by this request are so varied, I have, of necessity, had to make some decisions concerning both emphasis and scope. These decisions and the reasoning behind them should perhaps be explained at this point. With regard to what can be covered by the term "social structure," it is possible to isolate at least three separate levels of abstraction. One could, for example, focus on such subsystems as the family, and its associated social networks, and how these may be importantly linked to different levels of health status and the utilization of services.[2] On a second level, one could consider how particular organizations and broader social institutions, such as neighborhood and community structures, also affect the social distribution of pathology and at-risk behavior.[3] Third, attention could center on the broader political-economic spectrum, and how these admittedly more remote forces may be etiologically involved in the onset of disease. . . .

. . . [In this paper] I will argue, for example, that the frequent failure of many health intervention programs can be largely attributed to the inadequate recognition we give to aspects of social context. . . . The most important factor in deciding on the subject area of this paper, however, is the fact that, while there appears to be a newly emerging interest in the political economy of health care, social scientists have, as yet, paid little attention to the *political economy of illness.*[4] It is my intention in this paper to begin to develop a case for the serious consideration of this particular area.

A political-economic analysis of health care suggests that the entire structure of institutions in the United States is such as to preclude the adequate provision of services.[5] Increasingly, it seems, the provision of care is being tied to the priorities of profit-making institutions. For a long time, criticism of U.S. health care focussed on the activities of the American Medical Association and the fee for service system of physician payment.[6] Lately, however, attention appears to be refocussing on the relationship between health care arrangements and the structure of big business.[7] It has, for example, been suggested that:

... with the new and apparently permanent involvement of major corporations in health, it is becoming increasingly improbable that the United States can redirect its health priorities without, at the same time, changing the ways in which American industry is organized and the ways in which monopoly capitalism works.[8]

It is my impression that many of the political-economic arguments concerning develpments in the organization of health care also have considerable relevance for a holistic understanding of the etiology and distribution of morbidity, mortality, and at-risk behavior. In the following sections I will present some important aspects of these arguments in the hope of contributing to a better understanding of aspects of the political economy of illness.

An Unequal Battle

The downstream efforts of health researchers and practitioners against the upstream efforts of the manufacturers of illness have the appearance of an unequal war, *with a resounding victory assured for those on the side of illness* and the creation of disease-inducing behaviors. The battle between health workers and the manufacturers of illness is unequal on at least two grounds. In the *first* place, we always seem to arrive on the scene and begin to work after the real damage has already been done. By the time health workers intervene, people have already filled the artificial needs created for them by the manufacturers of illness and are habituated to various at-risk behaviors. In the area of smoking behavior, for example, we have an illustration not only of the lateness of health workers' arrival on the scene, and the enormity of the task confronting them, but also, judging by recent evidence, of the resounding defeat being sustained in this area.[9] To push the river analogy even further, the task becomes one of furiously swimming against the flow and finally being swept away when exhausted by the effort or through disillusionment with a lack of progress. So long as we continue to fight the battle downstream, and in such an ineffective manner, we are doomed to frustration, repeated failure, and perhaps ultimately to a sicker society.

Second, the promoters of disease-inducing behavior are manifestly more effective in their use of behavioral science knowledge than are those of us who are concerned with the eradication of such behavior. Indeed, it is somewhat paradoxical that we should be meeting here to consider how behavioral science knowledge and techniques can be effectively employed to reduce or prevent at-risk behavior, when that same body of knowledge *has already* been used to create the at-risk behavior we seek to eliminate. How embarrassingly ineffective are our mass media efforts in the health field (e.g., alcoholism, obesity, drug abuse, safe driving, pollution, etc.)

when compared with many of the tax exempt promotional efforts on behalf of the illness generating activities of large-scale corporations.[10] It is a fact that we are demonstrably more effective in persuading people to purchase items they never dreamt they would need, or to pursue at-risk courses of action, than we are in preventing or halting such behavior. Many advertisements are so ingenious in their appeal that they have entertainment value in their own right and become embodied in our national folk humor. By way of contrast, many health advertisements lack any comparable widespread appeal, often appear boring, avuncular, and largely misdirected.

I would argue that one major problem lies in the fact that we are overly concerned with the war itself, and with how we can more effectively participate in it. In the health field we have unquestioningly accepted the assumptions presented by the manufacturers of illness and, as a consequence, have confined our efforts to only downstream offensives. A little reflection would, I believe, convince anyone that those on the side of health are in fact losing. . . . But rather than merely trying to win the way, we need to step back and question the premises, legitimacy and utility of the war itself.

The Binding of At-Riskness to Culture

It seems that the appeals to at-risk behavior that are engineered by the manufacturers of illness are particularly successful because they are constructed in such a way as to be inextricably bound with essential elements of our existing dominant culture. This is accomplished in a number of ways: (a) Exhortations to at-risk behavior are often piggybacked on those legitimized values, beliefs, and norms which are widely recognized and adhered to in the dominant culture. The idea here is that if a person *would only do X*, then they would also be doing Y and Z. (b) Appeals are also advanced which claim or imply that certain courses of at-risk action are subscribed to or endorsed by most of the culture heroes in society (e.g., people in the entertainment industry), or by those with technical competence in that particular field (e.g., "doctors" recommend it). The idea here is that if a person *would only do X*, then he/she would be doing pretty much the same as is done or recommended by such prestigious people as A and B. (c) Artificial needs are manufactured, the fulfilling of which becomes absolutely essential if one is to be a meaningful and useful member of society. The idea here is that if a person *does not do X, or will not do X*, then they are either deficient in some important respect, or they are some kind of liability for the social system.

Variations on these and other kinds of appeal strategies have, of course, been employed for a long time now by the promoters of at-risk behavior.

The manufacturers of illness are, for example, fostering the belief that if you want to be an attractive, masculine man, or a "cool," "natural" woman, you will smoke cigarettes; that you can only be a "good parent" if you habituate your children to candy, cookies, etc.; and that if you are a truly loving wife, you will feed your husband foods that are high in cholesterol. All of these appeals have isolated some basic goals to which most people subscribe (e.g., people want to be masculine or feminine, good parents, loving spouses, etc.) and make claim, or imply, that their realization is only possible through the exclusive use of their product or the regular display of a specific type of at-risk behavior. Indeed, one can argue that certain at-risk behaviors have become so inextricably intertwined with our dominant cultural system (perhaps even symbolic of it) that the routine public display of such behavior almost signifies membership in this society.

Such tactics for the habituation of people to at-risk behavior are, perhaps paradoxically, also employed to elicit what I term *"quasi-health behavior."* Here again, an artificially constructed conception of a person in some fanciful state of physiological and emotional equilibrium is presented as the ideal state to strive for, if one is to meaningfully participate in the wider social system. To assist in the attainment of such a state, we are advised to consume a range of quite worthless vitamin pills, mineral supplements, mouthwashes, hair shampoos, laxatives, pain killers, etc. Clearly, one cannot exude radiance and success if one is not taking this vitamin, or that mineral. The achievement of daily regularity is a prerequisite for an effective social existence. One can only compete and win after a good night's sleep, and this can only be ensured by taking such and such. An entrepreneurial pharmaceutical industry appears devoted to the task of making people overly conscious of these quasi-health concerns, and to engendering a dependency on products which have been repeatedly found to be ineffective, and even potentially harmful.[11]

There are no clear signs that such activity is being or will be regulated in any effective way, and the promoters of this quasi-health behavior appear free to range over the entire body in their never-ending search for new areas and issues to be linked to the fanciful equilibrium that they have already engineered in the mind of the consumer. By binding the display of at-risk and quasi-health behavior so inextricably to elements of our dominant culture, a situation is even created whereby to request people to change or alter these behaviors is more or less to request abandonment of dominant culture.

The term "culture" is employed here to denote that integrated system of values, norms, beliefs and patterns of behavior which, for groups and social categories in specific situations, facilitate the solution of social structural problems.[12] This definition lays stress on two features commonly associated with the concept of culture. The *first* is the interrelatedness and interdependence of the various elements (values, norms, beliefs, overt life styles) that apparently comprise culture. The *second* is the view that a cultural system is, in some part, a response to social structural problems, and that it can be regarded as some kind of resolution of them. Of course, these social structural problems, in partial response to which a cultural pattern emerges, may themselves have been engineered in the interests of creating certain beliefs, norms, life styles, etc. If one assumes that culture can be regarded as some kind of reaction formation, then one must be mindful of the unanticipated social consequences of inviting some alteration in behavior which is a part of a dominant cultural pattern. The request from health workers for alterations in certain at-risk behaviors may result in either awkward dislocations of the interrelated elements of the cultural pattern, or the destruction of a system of values and norms, etc., which have emerged over time in response to situational problems. From this perspective, and with regard to the utilization of medical care, I have already argued elsewhere that, for certain groups of the population, underutilization may be "healthy" behavior, and the advocacy of increased utilization an "unhealthy" request for the abandonment of essential features of culture.[13]

The Case of Food

Perhaps it would be useful at this point to illustrate in some detail, from one pertinent area, the style and magnitude of operation engaged in by the manufacturers of illness. Illustrations are, of course, readily available from a variety of different areas, such as: the requirements of existing occupational structure, emerging leisure patterns, smoking and drinking behavior, and automobile usage.[14] Because of current interest, I have decided to consider only one area which is importantly related to a range of largely chronic diseases—namely, the 161 billion dollar industry involved in the production and distribution of food and beverages.[15] The present situation, with regard to food, was recently described as follows:

> The sad history of our food supply resembles the energy crisis, and not just because food nourishes our bodies while petroleum fuels the society. We long ago surrendered control of food, a vital resource, to private corporations, just as we surrendered control of energy. The food corporations have shaped the kinds of food we eat for their greater profits, just as the energy companies have dictated the kinds of fuel we use.[16]

From all the independent evidence available, and despite claims to the contrary by the food industry, a widespread decline has occurred during the past three decades in American dietary standards. Some forty percent of U.S. adults are overweight or downright fat.[17] The prevalence of excess weight in the American population as a whole is high—so high, in fact, that in some segments it has reached epidemic proportions.[18] There is evidence that the food industry is manipulating our image of "food" away from basic staples toward synthetic and highly processed items. It has been estimated that we eat between 21 and 25 percent fewer dairy products, vegetables, and fruits than we did twenty years ago, and from 70 to 80 percent more sugary snacks and soft drinks. Apparently, most people now eat more processed and synthetic foods than the real thing. There are even suggestions that a federal, nationwide survey would have revealed how serious our dietary situation really is, if the Nixon Administration had not cancelled it after reviewing some embarrassing preliminary results.[19] The survey apparently confirmed the trend toward deteriorating diets first detected in an earlier household food consumption survey in the years 1955–1965, undertaken by the Department of Agriculture.[20]

Of course, for the food industry, this trend toward deficient synthetics and highly processed items makes good economic sense. Generally speaking, it is much cheaper to make things look and taste like the real thing, than to actually provide the real thing. But the kind of foods that result from the predominance of economic interests clearly do not contain adequate nutrition. It is common knowledge that food manufacturers destroy important nutrients which foods naturally contain, when they transform them into "convenience" high profit items. To give one simple example: a wheat grain's outer layers are apparently very nutritious, but they are also an obstacle to making tasteless, bleached, white flour. Consequently, baking corporations "refine" fourteen nutrients out of the natural flour and then, when it is financially convenient, replace some of them with a synthetic substitute. In the jargon of the food industry, this flour is now "enriched." Clearly, the food industry employs this term in much the same way that coal corporations ravage mountainsides into mud flats, replant them with some soil and seedlings, and then proclaim their moral accomplishment in "rehabilitating" the land. While certain types of food processing may make good economic sense, it may also result in a deficient end product, and perhaps even promote certain diseases. The bleaching and refining of wheat products, for example, largely eliminates fiber or roughage from our diets, and some authorities have suggested that fiber-poor diets can be blamed for some of our major intestinal diseases.[21]

A vast chemical additive technology has enabled manufacturers to acquire enormous control over the food and beverage market and to foster phenomenal profitability. It is estimated that drug companies alone make something like $500 million a year through chemical additives for food. I have already suggested that what is done to food, in the way of processing and artificial additives, may actually be injurious to health. Yet, it is clear that, despite such well-known risks, profitability makes such activity well worthwhile. For example, additives, like preservatives, enable food that might perish in a short period of time to endure unchanged for months or even years. Food manufacturers and distributors can saturate supermarket shelves across the country with their products because there is little chance that they will spoil. Moreover, manufacturers can purchase vast quantities of raw ingredients when they are cheap, produce and stockpile the processed result, and then withhold the product from the market for long periods, hoping for the inevitable rise in prices and the consequent windfall.

The most widely used food additive (although it is seldom described as an additive) is "refined" sugar. Food manufacturers saturate our diets with the substance from the day we are born until the day we die. Children are fed breakfast cereals which consist of 50 percent sugar.[22] The average American adult consumes 126 pounds of sugar each year—and children, of course, eat much more. For the candy industry alone, this amounts to around $3 billion each year. The American sugar mania, which appears to have been deliberately engineered, is a major contributor to such "diseases of civilization" as diabetes, coronary heart disease, gall bladder illness, and cancer—all the insidious, degenerative conditions which most often afflict people in advanced capitalist societies, but which "underdeveloped," non-sugar eaters never get. One witness, at a recent meeting of a U.S. Senate Committee, said that if the food industry were proposing sugar today as a new food additive, its "metabolic behavior would undoubtedly lead to its being banned."[23]

In sum, therefore, it seems that the American food industry is mobilizing phenomenal resources to advance and bind us to its own conception of food. We are bombarded from childhood with $2 billion worth of deliberately manipulative advertisements each year, most of them urging us to consume, among other things, as much sugar as possible. To highlight the magnitude of the resources involved, one can point to the activity of one well-known beverage company, Coca-Cola, which alone spent $71 million in 1971 to advertise its artificially flavored, sugar-saturated product. Fully recognizing the enormity of the problem regarding food in the United States, Zwerdling offers the following advice:

> Breaking through the food industry will require government action—banning or sharply limiting use of dangerous additives like artificial colors and flavors, and sugar, and requiring wheat products to contain fiber-rich wheat germ, to give just two examples. Food, if it is to become safe, will have to become part of politics.[24]

The Ascription of Responsibility and Moral Entrepreneurship

So far, I have considered, in some detail, the ways in which industry, through its manufacture and distribution of a variety of products, generates at-risk behavior and disease. Let us now focus on the activities of health workers further down the river and consider their efforts in a social context, which has already been largely shaped by the manufacturers upstream.

Not only should we be mindful of the culturally disruptive and largely unanticipated consequences of health intervention efforts mentioned earlier, but also of the underlying ideology on which so much of this activity rests. Such intervention appears based on an assumption of the *culpability of individuals* or groups who either manifest illness, or display various at-risk behaviors.

From the assumption that individuals and groups with certain illnesses or displaying at-risk behavior are responsible for their state, it is a relatively easy step to advocating some changes in behavior on the part of those involved. By ascribing culpability to some group or social category (usually ethnic minorities and those in lower socio-economic categories) and having this ascription legitimated by health professionals and accepted by other segments of society, it is possible to mobilize resources to change the offending behavior. Certain people are responsible for not approximating, through their activities, some conception of what *ought* to be appropriate behavior on their part. When measured against the artificial conception of what ought to be, certain individuals and groups are found to be deficient in several important respects. They are *either* doing something that they ought not to be doing, *or* they are not doing something that they ought to be doing. If only they would recognize their individual culpability and alter their behavior in some approporiate fashion, they would improve their health status or the likelihood of not developing certain pathologies. On the basis of this line of reasoning, resources are being mobilized to bring those who depart from the desired conception into conformity with what is thouoght to be appropriate behavior. To use the upstream-downstream analogy, one could argue that people are blamed (and, in a sense, even punished) for not being able to swim after they, perhaps even against their own volition, have been pushed into the river by the manufacturers of illness.

Clearly, this ascription of culpability is not limited only to the area of health. According to popular conception, people in poverty are largely to blame for their social situation, although recent evidence suggests that a social welfare system which prevents them from avoiding this state is at least partly responsible.[25] Again, in the field of education, we often hold "dropouts" responsible for their behavior, when evidence suggests that the school system itself is rigged for failure.[26] Similar examples are readily available from the fields of penology, psychiatry, and race relations.[27]

Perhaps it would be useful to briefly outline, at this point, what I regard as a bizarre relationship between the activities of the manufacturers of illness, the ascription of culpability, and health intervention endeavors. *First,* important segments of our social system appear to be controlled and operated in such a way that people must inevitably fail. The fact is that there is often no choice over whether one can find employment, whether or not to drop out of college, involve oneself in untoward behavior, or become sick. *Second,* even though individuals and groups lack such choice, they are still blamed for not approximating the artificially contrived norm and are treated as if responsibility for their state lay entirely with them. For example, some illness conditions may be the result of particular behavior and/or involvement in certain occupational role relationships over which those affected have little or no control.[28] *Third,* after recognizing that certain individuals and groups have "failed," we establish, at a point downstream, a substructure of services which are regarded as evidence of progressive beneficence on the part of the system. Yet, it is this very system which had a primary role in manufacturing the problems and need for these services in the first place.

It is around certain aspects of life style that most health intervention endeavors appear to revolve and this probably results from the observability of most at-risk behavior. The modification of at-risk behavior can take several different forms, and the intervention appeals that are employed probably vary as a function of which type of change is desired. People can *either* be encouraged to stop doing what they are doing which appears to be endangering their survival (e.g., smoking, drinking, eating certain types of food, working in particular ways); *or* they can be encouraged to adopt certain new patterns of behavior which seemingly enhance their health status (e.g., diet, exercise, rest, eat certain foods, etc.). I have already discussed how the presence or absence of certain life styles in some groups may be a part of some wider cultural pattern which emerges as a response to social structural problems. I have also noted the potentially disruptive consequences to these cultural patterns of intervention programs. Underlying all these aspects is the issue of behavior control and the attempt to enforce a particular type of behavioral conformity. It is more than coincidental that the at-risk life styles, which we are all admonished to avoid, are frequently the type of behaviors which depart from and, in a sense, jeopardize the prevailing puritanical, middle-class ethic of what ought to be. According to this ethic, activities as pleasurable as drinking, smoking, overeating, and sexual intercourse must be harmful and ought to be eradicated.

The important point here is which segments of society and whose interests are health workers serving, and what are the ideological consequences of their actions?[29] Are we advocating the modification of behavior for the *exclusive* purpose of improving health status, or are we using the question of health as a means of obtaining some kind of moral uniformity through the abolition of disapproved behaviors? To what extent, if at all, are health workers actively involved in some wider pattern of social regulation?[30]

Such questions also arise in relation to the burgeoning literature that links more covert personality characteristics to certain illnesses and at-risk behaviors. Capturing a great deal of attention in this regard are the recent studies which associate heart disease with what is termed a Type A personality. The Type A personality consists of a complex of traits which produces: excessive competitive drive, aggressiveness, impatience, and a harrying sense of time urgency. Individuals displaying this pattern seem to be engaged in a chronic, ceaseless and often fruitless struggle with themselves, with others, with circumstances, with time, sometimes with life itself. They also frequently exhibit a free-floating, but well-rationalized form of hostility, and almost always a deep-seated insecurity.

Efforts to change Type A traits appear to be based on some ideal conception of a relaxed, non-competitive, phlegmatic individual to which people are encouraged to conform. Again, one can question how realistic such a conception is in a system which daily rewards behavior resulting from Type A traits. One can clearly question the ascription of near exclusive culpability to those displaying Type A behavior when the context within which such behavior is manifest is structured in such a way as to guarantee its production. From a cursory reading of job advertisements in any newspaper, we can see that employers actively seek to recruit individuals manifesting Type A characteristics, extolling them as positive virtues.[33]

My earlier point concerning the potentially disruptive consequences of requiring alterations in life style applies equally well in this area of personality and disease. If health workers manage to effect some changes away from Type A behavior in a system which requires and rewards it, then we must be aware of the possible consequences of such change in terms of future failure. Even though the evidence linking Type A traits to heart disease appears quite conclusive, how can health workers ever hope to combat and alter it when such characteristics are so positively and regularly reinforced in this society?

The various points raised in this section have some important moral and practical implications for those involved in health related endeavors. *First,* I have argued that our prevailing ideology involves the ascription of culpability to particular individuals and groups for the manifestation of either disease or at-risk behavior. *Second,* it can be argued that so-called "health professionals" have acquired a mandate to determine the morality of different types of behavior and have access to a body of knowledge and resources which they can "legitimately" deploy for its removal or alteration. (A detailed discussion of the means by which this mandate has been acquired is expanded in a separate paper.) *Third,* [it] is possible to argue that a great deal of health intervention is, perhaps unwittingly, part of a wide pattern of social regulation. We must be clear both as to whose interests we are serving, and the wider implications and consequences of the activities we support through the application of our expertise. *Finally,* it is evident from arguments I have presented that much of our health intervention fails to take adequate account of the social contexts which foster and reinforce the behaviors we seek to alter. The literature of preventive medicine is replete with illustrations of the failure of contextless health intervention programs.

The Notion of a Need Hierarchy

At this point in the discussion I shall digress slightly to consider the relationship between the utilization of preventive health services and the concept of need as manifest in this society. We know from available evidence that upper socio-economic groups are generally more responsive to health intervention activities than are those of lower socio-economic status. To partially account for this phenomenon, I have found it useful to introduce the notion of a *need hierarchy*. By this I refer to the fact that some need (e.g., food, clothing, shelter) are probably universally recognized as related to sheer survival and take precedence, while other needs, for particular social groups, may be perceived as less immediately important (e.g., dental care, exercise, balanced diet). In other words, I conceive of a *hierarchy of needs*, ranging from what could be termed "primary needs" (which relate more or less to the universally recognized immediate needs for survival) through to "secondary needs" (which are not always recognized as important and which may be artificially engineered by the manufacturers of illness). Somewhere between the high priority, primary needs and the less important, secondary needs are likely to fall the kinds of need invoked by preventive health workers. Where one is located at any point in time on the need hierarchy (i.e., which particular needs are engaging one's attention and resources) is largely a function of the shape of the existing social structure and aspects of socio-economic status.

This notion of a hierarchy of needs enables us to distinguish between the health and illness behavior of the affluent and the poor. Much of the social life of the wealthy clearly concerns secondary needs, which are generally perceived as lower than most health related needs on the need hierarchy. If some pathology presents itself, or some at-risk behavior is recognized, then they naturally assume a priority position, which eclipses most other needs for action. In contrast, much of the social life of the poor centers on needs which are understandably regarded as being of greater priority than most health concerns on the need hierarchy (e.g., homelessness, unemployment). Should some illness event present itself, or should health workers alert people and groups in poverty to possible further health needs, then these needs inevitably assume a position of relative low priority and are eclipsed, perhaps indefinitely, by more pressing primary needs for sheer existence.

From such a perspective, I think it is possible to understand why so

Figure 1.

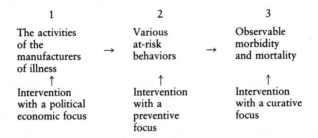

much of our health intervention fails in those very groups, at highest risk to morbidity, whom we hope to reach and influence. The appeals that we make in alerting them to possible future needs simply miss the mark by giving inadequate recognition to those primary needs which daily preoccupy their attention. Not only does the notion of a need hierarchy emphasize the difficulty of contextless intervention programs, but it also enables us to view the rejection as a non-compliance with health programs, as, in a sense, rational behavior.

How Preventive Is Prevention?

With regard to some of the arguments I have presented, concerning the ultimate futility of downstream endeavors, one may respond that effective preventive medicine does, in fact, take account of this problem. Indeed, many preventive health workers are openly skeptical of a predominantly curative perspective in health care. I have argued, however, that even our best preventive endeavors are misplaced in their almost total ascription of responsibility for illness to the afflicted individuals and groups, and through the types of programs which result. While useful in a limited way, the preventive orientation is itself largely a downstream endeavor through its preoccupation with the avoidance of at-risk behavior in the individual and with its general neglect of the activities of the manufacturers of illness which foster such behavior.

Figure 1 is a crude diagrammatic representation of an overall process starting with (1) the activities of the manufacturers of illness, which (2) foster and habituate people to certain at-risk behaviors, which (3) ultimately result in the onset of certain types of morbidity and mortality. The predominant curative orientation in modern medicine deals almost exclusively with the observable patterns of morbidity and mortality, which are the *end points* in the process. The much heralded preventive orientation focuses on those behaviors which are known to be associated with particular illnesses and which can be viewed as the *midpoint* in the overall process. Still left largely untouched are the entrepreneurial activities of the manufacturers of illness, who, through largely unregulated activities, foster the at-risk behavior we aim to prevent. This *beginning point* in the process reamins unaffected by most preventive endeavors, even though it is at this point that the greatest potential for change, and perhaps even ultimate victory, lies.

It is clear that this paper raises many questions and issues at a general level—more in fact than it is possible to resolve. Since most of the discussion has been at such an abstract level and concerned with broad political and economic forces, any ensuing recommendations for change must be broad enough to cover the various topics discussed. Hopefully, the preceding argument will also stimulate discussion toward additional recommendations and possible solutions. Given the scope and direction of this paper and the analogy I have employed to convey its content, the task becomes of the order of constructing fences upstream *and* restraining those who, in the interest of corporate profitability, continue to push people in. In this concluding section I will confine my remarks to three selected areas of recommendations.

Recommended Action

a. Legislative Intervention. It is probably true that one stroke of effective health legislation is equal to many separate health intervention endeavors and the cumulative efforts of innumerable health workers over long periods of time. In terms of winning the war which was described earlier, greater changes will result from the continued politicization of illness than from the modification of specific individual behaviors. There are many opportunities for a legislative reduction of at-riskness, and we ought to seize them. Let me give one suggestion which relates to earlier points in this paper. Widespread public advertising is importantly related to the growth and survival of large corporations. If it were not so demonstrably effective, then such vast sums of money and resources would not be devoted to this activity. Moreover, as things stand at present, a great deal of advertising is encouraged through granting it tax exempt status on some vague grounds of public education.[35] To place more stringent, enforceable restrictions on advertising would be to severely curtail the morally abhorrent pushing in activities of the manufacturers of illness. It is true that large corporations are ingenious in their efforts to avoid the consequences of most of the current legislative restrictions on advertising which only prohibit certain kinds of appeals.

As a possible solution to this and in recognition of the moral culpability of those who are actively manufacturing disease, I conceive of a ratio of advertising to health tax or a ratio of risk to benefit tax (RRBT). The idea here is to, in some way, match advertising expenditures to health expenditures. The precise weighting of the ratio could be determined by independently ascertaining the severity of the health effects produced by the manufacture and distribution of the product by the corporation. For example, it is clear that smoking is injurious to health and has no redeeming benefit. Therefore, for this product, the ratio could be determined as say, 3 to 1, where, for example, a company which spends a non-tax deductible $1 million to advertise its cigarettes would be required to devote a non-tax deductible $3 million to the area of health. In the area of quasi-health activities, where the product, although largely useless, may not be so injurious (e.g., nasals sprays, pain killers, mineral supplements, etc.), the ratio could be on, say, a 1 to 1 basis.

Of course, the manufacturers of illness, at the present time, do "donate" large sums of money for the purpose of research, with an obvious understanding that their gift should be reciprocated. In a recent article, Nuehring and Markle touch on the nature of this reciprocity:

> One of the most ironic pro-cigarette forces has been the American Medical Association. This powerful health organization took a position in 1965 clearly favorable to the tobacco interests. . . . In addition, the A.M.A. was, until 1971, conspicuously absent from the membership of the National Interagency Council on Smoking and Health, a coalition of government agencies and virtually all the national health organizations, formed in 1964. The A.M.A.'s largely pro-tobacco behavior has been linked with the acceptance of large research subsidies from the tobacco industry—amounting, according to the industry, to some 18 million dollars.[36]

Given such reciprocity, it would be necessary for this health money from the RRBT to be handled by a supposedly independent government agency, like the FDA or the FTC, for distribution to regular research institutions as well as to consumer organizations in the health field, which are currently so unequally pitted against the upstream manufacturers of illness. Such legislation would, I believe, severely curtail corporate "pushing in" activity and publicly demonstrate our commitment to effectively regulating the source of many health problems.

b. The Question of Lobbying. Unfortunately, due to present arrangements, it is difficult to discern the nature and scope of health lobbying activities. If only we could locate (a) who is lobbying for what, (b) who they are lobbying with, (c) what tactics are being employed, and (d) with what consequences for health legislation. Because these activities are likely to jeopardize the myths that have been so carefully engineered and fed to a gullible public by both the manufacturers of illness *and* various health organizations, they are clothed in secrecy. Judging from recent newspaper reports, concerning multimillion dollar gift-giving by the pharmaceutical industry to physicians, the occasional revelation of lobbying and political exchange remains largely unknown and highly newsworthy. It is frequently argued that lobbying on behalf of specific legislation is an essential avenue for public input in the process of enacting laws. Nevertheless, the evidence suggests that it is often, by being closely linked to the distribution of wealth, a very one-sided process. As it presently occurs, many legitimate interests on a range of health related issues do not have lobbying input in proportion to their numerical strength and may actually be structurally precluded from effective participation. While recognizing the importance of lobbying activity and yet feeling that for certain interests its scope ought to be severely curtailed (perhaps in the same way as the proposed regulation and publication of political campaign contributions), I am, to be honest, at a loss as to what should be specifically recommended. . . . The question is: quite apart from the specific issue of changing individual behavior, *in what ways could we possibly regulate the disproportionately influential lobbying activities of certain interest groups in the health field?*

   c. Public Education. In the past, it has been common to advocate the education of the public as a means of achieving an alteration in the behavior of groups at risk to illness. Such downstream educational efforts rest on "blaming the victim" assumptions and seek to *either* stop people doing what we feel they "ought not" to be doing, *or* encourage them to do things they "ought" to be doing, but are not. Seldom do we educate people (especially schoolchildren) about the activities of the manufacturers of illness and about how they are involved in many activities unrelated to their professed area of concern. How many of us know, for example, that for any 'average' Thanksgiving dinner, the turkey may be produced by the Greyhound Corporation, the Smithfield Ham by ITT, the lettuce by Dow Chemical, the potatoes by Boeing, the fruits and vegetables by Tenneco or the Bank of America?[38] I would reiterate that I am not opposed to the education of people who are at risk to illness, with a view to altering their behavior to enhance life chances (if this can be done successfully). However, I would add the proviso that if we remain committed to the education of people, we must ensure that they are being told the whole story. And, in my view, immediate priority ought to be given to the sensitization of vast numbers of people to the upstream activities of the manufacturers of illness, some of which have been outlined in this paper. Such a program, actively supported by the federal government (perhaps through revenue derived from the RRBT), may foster a groundswell of consumer interest which, in turn, may go some way toward checking the disproportionately influential lobbying of the large corporations and interest groups.

Notes and References

1. I.K. Zola, "Helping—Does It Matter: The Problems and Prospects of Mutual Aid Groups." Addressed to the United Ostomy Association, 1970.

2. See, for example, M.W. Susser and W. Watson, *Sociology in Medicine,* New York: Oxford University Press, 1971. Edith Chen, et al., "Family Structure in Relation to Health and Disease." *Journal of Chronic Diseases,* Vol. 12 (1960), pp. 554–567; and R. Keelner, *Family III Health: An Investigation in General Practice,* Charles C. Thomas, 1963. There is, of course, voluminous literature which relates family structure to mental illness. Few studies move to the level of considering the broader social forces which promote the family structures which are conducive to the onset of particular illnesses. With regard to utilization behavior, see J.B. McKinlay, "Social Networks, Lay Consultation and Help-Seeking Behavior," *Social Forces,* Vol. 51, No. 3 (March, 1973), pp. 275–292.

3. A rich source for a variety of materials included in this second level is H.E. Freeman, S. Levine, and L.G. Reeder (Eds.), *Handbook of Medical Sociology,* New Jersey: Prentice-Hall, 1972. I would also include here studies of the health implications of different housing patterns. Recent evidence suggests that housing—even when highly dense—may not be directly related to illness.

4. There have, of course, been many studies, mainly by epidemiologists, relating disease patters to certain occupations and industries. Seldom, however, have social scientists pursued the consequences of these findings in terms of broader political economy of illness. One exception to this statement can be found in studies and writings on the social causes and consequences of environmental pollution. For a recent elementary treatment of some important issues in this general area, see H. Waitzkin and B. Waterman, *The Exploitation of Illness in Capitalist Society,* New York: Bobbs-Merrill Co., 1974.

5. Some useful introductory readings appear in D.M. Gordon (Ed.), *Problems in Political Economy: An Urban Perspective,* Lexington: D.C. Heath & Co., 1971, and R. C. Edwards; M. Reich and T. E. Weisskopf (Eds.), *The Capitalist System,* New Jersey: Prentice-Hall, 1972. Also, T. Christoffel; D. Finkelhor and D. Gilbarg (Eds.), *Up Against the American Myth,* New York: Holt, Rinehart and Winston. 1970. M. Mankoff (Ed.), *The Poverty of Progress: The Political Economy of American Social Problems,* New York: Holt, Rinehart and Winston, 1972. For more sophisticated treatment, see the collection edited by D. Mermelstein, *Economics: Mainstream Readings and Radical Critiques,* New York: Random House, 1970. Additionally useful papers appear in J. B. McKinlay (Ed.), *Politics and Law in Health Care Policy.* New York: Prodist, 1973, and J. B. McKinlay (Ed.), *Economic Aspects of Health Care,* New York: Prodist, 1973. For a highly readable and influential treatment of what is termed "the medical industrial complex," see B. and J. Ehrenreich, *The American Health Empire: Power, Profits and Politics,* New York: Vintage Books, 1971. Also relevant are T. R. Marmor, *The Politics of Medicare,* Chicago: Aldine Publishing Co., 1973, and R. Alford, "The Political Economy of Health Care: Dynamics Without Change," *Politics and Society,* 2 (1972), pp. 127–164.

6. E. Cray, *In Failing Health: The Medical Crisis and the AMA,* Indianapolis: Bobbs-Merrill, 1970. J.S. Burrow, *AMA—Voice of American Medicine,* Baltimore: Johns Hopkins Press, 1963. R. Harris, *A Sacred Trust,* New York: New American Library, 1966. R. Carter, *The Doctor Business,* Garden City, New York: Dolphin Books, 1961. "The American Medical Association: Power,

Purpose and Politics in Organized Medicine," *Yale Law Journal,* Vol. 63, No. 7 (May, 1954), pp. 938–1021.

7. See references under footnote 5, especially B. and J. Ehrenreich's *The American Health Empire,* Chapter VII, pp. 95–123.

8. D. M. Gordon (Ed.), *Problems in Political Economy: An Urban Perspective,* Lexington: D.C. Heath & Co., 1971, p. 318.

9. See, for example, D. A. Bernstein, "The Modification of Smoking Behavior: An Evaluative Review," *Psychological Bulletin,* Vol. 71 (June, 1969), pp. 418–440; S. Ford and F. Ederer, "Breaking the Cigarette Habit," *Journal of American Medical Association,* 194 (October, 1965), pp. 139–142; C. S. Keutzer, et al., "Modification of Smoking Behavior: A Review," *Psychological Bulletin,* Vol. 70 (December, 1968), pp. 520–533. Mettlin considers evidence concerning the following techniques for modifying smoking behavior: (1) behavioral conditioning, (2) group discussion, (3) counselling, (4) hypnosis, (5) interpersonal communication, (6) self-analysis. He concludes that:

> Each of these approaches suggests that smoking behavior is the result of some finite set of social and psychological variables, yet none has either demonstrated any significant powers in predicting the smoking behaviors of an individual or led to techniques of smoking control that considered alone, have significant long-term effects.

In C. Mettlin, "Smoking as Behavior: Applying a Social Psychological Theory," *Journal of Health and Social Behavior,* 14 (June, 1973), p. 144.

10. It appears that a considerable proportion of advertising by large corporations is tax exempt through being granted the status of "public education." In particular, the enormous media campaign, which was recently waged by major oil companies in an attempt to preserve the public myths they had so carefully constructed concerning their activities, was almost entirely non-taxable.

11. Reports of the harmfulness and ineffectiveness of certain products appear almost weekly in the press. As I have been writing this paper, I have come across reports of the low quality of milk, the uselessness of cold remedies, the health dangers in frankfurters, the linking of the use of the aerosol propellant, vinyl chloride, to liver cancer. That the Food and Drug Administration (F.D.A.) is unable to effectively regulate the manufacturers of illness is evident and illustrated in their inept handling of the withdrawal of the drug, betahistine hydrochloride, which supposedly offered symptomatic relief of Meniere's Syndrome (an affliction of the inner ear). There is every reason to think that this case is not atypical. For additionally disquieting evidence of how the Cigarette Labeling and Advertising Act of 1965 actually curtailed the power of the F.T.C. and other federal agencies from regulating cigarette advertising and nullified all such state and local regulatory efforts, see L. Fritschier, *Smoking and Politics: Policymaking and the Federal Bureaucracy,* New York: Meredith, 1969, and T. Whiteside, *Selling Death: Cigarette Advertising and Public Health,* New York: Liveright, 1970. Also relevant are Congressional Quarterly, 27 (1969) 666, 1026; and U.S. Department of Agriculture, Economic Research Service, *Tobacco Situation,* Washington: Government Printing Office, 1969.

12. The term "culture" is used to refer to a number of other characteristics as well.

However, these two appear to be commonly associated with the concept. See J. B. McKinlay, "Some Observations on the Concept of a Subculture." (1970).

13. This has been argued in J. B. McKinlay, "Some Approaches and Problems in the Study of the Use of Services," *Journal of Health and Social Behavior,* Vol. 13 (July, 1972), pp. 115–152; and J. B. McKinlay and D. Dutton, "Social Psychological Factors Affecting Health Service Utilization," chapter in *Consumer Incentives for Health Care,* New York: Prodist Press, 1974.

14. Reliable sources covering these areas are available in many professional journals in the fields of epidemiology, medical sociology, preventive medicine, industrial and occupational medicine and public health. Useful references covering these and related areas appear in J. N. Morris, *Uses of Epidemiology,* London: E. and S. Livingstone Ltd., 1967; and M.W. Susser and W. Watson, *Sociology in Medicine,* New York: Oxford University Press, 1971.

15. D. Zwerling, "Death for Dinner," *The New York Review of Books,* Vol. 21, No. 2 (February 21, 1974), p. 22.

16. D. Zwerling, "Death for Dinner." See footnote 15 above.

17. This figure was quoted by several witnesses at the *Hearings Before the Select Committee on Nutrition and Human Needs,* U.S. Government Printing Office, 1973.

18. The magnitude of this problem is discussed in P. Wyden, *The Overweight: Causes, Costs and Control,* Englewood Cliffs: Prentice-Hall, 1968; National Center for Health Statistics, *Weight by Age and Height of Adults: 1960–62.* Washington: *Vital and Health Statistics,* Public Health Service Publication #1000, Series 11, #14, Government Printing Office, 1966; U.S. Public Health Service, Center for Chronic Disease Control, *Obesity and Health,* Washington: Government Printing Office, 1966.

19. This aborted study is discussed in M. Jacobson, *Nutrition Scoreboard: Your Guide to Better Eating,* Center for Science in the Public Interest.

20. M.S. Hathaway and E. D. Foard, *Heights and Weights for Adults in the United States,* Washington: Home Economics Research Report 10, Agricultural Research Service, U.S. Department of Agriculture, Government Printing Office, 1960.

21. This is discussed by D. Zwerling. See footnote 16.

22. See *Hearings Before the Select Committee on Nutrition and Human Needs,* Parts 3 and 4, "T.V. Advertising of Food to Children," March 5, 1973 and March 6, 1973.

23. Dr. John Udkin, Department of Nutrition, Queen Elizabeth College, London University. See p. 225, *Senate Hearings,* footnote 22 above.

24. D. Zwerling, "Death for Dinner." See footnote 16 above, page 24.

25. This is well argued in F. Piven and R. A. Cloward, *Regulating the Poor: The Functions of Social Welfare,* New York: Vintage, 1971; L. Goodwin, *Do the Poor Want to Work?,* Washington: Brookings, 1972; H. J. Gans, "The Positive Functions of Poverty," *American Journal of Sociology,* Vol. 78, No. 2 (September, 1972), pp. 275–289; R. P. Roby (Ed.), *The Poverty Establishment,* New Jersey: Prentice-Hall, 1974.

26. See, for example, Jules Henry, "American Schoolrooms: Learning the Nightmare," *Columbia University Forum,* (Spring, 1963), pp. 24–30. See also the

paper by F. Howe and P. Lanter, "How the School System is Rigged for Failure," *New York Review of Books,* (June 18, 1970).

27. With regard to penology, for example, see the critical work of R. Quinney in *Criminal Justice in America,* Boston: Little Brown, 1974, and *Critique of Legal Order,* Boston: Little Brown, 1974.

28. See, for example, S. M. Sales, "Organizational Role as a Risk Factor in Coronary Disease," *Administrative Science Quarterly,* Vol. 14, No. 3 (September, 1969), pp. 325–336. The literature in this particular area is enormous. For several good reviews, see L.E. Hinkle, "Some Social and Biological Correlates of Coronary Heart Disease," *Social Science and Medicine,* Vol. 1 (1967), pp. 129–139; F. H. Epstein, "The Epidemiology of Coronary Heart Disease: A Review," *Journal of Chronic Diseases,* 18 (August, 1965), pp. 735–774.

29. Some interesting ideas in this regard are in E. Nuehring and G. E. Markle, "Nicotine and Norms: The Reemergence of a Deviant Behavior" *Social Problems,* Vol. 21, No. 4 (April, 1974), pp. 513–526. Also, J.R. Gusfield, *Symbolic Crusade: Status Politics and the American Temperance Movement,* Urbana, Illinois: University of Illinois Press, 1963.

30. For a study of the ways in which physicians, clergymen, the police, welfare officers, psychiatrists and social workers act as agents of social control, see E. Cumming, *Systems of Social Regulation,* New York: Atherton Press, 1968.

31. R. H. Rosenman and M. Friedman, "The Role of a Specific Overt Behavior Pattern in the Occurrence of Ischemic Heart Disease," *Cardiologia Practica,* 13 (1962), pp. 42–53; M. Friedman and R. H. Rosenman, *Type A Behavior and Your Heart,* Knopf, 1973. Also, S. J. Zyzanski and C. D. Jenkins, "Basic Dimensions Within the Coronary-Prone Behavior Pattern," *Journal of Chronic Diseases,* 22 (1970), pp. 781–795. There are, of course, many other illnesses which have also been related in one way or another to certain personality characteristics. Having found this new turf, behavioral scientists will most likely continue to play it for everything it is worth and then, in the interests of their own survival, will "discover" that something else indeed accounts for what they were trying to explain and will eventually move off there to find renewed fame and fortune. Furthermore, serious methodological doubts have been raised concerning the studies of the relationship between personality and at-risk behavior. See, in this regard, G. M. Hochbaum, "A Critique of Psychological Research on Smoking," paper presented to the American Psychological Association, Los Angeles, 1964. Also B. Lebovits and A. Ostfeld, "Smoking and Personality: A Methodologic Analysis," *Journal of Chronic Diseases* (1971).

32. M. Friedman and R.H. Rosenman. See footnote 31.

33. In the *New York Times* of Sunday, May 26, 1974, there were job advertisements seeking "aggressive self-starters," "people who stand real challenges," "those who like to compete," "career oriented specialists," "those with a spark of determination to someday run their own show," "people with the success drive," and "take charge individuals."

34. Aspects of this process are discussed in J. B. McKinlay, "On the Professional Regulation of Change," in *The Professions and Social Change,* P. Halmos (Ed.), Keele: Sociological Review Monograph, No. 20, 1973, and in "Clients

and Organizations," chapter in J.B. McKinlay (Ed.), *Processing People— Studies in Organizational Behavior*, London: Holt, Rinehart, and Winston, 1974.

35. There have been a number of reports recently concerning this activity. Questions have arisen about the conduct of major oil corporations during the so-called "energy crisis." See footnote 10. Equally questionable may be the public spirited advertisements sponsored by various professional organizations which, while claiming to be solely in the interests of the public, actually serve to enhance business in various ways. Furthermore, by granting special status to activities of professional groups, government agencies and large corporations may effectively gag them through some expectation of reciprocity. For example, most health groups, notably the American Cancer Society, did not support the F.C.C.'s action against smoking commercials because they were fearful of alienating the networks from whom they receive free announcments for their fund drives. Both the American Cancer Society and the American Heart Association have been criticized for their reluctance to engage in direct organizational conflict with pro-cigarette forces, particularly before the alliance between the television broadcasters and the tobacco industry broke down. Rather, they have directed their efforts to the downstream reform of the smoker. See E. Nuehring and G. E. Markle, footnote 29, page 522.

36. E. Nuehring and G. E. Markle, footnote 29 above, page 524.

37. The ways in which large-scale organizations engineer and disseminate these myths concerning their manifest activities, while avoiding any mention of their underlying latent activities, are discussed in more detail in the two references cited in footnote 34 above.

38. For a popularly written and effective treatment of the relationship between giant corporations and food production and consumption, see W. Robbins, *The American Food Scandal*, New York: William Morrow and Co., 1974.

634

Acknowledgments (continued)

Peter Conrad and Joseph W. Schneider, "Professionalization, Monopoly, and the Structure of Medical Practice." Reprinted with permission from Conrad, Peter, and Schneider, Joseph W.: Deviance and medicalization, St. Louis, 1980, The C.V. Mosby Co.

Richard W. and Dorothy C. Wertz, "Notes on the Decline of Midwives and the Rise of Medical Obstetricians." Reprinted with permission of Macmillan Publishing Co., from Lying In: A History of Childbirth in America by Richard W. and Dorothy C. Wertz. Copyright © 1977 by Richard W. and Dorothy C. Wertz.

Eliot Freidson, "Professional Dominance and the Ordering of Health Services: Some Consequences." Reprinted from Professional Dominance: The Social Structure of Medical Care by Eliot Freidson. Copyright © 1970 by Atherton Press, Inc. Reprinted with permission from Aldine Publishing Company, New York.

Victor W. Sidel and Ruth Sidel, "Health Care and Medical Care in the United States." From A HEALTHY STATE by Victor W. Sidel and Ruth Sidel. Reprinted by permission of Pantheon Books, a Division of Random House, Inc.

Susan Reverby, "Re-forming the Hospital Nurse: The Management of American Nursing." An earlier version appeared in Health/Pac Bulletin, 66 (Sept./Oct.) 1975: 7–16. Reprinted with permission of Health/Pac and Human Sciences Press.

Vicente Navarro, "The Influence of Social Class Structure on the American Health Sector." Excerpted and reprinted with permission from "An Explanation of the Composition, Nature, and Functions of the Present Health Sector in the United States" in Medicine Under Capitalism. © Neale Watson Academic Publications, Inc. 1977.

James L. Goddard, "The Medical Business." Reprinted with permission from Scientific American, September 1973. Copyright © 1973 by Scientific American, Inc. All rights reserved.

Dorothy Nelkin and David J. Edelman, "Centralizing Health Care." Published by permission of Transaction, Inc. from Society, vol. 13, no. 6. Copyright © 1976 by Transaction, Inc.

Thomas Bodenheimer, Steven Cummings, and Elizabeth Harding, "Capitalizing on Illness: The Health Insurance Industry." Reprinted from the International Journal of Health Services, vol. 4 (April, 1974): 583–598, by permission of Baywood Publishing Company and the authors.

Sylvia A. Law, "Blue Cross—What Went Wrong?" Reprinted with permission of Yale University Press from Blue Cross—What Went Wrong? by Sylvia A. Law and published by Yale University Press.

Elliott A. Krause, "The Failure of Medicaid." Reprinted by permission of the publisher from Chapter 5, "The Medicaid Program: A Voucher Strategy," in Power and Illness: The Political Sociology of Health and Medical Care by Elliott A. Krause, pp. 168–173. Copyright 1977 by Elsevier North Holland, Inc.

Wornie L. Reed, "Suffer the Children: Some Effects of Racism on the Health of Black Infants," was written for this volume. Reprinted by permission of the author.

Barbara Ehrenreich and Deirdre English, "The Sexual Politics of Sickness." Extracts from "The Sexual Politics of Sickness" in *For Her Own Good* by Barbara Ehrenreich and Deirdre English. Copyright (c) 1978 by Barbara Ehrenreich and Deirdre English. Reprinted by permission of Doubleday & Company, Inc.

Diana Scully and Pauline Bart, "A Funny Thing Happened on the Way to the Orifice: Women in Gynecology Textbooks." Reprinted with permission of the authors.

Sandra Klein Danziger, "The Uses of Expertise in Doctor-Patient Encounters During Pregnancy." Reprinted with permission from *Social Science and Medicine,* vol. 12. Copyright 1978, Pergamon Press, Ltd.

Julius Roth, "Some Contingencies of the Moral Evaluation and Control of Clientele: The Case of the Hospital Emergency Service." Reprinted from the American Journal of Sociology 77 (1972):836–839 by permission of the University of Chicago Press. © 1977 The University of Chicago Press.

Judith Lorber, "Good Patients and Problem Patients." Excerpted and reprinted with permission of The American Sociological Association from the *Journal of Health and Social Behavior,* vol. 16, June 1975.

Marcia Millman, "Medical Mortality Review: A Cordial Affair." Reprinted with permission of William Morrow & Company from *The Unkindest Cut* by Marcia Millman. Copyright © 1976 by Marcia Millman.

Ivan Illich, "Medical Nemesis." Reprinted with permission of the author from *The Lancet,* May 28, 1974, pp. 918–921.

Paul Starr, "The Politics of Therapeutic Nihilism." Reprinted with permission from *Working Papers for a New Society,* Summer 1976. Copyright © 1976, Center for the Study of Public Policy.

John H. Knowles, "The Responsibility of the Individual." Reprinted by permission of *Daedalus,* Journal of the American Academy of Arts and Sciences, Boston, Massachusetts, Winter 1977, *Doing Better and Feeling Worse: Health in the United States.*

Robert Crawford, "Individual Responsibility and Health Politics." Reprinted from S. Reverby and D. Rosner (Eds.), *Health Care in America: Essays in Social History* (Philadelphia: Temple University Press, 1979) with the permission of Temple University Press and the author.

Richard J. Margolis, "National Health Insurance—The Dream Whose Time Has Come?" © 1977 by the New York Times Company. Reprinted by permission.

John Ehrenreich and Oliver Fein, "National Health Insurance: The Great Leap Sideways," from THE AMERICAN HEALTH EMPIRE: Power, Profits & Politics, prepared by John Ehrenreich, and Barbara Ehrenreich. Copyright © 1970 by Health Policy Advisory Center, Inc. Reprinted by permission of Random House, Inc.

Irving Kenneth Zola, "Medicine as an Institution of Social Control." Reprinted with permission from *Sociological Review,* vol. 20, pp. 487–504.

Renée C. Fox, "The Medicalization and Demedicalization of American Society." Excerpted and reprinted by permission of *Daedalus,* Journal of the American Academy of Arts and Sciences, Boston, Massachusetts, Winter 1977, *Doing Better and Feeling Worse: Health in the United States.*

Catherine Kohler Riessman, "Improving the Use of Health Services by the Poor." Reprinted with permission from *Social Policy*, published by Social Policy Corporation, New York, New York 10036. Copyright 1974 by Social Policy Corporation.

John L. McKnight, "Politicizing Health Care." Reprinted with permission of the Dag Hammarskjöld Foundation from *Development Dialogue*, 1978, no. 1, Upsala, Sweden.

Sheryl K. Ruzek, "Emergent Modes of Utilization: Gynecological Self-Help." Excerpted and reprinted from *Women and Their Health: Research Implications for a New Era*, edited by Virginia Olesen. DHEW publication no. (HRA) 77-3138, U.S. Government Printing Office.

Derek Gill, "A National Health Service: Principles and Practice," was written for this volume. Reprinted by permission of the author.

Victor W. Sidel and Ruth Sidel, "The Delivery of Medical Care in China." From *Scientific American*, Vol. 30, April 1974: 19–27. Reprinted with permission. Copyright © 1974 by Scientific American, Inc. All rights reserved.

John B. McKinlay, "A Case for Refocussing Upstream: The Political Economy of Illness." Copyright © 1974 by the American Heart Association. Reprinted with permission.

Index